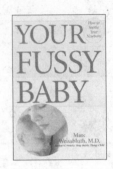
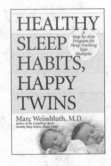

Healthy Sleep Habits, Happy Child

Fifth Edition

Healthy Sleep Habits, Happy Child

A NEW STEP-BY-STEP GUIDE FOR A GOOD NIGHT'S SLEEP

Fifth Edition

Marc Weissbluth, M.D.

 Ballantine Books • New York

2021 Ballantine Books Trade Paperback Edition

Published in the United States by Ballantine Books, an imprint of Random House, a division of Penguin Random House LLC, New York.

BALLANTINE and the HOUSE colophon are registered trademarks of Penguin Random House LLC.

Earlier editions of this work were published in the United States by Ballantine Books, an imprint of Random House, a division of Penguin Random House LLC, in 1987, 1999, 2003, and 2015.

Quotes by Carl D. Williams in chapter 5 are from "Case Report: The Elimination of Tantrum Behavior by Extinction Procedures" (*Journal of Abnormal and Social Psychology*, 1959).

"To White Noise" by Carrie Fountain © 2018 by Carrie Fountain. Originally appeared in *The New Yorker* magazine. Used by permission of Brandt & Hochman Literary Agents, Inc. All rights reserved.

ISBN 9780593158548
ebook ISBN 9780593356128

Printed in the United States of America on acid-free paper

randomhousebooks.com

9 8 7 6 5 4 3 2 1

Series book design by Mary A. Wirth

This book is dedicated, in loving memory, to Linda

As night falls, the weary creatures of earth,
And the woods and the frothing seas,
Grow calm like the stars as they circle their course,
And sleep with quiet ease.
And so all creatures far and wide,
From the craggy fields to the glassy lakes,
Stretch and live 'neath the silent night,
And sleep takes away their worries and aches.

—VIRGIL, *The Aeneid* (translation by Jed Weissbluth)

Contents

Foreword

A friend recommended this book to me when my first child, Presley, was seven months old. I was still nursing, but getting ready to stop, and definitely ready to stop the 4:00 A.M. feeding. Also, we had let Presley get into the bad habit of only wanting to sleep *on* someone. This was great when I needed an excuse for a nap, but not so convenient on busy days.

I devoured the book back then in a matter of hours and put the principles into practice immediately—with instant results. I especially liked how Dr. Weissbluth taught me to watch out for my child's sleepy signs and then encouraged me to get him to bed before he became overtired. I was also very comforted by Dr. Weissbluth's explanation of sleep as one of your child's basic needs. You offer healthy food to your child when she's hungry. You must also offer sleep when your child is tired—even if she doesn't know it or thinks she doesn't want it (just like my kids didn't usually choose the vegetable on their own!).

As a correspondent for *Good Morning America,* I had the good fortune to interview Dr. Weissbluth as part of a series called Baby's First Year. He became a trusted resource and adviser, not only on the topic of sleep, but also subsequently on potty training and discipline.

Dr. Weissbluth's philosophy that a well-rested family is the most important thing has stayed with us always. I can't say that my kids never woke up at night or always went to sleep without a power struggle. We had our ups and downs—that's parenthood. But from this book I learned the structure and rhythm of sleep and how to get back into it, an especially helpful skill when I was bleary-eyed at 2:00 A.M. or our schedule got out of balance after traveling or when someone had a cold.

Sixteen years have passed since I became a mother. In fact, my son just got his driver's license. Now, some nights, my husband and I lose sleep for different reasons. But what I have noticed is that even as teenagers both my children are good at reading their own sleepy cues. They seem to remember what it feels like to be well rested, know when they should go to sleep, and don't burn the candle at both ends. This makes for a much happier and harmonious family. I know we are all our best selves when we've given ourselves the gift of sleep. Fortunately, thanks to *Healthy Sleep Habits, Happy Child*, most days (and nights!) we do! Thanks, Dr. Weissbluth!

—Cindy Crawford

How to Use This Book

If you are a *sleep-deprived* parent:

Read chapter 1: Step-by-Step Program for a Good Night's Sleep and the age-appropriate chapter for your baby at this time. Perhaps, if you are severely sleep-deprived, only read the "Summary and Action Plan for Exhausted Parents" at the end of the chapter. If needed, follow up by reading chapter 5: Sleep Solutions. Skim or even skip the studies, numerical data, and parent reports as needed. They supply added context, but are not crucial to your understanding of this book.

If you are a *well-rested* parent:

Read chapter 1: Step-by-Step Program for a Good Night's Sleep, chapters 2–4, and the age-appropriate chapter for your baby. It may be useful to read the chapters for children younger and older than your child to help you understand how your baby's sleep developed and what changes are about to occur. If needed, follow up by reading chapter 5: Sleep Solutions.

If you are *not yet* a parent:

Read chapter 1: Step-By-Step Program for a Good Night's Sleep, and chapters 2–4 and 6.

Author's Note

Throughout the book, I use the terms *fathers, mothers, marriage,* and *marital problems* merely for convenience. I wish to embrace all partner and partner–child relationships.

Chapters 6–11 are partially *independent* so you will not need to search for information in other parts of the book. However, because some information applies to wide age ranges, there is some *repetition* of information in different chapters.

Through this text, I have often italicized key phrases (*SIDS*, for example). You can turn to the index for more information on these words.

Introduction

If you have not already done so, please go back and read the "How to Use This Book" section.

It's probably hard to think of a time when there were no parenting books about sleep—today, over a hundred books on children's sleep have been published containing widely varying and often conflicting advice. The marketplace is full of sleep aids, sleep apps, sleep trackers, special cribs, and other gadgets promising to help your baby sleep better. And then there's the internet. There are countless online forums, blogs, articles, and op-eds about children's sleep out there that aim to guide and comfort you—but they all have their own philosophies and, like all those new parenting books, contain conflicting advice that will create more confusion than comfort.

Once, there were no books for parents on helping children sleep. My first book, in 1984, focused on why babies cry and how to prevent post-colic sleep problems. Because there was no public discussion on how parents could help their children sleep, I made up the term *sleep training* to describe strategies for parents. At that time, there was no other parent-advice book on this subject.

Once, sleep for kids was easy. Our baby closed her eyes and she fell asleep. We hoped. Now the subject of children's sleep appears to be more complicated. When I published my first paper on children's sleep in 1981, there were only 141 scientific papers published that year on children's sleep. My first paper described a relationship between infant sleep and infant temperament. Over the next five years, I published seven more studies associating sleep-temperament with sleep durations, ADHD, SIDS, attention span, sleep apnea, and colic, but no other studies on this subject appeared until 1988. Since then, over a hundred studies linking sleep-temperament with different aspects of child development have been published. Now more than six hundred scientific papers on children's sleep are published *every year.*

Once, there were no pediatric sleep specialists or centers. Now professional pediatric sleep specialists, hospital sleep centers, and community sleep consultants are everywhere. In Australia, publicly funded and private residential Early Parenting Centers (EPC), also known as Sleep Schools, where mothers and unsettled infants stay for a few days and receive professional support are popular.

So much about the study of sleep has evolved since the first edition of this book was first published. In this new edition, I have included new research on how to help children sleep better. I have also added a brand-new, very short and easy-to-use Step-by-Step Program for a Good Night's Sleep to prevent and to treat sleep problems in children of all ages. The Step-by-Step Program is deliberately brief. After all, how much can you really read and remember when you might be very short on sleep?

There's a lot of untested, contradictory advice out there, but I promise you won't find that in my book. This book will provide you with new and trustworthy information. I will provide reassurance, support, and guidance to find the sleep solution that best fits your family values and lifestyle. Because every family is different, there isn't one best way to help children sleep; please don't judge yourself—or other parents.

Now, this book is long, but don't be intimidated by that. It is long because it includes details relevant to children of different ages and temperaments, as well as for different families. Only read the sections that you need (see "How to Use This Book"). Part I contains general advice and information that applies to children of all ages, while part II gives more detailed advice and information based on the age of the child.

Throughout the book I include many new studies and numerical data on how parenting helps or hinders the development of healthy sleep habits. Feel free to skip or skim them if you are sleep-deprived, as they are not crucial to your understanding of the material. I include them because having these new facts can strengthen your resolve to keep your child well rested when, for example, you are inevitably confronted by those who implore you to skip naps or keep your child up late for the convenience of their social event.

If you do read this new research, however, you'll be getting data that are vastly more accurate than what's found in older research studies (including my own) on children's sleep. This is because in the past, data were gathered mostly from mothers using sleep diaries in their homes. That is, mothers reported how a child's behavior, temperament, social or emotional development, or other items were thought to be related to the sleep data—whether the association was real or only a reflection of how the mother believed the two factors to be related. When there is only one source (for example, the mother) for different types of data (such as sleep durations or temperament ratings), it is referred to as *common method variance.* So the apparent association might be or might not be authentic. Another problem with older research was that there was no way to objectively know when the child actually fell asleep as opposed to when she was put in bed drowsy. Also, we did not know important details about children's sleep. For example, we did not know how often the child silently woke during the night and quietly went back to sleep without parental assistance, or how *long* she was up at night without fussing. A third problem was that many studies only captured a snapshot of children at one point in time, describing some association between sleep and something else without looking at what came before or after. Lastly, the role of the father was rarely studied.

During the past several years, studies have included the role of the father, not just the father's influence acting directly on the child, but also indirectly on the child as a partner supporting the mother. New research on how some fathers and mothers face challenges in helping their baby sleep well permits more evidence-based targeted advice and strategies to create a well-rested family despite these challenges. So what has changed since the 1980s? There is now a growing body of science that explains in detail how and in what ways quality sleep is beneficial and, conversely, how poor-quality sleep adversely impacts a child. More accurately, we now know in more detail how the entire family benefits or suffers when the child is or is not sleeping well. Not sleeping well or becoming overtired in childhood means different things at different ages and in different cultures. Biology, including genetics, plays an important role in how children sleep, but so do individual attitudes, family lifestyles, and cultural beliefs.

Now we have new technology to help us track the sleep habits and patterns of children. We have sleep trackers called *actigraphs,* worn by babies and parents to get objective data regarding actual sleep durations, measuring how long it takes for a child to fall asleep after being put in bed (*sleep latency*), how often she wakes at night, and for how long she is *wakeful after sleep onset (WASO)*. In homes, video cameras record parents' and children's behavior at bedtime and in the middle of the night so we have objective data on parents' and children's behaviors. In sleep laboratories, experimental night sleep restriction or nap restriction help tease out the different functions of nighttime and daytime sleep. In sleep labs, measurements include tests of memory, emotional responsivity, and behavioral regulation so we can better understand the specific benefits of specific aspects of sleep such as sleep duration, sleep consolidation, or the sleep schedule. Longitudinal studies of groups of children over long periods of time have recently been published. They help us understand what causes some children to develop sleep problems, and for children with sleep problems, what the adverse consequences are for the future.

While the technology to study sleep patterns has evolved since the first edition of this book in 1987, so have the challenges parents face today.

Single-parent families are far more common today. And these days, of course, work often follows parents home in the form of cell phones, email, and internet connections. Even when parents are physically present with their children, they may be distracted by digital screens. More and more parents work in a global economy that never sleeps. Online advice about parenting is often conflicting, creating more challenges. So it is not surprising that one or both parents may suffer from moments of inattentiveness to their child, uncertainty about parenting, inconsistency, and sleep deprivation.

Today's parents are exposed to daily reminders and images that magnify fearfulness about local, international, and environmental dangers impacting their children's safety now and in the future. Global climate change and pandemics affect everyone. On top of this feeling of physical insecurity is a heightened sense of academic competitiveness among some parents, who view preschool as but the first rung on a ruthless ladder of global competition for good jobs. Early education classes, enrichment programs, and scheduled activities to acquire knowledge and skills are increasingly popular among parents. And school itself has grown more demanding, with children expected to master more knowledge and skills at an earlier age than ever before, to say nothing of the demands placed on students by sports programs and other extracurricular activities. All of these factors run the risk of interfering with naps and early bedtimes for children, ironically making it more difficult for them to learn.

Sleep deprivation in parents and children alike, combined with the challenging, technologically complex modern world, has created even more anxiety about parenting. But you are not alone. I know from my practice that countless other parents are experiencing these feelings. I strongly wish to reassure you now that there will be much less worrying within a well-rested family. With healthy sleep, parents are better able to cope with many of the challenges they face. When families are well rested, they are more able to prevent and correct the inevitable problems that will develop. Becoming a well-rested family isn't really that difficult as long as we don't let our anxiety or exhaustion blind us. So please don't be scared by the topic of how or when your baby will sleep well. I know that you might be afraid or even desperate; haven't we all heard horror stories of babies who never sleep through the night, are cranky all day, and turn overwhelmed parents into nervous wrecks? The fact is, you *can* help your newborn to develop good sleep habits, even if she turns out to be colicky. Patience, practice, flexibility, and trial and error are the watchwords for success. Of course, because of new parents' inexperience and your baby's shifting sleep rhythms, there will be incidents when your timing will be off, and your baby will become painfully overtired. This is not your fault! It is inevitable.

The good news is that the harmful effects of unhealthy sleep are *reversible* when parents provide treatment. The younger the child, the more successful parents will be in reversing the ill effects of unhealthy sleep. A major treatment strategy that is emphasized in this edition and discussed in many of the stories by parents is: Move the bedtime a *few* minutes earlier. It is important to remember that the most common cause of sleep problems in children is a bedtime that is too late. To prevent a sleep problem, encourage an early bedtime based on drowsy signs. To treat a sleep problem, moving the bedtime just a few minutes earlier may help a lot. If it is unrealistic to establish an early bedtime based on drowsy signs, a bedtime that is a little too late is still better than a bedtime that is very late.

PART I

Sleep Strategies and Solutions— Understanding Healthy Sleep Habits

Chapter 1 Outline

PREVENT SLEEP PROBLEMS

HOW TO HELP YOUR CHILD FALL ASLEEP EASILY AT NIGHTTIME AND NAP TIME

Step 1: Younger than 6 Weeks: Encourage self-soothing
    A) Drowsy but awake
    B) Many hands
    C) Many naps
Step 2: At 6 Weeks: Early bedtime
Step 3: At 3–4 Months: Establish a nap schedule

HOW TO HELP YOUR CHILD SLEEP THROUGH THE NIGHT

Step 1: Based on your child's age: Steps 1–3 above
Step 2: After 2–3 months of age, do not always immediately respond to every sound your baby makes
Step 3: Do not always feed your baby whenever your baby makes any sound

TREAT SLEEP PROBLEMS

Step 1: Move bedtime earlier
Step 2: Encourage self-soothing
Step 3: Less attention during the night
Step 4: Protect naps

Step-by-Step Program for a Good Night's Sleep

If you have not done so, please read "How to Use This Book," page xv.

Are you sleepy? You might be feeling very sleepy because you are pregnant or you have a new baby, or your child is not sleeping well. If you are sleepy, of course, you want more sleep for yourself and you want your child to sleep well. Perhaps you just want me to tell you the right way to get better sleep for your child. In pediatrics, knowing the right thing to do is sometimes easy. For example, preventing infections may be as simple as handwashing; treating an ear infection may be as easy as prescribing an antibiotic. However, I am sorry to say that parenting decisions regarding sleep issues are not so straightforward. There isn't one right thing to do. There are so many different choices, so many opinions, and so very little strong science. Also, unfortunately, even if you know what to do, your own sleepiness might make it extra hard for you to actually do it.

But take heart; forget all the doom and gloom you probably heard about how kids always fight sleep and how all new parents become sleep-deprived zombies. Read this short recipe, follow the instructions, and you will make an angel-food sleeper! Or just jump in and get going. It's not rocket science, it's more like baking a cake; just remember that there are many different recipes, all of which will still make a sweet treat. To be safe, check out the American Academy of Pediatrics Safe Sleep recommendations for preventing *sudden infant death syndrome (SIDS)*. I have italicized key words and phrases (like *SIDS*) that are in the index, where you can find more information.

Chapter 1 outlines *what* you can do to help your child sleep better. The following chapters explain how these methods work and *why* sleep is important. Perhaps healthy sleep for your child is currently a low-priority item that you plan to work on in the future, or you think that healthy sleep isn't a big deal, or you want a quick preview of the proven benefits derived from healthy sleep. In the latter case, please look at my blog (marcweissbluthmd.blog) or read, in the very brief chapter 13, the US Department of the Army summary on *what* to do to promote healthy sleep and *why* healthy sleep is important. For the US Army, sleep is indeed a serious subject.

All right, here we go!

Prevent Sleep Problems

HOW TO HELP YOUR CHILD FALL ASLEEP EASILY AT NIGHTTIME AND NAP TIME

The most common pitfall parents encounter when trying to get their child to fall asleep is not recognizing subtle *drowsy signs*.

Drowsy signs are the early warning system, signaling that you need to find shelter and start the soothing process to sleep. Then sweet sleep is almost guaranteed. *Fatigue signs* occur when the storm has hit, you were too late; you can make the best of it, try to find safety, but finding sleep might be rough. If your child becomes overtired because your soothing was too late, expect him to have more difficulty falling asleep and staying asleep. The most common mistake made by parents is mistaking *fatigue* signs, which come late, with the *drowsy* signs that appear early and signal the rising of the sleep wave.

Now we can get to the three-step process to helping your child fall asleep at nighttime or nap time. The following three steps are *sequential* based on the *corrected age* (counting from the expected date of delivery, *not* the birth date) of your child.

STEP 1. YOUNGER THAN 6 WEEKS: ENCOURAGE SELF-SOOTHING

Do A, B, and C, below, when you come home from the hospital with your newborn or as early as possible:

A) Drowsy but Awake

Practice putting your baby down to sleep after soothing, when he's drowsy but still awake. If your baby has *colic,* try this at 2–3 months of age. Begin your *soothing* efforts at the onset of drowsy signs, not fatigue signs. Never forget the one sleep tip that will help all children sleep better. For all children, the single most important sleep advice can be stated in one word: *timing.*

You should try to start your soothing-to-sleep routine just as your child begins to become drowsy. You are using the start of his natural sleep rhythm as a *tool* to help him sleep better. When you do not let your child become overtired, then easier bedtimes, uninterrupted nighttime sleep, and better naps occur. Think of surfing: You anticipate the wave, you move as the wave approaches to catch it as it rises, and then you have a long, easy ride. Here the wave is drowsiness, the ride is slumber, and remember, the key to catch the wave is timing. Try to not miss the wave. Please be patient; it may take some practice.

Put your baby down, drowsy but still awake, as often as you feel comfortable. You may do this once a week, once a day, or more often. If your baby cries hard after being put down, immediately pick him up and resume soothing. Try again some other time, but this time, shorten the interval of wakefulness before the expected sleep period. If your baby quietly whimpers, immediately pick him up and resume soothing, or, if you are comfortable with this, wait a very brief moment to see if he drifts back to sleep. After you put your baby down, and there is no crying, you may wish to stay in the room awhile, but your baby will learn how to self-soothe faster if you leave the room.

Put your phone down; watch for drowsy signs. Be *emotionally available* when soothing to sleep.

B) Many Hands

Get Dad on board; try to have Dad and others soothe your baby to a drowsy state before your baby is put down to sleep. If you are breastfeeding, after feeding, sometimes pass your drowsy, but not completely asleep, baby to your husband for soothing before he puts your baby down. Fathers might be more successful than mothers in putting the baby down drowsy but awake. In addition to directly helping with nighttime parenting, during the day the father's support of the mother in general indirectly helps care for the baby. This general care, during the day, supporting the mother, may actually be more powerful regarding baby's sleeping than father's directly caring for the baby at night.

C) Many Naps

Brief intervals of wakefulness between naps prevents your baby from becoming overtired. Experiment with the first morning nap beginning after only one hour of wakefulness from night sleep. This will prevent a *second wind*. Brief intervals of wakefulness and brief nap durations will result in many naps each day. Parents have told me to emphasize the point that babies need many naps because it is not intuitively obvious. Babies need to return to sleep within one to two hours after waking from a nap.

STEP 2. AT 6 WEEKS: EARLY BEDTIME

Repeat the protocol outlined in step 1, plus create an *early bedtime* based on drowsy signs, not fatigue signs. Also, begin *bedtime routines,* and *be consistent*. After the bedtime routine and after your child has been put down to sleep, *leave the room*.

A common pitfall is to only pay attention to clock time instead of focusing on your child's drowsy signs. Perhaps it is late when you get home from work and/or you are tired and distracted at the end of the day, so it may be easier to quickly glance at the clock than to pay close attention to your child. Or perhaps you are innocently masking subtle drowsy signs with intense play or screen time.

STEP 3. AT 3–4 MONTHS: ESTABLISH A NAP SCHEDULE

Continue with protocols for steps 1 and 2, plus establish a *nap schedule*.

How to Help Your Child Sleep through the Night

All babies make vocalizations during the night. The sounds may be quiet and may or may not indicate distress. Some may sound like a quiet or intermittent whimper. Sometimes your baby will have a loud and persistent cry that might indicate that he is hungry, wet, soiled, or in distress.

All babies have moments of light sleep and moments of deep sleep. During a period of light sleep, your baby might drift toward being partially awake and then return to sleep unassisted (*self-soothing*) or call out for help from you to return to sleep (*signaling*).

STEP 1.

Based on your child's age, try drowsy but awake, many hands, many naps, earlier bedtimes, and establishing a nap schedule. Helping your baby learn self-soothing at sleep onset may help him self-soothe during the night.

STEP 2.

The First 2-3 Months of Life

A mother of a newborn might appropriately immediately respond to every sound the baby makes during the night because of complications or issues around the pregnancy, delivery, or breastfeeding. A first-time parent, because of inexperience, will likely have more uncertainty or anxiety about whether the sounds the baby makes indicate distress or non-distress and thus appropriately always immediately respond to every sound the newborn baby makes. A parent of a baby with *extreme fussiness/colic* might appropriately immediately respond to every sound to prevent full-blown crying spells. Babies vary in their capacity for self-soothing, and parents vary in how quickly they respond. Always immediately responding to every sound may be appropriate during the first two or three months and may not create any future sleeping problems in the baby, but it might exhaust a parent, with adverse consequences. Remember, get Dad on board! Dad might immediately respond with soothing but not feeding.

Alternatively, a parent of a newborn might try to discriminate between distress and *non-distress sounds* during the night and implement a very brief delay (maybe a minute or less) in responding to non-distress sounds.

After the First 2-3 Months of Life

During the night, after two or three months, do not always immediately respond to every sound your baby makes. A parent who always immediately responds to every sound the baby makes during the night interferes with the baby's learning how to self-soothe at night and thus might contribute to a night-waking habit (signaling). Try a differential response: Always immediately respond to distress vocalizations and always attempt a brief delay in your response to non-distress vocalizations.

STEP 3.

During the night, do not always feed your baby whenever he makes a sound.

To prevent a night-feeding habit, always feed your baby when you think he is hungry, but first try other methods of soothing when you suspect that he is not hungry. Even when breastfeeding, by using a test bottle of expressed milk or formula Dad can help determine whether the baby is truly hungry.

Treat Sleep Problems

The following four steps are best performed *together*.

Note: If you feel totally exhausted or discouraged, or if for whatever reason you are unable or do not wish to do all four steps, just do step 1.

STEP 1. MOVE THE BEDTIME EARLIER

This may seem counterintuitive if your child is having trouble sleeping, but dramatic improvements occur even when children get very small amounts of extra sleep. Hyperarousal in your child causes difficulties in falling asleep and staying asleep. Early bedtimes dampen or eliminate hyperarousal. Early bedtimes will not necessarily cause your baby to wake up earlier in the morning. Sleep begets sleep. More sleep at the front end makes it easier for babies to sleep in later in the morning. Because your child starts the day better rested, he is able to take longer naps. Remember, it is never too late to help your child sleep better by encouraging an earlier bedtime based on drowsy signs. So: *Just put your child to sleep twenty to thirty minutes earlier!* However, if you are only looking at clock time (instead of drowsy signs in your child), moving the bedtime from 8:30 to 8:00 P.M. might not help much if your child is becoming drowsy at 7:00 P.M. On the other hand, it may not be realistic for you to be able to put your child to sleep at night when drowsy signs appear; try your best, and know that a bedtime that is a only little late is still better than a bedtime that is way too late.

Choose an early bedtime based on your child's appearance in the late afternoon or early evening. Practice consistent and brief bedtime routines and leave the room after putting your child down. When an early bedtime is coupled with bedtime routines, dramatic improvement occurs over the first *three nights*. To help establish an earlier bedtime:

A. *Control the wake-up time.* Start the day earlier by waking your child in the morning in order to start naps and the bedtime earlier.
B. *Modify or eliminate nap(s) for a child older than 3–4 months.* Shorten or eliminate late-afternoon naps in order to achieve an early bedtime.

STEP 2. ENCOURAGE SELF-SOOTHING

A. Drowsy but awake.
B. Many hands.
C. Many naps if younger than 3–4 months; if older, schedule naps.

STEP 3. LESS ATTENTION DURING THE NIGHT

If your child cries, always respond immediately if you think he is hungry, wet, soiled, or in distress. Always delay your response if you think your child's vocalizations are non-distress sounds.

A. *Extinction.* Consider if *neither* parent has symptoms of anxiety or depression. Dramatic improvement occurs after *one or two nights.*

HOW MUCH CRYING OCCURS EACH NIGHT WITH EXTINCTION WHEN *ALL* FOUR STEPS ARE IN PLACE?

	Child Is Younger than 4 Months	Child Is 4 Months or Older
Night 1	30–45 minutes	45–55 minutes
Night 2	10–30 minutes	A little more or less than night 1
Night 3	0–10 minutes	20–40 minutes
Night 4	No crying	0–10 minutes
Night 5	No crying	No crying

There might be more crying each night and for more days when any of the four steps are *not* in place.

B. *Graduated extinction.* Consider if *either* parent has symptoms of anxiety or depression. If so, dramatic improvement occurs after *four to seven nights.*

C. *Check and console.* Minimal crying may occur.

D. *Fading.* Consider if *either* or *both* parents have symptoms of anxiety or depression. No crying occurs.

STEP 4. PROTECT NAPS

   A. Pitch-black and quiet room (if needed)

   B. Sound machine

   C. *Nap drill*

Understanding Differences among Families

Parents might ask which is the best method (extinction, graduated extinction, check and console, or fading—all are described thoroughly in chapter 5) to treat sleep problems. Actually, there is no best method, because different methods work better for different families because of differences among children and families. Hopefully, this outline will help you decide what is best for *your* family. Understanding some basic differences among children and parenting styles will help you make the most comfortable choice for your family.

Consider two groups of children and two parenting styles in order to better understand why there is no single "right" way to help *all* children sleep better.

Two Groups of Children: Common Fussiness/Crying and Extreme Fussiness/Colic

All babies sometimes fuss or cry, even when they are warm, dry, well fed, and in no distress (*common fussiness*), but some children fuss and cry much more and are more difficult to settle to sleep (*extreme fussiness/colic*).

	Common Fussiness/ Crying	Extreme Fussiness/ Colic
Prevalence	80%	20%
Symptoms of anxiety or depression in mother	Less	More
Maternal age at birth	Younger	Older

Maternal symptoms of anxiety/depression might cause or be caused by extreme infant fussiness/colic, or alternatively, because fathers were generally not included in many studies, the maternal symptoms might be the result of an absent, alcoholic, addicted, or abusive husband. Thus, there is *no* implication that mothers are directly causing extreme fussiness/colic in their babies.

Older mothers tend to be married to older fathers who are less involved in helping babies sleep well at night. So, again, it would be a mistake to think that there is something directly related to maternal age that is causing extreme fussiness/colic in babies.

	Common Fussiness/ Crying	Extreme Fussiness/ Colic
Unnecessary attention at night (unneeded feeding or picking up)	Less	More
Infant's capability to self-soothe	Easy	Difficult
"Start as you mean to go"	Yes	No

Consistency ("Start as you mean to go") in encouraging self-soothing applies mainly to the common fussiness group. Consistency may be difficult to accomplish because any parent might be extremely stressed from their own sleep deprivation; this is especially true for the parents of colicky babies. For extreme fussiness/colic infants, parents will struggle to cope with an unsettled infant and begin to try "drowsy but awake" at about 2–3 months of age.

WHEN TO START TO TEACH SELF-SOOTHING

	Common Fussiness/ Crying	Extreme Fussiness/ Colic
Drowsy but awake	Birth	Around 2–3 months
Many hands	Birth	Birth
Many naps	Birth	Birth
Earlier bedtime at 6 weeks	Yes	Yes
Protect naps at 3–4 months	Yes	Yes
Night waking or other sleep problems appear at 3–4 months	No	Yes*

* If self-soothing is not taught.

If you think that your baby has extreme fussiness/colic, the first few months will be extremely challenging, but have confidence that if you change your behavior to include drowsy but awake at around 2–3 months, you will help your baby sleep substantially better.

Two Parenting Styles: Limit Setting and Infant Demand

Professor Ian St. James-Roberts studied two different parenting styles: infant demand and limit setting. Parents who practice *infant demand parenting* want to hold their baby both when he's awake and when he's asleep and, in general, not allow their baby to be alone. They often will sleep with their baby, even though this is discouraged by the American Academy of Pediatrics because of the increased risk of sudden infant death syndrome. These parents might object to "drowsy but awake," "less attention during the night," or starting any of the steps to promote self-soothing at a very young age. They also might believe that always being close to their child, especially when very young, creates a stronger bond of "trust." They might accept some of these steps when the child is older or implement only some steps, such as "move bedtime earlier," when their child is 6 weeks old. Also, these parents might argue that their approach is right for all children because it is more natural or that giving less attention during the night when babies are very young harms the baby or the baby–parent relationship.

Parents who practice *limit-setting parenting* are more comfortable soothing their very young baby to a drowsy but awake state and then putting their baby down to sleep in a crib and leaving the room, even if some low-level whimpering or other sounds occur.

Let's try to clarify what is going on by looking at these two parenting styles.

	Limit Setting	Infant Demand
Hold your infant (hours per day)	7–8	15–16
Sleep with your baby (family bed)	Less	More
Breastfeeding duration	Shorter	Longer
Infant crying at 2 and 5 weeks	More (15 minutes more)	Less
Bouts of inconsolable crying	Yes	Yes
Extreme fussiness/colic	Yes	Yes
Infant crying at 12 weeks	More (5 minutes more)	Less
Night-waking problem at 12 weeks	Less	More
Infant wakes up parents at night at 10 months	Less	More

Some parents with the infant demand style are proactive and have chosen this style, even before their baby is born, because it lines up with their values, but other parents reactively fall into this style because their infant has extreme fussiness/colic. In either situation, the benefit might be more breastfeeding and a little less crying at 2, 5, and 12 weeks of age. However, the cost might be the failure to learn self-soothing, and if so, their child, starting at about 3 months of age, develops chronic sleep problems. One reason why this child may not learn self-soothing is that it is difficult to practice sleeping with your baby and also have an early bedtime. Another problem is that the child becomes dependent on parent soothing to sleep at the beginning of the night and does not have the opportunity to practice self-soothing at bedtime, so that later, in the middle of the night, he might have difficulty returning to sleep unassisted.

Among parents proactively using the infant demand style, some planned to practice consistent co-sleeping (bed-sharing or family bed) before their baby's birth and are described as "infant-cued."

INFANT FUSSINESS/CRYING AT NIGHT

	Limit Setting	Infant-Cued
Time to respond at night	3.5 minutes	Immediate
During the time to respond, at night, the infant fussed/cried	1 minute	None

MINUTES OF FUSSINESS/CRYING AT NIGHT

Age	Limit Setting	Infant-Cued
2 weeks	69	39
5 weeks	About 55	About 55
3 months	About 25	About 25
Sleeping continuously for 5 hours or more at night at 3 months (see below)	89%	37%

Some parents in the limit-setting group, at night, consistently introduced a short interval delay (about *one minute*) before feeding to see if the child might independently return to sleep. For those infants where the night feeding was slightly delayed, there was a longer interval between nighttime and daytime feedings at 5 weeks, and by 3 months twice as many (89 percent versus 37 percent) of these infants were sleeping continuously for five or more hours at night compared with the children in the infant-cued group (co-sleeping, no delay before feeding).

If your child has common fussiness/crying and your parenting style is limit setting—and only if you feel comfortable with this suggestion—consider slightly delaying a night feeding if your child is gaining weight appropriately, the interval from the previous feed is short, and you suspect that he might not be truly hungry because the whimpering or crying is very quiet. Then, because the vocalization might not really indicate hunger, your child is given the opportunity to practice some self-soothing and possibly return to sleep without requiring a feeding.

This brief delay in feeding might mean that you wait a moment before attending to your child—or alternatively, that you immediately attend to your child, but you change the diaper or soothe your baby first to see if he will settle to sleep without a feeding. Either way, your baby is more likely to have long sleep bouts at night by 3 months of age.

However, the inability to delay a response may be an innate trait in the parent and/or a response to their baby's fussiness/crying. So do what feels comfortable for you. I hope you will be comfortable with my advice, and please understand that there are no rigid rules regarding healthy sleep that apply to all children. For example, 80 percent of 6-month-olds sleep during the day between 2.5 and 4.0 hours, but my advice and guidelines might not apply to the 20 percent of 6-month-olds who sleep more or less than that during the day, especially if they are well rested. In other words, my suggestions might be appropriate for the majority of families but *not* necessarily for *all* families. Because your child may be well rested but sleep differently from the majority of children, please do *not* compare your child's sleep schedule with other children's sleep schedules. Your goal is a well-rested family, so watch your child and follow the advice in this book that is *helpful* to you and pay more attention to *drowsy signs* than to *clock time* when establishing sleep schedules for your child.

IMPORTANT POINTS

1. *Why it is not necessary to make your child cry to have a good night's sleep.* Sleep problems are preventable in the first place (chapter 4), and there are effective "no-cry" sleep solutions (chapter 5).

2. *Why a little earlier bedtime may have a great benefit.* Only a few minutes of extra sleep, over time, has been shown to be very helpful (chapter 2).

3. *Why it is wrong to judge another parent's parenting.* Parents have different values (chapter 1) and challenges (chapters 2 and 4). Parenting is different in different cultures.

4. *Why it is wrong to compare your child with other children.* Children are born with genetic differences regarding sleeping (chapters 2 and 6), and with different temperaments (chapter 8).

Conclusion

There is no one "right" way to help all babies sleep well. What works for one baby and one parenting style might not be right for you. What is best for *your* family is to identify *your* baby's capability to self-soothe, and to encourage that ability as soon as possible. If your child is not sleeping well, it is never too late to make changes.

The earlier you put forth the effort, the easier it is for you and your baby.

Moving the bedtime just a few minutes earlier can make a huge improvement, since small amounts of extra sleep can have a big impact. Remember, the most common cause of sleep problems in children is a bedtime that is too late.

Chapter 2 Outline

SLEEP DURATION: NIGHT AND DAY
Newborns and Young Infants
Older Infants and Children
Daytime Wakefulness, Sleepiness, and Hyperarousal
Witching Hour
Second Wind

NAPS

SLEEP INERTIA

MOTIONLESS SLEEP

SLEEP CONSOLIDATION AND FRAGMENTATION
Protective Arousals
Sleep Fragmentation

SLEEP SCHEDULE, TIMING OF SLEEP, BEDTIME
Bedtime
Proportion of Total Sleep Occurring during the Night or
Day
Night Sleep Organization
Day Sleep Organization

SLEEP REGULARITY
Biological Rhythms

What Constitutes Healthy Sleep?

If you have not already done so, please go back and read chapter 1. There are five main elements of healthy sleep for children:

1. Sleep duration: night and day
2. Naps
3. Sleep consolidation
4. Sleep schedule, timing of sleep, bedtime
5. Sleep regularity

When these five items are in proper balance, children get the rest they need. Let's first take a look at each one separately. Later, we will see how each element is not really independent of the others but simply part of a package called "healthy sleep." Other elements are the amount of time during the night that the child is wakeful after sleep onset and the proportion of total sleep that occurs at night.

There are five turning points in the sleep maturation process:

1. At 6 weeks, night sleep lengthens.
2. At 12–16 weeks, daytime sleep regularizes, with two major naps and a variable third nap.

3. By 9 months, night waking for feeding disappears, as does the third nap.
4. At 12–21 months, the midmorning nap disappears.
5. At 3–4 years, the midday nap becomes less common.

As your baby's brain matures, her patterns and rhythm of sleep change. If you adapt your parenting practices to these changes, your child will sleep well. Those parents who do not notice these changes or fail to make the proper adjustments have babies who become overtired. The biological development causing these changes is under the control of two regulatory mechanisms. (Things such as feeding routines, which vary from family to family, do not influence how the brain develops.) Understanding these biological controlling mechanisms will help you organize your thoughts and plan your actions to ensure healthy sleep for your child.

The first regulatory system controls the body's need for sleep and has been called the *homeostatic control mechanism*. This system keeps track of how much sleep you need. In a nutshell, it means that the longer you go without sleep, the longer you will subsequently sleep. If you lose sleep, the body tries to restore it. This automatic process reflects an internal biological mechanism that we do not control. It is similar to the body's regulation of temperature; when we get hot, we automatically sweat, and when we're cold, we shiver. It is no different with sleep needs. But since babies cannot use language to inform us of their needs, parents must be on their toes in order not to miss the signs of shifts in sleeping requirements.

The second regulatory system has been called the *circadian timing system*. It is also called the human body's inner clockwork or internal timing system and can be thought of as a dedicated regulatory program that switches specific genes on and off in response to the light–dark cycle. This regulatory apparatus is a molecular clock set to the proper time by sunlight. It automatically tries to ensure that the body is sleeping at the right time, and that when you are asleep, the timing and amounts of different stages and types of sleep are correct. Signals come from a specific area within the brain to make us feel sleepy or wakeful. These signals are present in babies as well as adults, but in babies the patterns change over the weeks, months, and years of growth and maturation. The pace of these changes is especially quick during the first several months, so it is easy for a parent to get a little off tempo. Just when you think you have figured out when your baby needs to nap or be put to bed at night, the circadian timing system sends her new instructions!

The internal timing system is under genetic control, so there is *individual variation*. It takes time for the internal timing system to express itself.

Genetic influences account for some of the individual differences in sleep measurements. Studies of twins, as young as 6 months, show that both genetic factors and environmental factors (parenting) are important.

Now let's get to the first pillar of healthy sleep.

Sleep Duration: Night and Day

If you don't sleep long enough, you feel tired. This sounds very simple and obvious, but how much sleep is enough? And how can you tell if *your* child is getting enough sleep?

The sleep patterns of infants under 3–4 months of age seem mostly to reflect the development of the child's brain. During these first few weeks, in fact, sleep durations equal sleep needs, since infant behavior and sleep durations are mostly influenced by biological factors. But after about 3–4 months, and perhaps even at about 6 weeks (or 6 weeks after the due date, for babies born early), parenting practices can start to influence sleep duration and, consequently, behavior. As I will discuss later in more detail, I believe parents can promote more charming, calm, alert behaviors by becoming more sensitive to their growing child's need to sleep and by helping to establish and maintain healthy sleep habits. The goal is to recognize and respect your child's need to sleep and not do things that interfere with the natural sleep process.

The natural process is under genetic control, but genes control more than the internal timing system. Genes also influence how individuals are affected by short sleep durations. For example, shorter sleep duration is associated with more negative emotionality, but only among some children with a variant of a gene. Also, some college undergraduates are genetically protected somewhat from the adverse effects from shifting sleep schedules on weekdays compared with weekends (*social jet lag*). Studies involving 13-year-old twins, using objective measurements of sleep, show a genetic influence on sleep durations, but only on weekends, not school days, when early wake-up times are required.

The take-home message is that some children *innately* need less sleep than others for optimal health or are more resilient to shifting sleep schedules. So just because your child is getting less sleep than others, it does not necessarily mean that she is sleep-deprived. Also, some children are more bothered by irregular sleep schedules than others. Sleeping out of sync with biological rhythms ("circadian stress" or "temporal friction") does not harm all children equally. In short, we have genetically driven individual differences regarding how much sleep we need and how much harm will be produced by short sleep or irregular sleep.

In this book, I will present a lot of information regarding durations of sleep and clock times for sleep, but please pay more attention to your child than these numbers. Please try to recognize and appreciate your own child's apparent need for sleep but try not to compare this amount with other children.

NEWBORNS AND YOUNG INFANTS

During their first few days, newborns sleep about sixteen to seventeen hours total each day, although their longest single sleep period is only four to five hours. It makes no difference whether your baby is breastfed or bottle-fed, or whether it's a boy or a girl.

> Nursing mothers often worry unnecessarily that long sleep periods deprive their baby of adequate breast milk. Weight checks with the doctor will reassure you that all is well.

Between 1 week and 4 months, the total daily sleep duration drifts down from sixteen and a half to fifteen hours, while the longest single sleep period—usually the night—increases from four to nine hours. We know from several studies that this development reflects neurological maturation and is *not* related to the start of feeding solid foods.

Some newborns and infants under the age of 4 months sleep much more and others much less. During the first few months, you can usually assume that your baby is getting sufficient sleep. But if your baby cries too much or has extreme fussiness/colic, you might assist Mother Nature by trying the helpful hints for "crybabies" described in chapter 6.

> When they are 1–2 weeks old, many infants begin to have periods of increasingly alert, wakeful, gassy, and fussy behavior. This continues until about 6 weeks of age, after which they start to calm down. This increasingly irritable and wakeful state is often misinterpreted as resulting from maternal anxiety or from insufficient or "bad" breast milk. Nonsense! The culprit is a temporarily uninhibited nervous system that causes excessive arousal. Relax; this developmental phase will pass as the baby's brain matures. It's not your fault.

Young infants are very portable. You can take them anywhere you want, and when they need to sleep, they will. I remember when, as a medical student at Stanford University, I was playing tennis with my wife one day and my first child was sleeping in an infant seat near the fence. A huge dump truck came crashing down the narrow street, making an awful racket. We ran over to our son, certain that he had been jolted from his peaceful sleep, only to be surprised that he slept on blissfully. After 6 weeks of age, he became more socially aware of people around him; after about 4 months of age, he, like all children, became interested in barking dogs, wind in the trees, clouds, and many other curious things, all of which could and did disturb his sleep, either by waking him up or by making him fight to stay awake.

In some cases, the time when the baby first makes a socially responsive smile (usually at 6 weeks of age, or 6 weeks after the due date for babies born early) is when social curiosity or social learning begins. However, under about 3–4 months of age, most infants, like my son, are not much disturbed by their environment when it comes to sleeping. When their body says it's time to sleep, they sleep. When their body tells them to wake up, they wake up—even when it's not convenient for their parents! This is true whether they are fed on demand or according to a regular schedule. It is also true even when they are continuously fed intravenously because of birth defects of the stomach or intestines. Hunger, in fact, seems to have little to do with how babies sleep. A much more likely candidate for influencing a baby's sleeping patterns is the hormone melatonin, which is produced by the baby's brain beginning at about 3–4 months of age. This hormone surges at night and has the capability to both induce drowsiness and relax the smooth muscles encircling the gut. So around 3–4 months of age, so-called day/night confusion and apparent abdominal cramps (colic) begin to disappear.

Furthermore, infants raised in an environment where the lights are constantly on evolve normal sleep patterns, just like babies brought up in homes where the lights are turned on and off routinely. Another bit of evidence to suggest that environment has little effect on sleep patterns in children under 3–4 months of age comes from infants born prematurely. A child born four weeks before her due date, for example, reaches the same level of sleep development as a full-term baby four weeks *later* than the child born on time. Biological sleep/wake development does not speed up in those preemies who are exposed to more social stimulation.

What we can conclude, therefore, is that for infants under 3–4 months of age you should try to flow with the child's need for sleep. Don't expect predictable sleep schedules, and don't try to enforce them rigidly. Still, some babies do develop regular sleep/wake rhythms quite early, at about 6–8 weeks. These babies tend to be very mild, cry very little, and sleep for long periods of time. Consider yourself blessed if you are the lucky parent of such an infant!

OLDER INFANTS AND CHILDREN

As children age, the amount of time they sleep tends to decrease. Figures 1 through 3 describe how much daytime sleep, night sleep, and total sleep occur at different ages for older children. The bottom curve in each graph means that 10 percent of children sleep less than the amount shown, while the top curve means that 90 percent of children sleep less than the amount shown for each age. These curves were generated by my own research using data collected from 2,019 children, mostly white, middle-class residents of northern Illinois and northern Indiana, in 1980. These graphs can help you tell whether your child's sleep is above the 90th percentile or below the 10th percentile. (Other studies have used only the 50th percentile, or average values, and do not tell you whether your child's sleep duration is slightly below average or extremely below average.) Interestingly, the results of studies of similar social classes in 1911 in California and in 1927 in Minnesota, also involving thousands of children, were the same as those in my study. In addition, studies in England in 1910 and Japan in 1925 showed identical sleep curves.

Thus, it seems that despite cultural and ethnic differences, social changes, and the impact of such modern inventions as television, computers, and cell phones on our contemporary lifestyles, the age-specific durations of sleep are firmly and universally rooted in our children's developing biology.

An exception to this generalization is that adolescents everywhere are now getting less sleep. During the second half of the twentieth century, a trend toward earlier start times for high school developed. This forced children to get up earlier during the school week and reduced the total number of hours available for sleeping. At the same time, it became more popular for teenagers to hold part-time jobs after school, and participation in extracurricular sports became more prevalent and demanding, so teenagers were going to bed later. Further, the amount of homework has increased.

But how long you sleep is not the whole story. In 9- to 16-year-olds, the timing of sleep, not just sleep duration, makes a big difference. Even when the sleep duration is the same, those children who went to bed later did less vigorous exercise each day and had more periods of physical inactivity than children with an earlier bedtime.

My study on sleep duration was in 1980. In 1990, less than 10 percent of children had a TV in their bedroom. However, beginning around 1990, the trend of having a TV in a child's bedroom developed, so that by 2007 about 20 percent of children under 2 years of age and 40 percent of children from 3 to 6 years old had a TV in their bedroom. Having a TV in the bedroom is associated with sleep problems and less sleeping (page 216). More recently, cell phone and computer use at night has pushed bedtimes even later. As noted previously, after about 4 months I think parents can influence sleep durations, and as you will see, sleep durations for these older infants, toddlers, and teens are especially important. One easy thing you can do is keep all screen-based media devices out of the bedroom at bedtime.

I studied sixty healthy children in my pediatric practice at 5 months of age and then again at 36 months. At 5 months, the infants who were cooing, smiling, adaptable, and regular (their sleep times and hungry times were around the same time every day) and who curiously approached unfamiliar things or people slept longer than infants with opposite characteristics. These easy and calm infants slept about three and a half hours during the day and twelve hours at night, for a total of fifteen and a half hours. Infants who were fussy, crying, irritable, hard to handle, irregular, and more withdrawn slept almost three hours less overall, almost a 20 percent difference (three hours during the day and nine and a half hours at night, or twelve and a half hours total).

In addition, for all the 5-month-olds studied, persistence or attention span was the trait most strongly associated with daytime sleep or nap duration. In other words, *children who slept longer during the day had longer attention spans.*

Figure 1

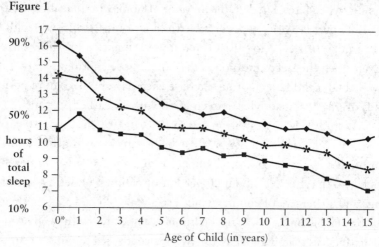

Age of Child (in years)

*Note: 0 represents children between 4 and 11 months of age.

As I will discuss in a later chapter, infants who sleep more during the day are better able to learn from their environment; this is because they have a better-developed ability to maintain focused or sustained attention. They soak up information about their surroundings like a sponge soaking up water. They learn simply from looking at the clouds and trees, from touching, feeling, smelling, and hearing, and from watching their mother's and father's faces. Additionally, we now know that naps have the ability to enhance cognitive development, because naps consolidate or strengthen memories of learning that occurred before the nap (page 45). Infants who sleep less in the daytime appear more fitful and socially demanding, and they are less able to entertain or amuse themselves. Toys and objects are less interesting to these more tired children.

Figure 2

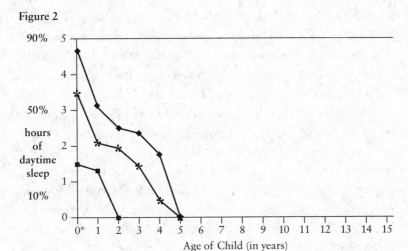

Age of Child (in years)

*Note: 0 represents children between 4 and 11 months of age.

Figure 3

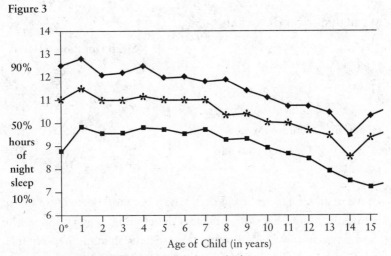

Age of Child (in years)

*Note: 0 represents children between 4 and 11 months of age.

By 3 years of age, the easier-to-manage children in my study—mild, positive in mood, adaptable, and more likely to approach unfamiliar people—slept twelve and a half hours total. The difficult-to-manage children—those who were intense, more negative, less adaptable, and withdrawing—slept about one and a half hours less, almost the equivalent of a daytime nap.

An important conclusion is that 3-year-olds who nap are more adaptable than those who do not. But napping did *not* affect the length of sleep at night. Comparing nappers and non-nappers, night sleep duration was ten and a half hours in both groups. Those who napped, however, slept about two hours longer during the day, so their total sleep was twelve and a half hours. Therefore, it simply is not true that children who miss naps will make up for it by sleeping more at night. In fact, the sleep they miss is gone forever.

Now, before you panic, I want you to understand that missing a nap here and there will probably cause no harm. But if this does become habitual, you can expect your child to lag further and further behind in her sleep and to become increasingly difficult to handle in this overfatigued state.

SLEEP DURATION OF 3-YEAR-OLDS

| | | Sleep Duration (Hours) | | |
		Day	Night	Total
Group A	Easy to manage	1.9	10.6	12.5
	Difficult to manage	0.9	10.4	11.3
Group B	Children who do not nap	—	10.5	10.5
	Children who nap	2.0	10.5	12.5

All in all, at age 3, the children who slept more were more fun to be around, more sociable, and less demanding. The children who slept less not only tended to be more socially demanding, irritable, and fussy but also behaved somewhat like hyperactive children.

One study examined the effects of a single night of sleep restriction in a group of children between 10 and 14 years old. The researchers noted that there were impairments in verbal creativity, abstract thinking and concept formation, and complex problem solving. These higher cognitive abilities appear to be essential for academic performance and success. In contrast, there were *no* deficits in rote performance or less complex memory and learning tasks. The ability to maintain routine performance despite being sleepy is familiar to every adult who sometimes gets very tired but nevertheless is able to perform the routine aspects of his or her job fairly well. My interpretation of this study is that chronic sleepiness in infants and young children impairs cognitive development, but this does not become apparent until the child is much older and challenged by more complex tasks. Of course, cognitive development starts in babies, not at 10–14 years of age, but the deficits from sleep deprivation remain *hidden* in young children. When children are younger, the challenges they face are at a much lower level, and these chronically sleep-deprived children may still do well with spelling, writing, reading, and simple arithmetic. Later, when they are older, more demanding academic challenges *unmask* the cognitive deficits lurking there all along.

Looking at our sleep curves again, we see that throughout early and middle childhood, the duration of sleep declines until adolescence, when the curve shown in figure 1 levels off and then slightly increases. This increase has been noted in some other studies and suggests that teenagers need more sleep than preteens. Yet, as noted previously, academic demands, social events, and school sports combine during adolescence to pressure teenagers to stay up later and later. Also, there are biological shifts in adolescents that seem to encourage more wakefulness in the evening. This is the time when chronic and *cumulative sleep losses* begin to take their toll and can make a normally rough period in life unbearably rocky for children and parents alike.

In general, do not pay too much attention to these graphs: They are only rough descriptions of age-specific groups of children. They are not prescriptions for *your* child. The fact is, for any specific age, there are short sleepers and long sleepers. You might wish that your child slept longer, but she might be a perfectly healthy short sleeper. It is much more important to watch your child than it is to watch the clock.

Daytime Wakefulness, Sleepiness, and Hyperarousal

Watching your child carefully allows you to become aware of subtle changes in her wakefulness or sleepiness. We tend to think superficially of being either awake or asleep, as if these two black-and-white states were the only possibilities. But there are gradations of sleep, and of wakefulness, too. Task performance, attentiveness, vigilance, and mood are influenced not only by the quality of our sleep at night but also by the quality of our wakefulness during the day. When we do not feel very awake during the day, we say that we feel "sleepy." Or, to be more precise, studies of adults show that most adults avoid the word *sleepy* and instead use the word *tired*, which implies previous effortful behavior or hard work—something to be proud of. It seems that the word *tired* is more acceptable in our culture, and an admission of feeling sleepy is something to deny, as if it were a weakness of character. I encourage parents to get into the habit of using the word *sleepy* for their child because it directly implies what is needed: more sleep. Think of excessive daytime sleepiness or impaired daytime alertness as a result of disturbed sleep.

The Stanford Sleepiness Scale is a self-rating instrument developed at Stanford University to describe the different states or levels of daytime sleepiness. Obviously, children who are depressed or irritable due to sleep deprivation will have high numerical ratings.

Level Description
1. Feeling active and vital; alert; wide awake
2. Functioning at a high level, but not at peak; still able to concentrate
3. Relaxed; awake; not at full alertness; responsive

4. A little foggy; not at peak; let down
5. Fogginess; beginning to lose interest in remaining awake; slowed down
6. Sleepiness; preferring to be lying down; fighting sleep; woozy
7. Almost in reverie; sleep onset soon; lost struggle to remain awake

The descriptions in this scale are self-assessments. Because young children cannot articulate what they are feeling, parents have to watch for signs of daytime sleepiness in their children. But what should you be watching for?

Dr. Murray Johns developed the Epworth Sleepiness Scale for Children and Adolescents. Although it is designed for children 12–18 years of age, you can also get a sense of how sleepy your younger child might be.

Chance of Falling Asleep
   0 = would never fall asleep
   1 = slight chance of falling asleep
   2 = moderate chance of falling asleep
   3 = high chance of falling asleep

Each numerical score is then assigned to the following activities:

Sitting and reading
Sitting and watching TV or a video
Sitting in a classroom at school during the morning
Sitting and riding in a car or bus for about half an hour
Lying down to rest or nap in the afternoon
Sitting and talking to someone
Sitting quietly by yourself after lunch
Sitting and eating a meal

Higher scores are associated with more daytime sleepiness. Cut-off values for the adult version are: mild (more than 11), moderate (more than 13), and severe (more than 16) excessive daytime sleepiness.

Daytime sleepiness resulting from disturbed sleep typically causes adults to feel a mild itching or burning in the eyes. Our eyelids feel heavy. As you become more sleepy, long eyeblinks and heavy eyelids are a result of the brain attempting to switch to the sleep mode. Our limbs feel heavy, too, and we tend to be lethargic. We are less motivated, lose interest easily, and have difficulty concentrating. Our speech slows; we yawn and rub our eyes. As we get sleepier, our eyes begin to close, and we may even find our head nodding. Are these the signs we should look for in our babies and young children?

No. This familiar picture of adult sleep is not usually seen in infants and young children who suffer from disturbed sleep. While it is true that infants who are usually well rested yawn on occasions when they are overtired, it seems that chronically sleepy infants do not yawn much or nod off. Instead, when most young kids get too sleepy, they get grumpy and excitable. At age 3, my first son coined the perfect word to describe this turned-on state: "upcited," a combination of "upset" and "excited," as in "Don't make me upcited!" when we admonished him for behaving like a little monster.

Two very interesting Australian studies on adults have helped to shed light on childhood "upcited" behavior. One study showed that the level of activation of the nervous system was associated with certain personality traits, sleep habits, and activity of the adrenal gland. Poor sleepers were more anxious and had higher levels of the hormone cortisol, which typically rises during stressful situations.

The second study was complex, but I think its results will better help you to understand your child's behaviors. In this study, adult volunteers reported their moods on four scales:

1. Tired to rested
2. Sluggish to alert
3. Irritable to calm
4. Tense to relaxed

The first two scales reflected degrees of *arousal*, while the third and fourth scales reflected degrees of *stress*.

The researchers measured four different hormones (cortisol, noradrenaline, adrenaline, and dopamine) that our bodies make naturally. These powerful chemicals affect our brain and how we feel, and they are related to the four scales in different ways.

For example, fatigue produces an increase in adrenaline concentrations. That is, when we are tired, our body chemically responds with a burst of adrenaline to give us more drive or energy. We become more aroused, alert, and excitable. Concentrations of cortisol also increase with increasing alertness. In children, cortisol concentrations remain high when they do not nap. Perhaps the nap allows the brain to be alert without needing the added boost cortisol provides. Increasing irritability and tenseness—stress factors—are also associated with increasing concentrations of adrenaline, noradrenaline, and dopamine.

These studies support the notion that when an overly sleepy child appears wired, wild, edgy, excitable, or unable to fall asleep easily or stay asleep, she is this way precisely because of her body's response to being short of sleep (page 120). Think of how you feel when you work hard and lose sleep in order to finish a major project. You are highly motivated and fight the daytime sleepiness. The impairments of performance and discomfort of sleepiness increase. After a while, you feel keyed up. Thankfully, modern adults are able to get out of this state by taking vacations. But have you noticed how, at the start of a vacation, it takes a few days to unwind? This is the time required for our accumulated nervous energy to dissipate.

REMEMBER
When your infant or young child appears wired, she may actually be tired.

This tells me that our lifestyle and sleep habits can affect our internal chemical machinery, which in turn causes us to feel certain ways. In a study at Dartmouth College, coronary-prone type A students had more night wakings than type B students. A vicious circle could develop whereby fragmented sleep causes increased arousal, the student feels more energized, and, sensing this greater level of energy, the student works even harder late into the night to achieve more, but at the same time loses more sleep. In a review of adult insomnia, Dr. Winkelman wrote, "Insomnia is commonly conceptualized as a disorder of nocturnal and daytime *hyperarousal* [emphasis added]." But distinct differences exist between adult insomniacs whose insomnia started in childhood and those whose insomnia started in adulthood. Childhood-onset insomniacs reported more nightmares as adults, and during childhood had more "fear of the dark" and nightmares. As adults, childhood-onset insomniacs take longer to fall asleep and sleep less than adult-onset insomniacs. However, objective sleep lab evaluations show that childhood-onset insomniacs' average total sleep time was only *twenty-nine minutes* less than that for adult-onset insomniacs. Additionally, among adults who had both insomnia and depression, comparing those who had childhood-onset insomnia with those suffering adult-onset insomnia, the group with childhood-onset was less responsive to all manner of treatments. I think these data support the hypothesis that the failure to establish good sleeping habits in infancy or early childhood has long-term harmful effects, such as adult insomnia.

IMPORTANT POINT

Loss of sleep produces central nervous system hyperarousal.

Infants over 4 months of age as well as older children can push themselves hard fighting sleep in order to enjoy the pleasure of their parents' company and play. The resulting sleep disturbances might produce fatigue, and the body would naturally respond by turning up production of those chemicals, such as cortisol, responsible for maintaining alertness and arousal. Perhaps researchers may someday find that different patterns of sleep deprivation (total sleep loss, abnormal schedules, nap deprivation, or sleep fragmentation) produce different patterns of chemical imbalances. Here are some terms used by professionals to describe the behavior of hyperalert children with disturbed sleep:

Physiological activation
Neurological arousal
Excessive wakefulness
Emotional reactivity
Heightened sensitivity

Parents simply call this behavior "wired."

IMPORTANT POINT
Some chronically sleepy children are always keyed up and never unwind.

So often I have heard comments like "She's so tired, she's running around in circles," or "She wants to fall asleep but can't." This is not a new observation; a classic paper published in 1922 described the "increased reflex-irritability of a sleepy child." In dramatic contrast, over and over again I have seen well-rested children in my practice who spend enormous amounts of time in a state of quiet alertness. They take in everything with wide-open eyes, never missing a thing. They find simple little toys amusing or curious. They never appear bored, even though the toy they pick up may be one they have played with many times.

The good news is that you can help guide your child to healthy sleep and make a big difference. Parents of children 4–12 months of age can *dramatically* and *quickly* change their children's mood and behavior depending on how much sleep they allow their kids to get.

For example, in a study published in 2002 of 4- and 5-year-olds, author Dr. John E. Bates stated, "In clinical treatment of young, oppositional children, we have seen some spectacular improvements in manageability associated with the parents instituting a more adequate schedule of sleep for their children. Our clinical impression in these cases was that the changes were too rapid to be accounted for by other changes, such as parental discipline tactics."

I think it worthwhile to remember that a calm alert state is a sign of sleeping well. Upon awakening, well-rested children are in good cheer and are able to play by themselves. I believe that in infants and young children, a cause-and-effect relationship exists between disturbed sleep and fitful, fussy behaviors. In addition, as described later, the harmful effects of excessive daytime sleepiness do not stay the same, but rather tend to accumulate (page 82). This means that there is a progressive worsening in a child's mood and performance even when the amount of lost sleep each day or night is constant. So a baby becomes increasingly crabby even if her nightly sleep is constantly just a little too brief. Another way to say this is that a constant small deficit in sleep produces a *cumulative* reduction in daytime alertness.

Here are some signs that your child is not getting quality sleep: She often falls asleep in the stroller or car when you are out doing errands; she often wakes up crying, grumpy, or painfully confused; and there is usually a "witching hour" in the late afternoon or early evening.

Witching Hour

After 3–4 months of age, if your baby is often fussy during the day, she is most likely short on sleep. But many children suffering from insufficient sleep appear fine during most of the day, only to exhibit the symptoms listed as the sleep tank begins to go dry near the end of the day (4:00 to 5:00 P.M. for children under the age of 3 years, and 5:00 to 7:00 P.M. for children 3 years and older). This is known as the witching hour, and a child experiencing it may be irritable, easily upset, clinging, whining, fussy, peevish, or, in the words of one mother, "clawing at my breast." She might have a short fuse, be rough around the edges, seem easily frustrated, or be less able than usual to entertain herself. She might be oppositional, defiant, uncooperative, or angry; she might throw tantrums, be aggressive, display a negative mood, be inattentive or distractible, exhibit learning difficulties, show decreased sociability and physical activity, and be generally depressed or anxious. This is quite a laundry list, but don't despair: Very few children demonstrate more than a handful of these symptoms at one time. But any of them, coming during the witching hour, can be a signal of sleep problems that parents should address.

Second Wind

The witching hour may be thought of as a second wind or pre-sleep arousal state. Dr. Alice Gregory studied pre-sleep arousals in 8- to 10-year-olds and showed that the arousal was both physical (rapidly beating heart) and cognitive (unable to stop thinking and worrying about falling asleep). In her study, cognitive arousal was associated with *sleep disturbances*. Also, Dr. Julio Fernandez-Mendoza studied 327 children age 5–12 years and showed that children with *short sleep durations* exhibited hyperarousal before sleep.

When you are short on sleep, your body reacts in a predictable way. As previously described, you get keyed up because your body produces stimulating chemicals such as cortisol, adrenaline, and noradrenaline. This results in a burst of energy commonly known as a second wind. When you catch your second wind, you are in a state of higher neurological arousal. You might feel more wired, turned on, or full of nervous energy. You also become more prickly or hypersensitive, just as a bad sunburn will make even a light touch painful. This state of hyperarousal is most obvious in a young child in the late afternoon or early evening when her sleep tank is almost empty and she is running on fumes because of missed naps, bedtimes that are too late, or both. Think of how your child might have a total meltdown late in the afternoon at a family holiday involving many hours of travel and many hours without sleep. But while the witching hour occurs near the end of the day, the second wind can occur whenever a period of wakefulness before a nap is too long. The result is difficulty falling asleep for a nap, or the nap is too short, or the nap is missed entirely. If this occurs only occasionally, it is probably not a problem for your child even though your nerves are frayed! But imagine what happens when your child usually goes to bed a little too late or too often misses naps.

When the bedtime is usually or often a little too late, the child wakes up too tired, and this higher neurological arousal then causes her to have difficulty napping well. Not napping well causes her sleep tank to tend toward empty by the end of the day and results in an even higher state of arousal, so it now becomes even more difficult for her to easily fall asleep and stay asleep at night. Parents might not appreciate that bedtime battles, long latency to sleep (taking a long time to fall asleep), or night waking result from a bedtime that is too late. Of course, the child eventually crashes. But before she does so, she is in an unhealthy state that gives rise to stressful parent–child interactions, stressful interactions between parents, and stress for each parent as an individual. Additionally, because the bedtime was too late, your child may not receive the benefits of healthy sleep—the very deep restorative sleep periods that naturally occur early in the evening.

Understanding how sleep deprivation causes a second wind that makes it more difficult to easily fall asleep and stay asleep also leads to a deeper appreciation of the opposite situation: Being well rested allows your child to more easily fall asleep and stay asleep.

It's a virtuous circle: Sleep begets sleep. It's also a vicious circle: Sleeplessness begets sleeplessness.

Naps

Having grown up in a highly achievement-oriented society, most American adults are likely to view naps as a waste of time. We tend to think that adults who nap are lazy, undermotivated, ill, or elderly. In turn, we do not attach much positive benefit to daytime sleep in our infants and young children beyond giving us, the parents and caregivers, a much-needed break. Let me explain why naps are indeed very important for learning, or cognitive development, in children. A study published in 2015 showed that naps enhance the consolidation of memory among infants at 6 and 12 months. Further, infants who have longer naps are better able to remember novel actions than infants who take naps for thirty minutes or less.

Naps are not little bits of night sleep randomly intruding upon children's waking hours. Night sleep, daytime sleep, and daytime wakefulness have rhythms that are partially independent of one another. During the first three to four months of life, these rhythms develop at different rates, so they may not be in sync. Only later do these sleep/wake rhythms become linked with fluctuations in body temperature and activity levels.

For example, most of us have experienced drowsiness in the afternoon. This sensation is partially related—but only partially—to how long you have been up and how long you slept the night before. Our mental state fluctuates during the day between alert and drowsy, just as fluctuations occur during the night between light and deep sleep stages. As adults, we find a midday nap most refreshing when we take it at the time when we are biologically most drowsy.

If you live in the siesta belt, afternoon drowsiness might prompt you to take a nap, but in the United States, it's time for a coffee break. In England, it's afternoon tea. Both rituals arose to help fight naturally occurring daytime drowsiness through the use of stimulating chemicals such as caffeine.

What happens when a nap is skipped? In toddlers of 30–36 months, Dr. Rebecca Berger experimentally eliminated a single nap. She noted that when only *one nap* is eliminated, "acute sleep restriction causes dampened positive emotion displays when positive responses are expected (solvable puzzle), as well as increased negative emotion . . . under challenging conditions (unsolvable puzzle)."

In other words, experimental acute nap deprivation revealed that "toddlers [were] neither able to take full advantage of positive experiences nor . . . as adaptive in challenging contexts. If insufficient sleep consistently 'taxes' young children's emotion responses, they may not manage emotion regulation challenges effectively, potentially placing them at risk for future emotional/behavioral problems. . . . Specifically, when children were given the opportunity to complete an age-appropriate puzzle, they showed *less joy and pride* when sleep restricted than when optimally rested. . . . [W]hen children were faced with a puzzle with no solution, they showed significantly *more worry/anxiety* when sleep restricted than when well rested. . . . In sum," Dr. Berger continued, "sleepy children may view and respond to the world differently than children who are well-rested: they may not be able to take full advantage of positive experiences and may not be able to manage challenges. . . . A lack of sleep in contexts that rely on young children's mastery of new information (e.g., preschool) may have significant and potentially dire long-term consequences."

The takeaway message is that if your child misses a nap now and then, it is not necessarily a big deal, but it will affect your child. Imagine, though, what happens when naps are routinely skipped!

Another study, by Dr. Janice Bell, showed that "insufficient nighttime sleep among infants and preschool-aged children may be a lasting risk factor for subsequent obesity. *Napping does not appear to be a substitute for nighttime sleep* [emphasis added]." One way to understand this better is to consider the components of the food we eat. Food contains carbohydrates, proteins, fats, minerals, and vitamins. At different ages, our children need different amounts of these components for healthy growth. But it is not simply a matter of counting calories, and you cannot substitute one component for another even though they may be equivalent in calories. Similarly, at different ages our children need different amounts of naps and night sleep, and it is not simply a matter of adding up the total number of hours asleep. You cannot substitute minutes of night sleep for minutes of naps even though the total sleep duration is equivalent. Whether it be food or sleep, different elements are required for health.

Another feature that distinguishes night sleep from day sleep is that cross-cultural studies show large differences for age-specific bedtimes and evening sleep but not for daytime sleep.

Not only are naps different from night sleep, but not every nap is created equal. There is more *rapid eye movement (REM) sleep* in the midmorning nap compared with the midday nap. During a nap, the duration of REM sleep within a nap, not simply the total duration of the nap, is related to creative problem solving (pages 117 and 137). Research also suggests that high amounts of REM sleep, under the influence of low melatonin levels, help direct the course of brain maturation in early life. Further, adult studies have suggested that REM sleep is especially important for restoring us emotionally or psychologically, while deep, non-REM sleep appears to be more important for physical restoration. Let's protect opportunities for naps in our children so they can get all the REM sleep they need!

Because naps have their own function and do their job best when they occur at the right time, I suggest that if a nap has been missed, try to keep your child up until the next sleep period in order to maintain the timeliness of the sleep rhythm. This suggestion has to be balanced with the general theme of avoiding the overtired state, so the next sleep period (nap or night) might begin a little earlier.

My studies show that at 4 months of age, most children take either two or three naps. The third nap, if taken, tends to be brief and in the late afternoon or early evening. But by 6 months of age, the

vast majority of children (84 percent) are taking only two naps; by
9 months of age, virtually all children are taking just one or two
naps. About 17 percent of children have started taking only a single
nap by their first birthday, and this percentage increases to 56 percent by the age of 15 months. By 21 months, most children are down
to just a single nap.

The midmorning nap develops before the midday nap, but it also
disappears before the midday nap. The single nap that is present by
21 months and resurfaces in adolescence or adulthood is always the
midday or later-afternoon nap. Infants and young children have
much more REM sleep at night than older children, and the midmorning nap has more REM sleep than the midday nap; this suggests that in some infants, the midmorning nap may be viewed as a
sort of continuation of night sleep. Later I will discuss how we can
help babies sleep better by keeping the interval of wakefulness between the wake-up time and the start of the first nap very short.
This strategy may work because we are really allowing night sleep
to continue longer.

WARNING
Not all sleep periods are created equal! Long naps do not
compensate for late bedtimes. Sleep *quality*, not just sleep
duration, is an essential component of healthy sleep.

Different studies show that longer naps may be associated with
later bedtimes even if the wake-up time occurs later. Depending on
the bedtime, the wake-up time, and the nap duration, total sleep
duration may be the same as, less than, or more than comparison
groups without later bedtimes. But despite longer naps, among children with later bedtimes, problems such as poor diet quality, obesity, and externalizing behavioral problems occur—even if total
sleep is unchanged or greater! Why? *Late bedtimes* rob your child of
deep, restorative sleep occurring before midnight, and this lost high-
quality sleep is not made up for by lighter early-morning sleep or

additional daytime sleep. Long naps are not a substitute for less night sleep.

Another thing I've discovered is that up until about 21 months of age, some babies are born to be short nappers and some are inherently long nappers. Some children with normal night sleep tend to have long naps naturally, but parents can interfere with a child's long naps by messing up her schedule. However, they cannot make short nappers into long nappers. Here are some important facts about short nappers: At 6 months of age, 80 percent of babies nap between two and a half and four hours total each day. Napping more than four total hours each day occurs in 15 percent of babies. However, in 5 percent of babies, the total daytime sleep each day is less than two and a half hours. If you look at brief naps slightly differently and include babies who sleep a total of two and a half hours or less each day, then 18 percent of babies fall into this category. These short nappers tend to keep this pattern for the next twelve to eighteen months! This truth is especially frustrating to parents and caregivers whose first child was a long napper, accustoming them to long breaks during the day. If their second child is a short napper, they may incorrectly think they are doing something wrong or that there is something wrong with the child.

If parents can cause problems that interfere with good naps, why can't parents make their babies sleep longer? This question provides a good example of the asymmetry between sleep and wakefulness. Sleep is not the absence of wakefulness; rather, the brain automatically and actively turns on the sleep process and simultaneously turns off wakefulness. You and your child can force wakefulness upon sleep, but you cannot force sleep upon wakefulness. You and your child can motivate or force yourself and her into a more wakeful or alert state, but you cannot will anyone into a deeper sleep state. So sleep and wake states are different but not opposite. Parents provide the *opportunity to permit* the maximum amount of sleep to occur; this amount reflects their child's actual need for sleep. As stated before, a baby's nap pattern is largely an individual

trait that stays stable until about 21 months. Evidence of the individuality of this trait comes from studies on twins and argues for a
strong genetic component to the control of sleep in babies.

At 21 months, the average nap duration is a little less than two
and a half hours, but the range is wide: between one and four hours.
At this age, some of the children who initially took brief naps are
now taking longer naps, and some who had been long nappers are
now taking briefer naps. My interpretation is that by 21 months,
biology is no longer the primary influence on napping; social factors begin to play a role. For example, events such as the birth of a
sibling, an older sibling starting preschool, or the child herself now
participating in organized and scheduled activities can cause children who have a biological need for longer naps to take shorter
naps. Often, no problems occur if catch-up days are provided, coupled with an extra-early bedtime.

The time of day when the nap occurs is also important. Some
studies have suggested that an early nap, occurring in the midmorning hours, is different in quality from a later nap, which occurs in
the midday. As mentioned before, there is more active REM sleep
than quiet sleep in the first nap, and this pattern is reversed in the
second nap. So naps occurring at different times are different! Even
for adults, a nap earlier in the day is lighter and less restorative than
a midday nap, which consists of deeper sleep.

Long naps occurring at the right time make the child feel rested.
Levels of cortisol dramatically fall during a nap, indicating a reduction of stress in the body. Not taking a needed nap means that the
body remains stressed. Brief naps or naps that are out of sync with
other biological rhythms are less restful, less restorative. But a short
nap is better than no nap. It still has a positive effect on alertness.

Children can be taught how to take naps. A nap does not begin
and end the way an electric light can be turned off and on. In fact, a
nap or night sleep involves three periods of time: the time required
for the process called falling asleep, the sleep period itself, and the
time required to wake up. One father complained to me, "I can't see

the pre-Z's coming out of his head," meaning he had difficulty see-ing the lull in activity or quieting that precedes sleep. In later chap-ters, I will show you how to recognize the pre-Z's and teach your children to fall asleep at the optimal time (page 167).

> Do not expect your baby to nap well outside her crib after 4 months of age. If you don't protect your baby's nap schedules, you can produce nap deprivation.

When children do not nap well, they pay a price. Infants between 4 and 8 months who do not nap well have shorter attention spans or appear less persistent when engaged in activities. By 3 years of age, children who do not nap or who nap very little are often described as nonadaptable or even hyperactive. Adaptability is thought to be a very important trait for school success.

One mother of a nonadaptable child said with a laugh that every morning she prayed to the "nap god" to give her a break. In con-trast, another mother described her son as a very easy child as long as she had a bed around. He was such a "rack monster" that she decided he just liked his own company best. Another mother de-scribed her son, who napped well, as the "snooze king."

Sometimes it appears that the older toddler needs exactly one and a half naps—while one nap is insufficient, two are impossible to achieve. These children are rough around the edges in the late after-noon or early evening, but parents can temporarily and partially compensate by putting the child to bed earlier on some nights.

An *earlier bedtime* may become a necessity when your child de-velops a single-nap pattern, between 15 and 21 months. Earlier bed-times help prevent bedtime battles, deter night waking, discourage extremely early-morning awakenings, and regularize and prolong naps. Why, then, do many parents resist the notion of putting their children to sleep when they first appear tired at night, even though it is clear that the brain is sleep-sensitive?

First, parents naturally want to be with their children and play with them. Second, there is a powerful inhibitory fear that if their child is put to bed very early when tired, she will get up extra early the next day. Third, because I recommend that, along with an earlier bedtime, the parents not go to the child at night except for feeding, parents are frightened about the possibility of prolonged crying when they put the child to bed or in the middle of the night. This fear of possible crying discourages parents from trying for an earlier bedtime. It is a natural fear . . . but in most cases a groundless one. These parents mistakenly think that a later bedtime will make the child more tired and resist sleep less.

Here is an example of how a family started early, at 8 weeks of age, to focus on an *earlier bedtime*. The baby was not overtired and did not have extreme fussiness/colic, so the transition went smoothly. But 20 percent of babies have extreme fussiness/colic, and for them, this change to an earlier bedtime at 8 weeks of age is not easy, as we shall see later.

When our daughter Jaden was born, we were anxious to start off on the right foot with her sleep habits. We immediately focused on no more than two hours of wakefulness with a bedtime around 10:00 or 11:00 P.M., which was very easy to accomplish. After a few weeks, though, we still weren't really seeing very long nighttime stretches. When Jaden was 8 weeks old, we visited Dr. Weissbluth to discuss her sleeping pattern. Dr. Weissbluth told us that at 6 weeks, we should have incorporated an early bedtime in addition to keeping shorter periods of wakefulness. We left wondering whether an early bedtime would really work for someone so young. We really expected that Jaden would be up within an hour or two after we put her down. We started off with a 7:00 P.M. bedtime. She still woke up in the late evening to eat, but we put her promptly back to bed. There were a few bumps in the road for the first couple of nights—sometimes she would wake up a few times and cry—but we kept at it.

After a few days, Jaden went from sleeping a four-to-five-hour stretch in the evening, to seven, then eight, then nine or ten hours a night. In fact, she seemed happy to be sleeping so much! If she woke up to nurse, she would eat and immediately fall back asleep as soon as we put her back in her crib. We couldn't believe how easy it was. The earlier we got her to bed, the better she slept. Her daytime naps even seemed longer and more restful. She is now 7 months old. We now try to get her down between 6:00 and 6:30 each night, and she is extremely happy about it. (So are we!)

Over and over again I have seen children who are put to bed too late. It becomes a vicious circle: The child's nap schedule is messed up, and the child is fussy in the late afternoon or early evening. This fatigue-driven fussiness ends in a wired state at bedtime, which interferes with the ability to go to sleep easily. As a result, in an attempt to avoid a bedtime battle, the parent keeps the child up until she crashes. The next day the child is still tired, the naps are messed up, and so on. The circle never ends.

The solution is obvious in Meg's story.

We had never been very consistent with Meg's bedtime. We would put her to bed when she appeared tired (rubbing eyes, yawning), anywhere from 7:00 to 7:45 P.M., but occasionally even later. It usually took her between fifteen and thirty minutes of crying to fall asleep. I thought this was normal. She had always gone to bed rather late, and she had always taken a while to fall asleep.

At Meg's 9-month appointment we asked Dr. Weissbluth about her night waking. He made a very simple suggestion. He told us that we should put Meg to bed twenty minutes earlier at night. He said that her night waking would disappear and she would still wake up at a normal hour in the morning. I told him that we had been putting her to sleep when she appeared tired, at around 7:30 P.M., give or take thirty minutes. He said that once she appears tired it is too late and she should already be in bed.

The first night we put her to bed at 6:45. We were very skeptical. We were sad to put her down so early when she seemed so wide awake and happy. She cried for about five minutes and then fell asleep, and with no night waking! The same thing happened the next night—about five minutes of crying and then asleep until morning. Sometimes she would wake up as early as 5:30, but we would give her a bottle and she would fall back to sleep, sometimes until almost 8:00!

It has been almost four weeks since our 9-month appointment. Bedtime is an absolute joy. Meg eats dinner, takes a bath, and is in bed about 6:30 P.M. Sometimes I hesitate to put her down so early when she seems to be in such good spirits, but she cuddles with her blanket and her doll, sucks her thumb, closes her eyes, and sleeps till morning. It's the sweetest thing I have ever seen.

As Meg's parents said about my recommendation for a much earlier bedtime, "He made a very simple suggestion." Sometimes simple approaches work better than complex solutions. And it's normal to be "skeptical" and "sad." Here's another example.

When we met with Dr. Weissbluth, Jared, now 19 months old, was waking up every hour and a half to two hours during the night. He would have to fall asleep while we were walking and carrying him on our shoulder. When placed in the crib, Jared would awaken and abruptly "pop up." He would only sleep in the bed "nest" we created for him on the floor of our family room. We endured three months of the night waking before we consulted Dr. Weissbluth.

We were instructed to place Jared in bed in an awake state between 6:00 and 7:00 in the evening and that we should leave him there until 6:00 in the morning. Our initial reaction was that Jared would carry on relentlessly when placed in his crib so early, and that the recommended approach was too strict and would never work. Much to our shock and delight, the first night we tried the new routine, Jared was asleep after five minutes of crying, and remained asleep for eleven hours, not waking until 5:30 the next morning. During the next two nights, Jared went to sleep on his own, with no episodes of crying. On the fourth night, he lay down in the bed with his favorite stuffed animal under his arm, as he has done since. Our baby was clearly overtired from going to bed at 8:30 P.M. and not being allowed to relax and go to sleep without interference. We never expected it to be so simple and provide such an immediate result. Jared wakes up happy, energized, and ready for a day full of adventures. Now, several months later, Jared is most happy when going to bed at 6:30 P.M., and will go to his bed himself if he is tired.

Probably the most common worry is that the earlier bedtime will produce an earlier wake-up time, as expressed by Anna's story.

At 18 months it became apparent that Anna was ready to make the transition from two naps to one, but would need some help because she fought the midmorning nap. We began, as Dr. Weissbluth suggested in his book, by gradually delaying the midmorning nap till 11:00 or so. Over a two-week window we were able to continue to push back the nap to sometime between noon and 1:00 P.M.

In his book, Dr. Weissbluth suggested an earlier bedtime to help prevent night waking or early-morning waking. Anna was going to bed at 6:30 P.M. and sleeping until 7:00 A.M., so we really questioned this theory. My husband and I agreed that Dr. Weissbluth's advice has always been right on the money, so we decided to put her down an hour earlier. We feared that she would wake up at 5:30 or 6:00 A.M. after her usual twelve or thirteen hours of sleep. To our surprise, she awoke at 9:00 A.M., and she was in the most cheerful mood to date!

Family, friends, even strangers constantly tell us what a happy, cheerful child we have. The reality is that she is a very well-rested child.

Not napping means lost sleep. Over an extended period of time, children do not sleep longer at night when their naps are brief. Of course, once in a while—when relatives visit or when a painful ear infection keeps the child awake—a child will make up for lost daytime sleep with longer night sleep. But day in and day out, you should not expect to satisfy your child's need to sleep by cutting corners on naps and then trying to compensate by putting your child to sleep for the night at an earlier hour. What you wind up with is a cranky or demanding child in the late afternoon or early evening. Your child pays a price for nap deprivation, and so do you.

Spending hours holding your child in your arms or in a rocking chair while she is in a light, twilight sleep also is lost sleep because you have delayed the time when she will fall into a deep slumber. It is similar to having a bedtime that is too late. It's a waste of your time as well. Brief catnaps during the day, motion sleep in cars or baby swings, light sleep in the stroller at the pool, and naps at the wrong time are all poor-quality sleep.

When your child does not nap well and you keep her up in the evening, she suffers.

SLEEP INERTIA

Beyond cultural conditioning, however, there is an important reason why some adults do not nap: *sleep inertia*. Sleep inertia is a feeling of disorientation, confusion, pain, discomfort, impaired mood, and the inability to concentrate or think well that occurs upon waking, especially from naps. Have you ever woken from a nap with a headache, mental fuzziness, or other unpleasant sensations? With sleep inertia, it appears that sleep is intruding into wakefulness, and this overlap state is painfully uncomfortable. In other words, we are partially awake and partially asleep at the same time. In fact, there is now more evidence that shows that part of the brain can be asleep while other parts are awake! I know this sounds strange, but the fact that part of the brain can be asleep while other parts are awake might explain the state called sleep inertia and also what has been called *local sleep*.

In children, sleep inertia appears to be more severe and more prolonged for those who are more overtired. One mother described it as a "fugue" state (neither fully awake nor fully asleep); another as a "demonic" state. The children are out of control, panicky, crying, or screaming hysterically. Parents would often call me after three-day holiday weekends, during which their children became severely overtired, and tell me that they were sure their child had a painful ear infection because she woke crying. They often added that they were sure their child was not overtired because she had just completed an extra-long nap! The ears were perfect; the child had simply missed some naps or had been allowed to stay up too late during the holiday, and as a result, sleep inertia was rearing its ugly head.

Sometimes a child shows sleep inertia after a single midday nap, suggesting that the bedtime is too late, but around the end of the day the child seems fine, suggesting that the bedtime is not too late. How to resolve this apparent contradiction? The culprit might be not the bedtime but an interval of wakefulness before the nap that was too long. Trial and error might be needed in adjusting either the bedtime or the nap time or both.

Here is a parent's report:

I was noticing occasional sleep inertia after naps. I assumed it was because the bedtime was too late. However, my sleep logs repeatedly showed that we only got sleep inertia when the wake-up time that day was too early. For example, for the last twelve days we have used super-early bedtimes (6:00–6:15 P.M.) to repay some sleep debt. It has started backfiring, though—this morning the wake-up was 4:45 A.M. And after the nap today—boom! Sleep inertia.

I have seen this again and again. Although sleep inertia might result from cumulative sleepiness from a too-late bedtime, my observation is that it can also result from a too-long interval of wakefulness before the nap.

Understanding that the rhythms of night sleep, daytime sleep, and daytime wakefulness are somewhat independent from one another leads to two important ideas. First, in a child under 3–4 months of age, these rhythms are not in synchrony, and the baby may be getting opposing messages from different parts of the brain. The sleep rhythm says "deep sleep," while the wake rhythm says "alert" instead of "drowsy." Wakeful but tired, the confused child cries fitfully; we might call this behavior colic or fussiness. Opposing or overlapping messages from different parts of the brain may cause ambiguous stages such as sleep inertia. In research with adults and animals, this has been called "dissociated states of wakefulness and sleep," or "status dissociatus." Thus, for example, narcolepsy can be seen as the intrusion of REM sleep into wakefulness, while sleepwalking, night terrors, and crying out at night occur during the overlap between wakefulness and non-REM sleep.

We know that adults may have overlapping sleep and wake states, experience incomplete sleep states, or switch rapidly between states. So it is entirely possible that during the first four months of a newborn's life, when sleep states are developing, partial states express themselves out of phase and in conjunction with other states, creating overlap problems that we refer to as fussiness, colic, or sleep inertia. For example, it is known that babies can suck, smile, and cry with their eyes open during REM sleep, so while they appear to be awake, they are actually asleep. We can call this indeterminate sleep or ambiguous sleep, reflecting the immaturity of the young brain. After about 4 months of age, these ambiguous states are less common.

Second, if these sleep/wake rhythms are somewhat independent, they may have different functions: learning for the wake cycle, physical and emotional restoration for the sleep cycle. Daytime sleep and nighttime sleep may be different in this regard. I believe that *healthy naps* lead to optimal daytime alertness for learning—that is, naps adjust the alert/drowsy control to just the right setting for optimal daytime arousal and consolidate memories for enhanced learning. Without naps, the child is too drowsy to learn well. Also, when chronically sleep-deprived, the fatigued child becomes fitfully fussy or hyperalert in order to fight sleep, and therefore cannot learn from her environment.

MOTIONLESS SLEEP

How well do you nap in a car or on a plane compared with in your bed? I think babies have better-quality, more restorative sleep when they are sleeping in a stationary crib, bed, or bassinet. Vibration or motion during sleep appears to force the brain to a lighter sleep state and reduce the restorative power of the nap. I explained to the mother of one child that her baby would not sleep well while she was shopping, walking in the park, or doing something active with her friends. The mother discovered that this was true, that her baby napped best at home, but she also found it very difficult to spend more time at home during the day, as she and most of her friends were outdoorsy people. On the positive side, after starting to nap at home, her child no longer cried before going down for a nap.

You may wish to use a moving swing or a calm ride in the stroller or car for a few minutes as part of the soothing-to-sleep process, but after your baby falls asleep, drive home, turn off the swing, or stop walking with the stroller. Although your baby may appear to be in an awkward position, don't disturb her if you notice that she always wakes as you try to move her to a crib. It doesn't hurt babies to nap in their swings or car seats. Your baby might also sleep well outdoors in a stationary stroller, especially if it's a quiet neighborhood. In general, however, as the brain matures, the child's increasing curiosity and social awareness make it more difficult to have good naps outside, so be careful.

When you maintain a healthy nap schedule and your child sleeps well during the day, well-meaning but clueless friends may accuse you of being overprotective. They'll say, "It's not real life," or "Bring her along so she'll learn to play with other children," or "You're really spoiling her." Remember: They are on the outside looking in. Only you know what works best for your baby and your family.

Sleep Consolidation and Fragmentation

Consolidated sleep means uninterrupted sleep, sleep that is continuous and not disrupted by awakenings. Slumber broken by awakenings or complete arousals is known as disrupted sleep or sleep fragmentation. Abnormal shifts of sleep rhythms toward lighter sleep, even if we do not wake completely, may also cause sleep fragmentation. Ten hours of consolidated sleep is not the same as ten hours of fragmented sleep. Doctors, firefighters, and parents of newborns or sick children who have their sleep interrupted frequently know this very well.

The effects of sleep fragmentation are similar to the effects of reduced total sleep: Daytime sleepiness increases and performance measurably decreases. Getting up four times at night, over an eight-hour time in bed, to care for your baby has the same effect as getting only four hours of consolidated sleep. Among healthy adults, even one night of sleep fragmentation will produce decreases in mental flexibility and sustained attention, as well as impairment of mood.

Adults with fragmented sleep often fight the ill effects of fragmented sleep with extra caffeine.

Let sleeping babies lie! Never wake a sleeping baby, except to maintain a sleep schedule. Destroying sleep continuity is unhealthy.

However, it is important to understand that our children, like ourselves, *normally* cycle between deep sleep and light sleep throughout the night. Babies often vocalize with quiet sounds during the light sleep period and then return to a deeper sleep by themselves. If a baby is unable to return to deep sleep unassisted, she may signal her awakening by crying or calling out. This signaling, as it is known, may disturb the parents and be considered by them to be a night-waking problem. The real problem is not the night waking per se but how the parents respond to it, as we shall see.

Protective Arousals

Some arousals from sleep are normal. Sometimes our brains wake us in order to prevent asphyxiation in our sleep. These awakenings, or protective arousals, occur when we have difficulty breathing during sleep, which can be caused by large tonsils or adenoids obstructing the air passage. Arousals may also prevent crib death, or sudden infant death syndrome (SIDS), which kills young infants. This tragedy might be caused by a failure to maintain breathing during sleep or a failure to awaken when breathing starts to become difficult.

Sleep Fragmentation

But after several months of age—beyond the age when crib death is most common—frequent arousals are usually harmful, because they destroy sleep continuity. Arousals are complete awakening from either a light, deep, or REM sleep.

Arousals can also be thought of as a quick shift from deep sleep to light sleep without a complete awakening.

Figure 4: Arousals During Sleep

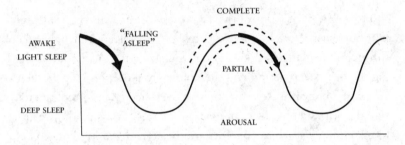

Figure 4 is a simplified illustration of the cycling from deep sleep to light sleep that normally occurs after about 4 months of age. During partial arousals, we stay in a light sleep state and do not wake. But during complete arousals, or awakenings, we might become aware that we are looking at the clock, rolling over, changing arm positions, or scratching a leg. This awareness is dim and brief, and we return to sleep promptly. The bold arrow in the figure indicates that the process of falling asleep at bedtime and after an arousal is similar and requires self-soothing skills. The most important way to encourage self-soothing skills at bedtime is to place your baby down to sleep drowsy but awake and then leave the room. In the middle of the night, when your baby quietly vocalizes and you suspect she is *not* hungry, self-soothing skills are encouraged by slightly delaying your response, and/or minimally soothing in the baby's crib, as well as not using feeding as a soothing technique. Then your baby learns to fall asleep unassisted at bedtime and in the middle of the night after a normal occurring arousal.

As we can see, arousals come in several forms, and depending on which types occur, how many times they happen, and how long they last, we pay a price: increased daytime sleepiness and decreased performance. For example, in a study by Dr. Anat Scher, children of 12–36 months with more fragmented sleep displayed higher cortisol levels upon waking. The elevated cortisol levels were associated with daycare teachers' reports of more negative emotionality and internalizing behaviors such as social withdrawal and appearing or feeling sad, lonely, nervous, or fearful. Another study of over one thousand children who were examined at 5, 17, and 29 months focused on those who had night awakenings of twenty or more minutes and compared them with children with no night awakenings or shorter night awakenings: "Our results indicate that, as early as 5 months, parental overprotectiveness scores were highest in parents with children waking 20 minutes or more at 29 months; they suggest that those children did not have an opportunity to learn self-regulation from an early age . . . regarding 29-month-old children's behavior, children in the extended night-waking group had highest scores on externalizing and internalizing behaviors (page 127). Girls had higher scores on shyness/inhibition and boys had higher scores on aggression/hyperactivity." They concluded, "Parental approaches (overprotectiveness) *predate* what parents might define as sleep problems [emphasis added]."

Some arousals, however, always occur naturally during healthy sleep. The brain, not the stomach, makes arousals. Please don't confuse arousals from sleep with hunger.

It's not just night sleep that can be fragmented. I believe naps can also be fragmented when parents rely on motion sleep in a baby swing or car, or when they allow catnaps in the stroller. Holding your dozing child in your arms in a rocking chair during the day also probably prevents good-quality day sleep. These naps are too brief or too light to be restorative. Motionless sleep is best. If you use a swing for soothing, turn it off once your baby falls asleep. After 4 months, naps of much less than one hour cannot count as "real" naps. Sometimes a nap of forty-five minutes may be all your child needs, but naps of less than thirty minutes don't help. By 4–8 months of age, infants should have at least a mid-morning nap and one at midday, and the total nap duration should be about two to four hours. If it is less and your child is well rested, do not worry. Remember, watching the child, not the clock, is most important.

Night sleep is ten to twelve hours, with one, two, or no interruptions for bottle-feeding. If you are breastfeeding and room sharing, you might feed your baby at night many times. In this situation, both mother and baby may be more asleep than awake during the feeding, and neither suffers from sleep fragmentation. As previously mentioned, some arousals or awakenings at night are normal, and a child returns to sleep unassisted. But in cases of signaling, when the child wakes and cries until the parent arrives for soothing, the real problem is the child's inability to return to sleep unassisted. Until the child learns self-soothing skills, the result will be fragmented night sleep for parent and child.

> Some arousals (or awakenings at night) from sleep are normal. Problems occur when children have difficulty returning to sleep by themselves. They "signal" because they have not learned the process of falling asleep.

Some older children continue to wake up during the night perhaps because they lack the capacity to soothe themselves back to sleep. A study of about one thousand children, in France, examined those with frequent night waking (the child waking every other night or more often) requiring parents to help soothe the child back to sleep. Frequent night waking occurred in 22 percent of children at two years, 26 percent at three years, and 9 percent at five to six years. The risk factors associated with frequent night wakings were passive smoking at home, daycare, watching television for extended periods, bottle-feeding at night, and a more difficult *temperament*.

Another study of children 6–36 months old showed an association of signaling more awakenings, shorter duration of night sleep, a later bedtime, an insecure *attachment* to their mother (page 339). It is not known whether the temperament or attachment issues were the result of fragmented sleep or whether these issues within the child caused the parents' behavior at night that led to fragmented sleep, or both. In other words, are the observations parent-driven, child-driven, or interactive between parent and child? A common problem involving studies that rely only on parents' reports is common method variance, which means that the association between sleep and temperament, for example, might really reflect only issues within the parent.

However, more objective and independent measurements such as direct observations by psychologists, video recordings, or actually measuring sleep with a motion sensor attached to the wrist (actigraph) support observations that fragmented night sleep is harmful.

Sleep Schedule, Timing of Sleep, Bedtime

Figures 5 and 6 show the times when most children wake or go to sleep. These graphs are based on data from the same 2,019 children referred to in figures 1 through 3 (pages 32 and 33). Looking at the graphs, you can see, for example, that 90 percent of preschool children (those under the age of 6) fall asleep before 9:00 P.M., and 10 percent of children between the ages of 2 and 6 fall asleep before 7:00 P.M.

> **MAJOR POINT**
> When our children are hungry, we feed them without delay. Just as you try not to let your child become overly hungry, so, too, you shouldn't let your child become overly tired.

Figure 5

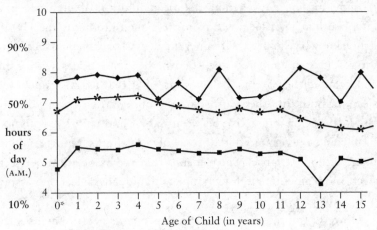

*Note: 0 represents children between 4 and 11 months of age.

Figure 6

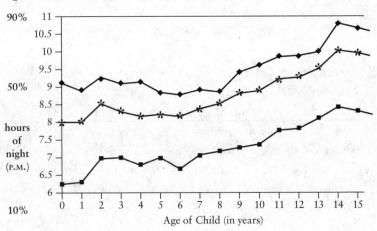

*Note: 0 represents children between 4 and 11 months of age.

When sleep/wake schedules are not in sync with other biological rhythms, attentiveness, vigilance, and task performance are measurably decreased and moods are altered. Jet lag syndrome is one example of this. Another is the poor sleep quality some shift workers suffer due to abnormal sleep schedules. Shift workers complain mainly of headaches and stomachaches. These are the most common complaints of older children with unhealthy sleep schedules. So if your child doesn't appear to be very sick but has frequent headaches or episodes of vague abdominal pain, especially near the end of the day, ask yourself if she might be overtired. A clue would be that she no longer has the energy or drive that she once had.

When thinking about sleep schedules in babies and toddlers, consider sleep to be food for the brain, just as breast milk or formula is food for the body. You don't breastfeed on the run while doing errands; instead, you find a reasonably quiet space. Same for naps. You don't withhold feeding because it is socially inconvenient; you anticipate when your child might become hungry. Same for naps. You don't try to force-feed your baby when she's not hungry; you know a hungry period will naturally come. Same for naps. A parent coming home late from work would not starve his baby by withholding food until he arrived and could feed the child. Same for the bedtime hour; don't "sleep-starve" your baby's brain by keeping her up too late.

BEDTIME

Early bedtimes are important. Often, moving the bedtime earlier, even if the child gets only a little more sleep (page 102), will dramatically help her sleep better. In general, earlier bedtimes might, or might not, be associated with longer night sleep, depending on the wake-up time. Also, earlier bedtimes might, or might not, be associated with longer total sleep duration, depending on the duration of naps in infants and young children. So an early bedtime might be beneficial because it might cause a *longer sleep duration*.

Separately, however, an early bedtime might result in *better-quality* sleep. For example, infants have much more REM sleep at night than older children. However, a late bedtime might cause an infant to get less REM sleep because of a short night sleep duration. But the infant still might have a normal total sleep duration because of long naps. *REM sleep* is especially important for learning. Also, for older children, more *deep sleep* occurs during the first half of the night, so when the bedtime is late, they might benefit less from this most restorative, high-quality sleep, even though they might sleep in late on weekends or school vacations. Lastly, more *growth hormone* is released during the first deep sleep period, which normally occurs early in the evening (page 133). Dr. Judith Owens emphasizes that when parents start the bedtime too late, children are being asked to stay awake and function at a time when their circadian rhythm is telling them to be asleep. Changing bedtimes earlier not only allows children to get more sleep but allows them to sleep at the optimal time. When they sleep may be equally important, if not more so, than how much sleep they get.

So early bedtimes might have an effect on sleep durations or the quality of sleep or both. Additionally, some studies suggest that early bedtimes are more important than sleep duration for some outcomes such as the development of *obesity*. Here are a few examples:

Preschool children, age 4–5 years, were divided into early bedtimes (before 8:00 P.M.), medium bedtimes (8:00–9:00 P.M.), and late bedtimes (after 9:00 P.M.). They developed adolescent obesity at rates of 10 percent, 16 percent, and 23 percent, respectively.

A 2020 study of children 2–6 years of age also showed that "more frequent exposures to late sleep were associated with greater increase in adiposity measures . . . [these children] had greater weight gain over time; this association was *independent* of sleep duration [emphasis added]." Unlike other studies that used sleep data from parents' reports, this study used objective measurements of sleep duration (night and day sleep) obtained yearly. Late bedtimes were defined as bedtimes later than 9:00 P.M. for all ages. The average bedtimes for children who did *not* have late bedtimes ranged from about 8:30 P.M. (age 2–4 years) to 9:00 P.M. (age 5–6 years). Bedtimes have tended toward a later hour in this age range in recent years (page 626), and later bedtimes, especially after 9:00 P.M., may explain the trend of increasing obesity in children.

Another study of over three thousand children assessed bedtimes at three points: 4–5 years, 6–7 years, and 8–9 years. At each point, children were grouped into either early or late bedtimes. At each time point, "our findings show that 6–9-year-old children who are early-to-sleep have better health-related quality of life, and their mothers have better mental health at 6–7 years compared with children who are late-to-sleep." However, children with late-to-sleep profiles at two or more time points "were more likely to have poorer BMI [higher body mass index], waist circumference, behavior, psychosocial quality of life, physical functioning, and maternal mental health at 8–9 years than children with no or one [point in time] late-to-sleep profile. . . . This suggests that there is a *cumulative* effect of late-to-sleep profiles on child and parent outcomes." Analysis of sleep durations did *not* show any such strong associations.

IMPORTANT POINT
Over time, the harmful effects of a late bedtime worsen.

A study of over two thousand children included assessments of bedtimes and sleep durations at 5 and 9 years. At age 15 years, they recorded BMI and made objective sleep recordings. They observed four groups of children:

1. No regular bedtime at age 5 years
2. No regular bedtime at age 9 years
3. Borderline bedtimes at age 5 (8:30–9:30 P.M.) and 9 (9:00–10:00 P.M.) years
4. Age-appropriate bedtimes at age 5 (before 8:30 P.M.) and 9 (before 9:00 P.M.) years ("the reference group")

At age 15 years, adolescents in the reference group (group 4) had longer sleep duration and *lower BMI* than the other groups. However, "Adolescents who had no [regular] bedtime at age 5 years but adopted borderline bedtimes at age 9 years did *not* have significantly higher BMI at age 15 than those in the reference group."

IMPORTANT POINT
The harmful effects of a late bedtime might be *reversible*. It is never too late to help your child sleep better by encouraging earlier bedtimes.

For children age 9–16, it was shown that if the bedtime is later, it is more likely that the child will have a *poorer-quality diet*. This observation was *not* related to sleep duration.

In addition to obesity, other studies have linked late bedtimes to negative emotionality, emotional distress, academic difficulties, ADHD, and sleep problems, even when the sleep duration might *not* be shortened. Here are a few examples:

In a study of over eight thousand children starting at 6 months and ending at 11.6 years, with six evaluations in between, later bedtimes at each measurement point were observed among those children who were diagnosed with ADHD at about seven years. They also had shorter sleep durations and more night wakings at each of the eight evaluations. Similarly, another study showed that late or irregular bedtimes among about forty-two thousand 2-year-olds predicted symptoms of ADHD at age 8 years.

Pediatric neurologists studied 18-month-old infants with typical or atypical development (impaired social and language abilities) and noted that those with *atypical development* had later bedtimes and shorter night sleep duration. There were *no* group differences in total sleep time because those with atypical development had longer naps.

At 6, 15, and 24 weeks of age, objective measurements of sleep using ankle-worn motion sensors (actigraphs) showed that "Infants who fell asleep earlier also slept longer at night . . . without compensating by sleeping less the next day [naps]. . . . For every one hour later in the infant's usual sleep onset, infants woke only eight minutes later the next morning. Keeping infants up later in hopes of them sleeping in longer may be counterproductive . . . and ineffective." In other words, later bedtimes reduce twenty-four-hour or total sleep time and will not make your baby sleep in much later in the morning. Among children 30 months of age measured with wrist-worn actigraphs, "The most consistent finding was the relation between parent-reported sleep problems and parent reports of bedtime and actigraph records of sleep onset time [the time actually falling asleep was later]." In other words, parents' reports of sleep problems and late bedtimes are validated by objectively measured late sleep onset time. In a separate study of children 4–6 years, actigraphs showed that later sleep onset times were associated with shorter night sleep durations.

PROPORTION OF TOTAL SLEEP OCCURRING DURING THE NIGHT OR DAY

As night sleep and day sleep become more organized, researchers studied the impact of the *proportion* of total sleep that occurs at night instead of simply the duration of sleep (day, night, and total). Parents' reports at 3 months and 8 months and objective sleep measurements at 8 months showed that a later bedtime was associated with shorter night sleep duration (even though the wake-up time was later), and the parents reported longer day sleep durations resulting in a *lower proportion* of total sleep occurring at night. The parents whose children had later bedtimes also reported at both time points increased difficulties for their infants settling to sleep, increased latency to sleep (time required to actually fall asleep after being put down), and more time awake during the night. Surprisingly, these parents also reported at both 3 and 8 months an increase of total (twenty-four-hour) sleep duration, but at 8 months, actigraph measurements were not obtained for day sleep so objective data for total sleep is lacking. Another study found that infants at 1 year of age who had a *greater proportion* of total sleep occurring at night scored higher, at age 4 years, on tests of *executive function,* reflecting higher abstract reasoning skills, concept formation, and problem-solving skills. This suggests that when a too-late bedtime causes a shorter duration of night sleep, babies may have poor-quality sleep—even those babies who have longer naps, and thus a normal or even a longer twenty-four-hour sleep duration. The two variables, the time of sleep onset (bedtime) and the proportion of total sleep occurring at night, seem to be associated with each other and/or might be individually important, or one variable might only be a marker for the other. Either way, *early bedtimes matter.*

In one study, children age 3–6 years with temperamental negative affect (a tendency to react to stressors with high levels of negative emotionality characterized by high discomfort, fear, anger/frustration, aggression, sadness, and low soothability) and late bedtimes were more likely to exhibit externalizing (attention problems or aggression) and internalizing (anxiety or depression) behaviors. The authors stressed that the relations between temperament and behaviors "were *not* moderated by sleep duration." Instead, the late bedtime "confers risk for maladaptive outcomes [because it alters] *the proportion of time spent in distinct sleep stages* [emphasis added]."

Among 15-year-olds with late bedtimes during the school year, worse educational outcomes and emotional distress were observed six to eight years later, but short sleep durations were *not* associated with changes in academic or emotional functioning.

IMPORTANT POINT
Late bedtimes may be harmful even if the duration of night sleep or total sleep is normal because of less REM sleep, less deep sleep, or a lower proportion of total sleep occurring at night.

Abnormal sleep schedules usually evolve in infants and young children when parents keep them up too late at night. Parents do this because they enjoy playing with their baby, they cannot put the child to sleep and instead wait for their child to crash from total exhaustion, or both. Some parents leave work late, have a long commute to the daycare site to pick up their child, and then arrive home even later. This lifestyle is extremely difficult for the child if naps are not regular at the daycare center and she is put down to sleep too late at night. If it is impossible to have an early bedtime under these circumstances, do the best you can. A bedtime that is only a little late is not as harmful as a bedtime that is way too late. Don't beat yourself up over this, but do your best to protect naps and early bedtimes on weekends.

Dr. Isabel Morales-Muñoz recently discovered another reason why some parents keep their child up too late. She studied about a thousand families before the child was born, and at 3, 8, 18, and 24 months, and observed that some children at each age have both a high proportion of day sleep compared with total sleep and late bedtimes; the mothers of these children tended to be "owls" instead of "larks." That is, these mothers preferred to go to bed later, woke up later, and felt better in the evening. As a group, the children of mothers with "eveningness preference" required more time to fall asleep after being put down and had more sleep difficulties. However, their total sleep duration was not different from children whose mothers with "morningness preference." The father's role was also studied, and his preference for eveningness or morningness had no effect. You might ask: Aren't some children owls who really come alive in the evening and thrive on late bedtimes? Some of my friends are owls and are just fine; others are larks. The answer is clear. Research using objective measures of sleep and salivary melatonin shows that in the age range of 30–36 months, the number of definite evening types (owls) is zero. Another parent-response study found evening types (owls) in this same age range to be 0.9 percent of children. In fact, they observed that between birth and 8 years of age, evening types occurred in less than 2 percent of children at every age. The vast majority of young children are larks. Larks sleep better with early bedtimes.

Bedtimes are based on *drowsy signs*, not clock times, so please do not compare your child's bedtime with that of another child. Also, realistically, as mentioned, circumstances may make it difficult for parents to synchronize soothing to sleep at night with the onset of drowsy signs. For some parents, the reality is that a bedtime that is too late is *unavoidable*. Even so, try to move the bedtime just a few minutes earlier. But an important point is that a little earlier bedtime, just a few minutes earlier (page 102), will benefit your child. A little bit of extra sleep goes a long way.

NIGHT SLEEP ORGANIZATION

Before 6 weeks of age, the longest single sleep period, unfortunately, is randomly distributed around the clock. In some babies, this longest sleep may actually be only two to three hours! But after 6 weeks of age (or 6 weeks after the due date, for babies born early), the longest single sleep period will predictably occur in the evening hours and last four to six hours.

> During these early weeks, you may find breastfeeding too demanding or too frequent and think that you might want to quit so that you can get some rest. On the other hand, you also may want to continue nursing because of its benefits. Hang in there until your baby is past 6 weeks of age. Then you, too, will get more night sleep.

After 6 weeks of age, the peak of wakefulness and fussiness passes, and babies sleep longer at night. So do moms! Also, babies start social smiling at their parents, and they become less fussy or irritable. Life in the family definitely changes after 6 weeks. One exception is the premature baby, whose parents might have to wait until about 6 weeks after the expected date of delivery. Another exception is the extremely fussy/colicky baby, whose parents might have to wait until their child is 3–4 months old.

DAY SLEEP ORGANIZATION

At about 3–4 months of age, daytime sleep becomes organized into two or three long naps instead of many brief, irregular ones. Mothers, especially nursing mothers, should learn to nap when their baby naps. You never know what the night will bring; you might be up a lot holding, walking, or nursing.

Unfortunately, if both parents are working outside the home, sometimes naps may suffer on weekends because the parents do too many errands with the child or attempt to spend too much time playing with her to make up for the minimal time together during the week. Sleeping well during the day may also suffer when parents skip naps in favor of organized, scheduled preschool activities. These baby classes are usually fun for both child and parent, but if they take up too much time, the child becomes overtired.

One common mistake is keeping bedtime at *exactly* the same hour every night. Usually this hour is too late and is based more on the parents' wishes than the child's sleep needs. It is important to have a fairly regular routine of soothing events before putting your child to sleep, but it makes biological sense to vary the bedtime a little because naps vary from day to day. The time when your child *needs* to go to sleep at night depends on her age, how long her previous nap lasted, and how long her wakeful period was just before the bedtime hour. The time when she *wants* to go to sleep may be altogether different! If your child is unusually active in the afternoon or if she misses a good midday nap, then she should be put to sleep earlier.

This is true even if a parent returns home late from work. A parent who arrives home late might walk into the house and immediately begin a twenty- to thirty-minute soothing-to-sleep routine without playtime. If the parent returns very late, the child should be put to bed as usual; keeping a tired child up to play with a tired parent does no one any good. At the cost to the parent of having less time with the child, the benefit is no bedtime battles, no night-waking habits, no early-morning arousals, good-quality naps, a well-rested child, a well-rested spouse, and relaxed private time for the parents in the evening. I encourage the parents to also go to bed early so that they are not rushed in the early morning with their baby. Morning time includes bathing, dressing, feeding, and playing, and may substitute for evening time. Because of the family's early bedtime, the weekends are enjoyably relaxed since everyone is well rested.

The completely opposite scenario occurs when one parent, usually the father, demands that the other, usually the mother, keep their child up late so that he can play with her. Not only does the child suffer, but it is the mother who is the unappreciated victim, because she is trying to maintain marital harmony and trying to keep her child well rested—and she can't do both. Obviously, this is not simply a child's sleep problem but a family problem.

> To establish healthy sleep schedules at 4–8 months of age, become your infant's timekeeper. Set her clock on healthy time.

Allowing brief naps in the early evening or long late-afternoon naps in order to keep a child up late at night will eventually ruin healthy sleep schedules. If your child misses her midday nap, it is better—in order for her to be able to fall asleep close to her biological bedtime hour and avoid the overtired state—to have no nap and an early bedtime than a late nap and a late bedtime. Similarly, you may occasionally need to wake your baby in the morning in order to establish an age-appropriate midmorning nap that is needed to set the sleep schedule for the rest of the day.

Sleep Regularity

The best time for your child to fall asleep at night is when she is just starting to become *drowsy*, before she becomes overtired. For young children in daycare, dual-career families with long commutes, and older children with scheduled activities, it may be impossible to catch that magical drowsy state. These children will be better off if the bedtime occurs at approximately the same time every night. In a study conducted by Dr. Yvonne Kelly, children with nonregular bedtimes examined at age 3, 5, and 7 years had more behavioral difficulties at age 7 than children with regular bedtimes. The effect of nonregular bedtimes was *cumulative*—the more years of nonregular bedtimes, the worse the behavior. So the effect of nonregular bedtimes builds up throughout early childhood. The good news is that the harm is *reversible.* That is, when children change from nonregular to regular bedtimes, they show improvements in their behavior. Additionally, behavioral difficulties were more common when the bedtime was after 9:00 P.M. As previously stated regarding late bedtimes and obesity, it is never too late to help your child sleep better by encouraging earlier and more regular bedtimes.

One study, by Dr. Bates, examined the sleep of 202 children between 4 and 5 years of age (page 42). He studied the home environment, behavior at preschool, and sleeping patterns. Here, variability in bedtime was associated with daytime problems described as "less optimal" behavioral adjustments in preschool. For example, these children did not "comply with teacher's urging to join an activity" or "show enthusiasm for learning something." They argued and fought more than other children. Dr. Bates hypothesized that those children with chronically variable sleep schedules might experience states similar to jet lag syndrome, characterized as nagging fatigue and cognitive disorientation. This particular study asked whether behavior problems at school and sleep behavior problems had a common denominator—that is, family stress—and the answer was no. The child's sleep problems seemed to directly cause the school behavior problems. Perhaps in other studies associating family stress with sleep problems, the sleep problems are directly caused by nonregular or too-late bedtimes.

In one study of about eleven thousand children at age 3, the lack of a regular bedtime was associated with obesity at age 11. In pre-teens, obesity is also associated with extreme differences in sleep between weeknights and weekends (social jet lag). For teenagers, this might occur with consistent bedtimes throughout the week but much later bedtimes on the weekends.

In another study, regularity of the bedtime schedule was assessed in 3,119 high school students. The researchers discovered that a more irregular sleep schedule was associated with more daytime sleepiness. These teenagers had lower grades, more injuries associated with alcohol or drugs, and more days missed from school.

Going to bed regularly around 11:00 P.M. might produce the same amount of sleep as a schedule in which bedtime is sometimes at 10:00 P.M. and sometimes at midnight, but the more regular schedule is probably better. Also, more digital screen time is associated with more irregular bedtimes. Among college undergraduates, irregular sleep patterns are associated with lower academic performance, but sleep irregularity was *not* related to the duration of sleep.

Either nonregular bedtimes or bedtimes that are too late can be corrected by parents. One study clearly showed that with parent-set bedtimes, teenagers went to bed earlier, obtained more sleep, and experienced improved daytime wakefulness and less fatigue compared with teenagers whose parents did not set bedtimes. Two other experimental studies on college students showed that regularization of sleep/wake schedules is associated with reduced daytime sleepiness (improvements in alertness) and a reduction in negative mood (tension-anxiety, anger-hostility, and fatigue). These studies prove that irregular bedtimes are harmful and correctable.

Yet some flexibility, especially with younger children, is often called for. For example, a bedtime that always puts a preschool child to sleep at exactly 7:00 P.M. does not take into account the biological variability, from day to day, of her activity levels or lengths of naps. So it makes sense to vary the bedtime by thirty to sixty minutes—but no more than that—based on how your child looks and behaves during the late afternoon. On the other hand, for older children who are not napping, having bedtimes that are hours earlier or later from day to day has been shown to be unhealthy.

A regular bedtime may vary by some minutes per night but not hours per night. Even if the bedtime is too late, a *regular* bedtime is better than an irregular bedtime.

BIOLOGICAL RHYTHMS

To better understand the importance of maintaining sleep schedules, let's look at how four distinctive biological rhythms develop. First, immediately after birth, babies are wakeful; they then fall asleep, wake, and fall asleep a second time over a ten-hour period. These periods of wakefulness are predictable and not due to hunger, although what causes them is unknown. Thus a partial sleep/wake pattern or rhythm emerges immediately after birth. Second, body temperature rhythms appear and influence sleep/wake cycles. Body temperature typically rises during the day and drops to lower levels at night. At 6 weeks of age, temperature at bedtime is significantly higher than later in the night. After 6 weeks of age, as temperatures fall more with sleep, the sleep periods get longer. By 12–16 weeks, all babies show consistent temperature rhythms. It is exactly at 6 weeks of age that evening fussiness or crying begins to decrease from peak levels and night sleep becomes organized, and it is at 12–16 weeks that day sleep patterns become established.

A third pattern is added by 3–6 months of age, when production of the hormone cortisol shows a similar characteristic rhythm, with peak concentrations in the early morning and lowest levels around midnight. Interestingly, a part of the cortisol secretion rhythm is related to the sleep/wake rhythm, and another part is coupled to the body temperature rhythm. I wish Mother Nature were simpler!

Melatonin rhythmicity is a fourth pattern to consider. Initially, a newborn has high levels of circulating melatonin, which is secreted by the mother's pineal gland and crosses the placenta. Within about one week, the melatonin that came from the mother has disappeared. At about 6 weeks of age, melatonin begins to reappear as the baby's pineal gland matures. But the levels are extremely low until 12–16 weeks of age. Then melatonin begins to surge at night, and the hormone appears to be associated with evolving sleep/wake rhythms by about 6 months of age. (Note: Melatonin supplements should not be given to healthy babies or young children to make them sleep better, as there is no evidence that this is safe.)

Even at only a few months of age, then, interrelated internal rhythms are already well developed: sleep/wake pattern, body temperature, and cortisol and melatonin levels. In adults, it appears that a long night's sleep is most dependent on going to sleep at or just after the peak of the temperature cycle. Bedtimes occurring near the lower portion of the temperature cycle result in shorter sleep durations.

Shift work or jet travel in adults, or parental mismanagement in children, might cause *disorganized sleep*. What is disorganized sleep? When you are awake but your body clock is in the sleep mode, or when you crash from exhaustion and your body clock is in the awake mode, then wakefulness or sleep is occurring out of phase with other biological rhythms. The result is poor-quality sleep or poor-quality wakefulness. Imagine a choir in which the individual voices, instead of blending harmoniously, blare out in strident dissonance! Many studies have been conducted with shift workers and in sleep labs on the internal desynchronization of circadian rhythms, the uncoupling of rhythms that are normally closely linked, and shifting rhythms that are out of phase with one another. The most common complaints in these adults are headaches and abdominal pain. Such people appear healthy and can function reasonably well except for the fact that they have pain in their head or stomach. Not surprisingly, headaches and stomachaches are the most common symptoms experienced by school-aged children whose busy schedules cause them to lose sleep. One parent told of gradually worsening stomachaches in their teen that necessitated repeated visits to the doctor and finally a trip to the emergency room. At no time was a physical cause or illness identified. The stomachaches subsided on their own; only later, when consulting me about sleep issues in a younger sibling, did the parent realize that the stomachaches had coincided with a stretch of difficult schoolwork that had resulted in the teenager staying up later and later, accumulating a substantial sleep debt that manifested itself in these unpleasant physical symptoms.

I always advise parents to become sensitive to their child's personal sleep signals. This means capturing that magic moment when the child is tired, ready to sleep, and will easily fall asleep. The magic moment is a slight quieting, a lull in being busy, a slight staring off, and a hint of calmness (page 167). If you catch this wave of tiredness and put the child to sleep then, there will be no crying. I like the analogy of surfing, because timing is so important there, too—you have to catch the wave after it rises enough to be recognized but before it crashes. If you allow a child to crash into an overtired state, it will be harder for her to fall asleep, because she is trying to do so out of phase with other biological rhythms. Her ride to sleep then will not be easy or pleasant. Timing is most important! Remember, not every sleep wave is the same, and not every child learns quickly how to ride her sleep wave. But as with everything else, after practice it occurs effortlessly.

More Healthy Sleep Issues

CUMULATIVE SLEEPINESS

It's been known for many years that the effect of lost sleep accumulates over time. In other words, your brain does not adapt to the challenge of short sleep. The sensation of sleepiness does not fade away over time. Instead, you might develop more subjective blind-

ness to your chronic state of sleepiness (page 101) and consume co-
pious amounts of caffeinated beverages. When you constantly have
insufficient sleep, the sensation of sleepiness when you should be
awake increases progressively. Lapses in behavioral alertness and
performance impairments increase. Let me explain what this means
by giving an example. When adult volunteers have their sleep shortened by a constant amount, impairments in their mood and performance can be measured during the day. If the sleep disruption is
repeated night after night, the actual measured impairments do not
remain constant. Instead, there is an escalating accumulation of
sleepiness that produces in adults continuing increases in headaches, gastrointestinal complaints, forgetfulness, reduced concentration, fatigue, emotional ups and downs, difficulty in staying
awake during the daytime, irritability, and difficulty waking. Not
only do the adults describe themselves as more sleepy and mentally
exhausted, but they also feel more stressed. The stress may be a direct consequence of partial sleep deprivation, or it may result from
the challenge of coping with increasing amounts of daytime sleepiness. Think how hard it would be to concentrate or be motivated if
you were struggling every day to stay awake.

If children have constant sleep deficits, do they show these same
escalating problems during the day? Yes! I believe the young child's
brain is as sleep-sensitive as an adult's, if not more so. It is also possible that severe or chronic sleep deficits occurring early during the
period of rapid brain growth might hardwire neurological circuits
to produce *permanent* effects (page 118). This would be difficult to
prove, because young children cannot report how they feel and we
assume it is natural for them to have difficult temperaments, have
tantrums, get frustrated, become easily angry, and so forth. In addition, in older children we have learned to accept as normal vague
neurological differences such as learning difficulties or attention
deficit hyperactivity disorder (which, oddly enough, we treat with
stimulant medications).

The problem with concluding that constant sleep deficits are associated with these problems is that early nighttime sleep deficits may be mild and masked by long naps. If the brain has been *permanently* changed due to severe or chronic sleep loss, then, when the naps disappear and school requires more mental vigilance and focused attention, preexisting problems may appear. It is not simply your child's academic performance that might suffer. We do not know the contribution of healthy childhood sleep toward creativity, empathy, a sense of humor, or adult mental health. Part of the problem is, of course, that we don't have yardsticks to measure items such as creativity or empathy, so we do not yet have a way to measure the contribution that healthy sleep during childhood might make.

I do know that many parents keep their child up an extra twenty or thirty minutes at night to have fun and notice no problems in the beginning. Later they call and ask why their "good sleeper" is now resisting bedtime or is cranky in the morning for "no obvious reason." Or their baby slept well for the first six weeks, but after this, "all of a sudden" has difficulty falling asleep at night. Because the change in routine was small and in the past, they don't even think about it. But during our conversation they will recall that because of the longer spring and summer days, or because "it didn't seem to cause any problems," they pushed the child's bedtime back. The interval between allowing the too-late bedtime and the emergence of sleep-related problems was months in young children who had always in the past been well rested and were taking good naps, or weeks in children who were always on the edge of being overtired anyway. When these parents were asked if they thought their child appeared able to go to sleep twenty or thirty minutes earlier, the answer was almost always yes.

MAJOR POINT

Small but constant deficits in sleep that *accumulate* over time tend to have escalating and perhaps long-term effects on brain function.

In older children who have outgrown naps, the interval before the effects of cumulative sleepiness show themselves may be very long because of high motivation in the child and many exciting parent-directed events such as classes, lessons, or excursions, which help mask impaired vigilance or performance. The right bedtime is based on your child's behavior, mood, and performance, especially in the late afternoon.

When parents make the effort to help the child get needed sleep, the child becomes better rested, and it becomes easier for her to accept sleep, to expect to sleep, to take long naps, and to go to sleep by herself. Some parents always have to endure days of disruption following trips, illnesses, or immunizations because any irregularity of schedule upsets sleep rhythms.

Slightly overtired children are more easily thrown off balance and take longer to recover. Well-rested children tend to be more adaptable and take occasional changes of routine in stride.

A well-rested baby with a healthy sleep habit wakes with a cheerful, happy attitude. A tired baby wakes grumpy.

Cumulative benefits from extra sleep also occur. Sleep extension studies using earlier bedtimes or longer times in bed and delayed middle and high school start times show that small amounts of extra sleep, over time, add up and produce substantial benefits (page 102).

GENETIC AND CULTURAL EFFECTS

Some adults claim that they do not need much sleep and do well on very little sleep. However, studies reveal that the vast majority of these adults not only consume a lot of caffeine, but also suffer impairments from chronic insufficient sleep. On the other hand, there are rare families that have inherited a "short sleep" gene so that they actually appear to do well on only four to five hours of sleep each night. Nevertheless, because this gene occurs in only about one in four million individuals and because it does not appear to manifest itself in childhood, please do not accept a common, but usually incorrect, belief that some children do very well on very little sleep.

Genetic influences account for some of the individual differences in sleep measurements. Studies of twins, as young as 6 months, show that both genetic factors and environmental factors (parenting) are important. This topic is extremely important but also complex so here is the gist from an expert, Dr. Robert Plomin, Professor of Behavioral Genetics at the Institute of Psychiatry, Psychology and Neuroscience at King's College London: "Estimates of genetic influence are called *heritability*, which has a precise meaning in genetics. Heritability describes how much of the differences between individuals can be explained by their inherited DNA differences. The word 'difference' is key to its definition. . . . It is not a constant like the speed of light or gravity. It is a statistic that describes a particular population at a particular time with that population's particular mix of genetic and environmental influences. . . . Genetics contribute substantially to differences between people. . . . Inherited DNA differences contribute substantially to your risk of being anxious or depressed but they do not specify whether you will be diagnosed as anxious or depressed. Whether you become anxious or you become depressed is caused by environmental factors." An environment risk factor is insufficient sleep. Sleep restriction increases anxiety symptoms in individuals who have inherited DNA differences that contribute to an increased risk of being anxious. The opposite is also true! If parents are able to help their children sleep well, then the parents are able to sleep better themselves, and some become less anxious themselves.

So when different cultures are studied, differences in how children sleep and how these differences affect them may reflect differences in the mix of genetic and parenting practices. For example,

Dr. Jodi Mindell described how predominantly Asian countries/regions had later bedtimes (attributed to placing a high value on academic accomplishment with studying late at night), shorter sleep durations, and more room sharing compared to predominantly Caucasian countries/regions. On the other hand, studies have documented later bedtimes and shorter sleep durations in Spain and Italy, attributed to placing a high value on having children participate in the family evening life, including a late dinner. So different populations may have different mixes of genetic influences and cultural values and parenting practices regarding children's sleep; importantly, it is also known that there are genetic differences regarding how an individual will react to short sleep durations. Therefore, recommendations regarding healthy sleep might *not* be generalizable across different cultures and certainly do not apply to *all* children within a specific region.

> Because all mothers and fathers are innately different, please don't judge other parents' parenting.
> Because all children are innately different, please don't compare your child with other children.

Differential Susceptibility: Intra-Individual

Usually, when we think of genetic influences, we consider individual variability in development or outcome such as eye color, the onset of puberty, or adult height. Also, we know from twin studies that there are genetically based individual differences among children at any given age regarding naps, bedtimes, and sleep durations. Separate from this narrow notion of individual variation is the wider concept of differential susceptibility. There are innate differences *between* individuals that might appear *only* when exposed to specific environmental events. For example, not everyone reacts the same way when fixed sleep deficits cause cumulative sleepiness. The differential susceptibility hypotheses states that there are genetic differences *between* individuals regarding how they react to specific environmental events, in either a positive or a negative fashion.

To restate, differential susceptibility means that individuals, under genetic influence, react differently to the same environmental event. The environmental event might be a short sleep duration, maternal sensitivity, maternal emotional availability at bedtime, the amount of infant crying, the composition and size of the population of microorganisms in the infant's gut, or a TV in the bedroom.

Here are some examples:

When a variant of a gene controlling circadian rhythmicity is present, in adults, there is less impairment of cognitive performance in response to sleep loss.

When a serotonin transporter gene variant is present, children between 6 and 36 months of age, with short sleep durations, developed negative emotionality (discomfort, fear, frustration, sadness, and shyness), but not if the gene variant was absent.

When a dopamine genetic variant is present, children at age 10 months with *insensitive mothers* (based on scoring videotapes of mother's awareness of her baby's signals, accurate interpretation of them, and appropriateness and promptness of response during feeding and free play) displayed more externalizing behaviors at 39 months compared with children who had sensitive mothers, but these effects did not occur when the dopamine genetic variant was absent.

High *negative* emotionality (whining, frustration, anger, hitting, kicking) in children at 36 months of age who experienced high maternal sensitivity (based on videotapes demonstrating sensitive, responsive, and child-centered interactions, providing encouragement if child is having difficulty in a controlled laboratory setting) compared with those whose mothers had low maternal sensitivity (showing overt anger or rejection toward the child) predicted fewer bedtime problems and longer sleep durations in sixth grade. But the effect of high maternal sensitivity was not observed for children with low negative emotionality at 36 months.

High *positive* emotionality (more expressive and warmer interpersonal interactions, more smiles and laughter) in infants 1–6 months who experienced high maternal emotional availability at bedtime (based on videotapes demonstrating sensitivity, structuring, nonintrusiveness, and nonhostility) correlated with children who were less distressed and slept more throughout the night (based on objective recordings). But the effect of high maternal emotional availability at bedtime was weak on infants rated low in positive emotionality.

The total of all the different species of gastrointestinal microorganisms is called the *gut microbiome (GM)*. Human genetics shape the GM; that is, the GM is influenced in part by the genetic makeup of the host. Also, environmental light/dark or day/night cycles cause a twenty-four-hour shift in some cells lining the gut. Having a large number of individual bacteria from each of the different bacterial species present in the GM is called *high diversity*. High diversity is associated with longer objective sleep durations and less time awake after sleep onset (page 91). Because some specific GM species produce neurotransmitters or serotonin, it is possible that the GM, under the influence of the host's genetic makeup, and light cues, influences the host's brain's control over sleep. The effect may be bidirectional because sleep fragmentation causes reversible harmful alterations in the GM. In a 2019 paper, Anna-Katariina Aatsinki observed, "Recent studies indicate that gut microbes play essential roles in the neurodevelopment and control of behavior. . . . [O]ur result [showed] greater gut microbiota diversity is associated with lower negative emotionality and fear reactivity" among infants at 6 months of age. Also, the abundance of one specific microorganism was demonstrated to be associated with more "surgency" (more positive emotionality, higher activity level, more smiling, higher-intensity pleasure, and more vocal reactivity). The association between having an abundance of this specific microorganism with surgency was observed for boys but not for girls.

For boys, at age 2 years, objective measurements of sleep showed that shorter sleep durations and lower sleep efficiency (less time actually asleep compared with total time in bed) predicted more externalizing symptoms (page 127) at age four years. But these results were not found for girls.

For boys at age 8 and 10 years, objective measurements of sleep showed that shorter sleep durations predicted more behavioral problems two years later. But these results were not found in girls.

Parents of sleep-disturbed infants have a lower tolerance for infant crying. Women without children, women with children that are not sleep-disturbed, and women with sleep-disturbed children all have lower tolerance for infant crying than men (page 418).

Surprisingly, there may be a genetic influence over the amount of *television* an individual watches, so the presence or absence of a television in the bedroom might be another example of differential susceptibility.

When studies on children's sleep reach different results, it may be due to comparing subjective parents' sleep diary reports with objective measurements of sleep; comparing populations of children from different socioeconomic groups; or having unappreciated differences among groups of children regarding differential susceptibility. Not only do children show individuality in whether they do or do not respond to a change in their environment (differential susceptibility), but the exact character of the response varies among those who do respond (differential sensitivity).

Differential Sensitivity: Inter-Individual Task-Dependent Resilience and Susceptibility

In addition to genetic differences among individuals regarding how they sleep and how their sleep is affected by environmental events, *within* an individual there are *task-dependent* differences in response to insufficient sleep. As described by Professor Tkachenko, "there are distinctive cognitive profiles of responding with differential vulnerability to sleep loss within the same individual." In adults, many studies have examined specific within-an-individual (inter-individual) differences in response to sleep loss: cognitive responses (alertness, vigilance, and sustained attention), tasks involving aspects of executive functioning (for example, speed of cognitive processing), and subjective response to sleep loss (for example, mood and daytime sleepiness). "While some individuals show no sign of impairment following sleep loss, others show significant decrements in performance on tasks of simple vigilance and attention as well as higher-order executive functions. Yet *resilience on one measure, such as lapses of attention or reaction time, does not necessarily carry over to other aspects of performance,* not withstanding the foundation criticality of vigilant attention for much of cognition. . . . Neurobehavioral vulnerability to sleep loss is a reality that appears to vary *depending on the task* and performance metric under consideration. . . . Vulnerability to sleep loss is reflected across multiple neurobehavioral facets that appear to function independently [emphasis added]." So how you, and your child, feel, behave, and perform when short on sleep is a highly individualized trait. Some individuals are more resilient, and some are more vulnerable to sleep loss, but this notion of how one reacts to sleep loss is *task-dependent.* "However, it appears that individuals with habitually higher homeostatic sleep pressure [individuals who need more sleep] are predisposed to greater vulnerability of accumulating deficits during sleep loss."

This last point might explain a curious observation I made after publishing my first paper in 1981 on sleep duration and infant temperament. Children with an easy temperament sleep longer than children with a difficult *temperament.* I noted that parents of children with an easy temperament described a much greater deterioration of their child's behavior and mood compared with parents of children with a difficult temperament when they both became short of sleep by the same amount. I originally thought that the difference was one of perspective: The mother of a child with an easy temperament was more likely to notice worsening of mood and behavior compared with the background of an easy temperament than was the mother of a child with a difficult temperament, who was more accustomed to deal with challenging moods and behaviors. But it is also possible that children who do need more sleep are predisposed to greater vulnerability in worsening mood, behavior, and performance during sleep loss, as described above. However, even among all children who do need more sleep, "differential sensitivity" tells us that some individuals might show greater or lesser deficits in either mood or in behavior or in performance ("task differences") because of inter-individual differences.

Individual children experiencing the same sleep loss might respond differently.

Don't assume that your child will behave like other children when she gets short on sleep because of late-night social events or missed naps. Try to watch her mood and behavior and respect her individual need for sleep.

WAKE AFTER SLEEP ONSET

When you put your baby in her crib, you may note her bedtime; when you go to her in the morning, you may note when she wakes up. So you can easily estimate the duration of her nighttime sleep. However, a researcher studying infant sleep might place a motion sensor, worn like a watch, on your infant's wrist or ankle. This device is called an actigraph. When your baby is asleep, there is much less movement compared to when awake. Now the duration of night sleep can be measured more objectively. Looking at the time between the mother's report of bedtime and wake-up time, a researcher can measure how long after "bedtime" it takes for your child to fall asleep (called latency to sleep), how many times your child wakes at night (independent of whether she cries or vocalizes), the proportion of time she is actually asleep between the mother's reported bedtime and wake-up time (called sleep efficiency), and lastly the amount of time she is actually awake after the onset of sleep (called wake after sleep onset or WASO). On the one hand, a parent might be aware of WASO because she is up with her child for prolonged periods of time trying to soothe her infant back to sleep. On the other hand, a parent, of course, might be unaware of quiet and calm wakefulness in their infant in the middle of the night. Even with a baby monitor, a parent might be dimly aware of this behavior, but it would be unreasonable to expect a parent to accurately measure its duration. Thankfully, the actigraph does it automatically.

Professor Michael Gradisar studied a group of infants (6–16 months) undergoing either graduated extinction or bedtime fading as an intervention to help a child sleep better at night (page 277). Both groups showed decreases in sleep latency, but only the graduated extinction group had large decreases in the number of awakenings and minutes of wake after sleep onset. In other words, graduated extinction, but not bedtime fading, produced more consolidated sleep, better sleep efficiency, and longer sleep durations. Another study, by Dr. Manuela Pisch (page 564), followed infants at 4, 6, 8, and 10 months. She showed that wake after sleep onset serves as a marker for different trajectories in cognitive development. She observed that less WASO, or more time actually asleep at night, is associated with enhanced cognitive development.

Taken together, the two studies suggest that WASO is an important element in the context of treatment of a sleep problem and enhancement of cognitive development, even though parents might not be directly able to appreciate it.

SLEEP POSITIONS AND SIDS

A common myth held by Western parents is that all children sleep better on their stomachs. Yet a Chinese mother whose baby preferred to sleep on her stomach said she knew something was very wrong with her infant, because all Chinese babies sleep on their backs! She truly worried that stomach sleeping was unhealthy.

The truth is that some babies seem to sleep better and fuss or cry less when asleep on their backs. Contrary to many parents' fears, sleeping on the back does not cause a misshapen skull. In the past, tradition and social circumstances dictated which sleeping position most parents selected. Now it appears that *sleeping on the back is healthier because it helps prevent sudden infant death syndrome (SIDS)*. Fortunately, most babies sleep just as well on their backs as on their stomachs.

A variant of the myth that babies sleep better on their stomachs is that when a 5-month-old child rolls over, away from the sleeping position selected by the parents, the parent has to intervene and roll the child back. Actually, leaving the child alone allows the child to learn to sleep in different positions. If you roll your child back and she instantaneously returns to sleep, obviously there is no problem. On the other hand, going to your child to roll her back can become a game for the infant by 5 months of age. Games should occur at playtime, not when it's time to sleep. Remember, not going to your baby allows her to learn to roll back alone, learn to sleep in the new position, and learn to remember the next night not to roll in the first place.

Likewise, when the older child pulls herself to a standing position in her crib, parents do not need to help her get down. A child might fall down in an awkward heap, but she will not hurt herself. Next time she will think twice about standing up and shaking the crib railings, or she'll be more careful when letting go.

Parents who rush in to roll the baby over or to help a child down run the risk of reinforcing this behavior, encouraging it to be repeated night after night. Children are very crafty and learn quickly how to get parents to give them extra attention. Don't deprive your child of the opportunity to learn how to roll over or sit down unassisted at night. These small triumphs of self-sufficiency set the stage for later behavioral accomplishments.

Prevent SIDS

The American Academy of Pediatrics 2016 recommendations for preventing sudden infant death syndrome are:

Place your baby to sleep on his back for every sleep up to 1 year. If he rolls onto his stomach by himself, he may be left in the position.
Place your baby to sleep on a firm surface with no bumper pads.
Breastfeeding is recommended.
Infants sleep in the parents' room, close to the parents' bed, but on a separate surface designed for infants, ideally for the first year of life, but at least for the first 6 months.
Keep soft objects and loose bedding away from the infant's sleep area to reduce the risk of SIDS, suffocation, entrapment, and strangulation.
Consider offering a pacifier at nap time and bedtime.
Avoid smoke exposure during pregnancy and after birth.
Avoid alcohol and illicit drug use during pregnancy and after birth.
Avoid overheating and head covering in infants.
Pregnant women should receive regular prenatal care.
Infants should be immunized.
Avoid the use of commercial devices that claim to reduce the risk of SIDS.
Do not use home cardiorespiratory monitors to reduce the risk of SIDS.

Some parents wish to co-sleep with their child but are worried about SIDS. There are bassinet-like stands, called co-sleepers, that abut the parents' bed. They allow the nursing mother to feed her baby at night without having to leave her bed. Please discuss safety concerns with your pediatrician. The last item on the above list is extremely important because of hazards of strangulation. For example, in 2014, there was a recall of a baby monitor because the wires could be separated from a sensor pad.

Separately, devices marketed to help your baby sleep better might be hazardous, such as a Rock 'n Play sleeper recalled in 2019 because it was linked to multiple infant deaths. In 2020, the federal Consumer Product Safety Commission recalled four different companies' infant incline sleepers due to a risk of suffocation.

SLEEP LOCATION: ROOM SHARING VERSUS SEPARATE ROOMS

Having your baby sleep in the parents' room for the entire first year is controversial because 90 percent of SIDS deaths occur in the first six months and the evidence, during the second six months, that room sharing helps prevent SIDS is weak. After the age of 6 months, evidence that independent sleeping arrangements increase the likelihood of SIDS is lacking. A 2020 nationally representative sample of mothers reported that 45 percent practiced room sharing without bed sharing between 2 and 6 months. Please discuss room sharing with your child's pediatrician.

In a study using nighttime video assessments that was conducted before the 2016 SIDS recommendations, infants were divided into three groups:

1. Early Independent Sleepers (sleeping independently without room sharing by 4 months)
2. Later Independent Sleepers (began sleeping independently between 4 and 9 months)
3. Still Room Sharing Sleepers at 9 months

At 9 months of age, the Early Independent Sleepers had longer sleep durations and fewer night wakings than the other two groups.

At 30 months of age, both Early and Later Independent Sleepers had longer night sleep than those who were in the Still Room Sharing group at 9 months. Further, the Early Independent Sleepers at 4 months had a more consistent bedtime routine and an earlier bedtime. In contrast, at 9 months, those who were Still Room Sharing had later bedtimes and were less likely to be put to sleep drowsy but awake. Also, those who were Still Room Sharing had more unsafe sleep practices such as soft objects on their sleep surfaces, and they were more likely to be brought into their parents' bed after a nighttime waking.

A separate study of about ten thousand children observed that infants 6–12 months old who slept in a separate room as opposed to room sharing had earlier bedtimes, shorter time to fall asleep, more nighttime and total sleep, increased sleep consolidation, more consistent bedtime routines, and better ability to fall asleep independently. These parents perceived bedtime to be less difficult and sleep to be better overall.

Using objective measurements of sleep at 3, 6, 12, and 18 months, another study, led by Dr. Ella Volkovich, classified families into two sleeping arrangement categories:

1. Persistent solitary sleeping (infants slept in a separate room on at least three out of four assessment times)
2. Persistent room sharers (infants sharing their parents' room on at least three assessment points)

Almost *no* objective differences in infant sleep quality were observed. However, among the room sharers, the mothers had lower objective and subjective sleep quality and reported more night wakings. They also had higher levels of maternal separation anxiety, while the *fathers' overall involvement during the day and nighttime involvement in infant caregiving was less.* These differences existed from the infant's age of 3 months and remained consistent until the age of 18 months. The authors did not know whether room sharing was planned or reactive but suggested this explanation: "Mothers with higher levels of separation anxiety and disturbed sleep are more likely to choose room-sharing arrangements *especially when their partner is not involved in caregiving;* these mothers are more likely to be vigilant to the infants' awakenings and are more likely to be awakened by the infants' sounds during the night; being awake during the night increases the likelihood of maternal active involvement in soothing the infant back to sleep when the infant wakes up; active nighttime soothing may reinforce the infants' signaling behavior, which in turn may affect the mother's sleep and separation anxiety, *the levels of paternal involvement* (page 410), and the decision to maintain room-sharing arrangements, and so on [emphasis added]."

Somewhat similar findings were observed by Dr. Douglas Teti, who studied families who practiced co-sleeping. Persistent co-sleeping was defined as room sharing or bed sharing beyond 6 months. Data were objectively recorded for sleep and nighttime video recordings, and home visits took place at 1, 3, 6, 9, and 12 months. "Persistent cosleeping was associated with sleep disruption in mothers but not in infants [or fathers], although mothers in persistent cosleeping arrangements reported their infants had more frequent night awakenings [which objectively did *not* occur]. Persistent co-sleeping was also associated with mother reports of marital and coparenting distress, and lower emotional availability with infants at bedtime. Persistent co-sleeping appeared to be a marker of, though not necessarily a cause of, heightened family stress."

Why would these mothers, as also in Dr. Volkovich's study, report frequent night wakings when objective measurements did not record them? Dr. Teti hypothesizes, "If persistent co-sleeping in a culture that does not support it is a marker of family and maternal distress . . . , one manifestation of maternal distress may be a hypersensitivity to and hyper-vigilance about infant night awakenings, leading distressed mothers to count even brief infant arousals and postural shifts as night awakenings. These very brief arousals may go unnoticed by nondistressed mothers, and they may be too brief and below threshold to be identified as wake activity by [objective] actigraphy." Further, "If mothers who engage in persistent co-sleeping do so because they are distressed, and if doing so places mothers at risk for sleep disruption, cumulative sleep debt, and relationship difficulties with their infants, such mothers comprise a high-risk group in need of intervention. The primary goal of intervention should not be, in our view, to advise against co-sleeping, but instead to improve the marital and coparenting relationship, particularly around but not limited to decisions parents make about infant sleep."

Researchers in Hong Kong examined *how* the child falls asleep ("falling asleep independently" referred to the ability to fall asleep without help by others, and reflects the child's ability to self-soothe versus falling asleep while being rocked, held, or fed by a parent) as well as sleep arrangements (bed sharing, room sharing, and separate room). They collected data on over a thousand children from birth to 36 months. They observed that "falling asleep independently was associated with longer nocturnal sleep duration and less sleep awakenings. . . . In Hong Kong room- or bed-sharing may sometimes even be unavoidable due to the small living spaces that many families live in. . . . Our data suggest that it is possible that whether or not the child develops sleep problems depends not so much on the sleep location, but the parental behavior at sleep initiation." Sleep location (bed sharing, room sharing, or a separate room) was not associated with better sleep. However, for all three sleep locations, the mean bedtime was very late, after 10:00 P.M. A much earlier bedtime, perhaps associated with a separate room, might have shown different results. In fact, in this study, the children in a separate room did have an earlier bedtime. So the three variables (encouraging self-soothing, an early bedtime, and a separate room, if possible) might act independently and each separately help children sleep better.

MODERN LIFE

The single most important fact to remember is that the time when sleep occurs may be more important than the duration of the sleep period. You can't fight circadian rhythms! We all have internal clocks that are genetically controlled and evolved from dark (night)/light (day) cues. These clocks create an internal timing mechanism for sleep. The power of this mechanism should never be underestimated, because it is very primitive and caused by the rotation of the earth on its axis. All living creatures are affected by it. Sleep that occurs in sync with circadian rhythms is more restorative and of better quality than sleep that occurs out of sync with circadian rhythms. Jet lag syndrome is an example of sleep not in sync with circadian rhythms. Additionally, a bout of sleep that is continuous (consolidated) is much more restorative than a bout of sleep that is interrupted (fragmented). *Quality sleep means consolidated sleep occurring in phase with circadian rhythms.*

None of this is new information. In 1927, Dr. Lewis Terman, who co-invented the IQ test that we still use today, wrote the following:

> Sleep is one of the many biological rhythms stamped into the organism by the movement of the planet on which we live. To interfere unduly with such an ancient and physiologically established rhythm would, theoretically, appear sufficient to menace the stability of the organism. Sleep is an instinct which involves the entire body, and is not simply a function of the brain. . . .
>
> An explanation for the lack of correlation we have found between school success and hours of sleep [is] that large quantitative differences in sleep may be fully offset by qualitative differences. If this is true then sleep cannot be accurately measured in units of time alone. . . . There can be little doubt that *qualitative* differences do exist.

He knew that sleep duration (quantity) does not tell the whole story about sleep quality. He also wrote:

> Many children secure insufficient sleep *merely because they are not put to bed early enough*. . . . The time lost in this way cannot be fully made up in the morning because of the disturbance caused by the early rising of parents and because of the necessity of getting to school at a given hour. In other words, the hours set apart for the sleep of children are not those best adapted to insure a sufficient amount. Even the families who set a reasonably early hour for the children to retire usually permit so many irregularities that, as one writer puts it, "the law is more observed in the breach than in the performance."
>
> Sleep ranks with food as one of the most imperative needs of the human organism, and like the latter it has its educational and economic aspects as well as its physiological and biological. But while diet has long received a liberal share of attention from economist, hygienist, and biologist, the scientific study of the hygiene of sleep has hardly more than initiated. We seem to have rested content in the supposition that sleep of satisfactory quantity and quality can always be had when needed. Theoretically, and under natural conditions, this may be true. *Under the conditions of modern life it is not true.* In this respect the problem is analogous to that of ventilation. The ocean of fresh air is always at hand, but the problems of the ventilating engineer are none the less real [emphasis added].

As early as 1927, "modern life" was being blamed for causing children's sleep problems. Consider that most of rural America did not have electricity until 1935! Even so, Dr. Terman noted that natural conditions were no longer of paramount influence in setting the sleep habits of children, and that "scientific study . . . of sleep has hardly more than initiated." Why, nearly a hundred years later, are we still struggling with sleep issues in our children? One answer is that when we are often mildly to moderately sleepy, we might not sense that we are short on sleep or appreciate the consequences of not being optimally alert. In other words, we tend to be subjectively blind to our own sleep deficits.

SLEEP BLINDNESS

A review article in 2013 described adults who were experimentally sleep-deprived and showed the expected decreases in performance, but they lacked subjective feelings of sleepiness. The authors, Drs. Hans Van Dongen and David Dinges, wrote that "those who are *chronically* sleep deprived may no longer be capable of reliably appraising their own sleepiness. . . . [This] may explain why sleep restriction is widely practiced: People have the subjective impression they have adapted to it because they don't feel particularly sleepy." If parents lack self-awareness about their own sleep loss, then it should come as no surprise that they fail to appreciate subtle harmful effects of sleep loss in their children.

This is such an important point, I wish to restate it: *It is possible that some parents are so unaware of how impaired they are by their own sleep deprivation, they are unable to appreciate the extent to which sleep deprivation is harming their child.* I suspect that this explains why otherwise observant and loving parents (who are nevertheless short on sleep themselves) allow their child to become sleep-deprived, with all of its attendant problems. And if the children are too often mildly short on sleep, they themselves might not develop a strong sense of how different it feels to be completely well rested versus mildly sleepy. This subjective blindness to one's own sleep deficit might continue as these chronically slightly sleepy children become adults, or it might be prevented by ensuring healthy sleep for your child. Reports by parents on their preteens and teens who successfully prevented subjective blindness to sleep deficits appear in chapter 3.

POWER OF SMALL CHANGES

Another answer to why sleep issues in children have been present for many generations may be that we tend to not appreciate the power of small changes. What we do day by day often has a rhythm, and there is a natural temptation to assume that small changes in our routines are probably not very important. It's human nature for adults to vary our patterns of behavior by twenty or thirty minutes and correctly think, *What's the big deal?* In our young children, however, this may be a fallacy, because biological processes often operate as if they were a finely tuned machine with many interacting parts. Like the famous "butterfly effect" in meteorology, in which the movement of a butterfly's wings in Asia produces a tornado in the Midwest, an extremely tiny change may produce dramatic damage.

Here is another helpful analogy. Our healthy body temperature is about 98.6 degrees Fahrenheit. When our temperature is greater than 104 degrees, it usually means that there is a serious or perhaps life-threatening illness. However, when our temperature is only slightly elevated, say 99.6 degrees—an increase of just over 1 percent—we still might have a life-threatening disease! A low fever does not necessarily mean a mild medical problem. The thermometer is a useful tool that measures body temperature, but it does not tell the whole story.

Unfortunately, we do not have a "sleepometer" to measure sleepiness. Nevertheless, consider that the work of healthy sleep is to keep the nerve cells in the brain functioning optimally. What happens if your child needs ten hours of sleep but you keep her up just an extra twenty minutes later every night? Twenty minutes seems like a small amount, but this represents a 3.3 percent loss of sleep every night.

Because I think an earlier bedtime will produce better sleep in children with sleep problems and perhaps avoid the need to try a sleep solution involving crying, I am presenting here some studies that show that a few extra minutes of sleep can make a big difference.

Delaying school start times caused 15-year-olds to sleep in, and five months later, they demonstrated improved mental health, better prosocial behavior, peer relationships, and attention level—and the average increase in night sleep was only *2.4 minutes*. Lower levels of sleepiness and improvement in alertness and well-being among 15-year-olds were observed in another study of delaying school start times, and the increase in night sleep time after nine months was just *ten minutes*. Similar results were observed in three other studies involving delaying school start times, with an additional *seventeen minutes, twenty-nine minutes,* and *thirty-four minutes* more sleep producing less sleepiness, less tardiness, and increase in grades (page 696).

In an additional study, a 15-year-old was "classified as having low mood if he answered "yes" to the following question: During the past twelve months, did you ever feel so sad or hopeless almost every day for two weeks or more in a row that you stopped doing some usual activities? Delaying the school start time caused a significant reduction of almost 5 percent of the prevalence of low mood with a *thirty-minute* increase in sleep duration. Also, in this study, among 13-year-olds, advancing school start time (school started earlier) caused a decrease of sleep duration of *fifteen minutes* and a 2 percent increase in low mood prevalence (page 696). So a few minutes *less* sleep every night also makes a big difference!

Experimentally extending sleep by adding one hour in bed for five nights caused adolescents to sleep *thirteen minutes* more at night with a reduction of insomnia and depressive symptoms. Separately, adding one hour in bed for five nights in children 7–11 years old provided an additional *twenty-seven minutes* of sleep with improvements in emotional lability and restless-impulsive behavior (page 128). Another study of those 7–11 years old showed that *eigh-*

teen minutes of extra sleep caused improvement in grades for mathematics and languages (page 128).

Parent-set bedtimes among 14-year-olds caused an earlier bedtime, which was associated with an extra *nineteen minutes* of night sleep and created improved daytime functioning (page 298).

Children at 3.5 years who slept about *seven minutes* less each night were more likely to develop symptom of bipolar disorder at age 11 years. Also, when 6- and 8-year-olds sleep *thirty minutes* less than their peers, they are more likely to have symptoms of psychiatric disorders two years later (page 132).

You have to ask yourself, can your child fall asleep a little earlier? Or the opposite, could a slight sleep deficit produce a chronic but mild impairment or blunting of function in your young child's developing brain?

But here's the good news: We now know that the brain primarily makes up for sleep loss by increasing sleep *intensity* (slow-wave EEG activity during non-REM sleep), and not necessarily by increasing sleep *duration*. Again, this suggests that sleep quality might be more important than sleep quantity. Nevertheless, if your child gets acutely short on sleep, sometimes a brief nap or an occasional super-early bedtime might be sufficiently restorative.

Dr. Terman blamed "modern life" as contributing to sleep problems in 1927; I just suggested that the real problem may be that we are subjectively blind to our own sleep deficits, and that it is part of human nature to simply not pay close attention to the details of our children's sleep. But there have been real changes in modern life since 1927. If we look closely at many published reports, it appears that children today are getting less sleep than in the past, even though that did not appear to be the case when I first studied this subject in 1981. More children have a *television* in their bedrooms now and use their computers or cell phones at night, causing the bedtime to be later. More mothers with young children are in the labor force, and the use of center-based daycare has increased, rendering quality naps and early bedtimes more difficult to obtain. So "modern life" today is really different from what it was in 1927, and it seems likely that many of these differences have had increasingly adverse effects on our children's sleep. *Adverse concerns* are more clearly recognized today, and thus we are better able to help families cope with common challenges in order to establish healthy sleep for their children.

RISK FACTORS

Research on why children do not sleep well focuses on risk factors. When risk factors are present, it means that there is a higher likelihood of sleep problems in some children. The mere presence of a risk factor does not automatically mean that your own child will have a sleep problem. If your child does have a sleep problem and some of these risk factors are present, please mention them when you discuss her sleep problem with your health care provider.

> *Family conflict* and *marital strife*. Family conflict at age 7–15 years predicts insomnia at age 18, and marital strife at age 9 months predicts a child's sleep problems at 4.5 years.
> *Intimate partner violence* (physical or sexual violence, stalking, or psychological aggression) during the first 12 months postpartum is associated with persistent children's sleep problems.
> *Low-quality co-parenting.*
> *Emotional unavailability* of the mother at bedtime (measured by using multiple video cameras) predicts poor infant sleep quality for children 1–24 months of age. The emotionally unavailable mothers gave stern directives regarding sleep, while the emotionally available mothers talked directly and gently while gazing at the child's face.
> *Parental presence in bedroom* until the child falls asleep (page 175).

Maternal and paternal smoking during pregnancy.

Maternal and paternal depression and *maternal separation anxiety* (chapter 4).

Maternal cannabis exposure during pregnancy.

Maternal eveningness preference ("owl").

Feeding or attending to the child whenever she vocalizes, even though she has recently been fed (chapter 4).

Television and digital screens in the child's bedroom.

Caffeine consumption in older children.

Eczema and *snoring* (chapter 12) should be discussed with your child's health care provider.

Bed sharing during the first six months is associated with chronic awakenings. The longer the infant shares a bed with a parent, the higher the risk of nightly awakenings one year later. Bed sharing is a risk factor for *SIDS*.

What is the most important thing parents can do to help their child sleep?

My opinion is that the most important thing parents can do to help their child sleep well is to focus on a regularly occurring *early bedtime* based on *drowsy signs*. I think an early bedtime allows a child to fall asleep quickly at night and have more consolidated night sleep with few or no awakenings requiring parental attention during the night and little awake time after sleep onset. Because of good-quality night sleep, the child wakes up well rested and is able to take optimal naps. Because of restorative naps, there are no meltdowns in the late afternoon or early evening. Because of an early bedtime, there are no bedtime battles or endless curtain calls and she can fall asleep, after soothing, drowsy but awake, without Mom or Dad in the bedroom.

Sleep Recommendations

Lisa Matricciani's 2013 review of the literature concluded that published recommendations for children's sleep are not based on empirical evidence. She wrote that "sleep timing [the time when sleep occurs] may be even more important than sleep duration."

There are several reasons why published recommendations for sleep are not very useful for your child. Genetics influence how much sleep your child needs and how she will respond when short of sleep (page 85). At every age, individual children vary widely regarding the duration of night and day sleep and bedtimes. Also, for young children, there is a wide range at many ages in how many naps occur per day and how many children are sleeping through the night. And for older children, there is a wide range at many ages in how many children are still napping and, for those who still nap, in how many naps occur per week. Furthermore, results from different studies vary widely depending on the social class of the families and whether they were conducted many years ago or more recently. There is even variation in results from country to country.

The take-home message is that what commonly occurs regarding sleep among your relatives, friends, and neighbors might not be what is right for your child. Ignore what they recommend and what you read about bedtimes, naps, and total sleep needs. Instead, *watch your child*. Remember, late bedtimes usually mean less night sleep. In addition, sleeping out of phase with the body's natural rhythms, as shift workers do or as travelers do when crossing time zones, is as unhealthy as jet lag syndrome.

Don't be surprised if your child needs an earlier bedtime and takes longer naps than other children. Also, don't be surprised if you are criticized by others for being too careful regarding early bedtimes and protecting naps.

Summary and Action Plan for Exhausted Parents

Think of healthy sleep as a collection of several related elements grouped together to form a package. All must be present to ensure good-quality, healthy sleep. The elements of healthy sleep are:

1. *Sleep duration: night and day.* Does your child sleep as long as she needs for night sleep and for naps? How long your child needs to sleep depends on her age and temperament. Restricted sleep impairs mood, performance, development, and cognitive ability.

2. *Naps.* Is your child taking naps, or do you sometimes or often skip naps? If a nap is missed, try to keep your child up until the next sleep period in order to maintain the timeliness of the sleep rhythm. If needed, move the next sleep period a little earlier before your child becomes extremely overtired. If the naps are too long because your child has become overtired, you might have to wake her from a nap in order to maintain the timeliness of the sleep rhythm at night. The midmorning nap develops before the midday nap and disappears before the midday nap. Not all naps are created equal. Babies are born to be short or long nappers. An earlier bedtime may be required when two naps are needed but you can get only one.

3. *Sleep consolidation.* Is the sleep interrupted (fragmented) or uninterrupted (consolidated)? Arousals from sleep are normal. Some arousals are protective. Too many arousals—for example, from unnecessary intervention by parents—fragment sleep, and this causes impairments in mood and performance.

4. *Sleep schedule, timing of sleep.* Do naps start and bedtimes begin just when your child is becoming drowsy? A bedtime that is too late will produce an abnormal daytime sleep schedule. Variability in activity and length of naps causes some

variability in the bedtime. Watch your child more than the clock.

5. *Sleep regularity.* Do naps or bedtimes occur at approximately the same times? Even if the bedtime is a little too late, regular bedtimes are better than irregular bedtimes.

These five elements are not independent of one another; each influences the others. So if sleeping is out of kilter, look at all five elements. If you focus on and correct only one element, you might not achieve permanent success, because another element that needed attention was inadvertently ignored.

6. *Prevent sudden infant death syndrome.* Recommendations by the American Academy of Pediatrics (page 94) include room sharing but not bed sharing, and having the baby sleep on her back, not her stomach or side.

Sleep is a natural process, and there will usually be few difficulties if we are patient and don't interfere. Timing is most important, but there are genetically controlled individual differences among children regarding when their sleep rhythms develop and how long they sleep, so don't compare your child with other children. Naps and night sleep are related, and both need to be in place to avoid sleep problems. Our goal is to have well-rested families. But always remember, the amount of sleep our children need is measured by mood, behavior, and performance, not by hours on a clock. The best advice I can give parents is this: Let your child's natural sleep rhythms do their job without unnecessary interference!

What a Parent Can Do

Encourage your partner to help care for the baby daytime and nighttime.

Encourage self-soothing; the earlier, the better.

Put your child to sleep drowsy but awake, then leave the room.

Set an early bedtime based on drowsy signs.

Provide opportunities for naps based on drowsy signs.

Avoid irregularity of sleep schedules, including between week-days and weekends.

Practice safe sleep recommendations.

No TV or screens in the bedroom.

Chapter 3 Outline

NATURE OR NURTURE

FUNCTION OF SLEEP

Local Sleep
Optimal Wakefulness
Personal Best

SLEEP IS BRAIN FOOD: HEALTHY SLEEP IS LIKE HEALTHY FOOD

Social and Emotional Development
General
Depression and Anxiety
Internalizing and Externalizing Behaviors
Medical Health
Obesity or Overweight
Temperament
Athletic Performance
Cognitive Performance
Infants and Naps
Preschool Children

SLEEP PROBLEMS AND BENEFITS PERSIST

HEALTHY SLEEP IN YOUNG CHILDREN HAS CARRYOVER BENEFITS IN ADOLESCENCE

HEALTHY SLEEP IN CHILDREN HELPS PREVENT MATERNAL DEPRESSION

Why Healthy Sleep Is So Important

Infants and children who are still of tender age [may be]
attacked by . . . wakefulness at night.

—Aulus Cornelius Celsus, A.D. 130

If you have not already done so, please go back and read chapter 1.

Sleeplessness in children and worrying about sleeplessness in children have been around for a long time. If you have not yet had your child and you feel fairly well rested, you may appreciate the detailed information in this chapter describing why sleep is as important to health as clean air and water. The information will motivate you to help stay the course when you are tempted to forgo naps or keep your baby up late for your own social convenience or because of pressure from family members. But if you are desperately exhausted because you and your baby are not sleeping well, skip this chapter for now and circle back to it later on when you feel better rested.

Healthy sleep appears to come easily and naturally to newborn babies. Effortlessly, they fall asleep and stay asleep. Their sleep patterns, however, shift and evolve as the brain matures during the first few weeks and months. Such changes may result in "day/night confusion"—long sleep periods during the day and long wakeful periods at night. This is bothersome, but it is only a problem of timing. The young infant still does not have any difficulty falling asleep or staying asleep. After several weeks of age, though, parents can begin to shape natural sleep rhythms and patterns into sleep habits.

It comes as a surprise to many parents that healthy sleep habits do *not* develop automatically. In fact, parents can and do help or hinder the development of healthy sleep habits. Of course, children will spontaneously fall asleep when totally exhausted—"crashing" is a biological necessity! But this is unhealthy, because extreme fatigue (often identified by "wired" behavior immediately preceding the crash) interferes with normal social interactions and even learning. You should not assume that it is natural for all children to get peevish, irritable, or cranky at the end of the day. Well-rested children do not behave this way.

Nature or Nurture

What do we mean when we say that a certain item is natural? For example, breast milk is natural and infant formula is not. So when thinking about rearing children, it might be useful to separately consider items based on biology—that is, your child's *nature*—and, in contrast, the variety of ways parents *nurture* children based on the customs of their society. Obviously, it would be false to assume that everything that is natural is healthy; think of naturally occurring poisonous plants. It would equally be false to assume that there is only one healthy way to nurture your child. Parenting customs change over time, and at any given time there are differences in parenting practices among societies and even within them.

For some parents, there is a temptation to judge some preindustrial parenting practices as more natural and therefore best for babies. But parenting practices performed in traditional cultures are not necessarily more biologically based or more natural simply because they have the weight of tradition behind them. For example, breastfeeding frequently day and night and sleeping with your baby, wearing your baby in a sling or soft carrier, always being close to your baby, and always responding to your baby may be common in some traditional societies, but there is no scientific evidence that they are superior to other, more modern parenting practices. In addition, modern science has shown that some traditions are potentially harmful: The increased risk of SIDS associated with bed sharing is a prime example. Further, traditional practices may not be practical for today's families.

Some parents may uncritically accept currently popular beliefs about child-rearing. Once, mistakenly, it was widely believed that fatter babies were healthier babies. At that time, the danger of obesity was not recognized. Today the harm from late bedtimes is not widely appreciated. Before the days of electricity, radio, television, computers, smartphones, or commuting long distances to work, some children went to sleep earlier than children do today. Our current popular late bedtimes are no more natural than the outdated and false natural belief that fatter babies are healthier babies.

Focusing on what is natural and on the challenges to nurture our children may clarify some of the goals and difficulties of child-rearing:

Universal Natural Factors

All babies have spells of fussing and crying.

These spells distress all parents.

All parents want to soothe their baby.

The more the baby fusses or cries, the less he sleeps.

The less he sleeps, the less the parents sleep.

The less the parents sleep, the harder it is for them to soothe their baby.

Relatives and friends want to help soothe the baby and are expected to assist parents.

Breastfeeding, rocking, and holding your baby closely are powerful ways to soothe him.

Challenges to Nurturing Babies

Urban stimulation (noises, voices, delivery trucks, shopping trips, errands) may interfere with the baby's sleeping.

Daycare (not being able to put your child to sleep when he is just starting to become tired, or too much stimulation) may interfere with the baby's sleeping.

Social isolation (forcing only the mother to be wholly responsible for the baby's soothing and sleeping) may cause intense stress for the mother.

Busy modern lifestyles mean that parents have many things to do and little time to do them; sometimes they have to take their baby with them even at sleep times.

Fathers or mothers who have a long commute and return home from work late want to play with their baby, and so they keep their baby up too late at night.

Digital and social media distraction interferes with healthy sleep routines.

Dr. Christian Guilleminault, who along with Dr. William C. Dement was the founding editor of the world's leading journal of sleep research, taught me, when I was in medical school, to consider five fundamental principles of understanding sleep:

1. The sleeping brain is not a resting brain.
2. The sleeping brain functions in a different manner from the waking brain.
3. The activity and work of the sleeping brain are purposeful.
4. The process of falling asleep is learned.
5. Providing the growing brain with sufficient sleep is necessary for developing the ability to concentrate and fostering an easier temperament.

Function of Sleep

Why do we need to sleep? Recent research by Dr. Giulio Tononi tells us that the purpose of sleep is to weaken or prune the unimportant noise coming into our brain so that important signals remain stronger. Think of pruning a tree: You selectively remove targeted branches to promote healthy growth. Nature also removes dead-wood. Here's an example of what pruning might look like in our brain. You are practicing a musical instrument and you hit the wrong note. The wrong note does not fit well with previous, older memories of hitting the right note, and sleep erases the memory of hitting the wrong note, leaving behind a stronger memory of hitting the right notes. During sleep the brain is refreshed by eliminating memories of insignificant events, but memories of more important or salient items will be preserved. A 2019 study, led by Professor Shuntaro Izawa, supports this idea that during sleep, pruning or active forgetting is vital for "helping the brain forget new information that is not important." This culling of information allows more memory resources to be available to us the next day. Izawa's research shows that only *during REM sleep*, certain nerve cells started firing the electrical signals necessary to effectively remove unimportant memories. In adults, experimental sleep restriction primarily leads to *deficits in REM sleep*, so maybe the brain gets cluttered with unimportant memories, making it hard for us to focus on the present.

This theory, in Dr. Tononi's words, "predicts that sleep is especially important in childhood and adolescence, times of concentrated learning. . . . In youth, [connections between nerve cells] are formed, strengthened, and pruned at an explosive rate never approached in adulthood. . . . One can only wonder what happens when sleep is disrupted or insufficient during critical periods in development. Might the deficit corrupt the proper refinement of neural circuits? In that case, the effect of sleep loss would not merely be occasional forgetfulness or misjudgment but a *lasting* change in the way the brain is wired [emphasis added]." Support for this idea comes from animal studies. "Consequences of [extremely stressful] early-life events . . . leave *permanent* changes in the brain. . . . This molecular *'scar'* may act as a predisposing factor in development of psychopathologies later in life. Sleep, *particularly REM sleep,* appears to be the most sensitive behavioral indicator of the early-life events in adulthood [emphasis added]." Sleep *quality,* not just sleep *duration,* is important. Indeed, some studies show that a *late* bedtime is harmful even when the *duration of night sleep* is normal because the child slept in longer and/or the *duration of total sleep* is normal because of longer naps.

LOCAL SLEEP

The targeted removal of irrelevant, redundant, or not useful memories explains a curious observation called *local sleep.* That is, a part of the brain may be asleep while other parts are awake. The more a portion of the brain is used in a task, the more likely it is that this particular area might need to shut down to take a break and do some pruning. So local groups of nerve cells in a tiny area might go offline—that is, go to sleep for a very short nap! This occurs when you *think* you are fully awake. Local sleep is a by-product of a local increase in learning. Local sleep occurs in adults and is more likely when we are short on sleep.

Dr. Tononi wrote, "One wonders how many errors of judgment, silly mistakes, irritable responses, and foul moods result from local sleep in the brains of exhausted people who believe they are fully awake and in complete control."

Perhaps local sleep occurs more commonly during childhood and adolescence, when learning is especially intense. Also, it is common for adults to be subjectively blind to their sleep deficits, so the attribution of errors of judgment, mistakes, irritability, or foul mood due to lack of sleep is unlikely.

Local sleep might explain why we sometimes feel uncomfortable or confused upon waking from a nap (*sleep inertia*). It might also contribute to *disorders of arousal (DOA)*—sleepwalking, sleep terrors, and confusional arousals. In both situations, there are aspects of sleep and wakefulness occurring at the same time. Dr. Anna Castelnovo wrote, "Human sleep is considered to be a global process orchestrated by central specialized neuronal networks that modulate whole-brain activity; however, some studies point to local regulation of sleep, whereby features of sleep and wakefulness can exist simultaneously in different cerebral regions, especially during DOA manifestations . . . sleep and wakefulness are not mutually exclusive, that sleep is not necessarily a global brain phenomenon and that dissociated (wake-like and sleep-like) [states] coexist with the sleeping brain . . . [these dissociative states during sleep] allows birds and dolphins to continue flying or swimming during sleep [implying] an adaptive role for this phenomenon. In humans [dissociative states] might have been selected during evolution because it enables a prompt motor response in life-threatening situations." Heightened vigilance during sleeping might be thought of as sleeping with one eye closed and the other eye open to make sure there are no lions nearby. In support of this view of brain-region-specific responses are sleep deprivation and sleep extension studies performed by Dr. Jelena Skorucak. She discovered that within the brain, there were "topographical differences in the response to sleep restriction and extension."

When you are short on sleep, the frontal brain regions are more protected from sleep loss—which makes sense since this is the region where more complex decision-making tasks are made, such as determining, when our ancestors were both hungry and sleepy, whether the rustling in the bush was prey or predator. A remarkable paper by Dr. Nicolas von Ellenrieder in 2020 added more insight, because he recorded not from the surface of the skull, but rather deep within the brain itself. Removing a portion of the scalp and recording intracranial EEGs, he documented the coexistence within the brain of wakefulness and sleep and regional variability of sleep.

Importantly, at the same time, different areas of the brain are not just asleep or awake like a light switch being on or off; instead, the electrical activity reflecting sleepiness is a graded or continuous variable, like a dimmer switch. So in addition to regional variation anatomically, for any specific region of the brain, variable electrical activity exists at different times during the sleep/wake cycle on a continuum between sleepiness and wakefulness.

OPTIMAL WAKEFULNESS

The point where you are not drowsy from insufficient sleep and you are not up so long that local sleep takes place may be described as *optimal wakefulness*, also called optimal alertness. As you will discover in reading this book, when children learn to sleep well, they also learn to maintain optimal wakefulness. The notion is important because we tend to think about the states of sleep and waking in polarized terms, as if people are either one or the other. But just as our twenty-four-hour cycle consists of more than the two states called day and night—dawn and dusk, for instance—so, too, are there gradations in sleep and wakefulness.

In sleep, the levels vary from deep sleep to partial arousals; in wakefulness, the levels vary from being wide awake to being groggy.

The importance of optimal wakefulness cannot be overemphasized. If your child does not get all the sleep he needs, he may seem either drowsy or hyperalert. If either state lasts for a long time, the results will be the same: a child with a difficult mood and hard-to-control behavior, unable to enjoy himself or get the most out of the myriad learning experiences placed before him.

Sleep is the power source that keeps your mind alert and calm. Every night and at every nap, sleep recharges the brain's battery. Sleeping well increases brainpower just as lifting weights builds stronger muscles, because sleeping well increases your attention span and allows you to be physically relaxed and mentally alert at the same time. Then you are at your personal best.

Personal Best

An athlete's best time in a particular event is called his personal best. Child development is not an athletic contest, and parenting is not a competitive sport, but all parents want to raise their children to achieve their own unique personal best.

At any age, different children will need different amounts of sleep to achieve their personal best. All children are born with different temperaments, skills, and endowments; ask any mother of fraternal twins! These individual differences are part of the joys and challenges of parenting. As previously discussed, there are also individual differences in nap duration, so that at 6 months of age some children take long naps and others take short naps, and these patterns are stable over time until about 2 years of age.

At any age, the effects of being a little short on sleep will affect different children differently. Adult research has shown there are individual differences in how resilient we are to performing on not enough sleep. A study by Dr. John Groeger found that "sleep deprivation-induced performance deterioration is more marked in some individuals than in others. These inter-individual differences in response to sleep deprivation have trait-like characteristics consistent with a genetic basis." We should assume that some children pay a higher price than others when they are short on sleep.

So in families or cultures where babies and children are allowed to sleep out of sync with biological circadian sleep rhythms (unhealthy sleep), I'm sure that this harms some children more than others. But I cannot imagine that unhealthy sleep, if chronic and severe, is good for *any* child. Sleep deprivation is never good for children. You can't fight circadian rhythms!

Without healthy sleep, all the resources of parents, family, and culture will not be sufficient to allow every baby and every child to be at his own personal best. Sweet, bright, and caring children who are receiving unhealthy sleep will become even sweeter, brighter, and more caring when they get healthier sleep. My research shows that sleep modulates temperament, so sleeping better makes children more adaptable, cooperative, and calmer.

With our busy lifestyles, how can we keep track of nap schedules and regular bedtime hours? Is it really true that I can harm my baby by giving him love at night when he cries out for me? How can I be sure that sleep is really that important? Am I a bad parent if my child cries? If he cries at night, isn't he feeling insecure? Many frustrated parents ask me these questions. They often mention that articles, books, or internet posts they have read advocate conflicting ideas, and so they conclude by throwing up their hands and saying that since the whole issue is "controversial," they might as well let matters stay as they are. But if your child is not sleeping well, how long would you be willing to wait for improvement to occur? Three months? Three years? If you are following the opinion of a professional who says you must spend more time with your child at night to make him feel more secure, and yet the results seem to be rather the opposite, ask that professional, "When will I know we are on the right track?" Don't wait forever! Consider what Dr. Charles E. Sundell, the physician in charge of the Children's Department in the Prince of Wales General Hospital in England, wrote in 1922: "Success in the treatment of sleeplessness in infants is a good standard by which to estimate the patience and skill of the practitioner." He also wrote: "A sleepless baby is a reproach to his guardians, and convicts them of some failure in their guardianship." Is this outmoded advice? Absolutely not. Sometimes scientific progress forces us to reevaluate the wisdom of the past. Other times, it reinforces it.

The truth is, modern research regarding sleep/wake states only confirms what careful practitioners such as Dr. Sundell observed about one hundred years ago. He wrote:

> The temptation to *postpone the time for a baby's sleep,*
> so that he may be admired by some relative or friend
> who is late in arriving, or so that his nurse may finish
> some work on which she may be engaged, must be

strongly resisted. A sleepy child who is *kept awake* exhausts his nervous energy very quickly in *peevish restlessness,* and when preparations are at last made for his sleep *he may be too weary to settle down.* . . .

Regularity of habits is one of the sheet-anchors by which the barque of an infant's health is secured. The reestablishment of a regular routine, after even a short break, frequently calls for *patient perseverance* on the part of the nurse, but though the *child may protest vigorously* for several nights, *absolute firmness seldom fails to procure the desired result.* . . . Our aim should be merely to re-establish the normal *habit* of sleep in the child [emphasis added].

So we see that healthy sleep habits were recognized all the way back in 1922! Each baby is unique. They're like little snowflakes. Babies are born with individual traits that affect the amount of physical activity, the duration of sleep, and the length of periods of crying they will sustain. But babies also differ in more subtle ways. Some are easier to "read"; they seem to have predictable schedules for feeding and sleeping. These more "regular" babies also tend to cry less and sleep more. They are more self-soothing; they fall asleep easier, and when they wake at night they are more able to return to sleep unassisted. But don't blame yourself if you have an "irregular" baby who cries a lot and is less self-soothing. It's only luck, although social customs may affect how you feel about it.

In societies where the mother holds the baby close all the time and her breasts are always available for nursing and soothing, there are still great differences among babies in terms of fussiness and crying. The mother compensates by increasing the amount of rhythmic, rocking motions or nursing. She may not even expect the baby to sleep alone, away from her body. As he grows up, a child might share the bed with his parents for a long time. So not only do babies sleep differently, but each society's expectations condition parents' feelings in different ways. Remember, there are no universally right or wrong ways, or natural versus unnatural styles, of raising children. Less developed societies are not necessarily more natural and thus healthier in their child-rearing practices. After all, strychnine and cow's milk are equally natural, but they have altogether different effects when ingested.

How much we are bothered by infant crying or poor sleep habits might partially reflect our own expectations about how to be "good" parents. Do we want to carry the baby all the time, twenty-four hours a day, or do we want to put the baby down sometimes to sleep while we carry on with our own responsibilities?

Here's a true story. A Saudi Arabian princess came to my office for a consultation, accompanied by her English-trained Saudi pediatrician, her English-trained Saudi nanny, and two other women, to discuss sleeping habits for the royal family's children. I listened in amazement as the pediatrician described the family's child care arrangements: They were identical to those popular among British aristocrats of the nineteenth century! Like trained baby nurses serving aristocratic families in Victorian England, the Saudi Arabian nanny was expected to hold the princess's baby while the child was asleep, in effect acting as a living cradle. The reason the nanny could do it was that she had servants of her own! These subordinate nannies, not as well trained, were assigned the menial domestic chores associated with child-rearing.

But the majority of parents do not have multiple nannies. They have to rely on their own skills. So if we are greatly bothered by our baby's crying or our guilt about not being good parents, this may interfere with our developing a sense of competence. We may feel that we cannot influence sleep patterns in our child. Unfortunately, this way of thinking can set the stage for future sleep disorders.

Sleep problems not only disrupt a child's nights, they disrupt his *days,* too, by making him less mentally alert, more inattentive, unable to concentrate, and easily distracted. They also make him more physically impulsive, hyperactive, or logy. But when children sleep well, they are optimally awake and alert, able to learn and grow up with charm and humor. When parents are too irregular, inconsistent, or oversolicitous, or when there are unresolved problems between the parents, the resulting sleep problems converge, producing excessive nighttime wakefulness and crying.

A common misconception among parents is that since children pass through different "stages" at different ages, each of these stages must inevitably create its own sleep problems. In fact, after 3–4 months of age, all children can begin to learn to sleep well. The learning process will occur as naturally as learning how to walk.

The bad news is that some *parents* create sleep problems. The good news is that parents can prevent sleep problems as well as correct any that develop.

Sleep Is Brain Food: Healthy Sleep Is Like Healthy Food

Food and sleep are similar. You would not starve your child by withholding food; try to not let him get short on sleep.

Think about food and food quality. Food is a biological need. Food is energy for the body. Poor-quality food or junk food damages the body by causing medical issues such as malnutrition, anemia, diabetes, heart disease, and obesity. A little junk food is okay. A lot is not. Fortunately, we can read the labels on our food in order to satisfy ourselves that we are eating healthily.

Now think about sleep and sleep quality. Sleep is also a biological need. Sleep is energy for the brain; poor-quality sleep harms the brain. Poor-quality sleep is junk sleep. Junk sleep is just as bad for our children as junk food. A little junk sleep is okay. A lot is not. However, unlike food, there are no labels to read with sleep. You have to watch your child, especially at the end of the day or in the early evening, for telltale signs of junk sleep. Junk sleep causes many problems.

Sleep deficiency is a serious medical problem. We should not be surprised that sleep deficiency is dangerous, because we know that iron deficiency in babies can cause permanent harm. Specifically, iron-deficient babies become adolescents with poorer cognitive functioning and then become adults with poorer emotional health, more negative emotions, and feelings of isolation. Sleep, like iron, is a biological necessity. Both are important for brain development.

Please do not worry if now and then your child gets a little short on sleep but is well rested most of the time. But I would worry if sleep problems are persistent and severe. In the extreme, long-term sleep deprivation in laboratory animals has been shown to permanently damage the brain and even cause death. Short-term sleep deprivation for airplane pilots, doctors in training, and truck drivers is so dangerous that sleep requirements for these occupations are highly regulated. And it's not just how much they sleep; it's also *when* they must sleep. For example, truck drivers opposed new sleep restrictions that were based on the body's natural tendency to sleep at night. The new regulations emphasized that while the duration of sleep was important, it was also important that some of the sleep take place in the evening hours. In 2013, they sued the government. But the United States Court of Appeals upheld the new federal sleep requirements that were based on solid scientific research. However, in 2014, for *commercial* reasons, the trucking industry successfully blocked some of the key regulations, and in 2020 the rules were further relaxed by the Federal Motor Carrier Safety Administration to extend driving from twelve to fourteen hours a day. This illustrates the practical difficulties that often accompany attempts to modify cultural or commercial behaviors based on scientific data. But that does not invalidate the data. And the data are clear that long-term and short-term sleep deprivation is at least as harmful to children as it is to truck drivers!

Here is a summary of some benefits of healthy sleep and problems associated with unhealthy sleep that cross over all ages. Although many studies focus on sleep *duration,* and the harm from short sleep duration, when short sleep duration is present it's usually because the *bedtime* is too late. So any observed adverse outcome might be due to short sleep duration or a late bedtime or both. Please note that all of these items are based on peer-reviewed published research and are not merely my opinion.

SOCIAL AND EMOTIONAL DEVELOPMENT

Because the contribution of sleep to your child's social and emotional development is powerful, but little appreciated by parents and professionals, I wish to share with you several studies that illustrate how sleep, especially a little extra sleep, helps your child. *Think of healthy sleep in your infant or young child as a buffer to prevent later problems or lessen their severity.*

General

Recent studies have given us startlingly clear evidence of how important sleep is for children's cognitive and behavioral functions. Not sleeping well in infancy might cause impaired brain development. Objective measurements of sleep in infants at 12 months of age showed that "lower quality of sleep in infancy significantly predicted compromised attention regulation and behavior problems" when the children were 3–4 years old. However, none of the sleep measures at 3–4 years was associated with the behavior scales at 3–4 years. Reflecting Dr. Tononi's view (page 117), the authors wrote, "our findings suggest that the impact of sleep deficits at critical stages of early brain maturation could potentially lead to long-term consequences." This notion that impaired sleep at an early age might "interfere with vulnerable brain maturational processes that later result in compromised regulatory capacities" is important because it may not be apparent to parents at 12 months that a real problem is silently developing.

Sleeping well appears to enhance brain maturation. In a study by Dr. Salome Kurth, connections between the right and left sides of the brain increased as much as 20 percent over a single night's sleep in a group of children 2–5 years old. Connections strengthened as the children aged. "Sleep is a key environmental contributor to brain optimization processes . . . [and] plays a crucial role in brain maturation," Dr. Kurth concluded. "In critical phases of development [walking, talking, problem solving], the maturation of skills not only require cortical activity during waking but also a subsequent period of sleep . . . There are strong indications that sleep and brain maturation are closely related. . . . I believe inadequate sleep in childhood may affect the maturation of the brain related to the emergence of development or mood disorders."

School-aged children who were taught the benefits of healthy sleep actually slept a little longer, and this extra sleep produced improved schoolwork. In children age 7–11 years, a study by Dr. Reut Gruber showed that teaching children about how and why to sleep better resulted in *eighteen minutes* of extra sleep, and report card grades in mathematics and languages improved. In another study of the same age group, she experimentally added or eliminated one hour of sleep over five nights and showed that fifty-four minutes of sleep restriction resulted in "a low threshold for expression of negative affect (irritability and frustration) and is associated with difficulty in the modulation of impulse and emotion . . . [and] a cumulative extension of sleep duration of *twenty-seven minutes* was associated with a detectable improvement of emotional lability and restless-impulsive behavior . . . and a significant reduction of reported daytime sleepiness. . . . Cumulative *small* additions to sleep duration potentially improve functioning in school [emphasis added]."

Gruber's study inspired another group of researchers, studying 15-year-olds, to gradually *move the bedtime earlier* by five minutes each night over a two-week period. This gradual sleep extension had beneficial effects on self-reported sleep problems (insomnia symptoms) and reduction of depressive symptoms. "Adolescents in the sleep extension group slept on average about *thirteen minutes* longer during the experimental week than during the baseline week." I know it goes against the grain of human nature to believe that such small changes could have such a profound impact, but the data bear it out (page 102).

A 2020 study of children age 7–11 years used objective measurements of sleep and experimentally controlled sleep duration in the laboratory under the conditions of either two nights of being well rested (seven hours in bed) versus sleep-restricted (six hours in bed). "On the whole, children's *positive* emotions appear to take the greatest 'hit' when sleep is inadequate. Two nights of partial sleep restriction adversely impacted subjective, physiological, and expressive responses to positive more so than negative emotional stimuli in prepubertal children [emphasis added]."

In a separate study of children 8–12 years old, experimentally changing the bedtime over four nights to be only *one* hour earlier or *one* hour later showed that the later bedtime caused impaired functioning on measures of *positive* affective response, emotion regulation, memory, and attention. Also, adolescents age 14–17 experimentally slept six and a half hours a night for three nights and demonstrated worsening of mood and decreased ability to regulate *negative* emotions. In adults, the results are marked as well: *One night* of short sleep results in increased impulsivity to *negative* stimuli, increased failure to inhibit a response, and faster incorrect responses.

Perhaps if your child does not seem to take joy in the simple pleasures of life, and/or seems unusually bothered by minor setbacks, he might not be getting healthy sleep.

Sleep continuity that is broken by frequent night wakings, like short sleep durations, is also harmful (page 60). Disrupted or fragmented sleep has been experimentally studied in adults by Dr. Patrick Finan. In one study, there was either restricted sleep or interrupted sleep for three consecutive nights. He observed that "sleep continuity disruption is more detrimental to positive mood than partial sleep loss from delaying bedtime." The same conclusion was reached in a separate adult study involving only *one night* of sleep continuity disruption by forced awakenings. Among 14-month-old infants, the day after a *single laboratory sleepover* during which sleep was interrupted, they demonstrated poorer emotional regulation and showed special difficulty in recovering from negative emotions.

Depression and Anxiety

Unhealthy sleep can also lead to an increase in depression and anxiety in young children that, if not addressed, can continue into adolescence and even adulthood. The research is clear on this.

A study of over two thousand students in high school found "evidence supporting an association between short sleep duration and depression," and a separate 2020 study of over fifteen thousand 15-year-olds showed that short sleep and poor sleep quality were predictive of anxiety and depression diagnoses and symptoms at age 17, 21, and 24 years. I say all this because it is *so* important to address sleep issues in the early years so that they do not continue into adolescence.

Internalizing and Externalizing Behaviors

When your child is not sleeping well, internalizing problems, externalizing problems, or both may develop.

From 12 to 36 months, children with more fragmented sleep displayed higher levels of the stress hormone cortisol. This was associated with teachers' ratings of more negative emotionality and *internalizing* (internalizing behaviors are directed inward such as social withdrawal and appearing or feeling sad, lonely, nervous, or fearful). In a study of about thirty-three thousand children, it was observed that sleep duration of ten hours or less and night wakings occurring three or more times each night at 18 months were associated with emotional and behavioral problems at 5 years. Those with mainly night wakings primarily had *internalizing* problems; those with mainly short sleep durations had both *internalizing* and *externalizing* problems. (Externalizing behaviors are directed against others or things and might manifest in such ways as overactivity, anger, aggression, impulsivity, tantrums, and annoying behavior.) Although these two studies suggest a link between fragmented sleep and internalizing problems, in contrast, a study by Professor Jodi Mindell that examined children initially between 3 and 18 months old and followed them until they were between 18 and 36 months found that *internalizing* problems were not associated with fragmented sleep but rather with later bedtimes and less total sleep duration. She wrote, "These findings are in contrast to a common perception that a child who is 'overtired' is overactive and noncompliant. Rather, these findings suggest that an 'overtired' toddler is more likely to be socially withdrawn and anxious." Another study showed that children exhibited *externalizing* behaviors when night sleep was short even though these children had longer naps, so their total sleep over a period of twenty-four hours was the same as for children without these problems. In other words, total sleep duration does not tell the whole story.

Helping children deal with these issues is a complex and highly individualized process, but helping them sleep better from the get-go with an *early bedtime* is a simple strategy that will pay big dividends in the future. Remember, Dr. Gruber's study (page 128) showed that sleep extension created improved emotional regulation! Small amounts of extra nightly sleep over time may really make a big difference (page 102).

Symptoms of Psychiatric Disorders

Children's unhealthy sleep patterns also forecast psychiatric symptoms described as either *emotional* (separation anxiety, generalized anxiety disorder, social phobia, specific phobia, major depressive disorder, and chronically mild depressed or irritable mood) or *behavioral* (ADHD, oppositional defiant disorder, and conduct disorder). Objective measurements of sleep durations and clinical interviews were performed at 6, 8, 10, and 12 years. "Clinical interviews allow probing for additional information concerning the intensity, duration, and onset of psychiatric symptoms to ascertain its actual presence." The results showed that at age 6 and 8 years, shorter sleep durations—as little as *thirty minutes* less—"forecasted symptoms of emotional disorders 2 years later."

A 2020 study of over seven thousand children observed that there was a strong association between shorter night sleep at 3.5 years and the development of symptoms of bipolar disorder at age 11 years. The difference in night sleep duration between those 3.5-year-olds who did and who did not develop bipolar symptoms at age 11 years was very small—*about seven minutes*!

These studies are remarkable because they show how losing just even a small amount of sleep can have a cumulative effect on the development of children.

Empathy

Emotional empathy is significantly lower in participants who are (experimentally) sleep-deprived. In young adults 18–25 years, experimental sleep deprivation in an affective face-recognition task clearly showed that sleep deprivation impairs the accurate judgment of human facial emotions.

Mood in Teenagers

Some things make you happy and some things make you sad. It appears that longer sleep and better-quality sleep *independently* improve mood. Positive affect and negative affect have been studied separately in teenagers in the context of how they sleep.

A group of adolescents about 15 years old were divided into a sleep-restricted group and a control group for *one* night. They were then shown color pictures from a standardized database that is used to measure emotion. Their responses to the pictures were sorted into either positive affect (joy, contentment, interest, engagement, or pride) or negative affect (anger, fear, anxiety, sadness, or depression). The sleep-restricted teens appeared to have "an impaired ability to experience pleasure from activities normally considered to be enjoyable." Have you ever felt that you were on autopilot and going through the motions in a dull, robotic, or mechanical way at a party when you were really short on sleep? Or not really feeling the joy at what should have been a pleasurable event because you were sleepy? In contrast, when coming back fully charged from a vacation, have you felt more engaged in and enjoyed more routine activities?

Another study of about 13-year-olds also divided them into a sleep-restricted group and a control group for *two* nights in a laboratory where their sleep was objectively recorded. Acoustic emotional stimuli were used in conjunction with measurements of pupil dilation. This study "demonstrated increased negative affect following sleep restriction, relative to extension, on self-report and pupil measures." Have you ever felt unusually sensitive or annoyed when short on sleep, such that little things bothered you a lot, the way a light touch on sunburned skin really hurts?

Both of these studies found the same result: Sleep restriction or short sleep duration decreases *positive* affect and increases *negative* affect.

MEDICAL HEALTH

Not only does a lack of sleep effect your baby emotionally, behaviorally, and cognitively—it can also affect his physical development. Growth hormone is released mostly during sleep, especially *early in the evening* during the first period of deep sleep. In one study, short sleep duration (less than twelve hours) at age 3 months was associated with short body length during the first two years. Among 17-year-olds, those with less sleep and later bedtimes were about one inch shorter. In 6-month-old infants, night sleep and physical growth were found to be related: The longer the objective night sleep duration, the lower the child's weight-to-length ratio. That is, the infants tended to be lighter or longer or both. No association between physical growth and parent-reported daytime sleep was observed. This study and another study on 6-month-old infants highlight the importance of *nighttime* sleep. In the second study, objective measurements of sleep over twenty-four hours showed that 6-month-old infants with less nighttime sleep took more naps and longer naps, but the sum of the naps did *not* compensate for the short nighttime sleep, so the total amount of sleep was less. Also, in this study, a longer night sleep duration was associated with a lower weight-to-length ratio. So if you want a tall and slim child, focus on night sleep (especially an *early bedtime*) and don't think that extra napping will compensate for short night sleep!

Short sleep duration in adolescents is associated with higher blood pressure, higher cholesterol, and higher insulin resistance (a risk factor for developing diabetes). Increased susceptibility to infection, increased stress hormone, and systemic inflammation also result from not sleeping well. Separately from short sleep duration, habitual loud snoring is associated with hyperactivity, depression, and inattention. Additionally, habitual snoring has been shown to be a factor in fragmented sleep. In another study of 17-year-olds, those with less sleep and later bedtimes were about one inch shorter. It is possible that earlier bedtimes and longer sleep durations are associated with a greater release of growth hormone, resulting in a taller child! Maybe an athletically inclined parent who wants a tall child will be motivated by this observation (also, see how sleep enhances athletic performance on page 136) to put forth more effort to promote early bedtimes.

One spurious link between lack of sleep and the physical health of your young child is the notion that growth spurts disrupt sleep. I consider this notion to be another handy excuse that parents use to explain why their child is not sleeping well. I say this because I don't want you to hide behind excuses; there will always be one handy! Some families use *extreme fussiness/colic* (birth–6 months), *teething* (6–12 months), *separation anxiety* (12–24 months), *"terrible twos"* (24–36 months), *fears* (36–48 months), and *acquiring a new motor skill* or imaginary *"sleep regressions"* (parenting.nytimes.com/sleep/sleep-regressions), one after another, to "explain" why their child wakes up at night and has trouble returning to sleep by himself.

OBESITY OR OVERWEIGHT

The percentage of children between 12 and 19 years old who were obese increased from 5 percent in 1980 to almost 21 percent in 2012. There is an epidemic of obesity and a famine for sleep these days, and it would appear that the two are not entirely unrelated! Most research papers describe short sleep duration as a risk factor for obesity or overweight (page 721). This is a major public health problem, because obesity may increase the risk for developing diabetes, heart disease, and stroke.

In a study led by Dr. Karr of over a thousand 6-year-old children, researchers tried to tease apart the contributions of diet (high or low fruit and vegetable, fast-food consumption, high consumption of sugar-sweetened beverages), physical activity, screen time, and short sleep duration. They observed that "sleep may be an important mechanism linking health behaviors to obesity" either directly or indirectly. In fact, in a small experimental study in which children age 3–4 years were denied a nap and had a delayed bedtime, sleep was objectively measured to be about three hours less, and the next day they consumed 21 percent more calories compared with baseline. Another study showed that short nighttime sleep under age 5 years predicts obesity by age 5–9 years. Also, among older children, in a study of over four thousand children 9–10 years old, blood samples showed higher risk markers for Type 2 diabetes and higher body fat mass to be associated with shorter sleep durations.

Dr. Racheal Taylor led a study to prevent obesity by advising the mother, both before delivery and when the infant was 3 weeks old, to develop appropriate sleep habits from birth. Emphasis was on recognizing tired signs, then putting the child down to sleep while awake without feeding in a quiet darkened room. At 6 months, about 27 percent indicated that their child's sleep was a problem, and these mothers then received personalized advice regarding graduated extinction to help their child sleep better. At age two years, there was less obesity in this group compared with control groups, and the "beneficial effect of sleep on weight status remained apparent at age five years."

Naps have no effect on the development of obesity, and long naps with short night sleep do not prevent obesity. But naps are beneficial in other ways. Naps reduce cortisol levels in infants. Naps in preschool children boost memory. In adults, naps enhance creative problem solving.

TEMPERAMENT

Temperament means behavioral style. Your child's temperament may be modulated by sleep in the same manner that adjusting the volume, bass, or treble controls makes a piece of music sound different—the basic musical composition has not changed, but the listening experience has. One study of infants at 3, 6, and 11 months of age showed that increased night sleep is associated with increased likelihood of approaching new and strange people and things. But fragmented sleep between 6 and 36 months of age is associated with a more difficult temperament.

Another study of infants at 4–10 weeks old observed that longer naps, but not night sleep duration, are associated with a more positive temperament (less active, more approaching, milder, and less distractible). You can ask yourself, what is the magical power of a nap that turns a raving, manic, out-of-control 2.5-year-old into a sweet Prince Charming?

ATHLETIC PERFORMANCE

College basketball players showed enhanced performance with a faster-timed sprint, better free throw percentage, and enhanced three-point field goal percentage with experimental sleep extension.

The opposite, experimental sleep restriction, impairs serving accuracy in tennis players and kicking skills in soccer players. In general, longer sleep durations improve athletic performance regarding reaction times, accuracy, and endurance.

COGNITIVE PERFORMANCE

Do sleep patterns really affect learning in children? Yes! Different studies of children at different ages all agree on this central point. As one study put it, "Sleep is universal, strictly regulated, and necessary for cognition. . . . Sleep consolidates memories, whereas sleep deprivation interferes with memory acquisition." Another study put it more succinctly: "Sleep is important for memory consolidation." Focusing on perfectly normal, healthy children, let's consider the data by age groups: infants, preschoolers, and school-aged children.

Infants and Naps

A study at the University of Connecticut showed that there was a strong association between the amount of time infants were in REM sleep and the amount of time they spent when awake in the behavioral state called quiet alertness. In the *quiet alert state,* babies have open, bright eyes, they appear alert, their eyes are scanning, their faces are relaxed, and they do not smile or frown. Their bodies are relatively quiet and inactive. One mother described her 4-month-old, who was frequently in this quiet alert state, as "a looker and a thinker." She's right! These infants don't miss a thing. Another study showed that naps with REM sleep enhance "the integration of unassociated information for creative problem solving." A separate study of sleep development at Stanford University showed that environmental factors, not simply brain maturation, are responsible for the proportion of time infants spend in REM sleep. Unfortunately, the exact environmental factors were not identified, but presumably parental handling could influence all of these items: sleep patterns, the proportion of REM sleep, and the amount of time the child is in the quiet alert state. *REM sleep* is especially important for learning. Also, as mentioned in chapter 2, naps longer than thirty minutes enhance the consolidation of memory among infants at 6 and 12 months.

Infants who are notoriously *not* quiet alert are those with *colic* or a difficult *temperament*. Their fussy behavior may be due to imbalances of internal chemicals such as progesterone or even cortisol. High cortisol concentrations in infants have been shown to be associated with decreased duration of non-REM sleep. So even in infants, as in adults, there seem to be connections between internal chemicals, sleep patterns, and behavior when awake. Also, these fussy children tend to have irregular schedules and short attention spans. Among 2- to 3-month-old infants, one study showed that the more irregular and less persistent the child was, the slower the rates of learning and the more difficulty in learning to fall asleep unassisted. Thus they easily could become sleep-deprived, fatigued, and hyperactive older children.

Two studies published in 2019 examined infant sleep and learning. The first by Dr. Tham divided 6-month-olds into habitual short sleepers (less than ten hours per day) and typical sleepers (ten to eighteen hours per day). Habitual short sleepers displayed impaired memory in a laboratory setting. The second, by Dr. Huhdanpaa, recruited pregnant women and followed their children from birth: "Our main findings suggest that [short] sleep duration at the age of 3, 8, and 24 months was associated with inattentiveness in 5-year-old children. Night awakenings (more than once per night) were associated with inattentiveness and hyperactivity-impulsivity at the age of 5 years." This study was based on the mothers' reports, and it's true that these types of studies can be criticized on the basis that the connection between sleep and inattentiveness might only reflect features within the mother (this is called common method variance).

However, objectively measuring infant night waking using a motion sensor worn by the child (actigraph) shows that after falling asleep infants, like adults, spend time quietly awake later during the night. The measurement of wake after sleep onset (WASO, page 91) is high when the infant is in bed at night but not sleeping. A group of infants were studied at 4, 6, 8, and 10 months with actigraphs and an eye-tracking memory test. The more time children spent awake in the night, the poorer they did on the memory task. Surprisingly, the duration of day sleep, night sleep, and how often the infant woke at night was not related to performance on the memory track. So less WASO might be more beneficial than long sleep duration. Another study, by Dr. Taveras, also recruited pregnant women and followed their children at 6 months, and yearly from 1 to 7 years. She observed that "Insufficient sleep in the preschool and early school years is associated with poorer mother- and teacher-reported neurobehavioral processes [executive function, behavior, and social-emotional functioning] in mid childhood."

Taken together, these studies, starting at 3, 4, and 6 months of age, highlight the importance of helping very young children sleep well—when healthy sleep habits persist, the benefits increase over time. On the other hand, it is possible that when children do not sleep well, the impaired sleep has adverse effects on the developing brain that persist. For example, in a study by Professor Sadeh, lower-quality objective sleep measurements on children at 12 months of age predicted compromised attention regulation and behavior problems at 3–4 years old, even though there was no significant contemporary association between sleep and attention regulation and behaviors at the age of 3–4 years. So if your 12-month-old is not sleeping well but is functioning well, it is possible that attention and behavioral problems will emerge a few years later. Professor Sadeh raised the tentative possibility that "it could be argued that sleep disruptions at an early age interfere with vulnerable brain maturational processes that later result in compromised regulatory capacities . . . [and] our findings suggest that the impact of sleep deficits at critical stages of early brain maturation could potentially lead to *long-term consequences* [emphasis added]."

While there may be some truth in this hypothesis, he does point out that "sleep patterns are still quite malleable during early childhood," and I would encourage parents to remember that it is never too late to help your child sleep better.

I think naps are especially important for infants. In my own studies, I've found that how long the infant sleeps during the day is strongly associated with persistence or attention span. Infants who take long naps have longer attention spans. They spend more time in the quiet alert state and seem to learn faster. Infants who do not nap well are either drowsy or fitfully fussy, and in either case they do not learn well.

Naps promote optimal alertness for children. Children who nap well spend more time in the quiet alert state when awake.

It is a myth that long naps interfere with acquiring socialization skills or infant stimulation. While it's true that "rack monsters" are less available for all the classes or activities that abound today—swim gym, mom-and-tot and pop-and-tot groups, or infant-stimulation groups—is that so bad? Do infants suffer because they don't participate in so many activities? Are they less likely to get into the right preschool, which feeds to the right nursery school, which feeds to the right private school? No.

Please do not confuse the quantity of time spent in these organized activities with the high-quality social awareness that well-rested children exhibit. The truth is that these infant-stimulation groups are often not important for infants but instead serve legitimate parental needs by allowing mothers and fathers to meet other parents and escape from their isolation at home.

Frequent Naps Longer than Thirty Minutes Enhance Learning

Preschool Children

My research has shown that when infants who are easy at 5 months of age develop into crabbier, more difficult 3-year-olds, it is because they have developed a pattern of brief sleep. In contrast, difficult infants who mellow into easier 3-year-olds have developed a pattern of long sleep. I think that parents' helping or hindering regular sleep patterns caused these shifts to occur. Three-year-old children who nap well are more adaptable. (*Adaptability* refers to the ease with which children adjust to new circumstances.) *Adaptability is the single most important temperament trait for school success.* The briefer the naps, the less adaptable the child. In fact, the major temperament feature of 3-year-olds who do not nap at all is nonadaptability. It is exactly these non-napping, nonadaptable children who also have more night wakings! A 2018 review of all relevant studies on children between 2 and 6 years old concluded that "higher quantity or quality of sleep was associated with better behavioral and/or cognitive outcomes."

Children age 1–3 years with more fragmented sleep had a higher cortisol level upon waking. Four-year-olds who, for at least a month, took more than thirty minutes to fall asleep or had five or more night awakenings (of a duration of at least ten minutes) a week or had difficulty waking up at least three times a week were found to be at an increased risk for psychiatric symptoms at age 6. When short on sleep, learning is impaired, even if your child does not feel or behave as sleepy.

Dr. Dean Bebe proved that the association "between sleep duration and academic performance reflect true cause-effect relationships." He studied 14- to 17-year-olds and compared their academic performance and videotaped behavior in a simulated classroom under the conditions of two sleep manipulations, each lasting five nights (Short Sleep of 6.5 hours versus Healthy Sleep of 9.1 hours, both for five nights). After "five nights of Short Sleep, adolescents showed diminished learning from lecture-format educational videos and also displayed evidence of increased sleepiness and difficulty paying attention while watching the lectures. . . . However, the [decrease] in quiz scores was not mediated by changes in attention or sleepiness." In other words, *sleep deprivation impairs learning whether or not you feel or behave as sleepy or inattentive.* If this is true for adolescents, it is also likely to be true for much younger children and infants, so even if an infant, toddler, or young child does not appear sleepy or inattentive, sleep deprivation still may interfere with learning!

SLEEP PROBLEMS AND BENEFITS PERSIST

Does extremely severe and chronic sleep loss starting early in life, or during critical stages, affect the development of the brain and thus cause permanent biological alterations leading to persisting adverse consequences? Experimental studies in laboratory animals strongly suggest that the answer is yes. How about for our children? Children do *not* suffer from the extreme sleep deprivation researchers employ in the lab. But it is possible that more mild and chronic impaired sleep in our young children does produce more subtle changes in the developing brain. Babies who do not sleep well might have problems later because of this direct effect of impaired sleep on the developing brain when young; or because persisting parenting/family issues causes both the impaired sleep when young and subsequent problems when older; or because genetic factors might cause both impaired sleep when young and subsequent problems when older. Prenatal factors (for example, alcohol or nicotine) during pregnancy might be salient. Also, any combination of these four factors is possible. Nevertheless, whatever the cause(s), a baby or child with impaired sleep might additionally cause sleepiness in parents, leading to challenges for them to figure out how to create and execute a plan to help their child sleep better.

If your child is not sleeping well and you do not see a sleep solution (chapter 5) that will work for you, seek help. Discuss this with your child's primary caregiver.

Sleep problems such as difficulty falling asleep at 6 months of age may persist to age 3 years and beyond. Different sleep problems are most prevalent at different ages. The most common sleep problem, as reported by parents, during the first three years is night wakings. Waking four or more times per week during this time predicted sleep problems continuing to age 6–7 years. Difficulty sleeping alone peaks at age 2–3 years. Difficulty falling asleep is most common at 10–11 years and when it occurs in infancy, it predicts sleep problems at age 8–11 years.

> **Difficulty falling asleep at bedtime, difficulty sleeping alone, and difficulty returning to sleep unassisted during the night might reflect less ability for your child to *self-soothe*.**

One study coded night waking three or more times per week, as reported by the mothers, to indicate frequent night waking and followed families at 3, 6, 9, and 12 months of age. Children who had frequent night waking at each age were considered to have *persistent* (and severe) sleep problems. These children were more likely to have emotional symptoms at age 4 years, as well as to meet diagnostic criteria for an emotional disorder and exhibit symptoms of separation anxiety, fear of physical injury, and overall elevated anxiety at age 10 years.

Another study showed that among children 3–6 years of age, sleep problems *persist* for at least four years, and those children with persisting problems were more likely to have aggressive symptoms, attention and social problems, and anxious or depressed mood.

Although these data suggest that biological maturation of sleep processes is fairly well established by age two years, please do not think that your young child's sleep issues will inevitability lead to future problems. My research suggests that when parents start early to help their child sleep better, there are better outcomes regarding *temperament* even when measured at age three years. And my experience is that it is never too late to help a child sleep better.

Healthy Sleep in Young Children Has Carryover Benefits in Adolescence

Benefits from early healthy sleep habits persist in preteens and teenagers, who continue, pretty much on their own, to get healthy sleep (page 704).

1. Because your older child appreciates how he feels better with healthy sleep, he strives for sleep.

   "[My children] feel the benefits and know the difference between being rested and being tired on their own because of the healthy sleep habits when they were young and strive for it even today."

2. Healthy sleep continues in the older child because the parents have established a foundation for it.

Family Routines

"It is inevitable they will have some late practices or games and the bedtime will get pushed out. What we learned very early on was to stick to a schedule a majority of the time, and when the exceptions happen, the healthy habits are still intact."

Establish Priorities

"There is an absolute carryover effect from the efforts we put forth during the early years to ensure healthy sleep. As parents, we were in 100 percent agreement that our children's sleep was the priority. We adjusted our dining and socializing and never regretted these changes for one minute. We

didn't lose any friends or miss any social opportunities that were important to us because of their napping or early bedtimes. In fact, we believe it helped us learn how to prioritize how, when, and where we spent our time. As a result, we see our children making similar choices on their own."

Family Values

"I do feel that getting the appropriate amount of sleep was instilled in them when they were young and the effects did and do carry through. It is almost as if getting appropriate amounts of sleep became a family value for us. I do not think that the importance of that can be overstated. When our daughters were able to catch up on sleep on the weekends, they always did so and were refreshed and ready to go. They both love their sleep and know how vital it is."

3. Among older children who appreciate feeling better when well rested and who have a family foundation for sleep, there is less resistance and more self-direction regarding sleep.

"I think that the carryover effect has helped somewhat, although I cannot imagine not getting any resistance from a preteen/teen on bedtime. Most of their peers do not sleep much. I do think that I get a lot less resistance because the healthy sleep habits were established when the children were so young and emphasized and maintained throughout their experience."

4. Helping older children sleep may be difficult, but it is not impossible. Early sleep training makes it easier to help older children sleep. Expect to experience resistance from friends and family.

"I observed and appreciated the enormous benefits of healthy sleep habits and a well-rested family from the be-

ginning. It was not always easy to follow the guidelines I had established, because I encountered significant resistance from family and most friends. Their routines and schedules were very different from ours. Our children, when very young, went to bed so early that few could relate to our schedule. I think that our healthy sleep habits helped our children in a myriad of ways: to explore school, to foster creativity, to face frustration, and develop adaptability."

"We have five children ranging in age from 8 to 18 years old. My husband and I were the first in our respective families to have children. Our family members gave us a hard time when we insisted on starting a gathering later or ending it earlier so that our children could take naps at the right time. After our siblings became parents themselves, however, they admitted to us that up until then they thought we were going overboard about protecting our children's nap times."

Healthy Sleep in Children Helps Prevent Maternal Depression

Three separate studies by Dr. Harriet Hiscock showed that healthy sleep in the child helps prevent depression in the mother. One study of 156 mothers of infants age 6–12 months with severe sleep problems used controlled crying (graduated extinction) to help solve the problems. This intervention improved sleep problems in the children and reduced symptoms of depression in the mothers. Unfortunately, the benefits for the child and the mother lasted only about two months.

Another study looked at 738 mothers of infants age 6–12 months, 46 percent of whom reported their infant's sleep as a problem. The researchers described a strong association between the maternal report of infant sleep problems and depression symptoms in the mother. After looking at all the variables that might have contributed to maternal depression and the observation that the better the child slept, the less likely the mother was to be depressed, they concluded that teaching mothers how infants sleep should decrease or help prevent maternal depression.

A third study consisted of 114 mothers enrolled when their infants were 8–10 months old; the mothers were again studied when their children were 3–4 years old. The researchers concluded that infant sleep problems tend to persist or recur in the preschool years and are associated with more child behavior problems and maternal depression. Analysis of their data led to the conclusion that the maternal depressive symptoms were a result, rather than the cause, of the children's sleep problems.

It is uncommon for so many studies to be in agreement! However, this conclusion that children's sleep problems might cause maternal depression has recently been challenged by studies that suggest the direction of effects might be the opposite, or perhaps really going both ways (chapter 6). Also, these three studies focused on infant sleep problems and maternal mood. But in the absence of sleep problems (bedtime resistance or difficulty falling asleep), simply not sleeping through the night at 6 and 12 months of age was shown to be common (chapter 8) and not to be associated with maternal mood. Additionally, in many studies regarding maternal depression and children's sleep, fathers were not included. So it is incorrect to assume that when a mother is depressed and a child is not sleeping well, there is necessarily a direct relation between these two observations. A third factor, such as a father's mental health problem or excessive drinking, might be the root cause (page 238).

Healthy Sleep and Public Awareness

Now that you understand why healthy sleep is so important for your child, I want to explain why many other parents and your relatives may not appreciate these benefits and why they may make it challenging for you to obtain healthy sleep for your child.

IT TAKES A LONG TIME TO APPRECIATE HEALTHY SLEEP BENEFITS

When there is a scientific observation regarding a health benefit from sleep, it may take a long time for the public to become aware of it, and even longer for the information to be acted upon. Here are three examples.

In 1914, a major medical textbook warned of the dangerous symptoms associated with snoring (page 715), and in 1976 *Pediatrics,* the official journal of the American Academy of Pediatrics (AAP), published a careful clinical study documenting the seriousness of the problem (hyperactivity, depression, and inattention). But it took until 2002, twenty-six years later, for the AAP to publish clinical practice guidelines regarding screening for snoring and sleep-related breathing problems. These guidelines were revised in 2012, almost a hundred years after the 1914 report!

In 1985, it was first observed that sudden infant death syndrome was less frequent in children who slept on their backs. The AAP waited until more evidence was available and finally recommended back or side sleeping in 1992; their recommendation for back sleeping alone did not come until 1996, eleven years after the original report. Over a fourteen-year period, from 1992 to 2006, the percentage of children put to sleep on their backs increased from 13 percent to 76 percent. Initial opposition that may have slowed widespread acceptance of this recommendation included an unwarranted fear that the baby might vomit and aspirate the vomit, or develop a flattened skull.

In 1998, it was first observed that a later start time for school for teenagers produced benefits for the children (page 696). But it wasn't until 2014, sixteen years after the original report, that the AAP finally recommended that all middle and high schools start later (at or after 8:30 A.M.). Initial opposition to this recommendation includes the unwarranted fear that teenagers will simply stay up later, that sports practices will be significantly disrupted, and that school bus schedules will be impossible to manage. In 2014, only 10 percent of high schools and 20 percent of middle schools had start times at or after 8:30 A.M. In 2019, California passed a law, to go into effect in 2022, that all high schools and middle schools will start no earlier than 8:30 A.M. and 8:00 A.M. respectively. However, schools may continue to offer optional class periods called "zero periods" that can start earlier. So there is progress, but it is very slow.

Separately, there are two well-documented sleep issues in children for which there are no strong AAP recommendations or acknowledgments by other professional organization. Hence, these issues are not widely recognized or acted upon:

1. In 2003, it was first observed that among children 5 years old and younger, there was a trend toward later bedtimes and less sleep that began between 1974 and 1978. The list of problems associated with chronic sleep loss in adolescents (page 696) led the AAP to recommend a later start time for schools. But there are no strong AAP recommendations regarding bedtimes in preschool or school-aged children. Hence, many parents do not appreciate the harm from chronic sleep loss caused by bedtimes that are too late.

   A little history might help explain why we are blind to this obvious problem. After the 1880s, when electric lights began to become commercially available, nighttime activities took off. Nighttime entertainment, sports, and socializing are so common today that we don't even think about it. But it wasn't always so. I suspect that most adults used to have an earlier bedtime, and I suspect that very young children who were too young to do chores or work by candlelight also went to bed earlier than today. Modern pressures on school-aged children and adults are real, and later bedtimes may be unavoidable, but how about our preschool children?

   It took eleven years to get the message out that back sleeping was good and sixteen years to recommend that school start times for teens should be later. Although seventeen years have passed since the first report regarding the development of later bedtimes in preschoolers, maybe in the future there will develop a more general awareness that late bedtimes and less sleep are harmful.

2. In 1988, it was reported that 10 percent of 3- to 10-year-old children had a TV in the bedroom. In 1999, it was reported that more television viewing was associated with less sleep and more sleep problems; also, 26 percent of 4- to 10-year-old children had a TV in the bedroom. The AAP recommended in 1999 that television should be limited to no more than two hours and no TV under the age of 2 years. But they did not discuss a television in the bedroom. By 2005, 40 percent of 3- to 6-year-olds and 18 percent of children under 2 years of age had a TV in the bedroom. The AAP in 2010 briefly mentioned at the end of a lengthy report that pediatricians should encourage removal of a TV from the bedroom, but the public focus was on the limitation of screen time. The AAP in 2011 again focused on discouraging media use younger than 2 years and barely mentioned placing a television set in the child's room. Studies published in 2013 confirmed that more television viewing was associated with less sleep and later bedtimes. This trend of more school-aged and preschool children having television in the bedroom began thirty-two years ago, and the fact that this is harmful was known twenty-one years ago, but this has not led to a general public awareness campaign that parents should not allow a television in their child's bedroom. The revised AAP recommendations in 2016 highlighted changes in the recommendations for screen time and again barely mentioned TV in the bedroom: "Designate . . . media-free locations at home, such as bedrooms." Having a TV in the child's bedroom is still quite common. For example, a 2019 study of children recruited from preschools showed that 36 percent had a TV in their bedroom. Furthermore, in this group of children who had TVs in

their bedroom, *33 percent* of the mothers had a college degree or higher education level! Hopefully in the future it will become common knowledge that television does not belong in your child's bedroom. In fact, *all* screen-based electronic media used by children at night may cause the bedtime to become later (pages 216 and 323).

CHALLENGES FROM FRIENDS AND RELATIVES

These examples show how long it can take for scientific findings to make their way into general circulation and result in widespread, commonly accepted behavioral changes. So do not be surprised if your friends or relatives do not agree with your practice of early bedtimes or limiting television and all other electronic screen-based media. Similarly, friends and relatives who are unaware of the health benefits from sleep might complain that you care too much about early bedtimes or naps.

Striving toward a balance between attending social events and keeping your child well rested may create tension between parents themselves or between both parents and their relatives and friends. Social events are important, family harmony is important, but a well-rested child is also desirable. So the goal is to include your child's sleep needs in the equation. Many parents in my practice who utilize early bedtimes feel like pioneers in their circle of friends and relatives because their desire to protect an early bedtime and naps may run counter to how other families live. Occasionally they feel a little like outcasts because they refuse to frequently socialize late at night with other parents or relatives with their child. Sometimes not attending late-night events or leaving early may have social costs. Similarly, parents may choose not to participate in playdates as frequently or go to family barbecues on weekends if they interfere with naps. These comments are not intended to suggest that you never allow your child to stay up late or skip naps; rather, look at the big picture of how well rested your child is most of the time and how disruptive a particular social event might be to his sleep schedule.

When in doubt about whether to attend a social event with your child that will cause a late bedtime or a missed nap, I always encourage a family to attend the event. After the event, I recommend they consider a super-early bedtime for one night only, to repay a sleep debt. Then I suggest that the parent observe how well rested the child is after the event or how long it takes to recover from the sleep loss from the event. Finally, I ask the parents to decide, "Was it worth it?"

Summary and Action Plan for Exhausted Parents

1. Good sleep quality permits optimal wakefulness, which allows you to be at your personal best.
2. Healthy sleep is good for the brain; junk sleep is bad for the brain.
3. Healthy sleep in children helps prevent maternal depression.

Sleeping is not a completely automatically regulated process, like the control of body temperature. Sleeping is more like feeding. We do not expect children to grow well if all they eat is junk food. Children need a well-balanced diet.

The same is true for sleep. Healthy sleep benefits the child socially, emotionally, medically, physically, athletically, and cognitively. Moreover, the benefits of sleeping well in early childhood carry over into adolescence and even beyond.

What a Parent Can Do
Encourage your partner to help care for the baby daytime and nighttime.
Encourage self-soothing.

Put your child to sleep drowsy but awake, then leave the room.

Set an early bedtime based on drowsy signs.

Provide opportunities for naps based on drowsy signs.

Avoid irregularity of sleep schedules, including between week-days and weekends.

Practice safe sleep recommendations.

No TV or screen in the child's room; limit screen time.

Chapter 4 Outline

ADVICE TO ALL PARENTS FOR ALL CHILDREN

TEACH SELF-SOOTHING

Start Early

Many Hands

  Father Care: Our Secret Weapon for Soothing

Drowsy but Awake

  Drowsy Signs and Fatigue Signs

  Parental Presence and Parental Response to
    Awakenings

Soothing

  Rhythmic Rocking

  Swing, Stroller, Car, and Carrying

  Sucking

    Non-Nutritive Sucking

  Swaddling

  Massage

  Sounds

  Other Soothing Methods

  Everything Works . . . for a While

  Soothing and Crying

  Resources for Soothing

Many Naps

BEDTIME ROUTINES AND BEDTIME PARENTING

Bedtime Routines

Bedtime Routines and Early Bedtimes

Bedtime Parenting

Preventing Sleep Problems

There never was a
Child so lovely but his
Mother was glad to see him asleep.

—Ralph Waldo Emerson

If you have not already done so, please go back and read chapter 1.

In 1957, a famous pediatrician, A. H. Parmelee, Jr., wrote, "Parents are never truly prepared for the degree to which the babies' sleep/wake patterns will dominate and completely disrupt their daily activities." That was then. Today I believe that parents *can* prepare and take charge to ensure a well-rested family. The good news is that most sleep problems in children can be prevented or treated. That does not mean that the road will be easy for all families, but be confident that we have learned a lot since 1957!

Let's start with a basic question: Why do some children have difficulty falling asleep or staying asleep? Temperament is part of the answer. In 1981, I discovered that 4-month-old infants with an easy temperament had long durations of sleep. Infants with the opposite temperament had short durations of sleep, and many of these infants had colic during their first few months. About 20 percent of all infants have colic, and they appear to be at a higher risk for the later development of sleep problems that persist well beyond early childhood. So colic, in addition to temperament, is part of the answer.

The fundamental problem is that colicky infants have difficulty falling asleep easily after several minutes of parental soothing with rocking or lullabies. This lack of self-soothing ability directly causes them to have difficulty returning to sleep unassisted when nighttime arousals naturally occur and parents are not present. Heroic parental efforts are required to soothe colicky babies to sleep and keep them asleep; the lucky parents of those 80 percent of babies that do not have colic have no clue how utterly exhausting this is. Parents vary in their ability to soothe their babies and cope with the stress of their own sleep deprivation. So when colic subsides at 3–4 months, some post-colic babies and their parents are well rested, while others are horribly sleep-deprived.

Around this time, in order to prevent subsequent sleep problems, parents need to allow their colicky babies to learn some self-soothing skills by reducing their efforts to soothe their babies to sleep and not responding to signaling behaviors. This reduction might be very gradual or abrupt and may or may not be associated with crying. Because parents are already familiar with the phrase *toilet training*, I call my suggestions to help babies learn self-soothing "sleep training." I made up the term *sleep training* because it seemed similar to other terms (*toilet training, Parent Effectiveness Training* to better communicate with our son, and *obedience training* for our dog to guard our son) used to describe a variety of activities to reach a desirable goal.

This phrase first appeared in 1987 in the first edition of *Healthy Sleep Habits, Happy Child*. Now, many years later, it has become popularly misunderstood to mean *only* a "cry it out" approach. Nothing could be further from the truth. But because controversy regarding this subject has overshadowed my original sleep-training suggestions, I think it's important to reintroduce these simple steps that parents can take—steps that have proven successful in preventing sleep problems in the 80 percent of infants without colic. *Our general goal for non-colicky babies is to prevent sleep problems by teaching self-soothing early.* The adage "start as you mean to go on" applies to these non-colicky babies, who are more able to learn self-soothing early; however, for babies with colic, teaching self-soothing when your child is older may be more appropriate and is discussed in chapters 6–8. However, because colicky behavior develops only after the first week and becomes more apparent after a few additional weeks, it makes sense to attempt to teach self-soothing early to *all* babies and, if needed, temporarily abandon these attempts if your child develops full-blown colic. Another reason it makes sense to try to teach self-soothing early in all babies is that there is no sharp distinction between babies without and with colic; rather, children lie along a spectrum of behaviors. Thus, early sleep training might prevent or ameliorate the development of colicky behavior in some babies.

Advice to All Parents for All Children

If you are too tired to read a lot and you are eager to do something, just review chapter 1. Or if your symptoms of sleep deprivation are severe, consider having your husband, wife, or partner read chapter 1 and temporarily put them in charge of helping your baby sleep. Perhaps, for now, continue to do everything that you are currently doing, but with one small modification: Just move the bedtime five to ten minutes earlier every three to four nights. Small amounts of extra sleep will have a big impact (page 102). This small amount of extra sleep will eventually make it easier for your baby to fall asleep and stay asleep. If you think that ignoring your baby's quiet cries is neglectful or insensitive and might cause you to feel shame or guilt, or that not always responding to every cry will harm your child or your relationship with your child, or that crying will disturb your other children or neighbors, consider *"no-cry" sleep solu-*

tions such as a *fade* procedure. A *community sleep consultant* might be helpful. If you have symptoms of anxiety or depression, they might worsen because all new parents become short on sleep, and these symptoms might interfere with your ability to guide your baby toward healthy sleep. If present, discuss this with your child's primary care provider.

Teach Self-Soothing

Self-soothing is the ability of your child to fall deeply asleep with or without a pacifier or swaddling after becoming drowsy from a parent's soothing efforts. The drowsy child is placed in a crib before she is in a deep sleep and allowed to fall asleep on her own, without parental intervention. A child who is not colicky will learn naturally how to self-soothe. All parents have to do is set up the proper conditions and get out of the way. Self-soothing is absent when your child *always* falls asleep at your breast, on your chest, in a parent's arms, or in a moving swing or car. By giving your baby the opportunity to learn self-soothing, you help prevent sleep problems. Parents who always soothe their baby into a deep sleep before putting her down to sleep deprive her of the opportunity to learn self-soothing skills. Not allowing your baby the opportunity to practice self-soothing will usually result in a baby or child who is entirely dependent on being parent-soothed. Subsequently, she may have difficulty falling asleep alone at sleep onset (bedtime battles) or during naturally occurring arousals at night (night awakenings).

It is common for most parents to spend ten to twenty minutes soothing before they put their baby down drowsy but still awake. However, the motion of rocking or pushing your baby for hours in a stroller for "soothing" might rob her of more restorative deep sleep even though she is in light slumber.

My impression is that self-soothing skills are a prerequisite for long-term healthy sleep habits, and the earlier they are developed, the easier it is for the entire family. But remember: About 20 percent of babies—those who are colicky—will likely have difficulty learning self-soothing until about 2–4 months of age. That is not your fault. That is not the babies' fault. It is just nature's roll of the dice.

START EARLY

The ability to fall asleep and stay asleep unassisted is learned behavior. The earlier you start to help your baby acquire these skills, the easier it is for her to learn them. Yes, initiating lactation or feeding your baby or perinatal issues such as prematurity are more important than thinking about sleep, but do not ignore sleep completely. Try the suggestions below as soon as you can—even, if possible, on the first day home from the hospital.

Waiting weeks or months to begin helping your baby learn self-soothing might result in her becoming accustomed to falling asleep only after feeding, or in your arms, a swing, or a stroller, or on your chest. When older, she will have to unlearn these expectations or associations. I cannot emphasize enough how important it is for parents to start early to help their child learn to sleep well.

In the late 1970s and early 1980s, to help direct my research career, I read all the papers published in English about children's sleep. This review led to this recommendation in my first book on colic, *Crybabies,* published in 1984: "The *three- or four-month birthday* appears to be an important milestone for sleep development. At this point, infants' sleep patterns tend to resemble those of adults," and parents can actively help their child learn to sleep well. For premature babies, it is three to four months after the expected due date. Subsequently, in 1987, in the first edition of *Healthy Sleep Habits, Happy Child,* the section "How to Teach Your Baby to Sleep or to Protect His Sleep Schedule" started at 4 months of age. This early approach was based on the fact that at that age the sleep machinery in the brain has developed to the point where parents need to pay closer attention to circadian rhythms for night and day sleep, or else the child would be more likely to develop a sleep deficit. When I did my research for *Healthy Sleep Habits, Happy Twins,* which was published in 2009, I used the 4-month mark to divide early and late parental efforts to help the twins sleep better. What I discovered was that parents who started helping their child sleep better at or before 4 months described better sleeping in their children than those parents who started after 4 months. This validates the notion that starting early is better than starting later.

Now we have research from 2010 by Dr. Jacqueline Henderson that more fully supports this concept. She discovered that "the longest self-regulated sleep period"—that is, the maximum length of night sleep plus quiet wakefulness plus reinitiation of sleep without parental intervention (self-soothing)—rapidly increases during the first three months. Dr. Henderson found that falling asleep before midnight and sleeping until 6:00 A.M. from "4 months of age also has implications for interventions intended to prevent infant sleep difficulties." She concluded: "Prevention should occur in synchrony with developmental tasks, which in this case is the task of self-regulating sleep throughout the night. . . . To achieve this, prevention interventions should target the management of infant sleep in the first 3 months of life . . . [because t]he most rapid consolidation in infants' nocturnal sleep occurs within the first 4 months of life. . . . *Prevention efforts should focus in the first 3 months, beginning as early as 1 month* for intervention to be synchronous with the onset of sleeping through the night [emphasis added]."

While it is never too late to help your child sleep well, research and experience demonstrate that it is also never too early. If your child is older and has more ingrained habits, it may take longer to unlearn the old habits and the process may be more stressful for the parents—but it can be done!

MANY HANDS

If your baby always falls asleep in her mother's arms after feeding, then she is less able to develop self-soothing skills because she learns to fall asleep only in association with her mother's body odor, skin contact, heartbeat, breathing rhythm, and rocking motions. After breastfeeding, the mother should sometimes pass her child to someone else for soothing to sleep—or, if the child is bottle-fed, allow others to feed her before soothing to sleep. Try to get both parents as well as grandparents, aunts, uncles, friends, or nannies involved in soothing before sleep.

Father Care: Our Secret Weapon for Soothing

How important is the father? Very! A 2020 study from Italy noted that "Italian fathers have been compared to fathers in Sweden, France, and the UK. Results from this study showed that in Italy and France, fathers show the lowest commitment to fathering activities. [In our study] we found that when fathers are involved in their children's sleep care, the number of night awakenings decreased, even in infants aged 8–12 months." Another scientific paper, by Dr. Liat Tikotzky, also emphasized the role of the father and concluded, "Paternal involvement in infant care may contribute significantly to the development of infant sleep . . . because fathers in general may endorse to a higher degree of limit-setting approach that encourages the infant to self-soothe. . . . A higher involvement of fathers in infant care predicted and was associated with fewer infant night wakings and shorter total sleep time," perhaps because the children spent more time asleep at night with better-quality consolidated night sleep. Also, she studied how rapidly fathers and mothers responded to intervene when watching a video of a child (not their own) displaying increasing amounts of distress (page 417). Fathers demonstrated higher tolerance for infant crying than mothers. In a separate study, she observed, "Greater paternal involvement in infant daytime and nighttime caregiving at 3 months significantly predicted more consolidated maternal and infant sleep at 6 months." So when Dad gets on board, not only does the baby sleep better, so does the mother! In one study, by Dr. Klaus Minde, of children 1–3 years of age, sleep problems were solved when fathers took over the management of the bedtime routine and night awakenings: "The reason for this suggestion [that fathers manage the bedtime routine and night wakings] came from clinical experience which indicated that fathers, partly because of their overall designated caretaking role in the family, and partly because of their more limited contact with their children during the day, were able to relate to them in a more forthright and authoritative fashion. In contrast, mothers often felt tired and spent in the evening and perceived their toddlers as particularly difficult at that time. It was of interest that most fathers were willing and even enthusiastic about this new role. Mothers were initially sometimes doubtful either of their husband's coping or of their own ability to tolerate these new arrangements." Studies have shown that fathers have a higher tolerance for mild or low-level fussing/crying than mothers and as a result, are more willing to delay their response, with the hope that their child will independently self-soothe back to sleep (page 419). Research suggests that mothers play the role of "gatekeeping," either encouraging or inhibiting the father's involvement.

But many mothers may say, "I want to do it all by myself because I can do it better than anyone else." It is completely normal for mothers to feel uncomfortable with fathers playing a major role at bedtime. As one mother stated, "I struggled to trust other people to put my baby to sleep." But remember, falling asleep under different conditions promotes the learning of self-soothing skills. Dads might be available only on weekends and only for naps. No matter. Some attempts are better than none. So get dads, or others, on board!

Before the baby is born, fathers should make the decision to become involved in child care right from the start. Some fathers hold back initially, afraid they might "do the wrong thing" when holding, burping, bathing, changing, or feeding the baby. After mothers get their strength back, they should deliberately leave the house on a weekend, when Dad pulls nap duty, for a few hours to visit a friend, hang out with the older kids, go to a movie, or exercise at a time when they expect the baby to go through a cycle of feeding, changing, bathing, and putting to sleep. Guess who has to do the work then? Often a father will feel more comfortable doing these things when the "expert" is not looking over his shoulder. Moms deserve to take breaks to get their batteries recharged. This strategy is smart, not selfish, because moms do the heavy lifting when it comes to baby care, and a sleep-deprived mom is not at her personal best. Remember the safety advice on the airplane: You put on your oxygen mask first so you can take care of your child second. So the first point is for fathers to start early in practicing baby care.

Second, fathers should plan for the six-week peak of fussing/crying that occurs in all babies. They should come home early or take a few days off from work if they are able. Make adjustments if your baby is born before or after the expected date of delivery, because the six-week peak is counted from the due date. At 6 weeks of age, babies fuss/cry more and sleep less. Less sleep for the baby means less sleep for the mother. All mothers need help in caring for their 6-week-old and themselves. Fathers should give mothers a well-deserved break at this time by taking the baby out for long walks or car rides in the evening or night. The baby might not sleep well during these outings, but at least the mother gets a break.

The third point is that fathers can practice and learn how to help their baby fall asleep. For example, after nursing her baby, the mother could pass her daughter to the father, who then rocks his baby gently for a while and puts her down to sleep or lies down with her in their bed and they both snooze. This may only occur on weekends, when the father is around at nap times. The participation of fathers in putting their babies to sleep will help them gain confidence in becoming a parent. If the mother is giving expressed breast milk in a bottle, fathers and babies may have an easier time accomplishing the feeding if the mother actually leaves the house. This is because the baby can smell the mother's presence and might resist taking the bottle if she knows her mother is home. So, maybe on weekends, when it's time for the baby's nap, Mom leaves the house and has fun while Dad gives the bottle and puts his baby down to sleep.

Fourth, fathers can learn how to soothe baby fussiness and crying and spend lots of time doing the soothing. For example, fathers can learn infant massage. Classes are offered everywhere; call your local maternity hospital or go online. Fathers can learn lullabies (your baby will not care how well you sing). A baby bath might be especially soothing, and fathers can spend time letting the warm water calm the baby. A father can learn to do everything a mother does to soothe the baby except breastfeed. For babies 6 months of age or older, fathers can attempt to help lengthen naps by responding immediately as a mini nap nears its end (the baby just begins to whimper or cry) by attempting to soothe her back to sleep for a nap extension. If mothers do this, it might be more stimulating than soothing and lead to an unnecessary feeding that is more likely to wake the child.

Lastly, a father can request to help feed or soothe the baby in the middle of the night when the mother needs extra sleep. This is a little bit tricky, because many mothers have the attitude that nobody can do the soothing as well as they can, and also that dads need their rest so they can go out to work well rested in the morning. With this attitude, the mother rejects or resists the idea that baby care in the middle of the night should be a shared experience. For some families, this might be the right course of action. But if the mother is distressed, exhausted, sleep-deprived, or going through baby blues, then extra help at night from the father is absolutely needed to give the mother a little more sleep. After all, no matter how stressful his job might be, the father at work always gets some breaks. A mother with a baby might not get any breaks during the day.

Fathers need to understand that when children are overtired and not sleeping well, it is sometimes useful to go to a *temporarily* ultra-early bedtime to repay the sleep debt. The child wakes better rested, then learns to nap better, and later is able to have a later bedtime. If fathers refuse to help prevent and solve sleep problems, then they have to accept responsibility for their overtired child's behavior—and not blame the mother!

Sadly, some fathers are unwilling or unable to be helpful partners due to their own *issues*. Mothers might have to look for community services, relatives, or friends for support.

The contribution of the father is especially important if your baby develops extreme fussiness/colic. Here is one parent's explanation of why fathers are helpful:

> I think part of the reason that dads can be so good at soothing is that they, especially with newborns, often have greater internal resources for it. If a mother is nursing, she is up often, and is "on call" 100 percent of the time for months on end. Dad is not worried about being on call with baby all the time. He's not worried that baby might cry all night and keep him up for hours and hours when he's already been up for the last month! Dad isn't worried that he's going to have to nurse, and nurse, and nurse (sometimes painfully, in the beginning!) if there is no other way to soothe the baby. Dad is often pretty logical and unemotional—babies cry, babies are soothed, babies sleep. If babies are not ever soothed, maybe they are sick. This is not true for all dads and all moms, of course! But it is my observation that the combination of male tendencies toward logic/unemotionalness + not being awake since the birth + not nursing + not being on call for baby 100 percent of the time = greater ability to calmly, successfully soothe a baby.

DROWSY BUT AWAKE

As your baby begins to show signs of becoming *drowsy*, you should begin a soothing-to-sleep routine in any way that calms her. These signs usually appear after one or two hours of wakefulness, or sooner following a very brief nap. The 20 percent of babies that have colic may not show these drowsy signs, so you have to watch the clock more carefully with them. If your child often shows signs of fatigue, note how long she has been awake and the next time begin the soothing-to-sleep routine about twenty minutes earlier. It is not necessary for your child to always be drowsy but still awake when you put her down. Sometimes she goes from drowsy to asleep very quickly, and there is no reason why some books suggest that you should then wake up your baby and put her down in a more wakeful state. Your baby may become drowsy after being awake only forty-five minutes; if so, begin your soothing-to-sleep routine then.

If she makes quiet sounds such as whimpering or low-level fussing, wait and watch as long as you feel comfortable. She might fall deep asleep. Or instead of just waiting, send in Dad for brief and minimal soothing such as gently patting or rubbing the baby, jiggling the crib, or shushing, but not picking up. There is nothing wrong if your newborn sometimes or usually falls asleep at your breast, in your arms, on Dad's chest, or in the swing, car, or stroller. If she falls asleep during feeding, do not wake her.

But here is the problem: If she is *always* in a deep sleep state when you put her down, then she has no opportunity to learn self-soothing skills. So I suggest that you sometimes put her down after soothing, drowsy but awake. You might be comfortable trying it only once a day. That's okay. Maybe you will have to shorten the duration of soothing to accomplish this. There is no rule regarding the time of day when you should attempt this or how many attempts you should make in a day.

However, you might be more successful if you try this *within one hour of the baby waking in the morning*, because she will be best rested from night sleep. That is, do the changing, feeding, a little playing, and soothing *all within one hour*. Look at the clock when you think your baby wakes to start the day; this time may vary from day to day. On a weekend, have Dad, if available, put her down in a dark and quiet room, drowsy but awake. For these attempts, maybe Mom should leave the house. This often produces more sleep and less crying.

Think of "drowsy but awake" as somewhere between the extremes of fully awake and completely asleep. Please don't overthink or obsess about the exactitude of what "drowsy but awake" means. Just watch your baby for drowsy cues.

Here is a report by a parent who usually had good timing, so most drowsy cues were absent:

> Drowsy in this context doesn't mean about to fall asleep (half-closed eyes, barely able to keep open). When my son was a baby he would become very still about 10 minutes before he fell asleep—he is a wiggle worm, so it was noticeable. He would also gaze for long periods of time at something. This was the window when he needed to be put down for his nap. If I waited until it passed and he was really tired, he would fight sleep. So when "the stare" appeared, I would check his diaper, swaddle him, and put him down. He would gaze at his mobile for a while and then fall asleep.

The baby should be awake when you put her down for her nap. You aren't trying to ease her down and then sneak out—you want her to be able to fall asleep on her own, without rocking, patting, and so on. Try to catch her in that drowsy pre-sleep period—for many babies it is right around one to two hours after waking for the day. Start watching for signs at around thirty to ninety minutes, and I bet you will soon be able to tell when she is ready to go down. Good luck!

DROWSY SIGNS AND FATIGUE SIGNS

Drowsy Signs

Here are some of the drowsy cues or sleepy signs as your baby becomes drowsy—moving into the Sleep Zone, moving away from alert, calm, and relaxed:

Decreased activity, less animated, becomes quieter.
Slower motions, less social, less vocal.

Less interested in toys or people.
Sucking is weaker or slower.
Yawning.

These behaviors are most noticeable when the child is in a quiet and relaxed environment—for example, when being read to. They might be less apparent in a stimulating environment such as a busy mall or when she is in front of a television or screen-based media device. Or they might not be noticed because you are distracted by looking at a screen or on a phone call.

IMPORTANT POINT
Try to begin soothing *before* you notice changes in the eyes.

Pay close attention to the *eyes* and *eyelids* as she transitions from mild to deeper drowsiness to almost a sleep state:

Eyes become *less focused* on surroundings, eyes appear *glazed over*, staring, or not as sparkling.
She may seem to look "through you" and not socially "at you."
Eyelids *drooping,* eyelids come down slowly, *long blinks.*

Fatigue Signs
Think of fatigue signs as signaling the distress of being short on sleep (SOS): "Help me, I need to sleep." She's entering the overtired zone, moving toward irritable and tense.

Mild fussiness, irritability, cranky, moodiness, pulling ears, drooping head, *rubbing eyes*
Easily upset, clinging, peevish, easily frustrated, short-fused, rough around the edges
Whining, crying, slightly "wired," less cooperative, less able to entertain herself

Older children might also be oppositional, defiant, uncooperative, angry, aggressive, or complain of headache or stomachache.

Adults might also complain of depressed mood, mental fog, inability to concentrate, lack of motivation, or a sensation of just going through the motions, like a robot, without much feeling or sense of vitality.

As mentioned earlier, the most common mistake made by parents is mistaking *fatigue* signs, which come late, with *drowsy* signs, which appear early and signal the rising of the sleep wave. I know this subject is confusing because I often speak to groups of parents and ask them to describe how their child looks when starting to become drowsy. Always, most parents describe fatigue signs, not drowsy signs. A good way for parents to familiarize themselves with their baby's drowsy signs is to make a video recording of their baby from waking to falling asleep. When watching, they should look for changes in their baby during the time period around falling asleep.

The importance of initiating soothing to sleep at the onset of drowsy signs cannot be overemphasized, because once your child is allowed to become overtired, she is in a state of hyperarousal and is less able to easily fall asleep and stay asleep. In addition to parents not appreciating the importance of acting when subtle drowsy signs begin to appear, sleep researchers sometimes mix together drowsy signs and fatigue signs. This is an honest mistake, because appreciating early-onset drowsy signs is not widespread. Here is an example of how and why an attempt to help children sleep better *failed*, because the children were unintentionally allowed to become overtired:

A meticulous study of anticipatory guidance by Dr. Barbara Galland measured objective sleep data on infants at age 6 months and made home visits to gather data on both mothers and partners. Some families were randomized to receive sleep intervention: They received sleep advice information before the child was born and at a home visit at 3 weeks postpartum. Although not in the published paper, the online supplements appendices 1 and 2 summarized the topics covered in the parent advice package intended to promote healthy sleep practices. Appendix 1 included items such as: "Notice and act on baby's tired signs early. Signs of tiredness outlined. Act on tired signs to prevent overtiredness. Notice tired signs early." The last item in appendix 2 was: "Baby's tired signs: Important to learn baby's tired signs." However, the "baby's tired signs" were not actually described. Dr. Galland graciously put me in touch with the research aide who conducted the education sessions, and she shared with me the two PowerPoint slides used before the baby was born and at the 3-week home visit which she used to illustrate "baby's tired signs." From these slides, parents learned that "Your baby may also tell you they are tired by showing, one or more of the following 'tired signs': Yawning, Staring, Jerking arms or legs, Arching their back, Rubbing their eyes." Well, in my opinion, any baby who is staring, jerking, arching, or rubbing eyes is way overtired. One slide did state, "Babies need to go to bed when they are tired. Without enough sleep they become *overtired* and will be very hard to soothe, put down and then settle to sleep [emphasis added]." But no mention is made of what an overtired baby looks like.

Unsurprisingly, because little emphasis was placed on watching for early and subtle signs of drowsiness and signs of fatigue/overtiredness were presented as drowsy signs, the entire sleep education project was found to be ineffective. Unfortunately, a reader of the published report, not having this additional information, would erroneously conclude that anticipatory advice such as "Notice and act on baby's tired signs early" is not helpful.

Effective parent advice should include more focus on the *subtle signs of drowsiness that develop early* and advise shortening the intervals of wakefulness in the future if signs of overtiredness had previously developed.

Parenting would be so much easier if we had a "sleepometer" that objectively measured sleepiness like a thermometer measures temperature! Even without a thermometer, when we feel the hot skin on our child's forehead, we know there is a problem. Other problems we can actually directly see, such as a very overweight child. But we don't really directly see sleepiness, we see the behavioral consequences of sleepiness. With an overweight child, our thoughts go to food quantity and food quality. Remember, to avoid junk food, you read the nutritional label. Junk sleep has no label to read, so instead you must learn to "read" your child. Even when there is not a full-blown "witching hour," a child might often have mild fussiness or irritability in the late afternoon. Why is this deterioration in behavior and mood at the end of the day often not recognized by some parents as being directly caused by junk sleep or lack of sleep?

Some parents deny their child is suffering from SOS distress because they are not present when it is full-blown in the late afternoon and she is in daycare or nanny care. When parents return home from work, naturally there is intense excitement as they reconnect with their children, play, and have dinner, so some of these distress items are masked. Other parents do not see these SOS signs because their child is pacified and distracted by being parked in front of television or a videogame. Or the parents are digitally distracted. Other parents have been sleep-deprived themselves for much of their life and do not appreciate the power of healthy sleep because they have not experienced it (page 101). Or they think it is normal for children to have a witching hour.

What if your baby cries when you put her down drowsy but still awake? When you first try to put her down drowsy but awake, she might be almost completely asleep, but with practice you will be able to put her down in a more wakeful state. When you put her down drowsy but awake and she cries hard, immediately pick her up for more soothing and try again some other time that day or the next day. If she makes very quiet sounds, wait and see. She might drift off to sleep or begin to cry hard. If she now begins to cry hard, quickly pick her up. Don't be disappointed if she does not fall asleep when you first start to practice putting her down drowsy but awake; it just takes practice. Expect to become frustrated, because you may be successful only about 10 percent of the time during the first week. But by the end of the second week, you may be successful 20 percent of the time. This percentage may double each week, so after a few more weeks it becomes much easier. Be optimistic! After a few months of practice and the maturation of sleep rhythms, you will develop an anticipatory sense of when she will need to sleep. Later, when she is completely well rested, don't be surprised if drowsy signs disappear altogether because you have successfully synchronized the timing of your soothing to sleep with the beginning of her emerging sleep wave. It's like being good at surfing; you catch the wave for a long ride. Patience, practice, timing, and trial and error will guarantee success.

Here is a simple example. You go outside with your baby for some fresh air and walk to the park. After a while, you decide to go home to nap your baby but on the way home, she becomes mildly fussy or quietly cries. You say to yourself, *Whoops, I blew it this time; next time I'll head home ten minutes earlier,* as you glance at your watch to estimate how long your baby has been up. Watching your child and practicing brief intervals of wakefulness will guarantee success.

An important point worth restating is that you might be more successful with putting your child down drowsy but awake in the early morning, when she is best rested from the previous night's sleep, especially if the interval of wakefulness between the wake-up time and the first nap is very brief (thirty to ninety minutes). Nursing mothers might have more success if they leave the home and let the father put the baby down drowsy but awake with a bottle of expressed breast milk. The baby senses that Mom is gone, and she knows that Dad cannot breastfeed. She is tired anyway, so she might as well go to sleep. Why not?

Drowsy signs might be absent when a child has colic or is extremely overtired and instead crashes directly from a wakeful state to showing fatigue signs. Also, drowsy signs might be absent in the well-rested child with good self-soothing skills who is put down to sleep just as she is becoming sleepy. This suggests that drowsy signs really are mild expressions of becoming overtired (sleep-deprived), not simply tired.

As previously mentioned, drowsy signs might not be noticed by parents because of their own digital distractions (TV, smartphone, or computer). Maybe take a weekend break from all such distractions and simply watch your child for drowsy signs.

Also, signs of drowsiness and fatigue may be masked by parents' intensive play or the child being distracted with videogames, TV, or a DVD. Please observe how your child appears and plays independent of digital distractions, especially near the end of the day.

Why Does a Child Become Parent-Soothed and Not Learn Self-Soothing?
Parental sleep deprivation, excitement, or medical conditions push the topic of sleep for the child off the parent's radar.

Thinking that feeding directly causes sleeping causes parents to focus only on feeding.

Distraction interferes with appreciating signs of drowsiness.

Colic interferes with learning self-soothing.

Parental Presence and Parental Response to Awakenings
After a *bedtime routine* and *soothing*, you put your baby down drowsy but awake. Do you then leave the room or stay until your child is in a deep sleep state? If you strongly feel that you are or that your child is more comfortable with you staying for a while, then do so. Otherwise, it is probably better to leave the room. Leaving the room at bedtime when bed sharing or room sharing may not be practical because there no separate room for your child, and it may not be desirable for SIDS prevention, but leaving the room after soothing could be practiced at nap times.

One research study by Professor Mindell noted that parental presence at sleep onset is much more common in Asian than English-speaking countries. *"Parental presence in the room at bedtime* was the most potent predictor in explaining the number of night wakings, longest sleep interval, and total sleep time . . . The results also support the common recommendations made to parents for an *early bedtime,* consistent bedtime routine, and *encouraging children to fall asleep independently to learn self-soothing skills* [emphasis added]." Separately, in a study of 3-year-olds, shorter night sleep duration was linked to parental presence when falling asleep; further, children with short sleep durations, when young, have a tendency to maintain short sleep durations when older, sometimes with significant *adverse* outcomes.

Other research studies support the recommendation that your child will learn self-soothing better if you leave the room after you put your child down (pages 175 and 225). When thinking about encouraging self-soothing to prevent sleep problems, leaving the room might be something you routinely practice from the get-go. However, you might feel more comfortable doing this in a gradual fashion (page 240) in the context of implementing a sleep solution to help your child sleep better.

After she has fallen asleep at night, your child, while *asleep* or after waking, may make *non-distress* sounds or movements. Do you leave her be for a short time or do you respond immediately (see chapter 1 and page 417)?

Before answering this question, it is important to describe *non-distress* sounds and why they occur. I am talking about harmless sounds that all babies make that do *not* indicate distress and, if you feel comfortable, can usually be safely ignored. You will hear sounds creating the false impression that your healthy baby has a cold (mucous, gurgling, nasal congestion) because, for all babies, the nasal passage is narrow, and a little fluid there vibrates when your baby breathes through her nose. You will hear quiet wheezing, whistling, and noisy respiration sounds because, for all babies, the muscles lining the airway are not well developed; during inhalation, the airway narrows slightly. You will hear coughing because, for all babies, saliva pools at the back of the mouth and stomach contents normally reflux a little up the esophagus; the cough thus protects the lungs by clearing the back of the throat.

Also, there may be some low and feeble noises that sound like a whimper, or a quiet moan or groan, which may or may not indicate distress. If you go to her because you hear a quiet whimper, moan, or groan, and it appears that she is not having difficulty breathing but is calmly asleep without signs of distress such as grimacing, vomiting, or diarrhea, and her forehead does not feel warm or hot, and she showed no signs of illness during the day, it is probably safe to practice watchful waiting. That is, closely watch but do not intervene, even if she appers to be partially or completely awake.

So do you delay your response or respond immediately? Using video cameras in the child's bedroom, it was observed that often the infants self-soothed back to sleep unassisted. At 3 months of age, the average number for parental checks was one or two times each night, but the range was wide (zero to twelve). The average parental delay time was about three minutes. Although not given for 3 months of age, for 6 months of age, the range for the delay time was wide, 0.5 to 27 minutes. "The children of parents who waited longer to respond to their awakenings at 3 months were more likely to be self-soothers by 12 months of age."

It is not known whether these associations regarding parental presence and response to awakenings around bedtime or during the night are parent-driven (less parental attention encourages more self-soothing in the infant), infant-driven (infants with more self-soothing capability need less parental attention), or both. Also, it is not known whether these associations apply in general or they vary depending on specific circumstances. For example, before and during pregnancy, some mothers have anxiety or beliefs that their child must always be attended to immediately at night to prevent infant distress (page 218), and some infants have difficulty self-soothing because of *extreme fussiness/colic*. So waiting a minute or two to respond at night during the first three months for non-distress sounds might be a general recommendation but not when there is maternal anxiety, infant colic, or other circumstances.

Soothing

What exactly is soothing to a drowsy state? Soothing is restoring a peaceful state. To soothe your newborn is to render her calm or quiet, to bring her to a composed condition by reducing the force or intensity of fussiness or crying. Soothing brings comfort to your baby, a cessation of agitation. Snuggled close to your body, she feels your warmth and senses your affection and protection. Cuddling is the close embrace you do with someone you love. Sometimes you just want to nestle with her as you take a cozy position and press her close to you or lie down close to her. At best, when a child is tired, we hope to lull her into a relaxed, sleepy state.

Bodily contact, sucking, and gentle rhythmic motions over long periods of time seem to work best for soothing. Sometimes loud mechanical sounds like the garbage disposal or hair dryer seem to help. Be careful, however, not to bombard your baby with stimuli. Initially, try to appeal to one sense at a time: tactile (massaging, rubbing, kissing, rocking, patting, changing from hip to shoulder), auditory (singing, humming, playing music, running the vacuum cleaner), sight (bright lights, mobiles, or television; or dim light or darkness when drowsy), or rhythmic motion (swings, cradles, car rides, going for a walk). Sometimes doing too many of these things simultaneously or with too much force has a stimulating effect rather than a relaxing one. However, if your baby remains fussy, try combinations of these different modalities.

Try to synchronize your actions with your baby's rhythms. If she is tense and taut, with deep exhausted heaving sobs and little physical movement, try rubbing her back ever so gently or moving your cheek over hers in a slow rhythm that coincides with her breathing pattern. If she is boxing with her fists, jerking her legs, and arching her back, maybe a ride on your shoulders will grab her attention and arrest the spell. You will find that after a while you become attuned to the nuances of your baby's rhythms and respond accordingly.

Each parent should experiment to see what soothing method

works best and then try to be somewhat consistent so that your child learns to associate certain behaviors with falling asleep. But it is not necessary that Mom and Dad have the same soothing style.

Rhythmic Rocking

Rhythmic motions are one of the most effective methods of soothing your infant. Use a cradle, rocking chair, baby swing, or Snugli; take the baby for automobile rides, dance with her, or simply walk with her. Rocking motions may be gentle movements or vigorous swinging, depending on what your child responds to. Gently jiggling or bouncing may calm your baby. Some parents claim that raising and lowering the baby like an elevator is effective. Perhaps these rhythmic movements are comforting because they are similar to what the baby experienced in the womb.

Swing, Stroller, Car, and Carrying

Rhythmic rocking motions might occur in an old-fashioned cradle, a swing, a stroller, your car, or when your baby is carried in your arms or an infant carrier. These activities are fine for soothing, but not for sleeping. Sure, your baby can fall asleep in the moving cradle or swing. But it will probably be a light sleep, and your child will miss the full restorative benefit of deeper sleep. Remember, think of sleep *quality*, not just sleep *quantity*.

In your home, perhaps napping in a gently moving swing in a dark and quiet room is very similar to motionless sleep in a crib. If this is the only way your child will nap, then sometimes turn off the swing after your child falls asleep and leave her there until she wakes. Later, try to make a transition to placing her in her crib without the swing. For a colicky child, this might only work around 3–4 months of age, when the colic is winding down.

Outside your home, the rhythmic rocking motion of a stroller might lull your child to a drowsy state, and you might find a quiet park to stop to let her enjoy motionless sleep while you enjoy the fresh air. But in a bright and noisy shopping environment or public place, I suspect that the naps might be less restorative and maybe shorter.

As a generalization, I think that planning for naps at home helps parents organize schedules and think about consolidated sleep, naps in sync with biological rhythms, and reasonably early bedtimes. In contrast, I think that frequent napping in shopping malls and other busy places is associated with children who tend to be chronically mildly short on sleep, so they crash despite all the stimulation around them. So when I encourage motionless sleep in the crib or bed over sleep in motion, I am thinking more about discouraging sleeping outside than swings at home.

Sucking

Anything you can do to encourage your baby to suck will help soothe her. Offering the breast, bottle, pacifier, finger, or wrist usually helps calm your baby. If you are breastfeeding, one way to help distinguish between sucking for soothing and sucking for hunger is that the sucking for soothing is often rapid, repeated sucks with very little swallowing. If your baby is hungry, the pattern is usually a rhythmic suck-swallow, suck-swallow, and so forth. But the fussy baby does not suck-swallow in a rhythmic steady fashion; she sucks more than swallows; she starts and stops, twists and turns. If you are bottle-feeding, do not always assume that when your baby eagerly takes several ounces, this means she is hungry. Many babies with extreme fussiness/colic suck more than they need and spit up a lot.

Because sucking is such a powerful way to calm a baby, and babies often fall asleep with sucking, I think it is unnatural and unhealthy for parents to deliberately do things that interfere with sucking. One popular book that promotes "no-cry sleep solutions" tells parents to remove the breast while the baby is sucking, before she falls asleep, and if she continues to want to suck after the removal, the book tells parents to hold her mouth closed to prevent it! Another popular book describes sucking as one of the major ways that babies can calm themselves, but then goes on to recommend that you wake your baby up during sucking if she falls asleep at the breast. Furthermore, the author instructs you to begin this practice at 1 month of age! Both books make the assumption that if the baby falls asleep while sucking, you will be creating a sleep problem. There is no good evidence to support this assumption. Mothers in my practice do not deliberately interfere with sucking at the time of soothing to sleep, and their babies sleep well. Both books also incorrectly assume that feeding and sleeping are tightly linked. So both encourage you to force-feed your baby in order to help her sleep longer. Phrases like "cluster feed," "top off the tank," or "awake when hungry and asleep when full" reveal a profound ignorance about how the developing brain, not the stomach, controls sleep/wake rhythms. I believe it is much healthier and more effective to follow your baby's needs. If your baby is hungry, feed her. If your baby is fussy, soothe her. If your baby is tired, put her to sleep. If you're not sure what she needs, encourage sucking at the breast or bottle until she seems satisfied because she is full or calm or asleep.

Non-Nutritive Sucking

Sometimes, try to give your baby a chance or chances to self-soothe to sleep without feeding during the day or night: This means that you do some soothing, and then your baby is put down drowsy but awake before falling asleep. Some mothers feel more comfortable trying this than others, and some babies accept this more than others, so try to do what feels right for you and your baby without making comparisons to others. Try to remember that breastfeeding is first of all feeding.

But as long as some chances to self-soothe are offered, I do not think there is a problem using the breast to soothe to sleep when necessary, especially when other soothing methods are not effective. This might occur when your child develops a second wind and becomes overtired, your baby is about 6 weeks old and at the peak of fussiness/crying, or your baby has colic—or anytime Mom is desperate for sleep herself. So what if sometimes you might be soothing to sleep using breastfeeding and sometimes you might use other methods to soothe to a drowsy but awake state? This is parenting, not the military!

Pacifiers may help babies sleep and reduce the risk of SIDS. If you have to replace the pacifier once or twice during a night to get great sleep, do it. But if replacing pacifiers occurs many times throughout the night, then one or both parents will be short on sleep. Maybe it is time to teach more self-soothing skills. When your child is older and throws the pacifier out of the crib, instead of going back in to pick it up and return it, just buy a dozen pacifiers, or use one with a ribbon substantially shorter than the circumference of your child's neck (to prevent strangulation) that has an alligator clip allowing you to attach it to your child's pajamas. That way the child will learn self-soothing with the aid of a pacifier.

Swaddling

Gentle pressure, such as that experienced when embraced or hugged, makes us feel good. Swaddling or gentle wrapping, sleeping in a car seat, and being held in a soft baby carrier or sling are other ways to exert gentle pressure. Here, too, perhaps the sensation of gentle pressure resembles a state of comfort that the baby feels before she is born. Both rhythmic motions and gentle pressure may be effective because human babies are born too early. Wait a minute: Of course premature babies are born early! No, not just premature babies—*all* babies. The theory is that human babies are born earlier compared with other primate babies because as human pelvic bones evolved to support an upright posture, they became narrower. Thus human babies had to be smaller at the time of birth in order to pass through the pelvic opening. If this theory is correct, then it is likely that rhythmic motions and gentle pressure exert their soothing effects because they partially re-create the sensations experienced by the baby in the womb.

Swaddling should be attempted if it appears to help your child sleep better. Just as with pacifiers in the preceding section, if you have to reswaddle a baby once or twice a night in order to get great sleep, it is worth it. But if swaddling occurs many times throughout the night, then one or both parents will be short on sleep, and this is not good. It is time to allow your child to learn some self-soothing. When your child appears to want to kick free and not be swaddled, then stop.

Massage

Massaging babies has been practiced in many different cultures and has a long history. It is not just a new fad. One particular advantage to massaging your newborn is that the mother or father also directly benefits from this activity. While lovingly stroking your baby, you smile at her, talk softly, or sing or hum. These efforts, while focused on your baby, relax you, too! As your child bonds with you through the close contact, you bond with your child. Since fathers cannot breastfeed their babies, I encourage them to develop an intimate bond with their newborn by practicing baby massage right away— even before any fussiness begins. Using a natural cold-pressed fruit or vegetable oil, gently stroke the skin and gently knead your baby's muscles. All the movements are performed gently—books with pictures and online videos are available to assist you. Baby massage is not a gimmick. Nor is it a cure for extreme fussiness. But it does soothe babies. Equally important, it provides you with a singular opportunity to be completely focused on your baby—turn off the phones. Both you and your baby might even enjoy listening to relaxation music at this time. You are doing something quite different from feeding, changing, and bathing. Comforting your baby this way will give you an inner calmness that will help you get through possible rough times when your baby is extremely fussy and not very soothable. Think of it as making deposits to an interest-bearing account that you will need to draw upon in more difficult times. Only instead of money, it is love that you are putting in the bank. A recent study among children age 3–18 months without significant sleep problems showed that including a massage into the child's usual bedtime routine reduced the number of night wakings in the child and improved the quality of *maternal* sleep.

Sounds

What is the power of a lullaby? Babies calm down and slip into slumber; parents relax and feel more at peace with themselves and their baby. Lullabies, such as those found on my CD *Sweet Baby: Lullabies to Soothe Your Newborn,* are the universal language of parents loving babies. Lullabies, music, songs, humming, reading, talking, or nature sounds may have a soothing effect on your baby. One study suggested that music that has a wide dynamic range with lots of loud and quiet elements was not as soothing as music that varied little in intensity, such as harpsichord or guitar pieces. Noise machines may be useful for soothing and for masking street noises. For safety, noise machines should be on their lowest setting and as far away from the child as possible. Maybe gently stroke or massage your baby when listening.

Other Soothing Methods

Be skeptical about the supposed miracles accomplished with crib vibrators, hot-water bottles, herbal teas, or recordings of heartbeat or womb sounds. There has been a great deal of nonsense written about burping techniques, nipple sizes and shapes, baby bottle straws, feeding and sleeping positions, lambswool pads, diets for nursing mothers, special formulas, pacifiers, and solid food. There is no good evidence that chiropractic spinal manipulation helps babies. These items have nothing to do with extreme fussiness, crying, temperament, or sleeping habits.

Many useless remedies can be purchased without a prescription. Anti-gas drops, such as simethicone, have not been shown to be more effective than a placebo in well-conducted studies. One popular pellet contains chamomile, calcium phosphate, caffeine, and a very small amount of active belladonna chemicals (0.0000095 percent). Another remedy contains natural blackberry flavor, Jamaica ginger, oil of anise, oil of nutmeg, and 2 percent alcohol. Maybe enough alcohol will sedate some infants! Please read labels carefully—any natural substance, flavoring agent, or herb can have pharmacological effects. Call a school of pharmacy or a medical school to locate experts in pharmacognosy, the study of natural herbs and plants, to find out if a particular plant or herb is dangerous. Don't assume that if it is safe for adults, it must be safe for infants.

Beware of gimmicks. Newborns have been drowned in rocking waterbeds, strangled in trampoline-like crib platforms, and suffocated by pillows. Beware of prescribed drugs. A London *Times* headline of May 22, 1998, screamed, "Baby Died after Drop of Medicine for Wind." A midwife had "diagnosed trapped wind" and prescribed what was thought to be peppermint water.

Also be cautious in using home remedies. One mother almost killed her baby by giving a mixture of Morton Salt Substitute with *Lactobacillus acidophilus* culture, as prescribed in a popular book. A good rule of thumb here is: When in doubt, don't!

Everything Works . . . for a While

When you believe that something is going to calm your baby— herbal tea, womb recordings, lambswool blankets, you name it— often it appears to work . . . for a while. You are emotionally expecting relief because you trust the advice of an authority. Your

fatigue may breed inflated hopes for a cure, and the day-by-day variability in infant crying creates the illusion that a particular remedy
works. What is really happening is a placebo effect, the emotional
equivalent of an optical illusion.

Mothers may initially fool themselves into believing their babies
are better because of a new formula or special tea. Of course, reality sets in after a few days and shatters the illusion. Some doctors
believe the mothers' reports and agree that the babies really did
improve for a day or two because the babies received novel stimulation.

Novelty is unlikely to be important, because parents report that
upon reintroduction, weeks after the special tea or gimmick was
discarded, they see no improvement. In other words, there was no
placebo effect the second time around. Naturally, if the baby coinci-
dentally outgrows extreme fussiness/colic when a useless remedy is
introduced, the mother, the family, and even the doctor might become convinced that the useless remedy actually cured the extreme
fussiness/colic!

SOOTHING

There are many ways to soothe babies, but only a few major
themes.

1. Rhythmic rocking: swings, cars, arms, rocking chairs, stroller
   rides, crib, swaying to and fro
2. Sucking: breast, bottle, pacifier, wrist, fingers
3. Gentle pressure: swaddling, massage, soft cloth carriers
4. Sounds: lullabies (for example, my CD, *Sweet Baby: Lullabies
   to Soothe Your Newborn*), nature sounds, music, quiet talking,
   shushing

Soothing and Crying

I asked a group of new parents in my practice how they soothed
their babies when fussy or soothed them to a drowsy state before
sleep. The group seemed to agree that slow, rhythmic stroking and

rocking was usually more effective than rapid bouncing or patting. But one mother described how the intensity and rapidity of her movements increased when her baby became fussier. This seemed to help calm her baby, and the mother felt this was because she had become more attuned to her baby. However, other new parents in the group did not find this helpful. One mother felt that she increased the intensity and rapidity of her movements when her baby became fussier because she was becoming more stressed herself, not because it was helping her baby calm down. Another mother said that she felt her style of soothing was organically part of who she was, and although she had tried different methods suggested by books and friends, she ultimately did what felt comfortable to her. Perhaps there is no "best" way, but every mother and baby discovers what works for them.

The group also agreed that dads sometimes seemed more effective in soothing because they had a more matter-of-fact approach and talked to the babies as if they were adults. "Here's the deal: I'm going to rock you for a while and then you're going to be put down to sleep because it's time to sleep. Got it? So don't give me any problems."

Some mothers in the group started teaching self-soothing when their babies were only a week old, after hearing from other moms how they had also started early. One mother described how, after feeling comfortable with some successes, she decided that she would let her baby cry at night to learn some self-soothing for night sleep. Her baby cried quietly one night only for twenty minutes and then slept well at night and has slept well since. She did this at age *4 weeks,* and her baby was now 5–6 months. There were no gasps or astonished looks but simply smiles and nods from the more experienced mothers. I think that more mothers and fathers might experiment with a few minutes of quiet crying to allow self-soothing at night in the newborn period if they feel comfortable. I pointed to a couple present with 38-week newborn twins and described how when attending to one twin, the other might cry and then stop crying and fall asleep before you could get to the crying twin. My impression is that ten to twenty minutes of low-level or quiet crying cannot be harmful.

But here is a curious observation: In the office, after soothing a 2-week-old following an exam, I put the baby down on the examination table, and the baby began whimpering and quietly crying. I said to the mother, "Let's watch the minute hand and leave your baby for one to two minutes, as long as the crying does not become loud or strong, to see if she might fall asleep." Her immediate response was, "Isn't she crying hard?" I pointed out that hard crying occurs after an immunization, and this was quiet crying. So it appears possible that some mothers, in the beginning, are less able to make the distinction between very quiet crying or whimpering and hard, loud crying and are therefore loath to allow any crying to occur in the context of allowing a child to learn self-soothing. I asked the parents in the group about this and their experiences with teaching self-soothing, and here are some representative responses:

I wanted to respond to your comment about the mother who felt her baby was crying hard. I can relate to this and found with my baby at the start that his crying would actually "hurt" me. My partner, in contrast, didn't know what my problem was and didn't feel he was crying particularly hard (other people also commented that he didn't sound very loud or upset). For me, I feel that the combination of sleep deprivation, hormones, and the overwhelming responsibility of being a first-time mum meant that I overreacted to every single cry, and this has gradually reduced with time and experience.

I am a frequenter of the new parent group at Dr. Weissbluth's office and have had tremendous success with letting my now 11-week-old daughter cry it out. I let her do it the first time for twenty minutes at 4 weeks of age and had success pretty immediately. After about four nights the crying was either extremely limited or nonexistent. Some people might think it's crazy or terrible, but I feel as though I was able to help my daughter sleep and feel better. I limit her to short periods of wakefulness (thirty to forty-five minutes usually), put her to bed early (5:30-6:30 P.M.), and let her cry it out when she needs to. She is now 11 weeks, sleeps twelve to fourteen hours each night, naps really well, and is just the happiest little girl. In addition, I am well rested, happy, and am able to give her my best self. I think you need to be comfortable and do what you believe is the right thing. But no, I don't think it's too early to let her cry it out. My opinion is to put her to bed in a dark, quiet room well fed with a clean diaper and close the door. Turn the baby monitor off and the TV up for twenty to thirty minutes and see what happens.

Resources for Soothing

Some families have vast resources to invest in soothing their babies, but other families are not so fortunate. Twenty percent of babies have colic and require much more soothing, and families with a colicky baby and limited resources to soothe might easily become overwhelmed and frustrated. The other 80 percent of babies are more easily soothed and usually do not overly stress their parents. So you want to pay attention to whether your child has colic or not, and take some time to reflect on how able you will be to enlist help to soothe your baby. It is often more than a one-parent job! If you have a baby who fusses and cries a lot and is difficult to console, and your available resources for soothing are limited, you might modify some of the plans you made before your child was born regarding a family bed or crib.

Consider a balance between the baby's disposition to express distress and the parents' capability to soothe their baby. Not only do babies vary in their expression, but parents also vary in their capability to soothe (page 218). The resources for parents' ability to soothe fussiness and crying and promote sleep in their baby include the following.

RESOURCES FOR PARENTS' ABILITY TO SOOTHE
- Father involvement versus absent father
- Agreements or disagreements between parents regarding child-rearing, such as breast- versus bottle-feeding or crib versus family bed
- Absence or presence of marital discord
- Absence or presence of intimacy between wife and husband
- Absence or presence of baby blues or postpartum depression
- Absence or presence of other children requiring attention
- Ease or difficulty in breastfeeding
- Absence or presence of medical problems in child, mother, father, or other children
- Number of bedrooms in the home
- Absence or presence of relatives, friends, or neighbors to help out
- Help or interference with sleep routines from grandparents
- Ability or inability to afford housekeeping help
- Ability or inability to afford child care help
- Absence or presence of financial pressures such as mother having to return to work soon

MANY NAPS

Immediately after the baby is born, you will see what people mean when they say "sleeping like a baby." For a few days, babies sleep almost all the time. They barely suck and normally lose weight during this time. (If your baby was born early, this very drowsy time might last longer; if your baby was born past the expected date of delivery, the drowsy period might be brief or nonexistent.)

A few days later, babies begin to wake up more. This increased wakefulness reflects the normal maturation of your baby's nervous system. I tell families that the brain wakes up after three or four days, just in time to catch the breast milk that is now available in ample amounts. The baby looks around more with wider eyes and is able to suck with more strength and for longer periods. Within days, the weight loss stops and a dramatic growth in weight, height, and head circumference begins. Also, slightly longer periods of wakefulness begin to appear after a few days. Although your baby is intently interested in you and is quickly able to recognize your face and voice, she is not yet curious about objects such as toys or mobiles. She does not appear to care about the general buzz or noises, colors, or other activities surrounding her, and therefore she falls asleep almost anywhere. The extremely fussy/colicky baby is not like this and appears to have difficulty falling asleep and staying asleep even at only several days of age. All babies gradually seem to become more aware of action, motion, voices, noises, vibrations, lights, wind, and so forth as they become more curious. At that point they often do not "sleep like a baby."

During the day, your baby will have a one- to two-hour window of wakefulness, and then become drowsy and want to go to sleep. Some parents mistakenly think that you must always keep the baby up for one to two hours before putting her to sleep. Remember, the one- to two-hour guideline is a ceiling, not a floor.

I discovered this window during my research on naps. Because most naps are quite brief, your baby may need to go back to sleep after being up for only thirty to ninety minutes. Other children might have long naps and can comfortably be up for an hour to two hours. Respect your baby's need to nap and avoid keeping her up too long.

Watch your baby closely for *drowsy signs*. If you soothe her during the beginning of drowsiness, most likely she will easily fall asleep. The exception is the extremely fussy/colicky baby, who might fall asleep, but not easily; these babies need longer and more complex soothing efforts to help them fall asleep. The other exception is during the evening fussy periods and especially around 6 weeks of age.

Here are some ways to note that your baby is becoming drowsy. Watch for the early signs of drowsiness—quieting of activity, less movement of the arms and legs, and sucking that may be weaker or slower. If your baby is over 6 weeks old, you may notice less socially responsive smiling, or she may be less engaging. This is the time to begin soothing to sleep. All babies become this way within one to two hours of waking.

You might miss signs of drowsiness if you are digitally distracted. If the intervals of wakefulness are too long because grandparents keep the new baby up too long or you run too many errands with her, then she gets keyed up (a second wind) and has difficulty self-soothing to sleep. Instead of thinking of overstimulation as very intense or active play, think of it as *an interval of wakefulness that is too long*. Don't beat yourself up if real-life circumstances occasionally or frequently interfere with brief intervals of wakefulness. It is a fact of modern life that daycare and nanny care have become more common. Thus, older infants and children are experiencing more missed naps, brief naps, or naps not in sync with circadian rhythms. What can be done about this? An extra-early bedtime partially compensates for poor-quality naps, and being vigilant about good-quality sleep on weekends helps keep your child well rested.

What happens if you miss this window of drowsiness? Your baby will become overtired if she cannot fall asleep because of too much stimulation around her. When you or your baby becomes overtired, the body is stressed. Chemical changes then occur to fight the fatigue, and this interferes with the ability to easily fall asleep and stay asleep—that is, the baby gets a second wind. Babies vary in their ability to self-soothe and deal with this stress, and parents vary in their ability to soothe their babies. Not all babies go bonkers if they are kept up a little too long. But you will have a more peaceful and better-sleeping baby if you respect her need to sleep again within one to two hours after waking. I consider this to be the beginning of teaching self-soothing for babies.

Teaching self-soothing starts with developing a sense of timing, so that you are trying to soothe your baby at the time when she is naturally getting drowsy before falling asleep. Some young babies will need dark and quiet environments to sleep well, and others will appear to be less sensitive to what is going on around them. Respect your baby's individuality and do not try to force her to meet your lifestyle. I like the analogy with feeding: We do not withhold food when our baby is hungry. We try to anticipate when she will be hungry, so that we will be somewhere calm where we can feed her. We do not feed her on the run. The same applies for sleeping.

If your newborn does not fall asleep, continue trying to soothe. Do not let her cry or ignore her. Mothers' reports of allowing their 4-week-olds to cry are described on page 187. Elsewhere, I might advise letting infants cry in order to teach them self-soothing skills, but newly born infants are a different matter. You cannot spoil a newborn. You cannot teach a newborn a crying habit.

Bedtime Routines and Bedtime Parenting

BEDTIME ROUTINES

Just as soothing helps your child feel safe and secure, bedtime routines help all children calm down before falling asleep, because both are associated with the natural state of relaxed drowsiness. As with soothing, bedtime routines should be started early, before sleepy signs change into overtired fussy signs. Older children and more regular babies will develop predictable sleep times, and these children might be "slept by the clock." Pick and choose from the following list based on your child's age and your personal preference. Try to follow the same sequence at all sleep times, because a consistent bedtime routine has been found to be a predictor of better sleep, including, specifically, fewer night wakings. Follow any routine that you feel comfortable with and stick with it. Don't worry if Mom and Dad have different routines. Your baby will learn to associate each routine with each parent.

BEDTIME ROUTINES

Before sleep times, reduce stimulation: less noise, dimmer lights,
    less handling, less playing, lower levels of activity.

The bedroom should be quiet, dark (use room-darkening shades),
    and warm, but not too warm.

Bathe.

Massage after the bath with smooth, gentle motions (page 183).

Dress for sleep.

Swaddle if it comforts and relaxes your baby; use a blanket warm
    from the clothes dryer for older children.

Lullaby, quiet singing, listening to music, or humming words, sounds,
    or phrases.

Rock.

Cuddle.

Feed, but do not rush in to feed again at the first sound your baby
    makes.

You may put down your baby drowsy but awake (this often fails for
    colicky babies and all 6-week-olds in the evening).

Read books to the baby.

Quiet play.

Say prayers.

Brush teeth.

After soothing and a bedtime routine, place your baby down to
sleep, and leave the room.

Staying in the room with your baby interferes with the development of self-soothing skills.

In addition to being consistent in your bedtime routines, try to cultivate patience, because it may take time for your child to get the message that this is not playtime. I would also add that, except for premature babies (for feeding) and trying to correct a sleep problem, you should never wake a sleeping baby.

Professor Jodi Mindell has recently published several papers regarding bedtimes. Bedtimes can be viewed as a daily routine to promote a variety of positive developmental outcomes such as improving your child's hygiene (bathing and brushing teeth), language development and literacy (reading, singing, or lullabies), positive mood, emotional-behavioral regulation, parent–child bonding or attachment (cuddling, rocking, or massage), and improving mother's mood and sleep quality. She studied over four hundred children 7–36 months old and compared half whose mothers followed their child's usual bedtime practice but were instructed to also institute a new nightly bedtime routine consisting of a bath, massage, and quiet activities (cuddling, singing, or lullaby). During the next two weeks, compared with those not receiving the bedtime routine instructions, the children experiencing the new bedtime routine fell asleep faster, had less wake time after falling asleep, and experienced fewer night wakings. Remarkably, these improvements in sleep developed over only *three days*!

In a separate study involving over ten thousand children (age 0–5) from thirteen countries, she asked how many times per week there was a bedtime routine. The striking results showed "that having a regular nightly bedtime routine is associated with improved sleep in young children, and that the more consistently a bedtime routine is instituted and the younger started the better." Furthermore, *as the bedtime routine increased in frequency, sleep improved more.* In other words, bedtime routines practiced every night produce the best improvements and, in a stepwise fashion, lower "doses" of bedtime routines produce lesser improvements. Improvements were an earlier bedtime, falling asleep faster, fewer night wakings, and increased sleep duration. So bedtime routines have powerful effects, especially if they are performed nightly or almost nightly.

Bedtime Routines and Early Bedtimes

I asked Professor Mindell about the bedtimes among those children who had a routine every night. She graciously did a detailed analysis that showed, among the almost five thousand children who had a bedtime routine every night, *those who had an earlier bedtime also had even longer nighttime sleep durations.* I think this is an important observation because if the bedtime is way too late, the power of a bedtime routine to help the child sleep better may be significantly diminished. Another way to look at this is to say that there are many benefits of bedtime routines, but as Professor Mindell told me, data from this study show that the "biggest driver of nighttime sleep duration is what time a child goes to bed." So. Bedtime routines are important, but *early bedtimes may be more helpful for longer, healthier sleep.*

Now, because data showing the importance of early bedtimes were not included in the published paper, a reader might not appreciate the possibility that parents who employ bedtime routines also put their child to sleep at night earlier than those who do not. In addition to bedtime routines and early bedtimes, there are studies describing how healthy sleep results from high maternal emotional availability at bedtime (page 195), parents leaving the room after the child is put down to sleep at night (page 175), and more involvement of the father (page 163). In some studies, the benefits include objective measurements of less time awake after sleep onset (page 91), or a higher proportion of total sleep occurring at night (page 71). However, it should be noted that while high maternal emotional availability at bedtime, parents leaving the room, and involvement of the father may be valuable for a variety of reasons, in many of these studies subjective parent reports of the *bedtime* or objective reports of *sleep onset* are not presented. Thus, as with bedtime routines, while each item might be worthwhile for different reasons, all these items might enhance sleep if they are associated with *earlier bedtimes.* There are many reports showing that early bedtimes are associated with longer sleep durations and fewer night wakings, creating better developmental outcomes, and there are some reports showing that early bedtimes are important *independent* of other sleep measurements in producing better outcomes (page 127). Remember, early bedtimes permit the sleeping child to enjoy more deep sleep occurring early in the sleep cycle, and more of this high-quality sleep might make a world of difference!

Additionally, although I discuss the importance of putting your child down to sleep drowsy but still awake to develop self-soothing skills when you come home from the hospital, after 6 weeks of age it appears that the success in doing so might be dependent upon having an early bedtime, before the child develops a second wind. Well, it is also possible that an early bedtime alone, without using the strategy of "drowsy but awake" at bedtime, will promote self-soothing skills *in the middle of the night* and reduce signaling and promote more consolidated, better-quality night sleep. Indeed, I published a case report in 1982 that proved that a new earlier bedtime could be established by awakening the child at 7:00 A.M. and not permitting naps to begin late in the afternoon. This new earlier bedtime produced a significant, abrupt, and rapid decrease in night waking. The parents did not change any other sleep behaviors or routines, so it is clear that this modification of the sleep schedule alone was beneficial.

BEDTIME PARENTING

Related to the notion of bedtime routines is the topic of bedtime parenting. Previously, I have discussed *what* a bedtime routine is and *when* to start it. Now we have information on *how* to do it. Because the data are objective and the concepts perhaps unfamiliar to most parents, I will share with you some of the details of the studies by Dr. Douglas Teti. He used in-home audio-videos and motion-sensing sleep recordings to objectively investigate how parents behave around bedtime and how their behavior affects children's sleep. Fathers were not included in these studies so it is not known how they may or may not have influenced the results. An important concept in his research is *emotional availability* (EA) of the mother at bedtime, which comprises four items:

1. *Sensitivity* ("rated high when the mother detected immediately, interpreted accurately, and responded promptly and appropriately to the infant's signals by fulfilling the infant's needs such as feeding, soothing, and diaper changing, but it was rated low when the mother did not respond to the infant's signals quickly, did not understand what the infant wanted, or her response did not reduce the infant's distress for a long time").

2. *Structuring* ("rated high when the mother engaged with the infant in bedtime routines in a quiet, soothing, and organized manner that gently induced the infant to sleep, but was rated low when the infant's bedtime was interrupted by activities unrelated to them or when they were left unattended for a long time").

3. *Nonintrusiveness* ("rated high when the mother did not initiate arousing activities with the baby or other family members, such as tossing the baby in the air, or yelling/talking loudly to the baby or family members, or did not insist that the baby fall asleep when the baby was not ready").

4. *Nonhostility* ("rated high when the mother did not display covert or overt impatience, frustration, or anger at bedtime").

Dr. Teti refers to EA as "parenting quality" at bedtime. In one study, he followed a group of eighty-two infants at 3, 6, and 9 months of age. He observed that mothers ranked high on EA had infants with lower bedtime and nighttime cortisol levels (indicating less stress) compared with infants whose mothers ranked low on EA.

Separately, he discusses "parenting practice" at bedtime. Parenting practice means:

1. Whether or not, after soothing and putting down the child, *the parent stays in the room until the child falls asleep* (page 175)
2. *How long the parent is in contact with the child,* such as for feeding or co-sleeping

When infants consistently fall asleep with their parents present, it is thought that they might not learn how to settle themselves to sleep on their own (self-soothing), so during the night, when a normal arousal occurs, they have difficulty returning to sleep unassisted.

Dr. Teti studied a group of infants 1–6 months old. At bedtime, "When mothers were more emotionally available (EA), infants were less distressed and slept more throughout the night. . . . Higher maternal EA in combination with *less* close contact at bedtime [parenting practice] was associated with more infant sleep across the night. . . . [T]here was evidence of infant-driven effects, as higher infant nighttime distress predicted lower EA at subsequent time points. . . . Finally, neither infant nighttime distress nor sleep predicted *parenting practices,* and thus there was no evidence supporting an infant-driven model of bedtime *parenting practices* [emphasis added]." So infant distress and sleep has an effect on parenting quality (EA) but not on parenting practice at bedtime.

The point is quite clear: It's not only *when* (appearance of drowsy signs), but also *how* (parenting quality plus parenting practice) you put your child to sleep makes a difference. But the power of good bedtime parenting (parenting quality plus parenting practice) is not equally apparent among all infants. Dr. Teti observed that high EA had a strong effect on infants rated high in "surgency," defined as enthusiastic positive affect (more expressive and warmer in interpersonal interactions, more smiles and laughter) and a weak effect on infants rated low in surgency or positive affect.

Some refer to this as a differential susceptibility based on *infant temperament*, and genetic studies support this notion that not all children will react the same to the environment in either a positive or negative fashion (page 86). For example, short sleep durations adversely affect infant temperament, but this is especially true if the infant has a specific genetic variant.

So we now have a clear picture of *when* (see "*Drowsy Signs,*" and *how* (parenting quality plus parenting practice) to put our children to sleep, but because not all children are the same, even when we have the *when* and the *how* spot-on, there is no guarantee that it will all be smooth sailing ahead! But the seas will be calmer if our children are better rested.

Bedtime parenting was examined in another study led by Burt Hatch, which was notable because it included randomization of children into control and intervention groups and objectively measured sleep duration. Expectant mothers were allocated to four groups:

Usual care (Control)
Additional support regarding Food, Activity, and Breastfeeding (FAB)
Advice on infant sleep (Sleep)
Both FAB and Sleep

Parents assigned to the Sleep interventions received a group education session during the pregnancy and a one-hour home visit by a trained nurse when the infant was around 3 weeks of age. An emphasis was placed on four strategies:

1. Putting the infant down to sleep when tired but still awake
2. Allowing the infant to fall asleep on her own (without touching or feeding her)

3. Providing a consistent environment for the infant to sleep in
4. Minimizing parents sleeping with their infants on the same surface

"An index relating to parent's consistent use of strategies to encourage infant sleep self-settling was developed from data when infants were 4 and 6 months of age. Child sleep self-control was measured at 3.5 years of age through a behavior rating scale [bedtime resistance, difficulty falling asleep, night wakings]." Objective recordings of night sleep duration were made at 1, 2, 3.5, and 5 years of age.

Compared with Controls, Sleep group parents' *consistent* use of bedtime sleep strategies at 4 and 6 months was associated with a decrease in child bedtime behavioral difficulties at 3.5 years and increased sleep durations from 1 to 5 years of age. "Notably, bedtime parent strategies *consistently* implemented acted as a mediating mechanism between the intervention and [better sleep] . . . *Consistent* use of appropriate bedtime strategies in *infancy* is an important factor that influences child sleep self-control *in later development* [emphasis added]."

So the take-home message is that early bedtimes, bedtime routines, emotional availability of the mother, and leaving the room after putting the baby down drowsy but awake help babies learn healthy sleep habits so that when they're older, they fall asleep easier and sleep longer.

Breastfeeding versus Formula, and Family Bed versus Crib

Because breastfeeding and a family bed often go together, the topics of how to feed your baby and where to put your baby to sleep are linked.

How you feed your baby and where you sleep with your baby might depend on many factors, including whether the baby is easy or difficult to soothe and whether you and your baby are well rested or not. Ask yourself these questions:

1. Do you spend a total of more than three hours per day soothing your baby to prevent crying? That is, when you add up the total amount of minutes spent walking, rocking, driving around in the car, swaddling, singing, humming, running water, offering the breast or bottle even when not hungry, using a pacifier, and so forth, does the total exceed three hours?
2. Do you behave this way more than three days per week?
3. Have you been doing this for more than three weeks?

If you answered yes to all three questions, then your baby has colic. These diagnostic criteria focus on the behavior of the infant. Because of your soothing efforts, there may be no crying, just endless fussing. Or she might sometimes cry anyway despite your soothing efforts. If your baby has colic, please stop here and skip ahead to chapter 6 to better understand the challenges you will be up against. If you answered no to some of the questions (and your baby is often consolable), but your baby fusses often, especially in the evening and especially around 6 weeks of age, then your baby has common fussiness.

Another, more recent, definition of colic focuses on the notion of *inconsolability,* which might reflect features within the infant and/or parental soothing skills. For this definition, the infant exhibits recurrent and prolonged periods of infant crying, fussing, or irritability reported by the caregiver that occurs without obvious cause and *cannot be prevented or resolved by caregivers.* These symptoms begin and end during the infant's first five months.

BREASTFEEDING VERSUS FORMULA

Breastfeeding is considered best for baby and mother. The mother's decision on how to feed her baby may be influenced by the support or lack thereof from her husband, her mother, or other family members, along with other issues such as prematurity, twins, or perinatal complications. However, many babies are formula-fed because of adoption, prematurity, or medical problems with the baby or mother. Bottles can contain expressed breast milk or formula, so "bottle-feeding" may include feeding breast milk or formula. Formula-fed babies grow up to be just as healthy as breastfed babies. Many studies have shown that breastfeeding does not prevent extreme fussiness/colic, and does not prevent or cause sleep problems. At night, breastfed babies are often fed more frequently than formula-fed babies, but it is not known whether this is caused by the breastfeeding mother responding more promptly to her baby's quiet sounds or whether breast milk is digested faster, causing the baby to wake up more often. In general, research has shown that sleep/wake rhythms evolve at the same pace whether the baby is breastfed or formula-fed, whether the baby is demand-fed or schedule-fed, or whether cereal is given in the bottle or by spoon. Some babies with a birth defect of the digestive system are fed continuously by vein or tube in the stomach. Because of the constant feeding, they are never hungry. These babies develop the same sleep/wake rhythms as all other babies. This is why I tell parents that "sleep comes from the brain, not the stomach." Although there are rare medical exceptions, changing formulas will not reduce fussiness/crying or promote better sleeping.

How Do You Know if Your Child Is Getting Enough Food?

Your baby's pediatrician will check her weight at each office visit, and seeing that weight gain will reassure you that your baby is getting enough food overall. But sometimes you might not be sure on a particular night or at a particular feeding whether she is really hungry. She will suck at the breast or bottle even when she is just fussy but not hungry, because sucking is soothing. There are three ways to tell if your baby is truly hungry at night:

1. *Pay attention to the suck-swallow pattern.* A hungry baby sucks, fills up her mouth, and swallows, so the pattern is suck-swallow, suck-swallow, suck-swallow, and so forth. A swallow usually follows almost every suck. A fussy baby in the middle of the night will have a different pattern: suck-suck-suck-swallow, suck-suck-suck-swallow. There will be many more sucks before each swallow.

2. *Offer a bottle immediately after breastfeeding in the middle of the night.* The well-fed breastfed baby will not take much from the bottle. If your baby takes a small volume slowly, this tells you that you have sufficient breast milk and your baby is not hungry even though she wants to suck more at the breast. If your baby takes a large volume quickly, this tells you that your breast milk supply is low. An exception might be a colicky baby who does rapidly suck down more (for soothing, not hunger) and then spits up.

3. *Once, have Dad offer a bottle instead of Mom breastfeeding in the middle of the night.* If your baby is truly hungry or thirsty, she will take a large volume quickly. If not, this tells you that your baby is up at night but not hungry.

It is important to resist the temptation to always feed your baby whenever she vocalizes at night, because this particular behavior partially or fully wakes your baby. This may cause fragmented sleep or encourage a night-crying habit whereby your baby learns to cry more frequently and louder at night for the pleasure of your company, not because she is hungry. This might not occur when the breastfeeding mother is bed sharing, because both she and her baby may be more asleep than awake at these frequent feedings (please see page 94 for why bed sharing is discouraged).

Of course, if your baby is not being fed enough, then she might be too hungry and fuss/cry or not sleep well. In this situation, the child will not be gaining weight, and some help will be needed to establish a better breast milk supply, or an evaluation made for medical problems that are causing poor weight gain. In my practice, I encourage first-time mothers to give a bottle of expressed breast milk or formula once per twenty-four hours beginning when their baby is 2–3 weeks old. A single bottle given at night is not a "gateway drug" that will hook your baby on bottles and interfere with breastfeeding. The single bottle allows fathers and other family members to have the pleasure of feeding the baby, as well as giving the mother a mini break once a day to rest and allow for the healing of cracked or painful nipples. It also gives the parents the chance to have a date to recharge their batteries. Fathers can be more helpful during fussy/crying periods or middle-of-the-night feedings to allow mothers a little more sleep.

Some experienced mothers, who have previously breastfed successfully, give the single bottle sooner. They have confidence in their ability to breastfeed and either give formula in the hospital or start pumping sooner. They know that the single bottle does not confuse the child or interfere with breastfeeding. They instruct the maternity nurses to give one, and only one, bottle of formula in the nursery and bring the baby to them at all other times for breastfeeding.

The reason the bottle is given once every twenty-four hours is to keep the baby adapted to taking the bottle. Some babies do well with less frequent bottles, but others will reject all bottles if days go by without having had one. A popular view is that the single bottle will cause your baby to prefer the bottle going forward and not suck at the breast because less energy is required to suck from a bottle. Therefore, giving bottles will cause "nipple confusion" and prevent successful breastfeeding. There is no scientific support for this opinion.

FAMILY BED VERSUS CRIB

Our goal is a well-rested family, and a family bed—sometimes described as co-sleeping or bed sharing—may be something you have considered (again, please see page 94 for why co-sleeping is discouraged). The decision to sleep with your baby might be made before the child is born, because this is what you want for your family. You might decide that unrestricted breastfeeding day and night, always caring for your baby, and sleeping with your baby at night, or day and night, will promote a tighter or more sensitive bond between you and your baby. Parents then begin the practice of co-sleeping as soon as the baby is born. Researchers use the term *early co-sleepers* to describe these children. Alternatively, you might not have thought about or not really wanted to have a family bed, but you discovered that because your baby was so fussy/colicky, or because she grew older and not sleeping well, the only way anyone got any rest was to sleep with your baby in your bed. Researchers use the term *reactive co-sleepers* to describe these children. Scientific studies have shown that co-sleeping in infancy is often associated with the later development of sleep problems. I suspect that the majority of these problems occur among former reactive co-sleepers. In other words, some parents find that the family bed is a short-term and partial solution to sleep problems, and the sleep problem continues long after the child has been moved to her own crib or bed because she was not given the opportunity to learn self-soothing skills.

Many families in different cultures frequently sleep together in a family bed for all or part of the night. By itself, this is neither good nor bad. Studies in the United States suggest that the family bed might encourage or lead to a variety of emotional stresses within the child; opposite results were found in studies conducted in Sweden. This probably reflects differences in social attitudes toward nudity, bathing, and sexuality. Think of it as a family style, one that does not necessarily reflect or cause emotional or psychological problems in parents and children.

One exception might be the situation where the infant consistently is bed sharing or room sharing during the first twelve months. In a study using video recorders and objective measures of sleep on the mother, father, and infant at 1, 3, 6, 9, and 12 months of infant age, Dr. Douglas Teti made the following observations regarding these families. Mothers', but not infants' nor fathers', sleep was disrupted in persisting co-sleeping arrangements. Mothers who were persistent co-sleepers (co-sleeping for the entire 12 months), compared with mothers who never co-slept and those who stopped co-sleeping by 6 months, reported heightened marital and co-parenting distress. Fathers did not report heightened marital or co-parenting distress. Among these mothers, because the distress was reported as early as 1 month, "persistent cosleeping throughout the infant's first year, particularly in a culture in which persistent cosleeping is not supported, may be symptomatic of preexisting heightened marital and family stress that is evident very early in the life of the infant." When someone is not getting enough sleep, either parent or child, the family bed can reflect or cause marital or family problems. By the age of 1–2 years, sleeping together is often associated with night waking. Once there is a well-established habit, the child is unwilling to go to or return to her own bed.

So if you want to enjoy a family bed, fine. But understand that your cuddling in bed together may make any future changes in sleep arrangements difficult to execute. Remember, while it sounds like an easy solution to a baby's sleep problems, you may wind up with a twenty-four-hour child even when she gets older.

In contrast, many families use a family bed overnight only during the first few months, then shift the baby to her own crib for overnight sleep. Then at 5:00 or 6:00 A.M., parents might bring their older infant or child into their bed for a limited period of warm cuddling.

Sleeping with your baby might include both day and night or just night, and all night or part of the night, in your bed or using a small crib attached to your bed, with other children in your bed or other children in your bedroom but not in your bed. All of these variations are collectively called "family bed." In many cultures, families sleep together because of tradition or a limited number of bedrooms. It is rare in Japan or in traditional or tribal societies for children to sleep apart from their parents. There is a great appeal for sleeping together. A powerful word to describe soothing is *nesting*, and this easily brings forth the image of creating a nest for your baby in your bed.

However, it is important to note that both the US Consumer Product Safety Commission and the American Academy of Pediatrics actively discourage the family bed because of the risk of entrapment between the mattress and the structures of the bed (headboard, footboard, side rails, and frame), the wall, or adjacent furniture. There is the hazard of suffocation or overlying by an adult who is in an unusually deep sleep caused by alcohol, mind-altering drugs, or a medical condition. Also, soft surfaces or loose covers can cause suffocation. They point out that there is no evidence that bed sharing protects against sudden infant death syndrome. Nor is there any evidence that bed sharing prevents extreme fussiness/colic.

So if you want to use a family bed, try to make it a safe environment by not drinking or taking drugs at night and by making sure your baby is always sleeping on her back. Also, fill in the spaces between the bed and any walls or furniture and eliminate loose bedding.

SOLID FOODS AND FEEDING HABITS

Big meals make us sleepy, so shouldn't solids make babies sleep better? Wrong. Feeding rhythms do not alter the pattern of waking and sleeping.

Sleeping for long periods at night is not related to the method of feeding, whether it be breast or bottle. The studies I think are the most convincing involve comparing the development of sleep/wake rhythms of infants fed on demand with those who are continuously fed intravenously because of birth defects involving their stomachs or intestines. The babies who were fed on demand cycled between being hungry and being full. The other babies were never allowed to become hungry. Objective recordings in sleep laboratories show that there were no sleep differences between these groups of infants. Other studies involve the introduction of solid foods; they all show that solid food, such as cereal, does not influence nighttime sleeping patterns. No well-controlled published studies have ever shown that the method of feeding (breast milk versus formula, or scheduled feedings versus demand feedings) or the introduction of solids affects sleep.

One study involved mixed breast- and formula-fed infants who were randomly given a bedtime cereal feeding either at 5 weeks of age (early group) or at 4 months of age (late group). "The timing of the introduction of cereal in the bedtime bottle was not related to total hours of sleep, number of sleeping periods, longest duration of sleep, or the time interval in which sleeping occurred . . . no relationship was found between sleeping through the night and introduction of cereal at 5 weeks vs 4 months of age." Another study looked at exclusively breastfed infants, some of whom received solid foods at 3 months of age. They observed that those who received solids slept longer and woke less often; in addition, fewer parents believed their children's sleep habits were a serious problem at 6 months of age. Neither study objectively measured sleep, so which is correct? Children who are *room sharing* (more common with exclusive breastfeeding) do not sleep as well as children who are in a *separate room* (page 95). Perhaps in the second study, more of those children who received solids at 3 months of age were moved to a separate room and that is the real reason they seemed to sleep better. The researchers did not control for sleep location.

Some studies, however, do indicate that formula-feeding is more popular than breastfeeding among mothers who are more restrictive. Mothers who feed their babies formula tend to be more interested in controlling their infant's behavior and like being able to see the number of ounces of formula given at each feeding. These parents are more likely to perceive night waking in a problem/solution framework and consider the social wants of the child instead of nutritional needs. In contrast, the nursing mother, perhaps more sensitive to the health benefits of nursing, might respond to night waking more often or more rapidly because she perceives herself as primarily responding to her infant's need for nourishment. After a while, of course, the child learns to enjoy this nocturnal social contact. Over time, the baby learns to expect attention when she wakes.

This explains why there is no difference in night waking between breast- and formula-fed infants at 4 months, but by 6–12 months night waking is more of an issue among breastfed babies. Babies learn quickly!

The bottom line is that cereal does not appear to make babies sleep better. Formula may appear thicker than breast milk, but both contain the same twenty calories per ounce. Giving formula to breastfed babies or weaning them also will not directly cause longer sleeping at night, although it is possible that attitudes toward breastfeeding may indirectly foster a night-waking habit.

Earlier Bedtime Around 6 Weeks Old

Around 6 weeks after the due date, a baby's brain develops the capacity for specific social smiling, more calmness in the evening, longer blocks of sleep at night (four to six hours), and an earlier bedtime. All of these wonderful changes will occur independent of parenting. Six weeks is the time when moms start to get more night sleep and maybe get their sanity back! So hang in there.

After 6 weeks of age, it is possible to inadvertently put your baby

to sleep past the time of her biological drowsiness, with the unwanted consequences of accumulating a sleep deficit. The biological bedtime is based on a night sleep circadian rhythm and is
signaled by changes in the baby's mood and behavior in the late afternoon and early evening. Watching her is more important than
watching a clock. Synchronize your soothing to sleep with her
emerging drowsy cues before fatigue signs appear (page 167). Catch
the wave. Digital distraction might cause you to miss her emerging
subtle drowsy cues. A parent returning home from work might
mask the baby's drowsy signs with intense social stimulation. So
watch her carefully when she is more on her own. Her bedtime is
not a fixed clock time, because of her variability in daytime sleep.
Occasionally keeping your baby up late for special events is fine, but
if her behavior suffers the next day, please ask yourself whether it
was worth it. If she is frequently allowed to stay up too late, the ill
effects of *cumulative sleep loss* will definitely appear.

I have had many sleep consults with parents of children around
3–4 months of age in which I am told that their child slept well until
about 6–8 weeks. Thereafter, the child had trouble falling asleep or
staying asleep at night. I always ask these parents to remember how
their child looked in the evening before bedtime, before the sleep
problem began, around 2 months of age. I ask them: "Do you think
your child could have gone to sleep a little bit earlier?" The answer
is always yes.

One parent put it this way: "The early bedtime is a non-negotiable
component of healthy sleep training. If you want your child to sleep
soundly, wake up well rested, you have to marry the idea of an early
bedtime."

Naturally, all parents want to spend time with their children in
the evening. But I encourage families to try to avoid a bedtime that
is chronically too late and instead focus on morning activities with
their baby: bathing, changing, feeding, and playing. Parents are also
encouraged to go to bed earlier themselves so they feel less rushed in
the morning. Sadly, this means that some parents will not see their

baby when they return home from work. But they will have the opportunity to thoroughly enjoy their calm baby every morning. And because the family is well rested during the week, weekends are relaxed and fun.

An early bedtime might be resisted by parents because they do not appreciate the power of healthy sleep or that sleep problems are directly caused by a too-late bedtime. Therefore, I would tell both parents that one possible benefit of an earlier bedtime was that their child might grow taller due to increased exposure to growth hormone, which is secreted only during sleep and especially before midnight (page 133).

My impression is that sleep problems caused by bedtimes that are too late are now more common than colic-related sleep problems. Some modern reasons for a bedtime that is too late include more dual-career parents returning home late and more parents who do not notice the baby's drowsiness in the early evening because they are distracted by digital devices.

For 80 percent of parents, sleep training is a process of helping your baby learn to sleep that *never requires you to let your baby cry*. But for 20 percent of all parents, their colicky baby needs constant soothing during the first few months to prevent crying and to encourage some sleeping. For these colicky babies, the phrase "start as you mean to go on" does not make sense regarding "drowsy but awake," but you can still try for earlier bedtimes at 6 weeks of age.

Do not worry during the colicky phase if, despite your best efforts, you think your baby is not getting enough sleep. Do whatever works to maximize sleep and minimize crying for the first few months, even though she may later be described as parent-soothed and lacking in self-soothing skills. It is extremely important for parents of colicky babies to get help and take breaks without guilt. Around 3–4 months of age, parents of colicky babies should begin to change gears and employ methods such as check and console, graduated extinction, or extinction to allow their baby to learn self-soothing skills (chapter 5). Actually, *colic* is ending around 2 months of age in 50 percent of infants, so you could give it a try even then, with the understanding that if you see no improvement in one or two nights, you abandon the effort and try again in a month or two. The well-rested post-colic baby may make this transition with little or no crying, as described in my book *Your Fussy Baby*. The somewhat sleep-deprived post-colic baby may cry during this transition. Crying is hard, but sleeplessness is harder.

Colicky babies who fail to make this transition from parent-soothed to learning self-soothing at 3–4 months are at risk of accumulating a sleep debt and becoming chronically sleep-deprived. If you think that your post-colic child is short on sleep, try to fix her sleep problem around or soon after 3–4 months of age.

On the other hand, even for the colicky baby, there is nothing wrong with trying an earlier bedtime around 6 weeks of age. This is tricky because the colicky baby might not show drowsy signs. So if you want to try this, start on a Saturday when both parents are home to support each other and you are able to try a really early bedtime. Label her last nap as the sleep period that starts between 4:00 and 5:00 P.M. When she wakes up from this nap, depending on its duration, plan for a bedtime thirty to ninety minutes later. Then attempt to put her to sleep drowsy but awake even though she may be much more drowsy than awake! If she cries hard, pick her up immediately; otherwise you might decide to leave her alone for a short period of time to see if she nods off. Repeat this plan on Sunday night, and based on what happens and your own feelings, you might decide to abandon this effort completely and wait it out until she is 2–4 months of age—or you might want to try again after a couple of weeks.

WHEN THE BEDTIME IS EARLY AND SELF-SOOTHING IS ENCOURAGED

Dr. Ian Paul studied almost three hundred children in their homes at 3, 16, 28, and 40 weeks and at a research center at 1 year. Half of them received detailed information at 3 weeks regarding "the importance of consistent, short bedtime routines that do not finish with feeding, early bedtimes, and the importance of self-soothing to sleep [at bedtime] and after night wakings." The other half received information on home safety and prevention of SIDS. All of the infants who had received the advice regarding sleep had longer sleep durations at night (*twenty-two to thirty-five minutes,* at different ages). However, among those infants receiving advice regarding sleep who also had an *early bedtime* (before 8:00 P.M.), compared with the control group, the difference in sleep duration was more dramatic: *fifty-seven* minutes at 16 weeks and *seventy-eight* minutes at 40 weeks! So it appears that the benefits of an early bedtime and learning self-soothing are *additive.* Also, at 16 weeks, those infants with an early bedtime plus self-soothing compared with those with a later bedtime who did not self-soothe, woke and fed half as often! "Across study groups, self-soothing [allowing infants to fall asleep without being held, rocked, or fed] and earlier bedtimes predicted fewer night wakings, fewer nighttime feeds, and less time awake at night."

WHEN THE BEDTIME IS TOO LATE

What occurs when children are allowed to fall asleep too late at night? They wake up short of sleep in the morning in a state of higher neurological arousal that in turn makes it harder or even impossible for them to nap well. The consequences of not napping well are that by the end of the day a child's sleep tank is empty (the witching hour, page 42) and she is in an even higher state of arousal, which makes it even more difficult for her to easily fall asleep and stay asleep at night. A vicious cycle is generated.

In contrast, an *early bedtime* permits long naps to occur because the child wakes in a lower state of neurological arousal. It is easier for parents to catch the wave of drowsy signs, and there is no witching hour. It becomes a *virtuous* cycle: Sleep begets sleep.

Thus, begins the long arc of *sleep begets sleep*, from infancy to adolescence and beyond.

Parents might not appreciate that bedtime battles, long latency to sleep (time needed to fall asleep), or night waking result from a bedtime that is chronically too late. Of course, the child eventually crashes late at night. But this bedtime is preceded by an unhealthy state for the child, stressful interactions with her, stressful interactions as a couple, and stress for each parent as an individual.

Sometimes naps are very long and late (say, 1:00–4:00 P.M.) because the bedtime is too late; this makes a witching hour less likely but also makes a reasonably early bedtime difficult to achieve. Also, the child's sleep deprivation at the end of the day may be masked by parents returning home from work and playing with her. Some parents do not believe that their child's bedtime is too late, because when they moved the late bedtime from 9:00 P.M. to 8:00 P.M., they saw no benefit; but what these parents fail to appreciate is that their baby was starting to get drowsy around 7:00 P.M., so a second wind had already developed by 8:00. Obviously, watching your child closely for drowsy signs in the late afternoon and early evening is more valuable than watching the clock. If this is impossible due to the parents' work schedule, have a trustworthy caretaker look for the signs, or the parents themselves can do it on weekends, where there is more time.

Protect Naps Around 3–4 Months of Age

As your baby becomes more aware of her environment, she is less likely to sleep well in brightly lit or noisy places in the stroller. A goal is to use her emerging nap rhythms as an aid to obtain long periods of deep day sleep. Nap rhythms begin to emerge around 3–4 months of age. Now parents have the opportunity to "catch the wave" of developing drowsiness and synchronize their soothing to a drowsy-but-awake state with the wave before it crashes into a second wind. The midmorning nap becomes more regular before the midday nap. Typically, the approximate times are around 9:00 A.M. and between 12:00 and 2:00 P.M. An additional nap or naps occur in the late afternoon or early evening. The midmorning and midday naps may be brief at first, but between 4 and 6 months of age they become more predictable and longer, so that each is one to two hours long. Often there is one late-afternoon nap that may not occur every day and is usually briefer than the midmorning and midday naps.

After 3–6 months of age, it is possible to inadvertently put your baby to sleep for a nap before or past the time of her biological drowsiness, with the unwanted consequence of accumulating a sleep deficit from no naps or poor-quality naps. Please remember that good-quality naps are those that occur during the biological rhythm of daytime drowsiness, and naps while you are outside and in motion might be less restorative than motionless naps at home or in a quiet park.

One parent wrote, "My 4-month-old is still getting the kinks out of cycles, and so I am starting to go by the clock more for his midday nap. But I am still going by sleep cues for the midmorning nap."

No Television or Other Digital Media Devices in the Bedroom

Having a television in your child's bedroom is an invitation for sleep problems. A nationally representative 2007 survey showed that 18 percent of children under 2 years of age had a television in their bedroom. This number rose to 43 percent for 3- and 4-year-olds and to a whopping 75 percent for 5- and 6-year-olds. If these statistics are true, and there is little reason to doubt them, an entire generation of children is at risk of the serious developmental and other health-related problems that cluster around the failure to learn proper sleep habits at a young age. Much attention has been focused recently on the subject of childhood obesity, and rightly so, but our modern lifestyle is contributing to another epidemic, one less visible, perhaps, than obesity, but no less pernicious in the long run.

Limit Screen Time

In the United Kingdom, 75 percent of children age 6–36 months use a touchscreen on a daily basis for about twenty-four minutes with increasing touchscreen use associated with decreasing nighttime sleep. Children between 2 and 4 years or 6 and 9 years with longer periods of television viewing had shorter sleep durations. Among children 11–12 years, increased screen-based media time was associated with poor sleep outcomes. One study of over five hundred 5-year-olds highlighted the fact that when electronic devices are in the child's bedroom, parental restriction partially alleviated the harmful effects.

A recent study, by Professor Przybylski, analyzed a large sample (50,212) of American children 6 months–17 years old and concluded that increased digital screen time was associated with more inconsistent bedtimes and shorter durations of sleep. Children who followed the older (2010) American Academy of Pediatric guidelines (no screen time under age 2 years and restriction to fewer than 2 hours each day for older children) slept for an average of *twenty* additional minutes compared with children who did not follow these guidelines.

A school-based forty-minute sleep education workshop and a two-week intervention phase where 12- to 19-year-olds were asked to stop using screens after 9:00 P.M. produced a post-intervention objective earlier sleep onset and increased total sleep duration. The increased sleep duration resulted in improved daytime vigilance.

Prevention Versus Treatment of Sleep Problems

There sometimes appears to be a contradiction about whether or not to let your child cry. For the 80 percent of babies who have common fussiness, if the parents have ample resources for soothing, sleep solutions that involve *no crying*—such as starting early to teach self-soothing, utilizing many hands (that is, enlisting the help of the father and others), putting the baby down drowsy but awake, providing the opportunity for many naps, feeding at night only when hungry, instituting bedtime routines, starting an earlier bedtime around 6 weeks of age, and protecting naps around 3–4 months of age—should work to *prevent* sleep problems. A few of this group of common fussy babies (5 percent of this group or four babies out of a hundred unselected babies) do become very overtired 4-month-olds. When you try to treat or correct the sleep problem, some crying might occur. However, in this group, improvements in sleep patterns and in the child are often dramatic and rapid.

For the 20 percent of babies with extreme fussiness or colic, however, if the parents have enormous resources for soothing, sleep solutions that involve no crying—such as always holding your baby, always promptly responding, and soothing your baby as long as needed to induce sleep—might work to *prevent* sleep problems. But about 27 percent of these extremely fussy/colicky babies (or five babies out of a hundred unselected babies) do become very overtired 4-month-olds. *Treatment* to correct the sleep problem might involve more crying, and improvements in sleep patterns and in the child are often slow and not dramatic. This is especially hard for parents because they have already endured four months of sleep deprivation associated with the child's constant fussiness, crying, and not sleeping.

Some parents allow their child to cry to help her sleep before 4 months of age (see page 187, and chapters 5–7). Perhaps they started to encourage self-soothing when their baby was several weeks old, saw improvement, and wanted to quickly end the sleep deprivation that they and their child have experienced. Another example is the mother who has to return to work and desperately wants to see if her child will sleep better at night with less attention. Another example is the exhausted and overwhelmed mother who is becoming depressed or getting angry or resentful toward her baby. Under these and similar circumstances, I usually try to enlist the father to help his wife put the baby to sleep, to feed and soothe the baby at night, and to try to give the mother a well-earned break by making her go somewhere for several hours or a night to get some uninterrupted sleep. Obviously, these suggestions are impractical for some families. Nevertheless, the instructions are to give the child less attention at night, perhaps feeding only twice at night, and ignoring crying for either brief or long periods of time, and to do this for only four or five nights. Sometimes the crying quickly diminishes, especially in the child who had common fussiness. Sometimes the crying does not decrease, especially in the child who had extreme fussiness/colic, and the plan is abandoned. Parents then resort to whatever method maximizes sleep and minimizes crying until the child is older.

Parent Issues or Barriers That May Make Prevention or Treatment of Sleep Problems More Challenging

Parents can *prevent* sleep problems in their children by encouraging them to learn self-soothing skills. Some parents find this endeavor to be fairly straightforward, especially if their child has an easy temperament. Others struggle to accomplish this, especially if their child has a more difficult temperament. Putting aside the issue of *infant temperament* for now, you might ask why it is that some parents appear to find the teaching of self-soothing fairly manageable, while others find it an ongoing, frustrating challenge. In fact, allowing their child to learn self-soothing skills is simply too tough for some parents, and they give up completely. The short answer is that parents vary enormously in their ability to restore a calm balance to their lives after the baby is born (page 190), assuming that their lives were reasonably stable beforehand.

Imagine an idealized family in which there were no complications around the delivery for baby and mother. The marriage is strong, both parents are actively involved in parenting and agree on how to care for their child, there is no postpartum depression or baby blues, there is only the one child, breastfeeding is easy, there are no medical problems in the family, extra bedrooms are available for the child and those relatives and friends who want to help, there is adequate housekeeping and child care assistance, and the mother is under no financial pressure to return to work soon. In this lucky family, we might say that the parents have many resources to support them in their effort to teach self-soothing skills to their baby. Of course, most of us are not so fortunate! But even these parents might find themselves faced with unanticipated real-life challenges that would interfere with their ability to teach their child self-soothing skills. Job pressures, family emergencies, distractions large and small: All these and more can cause parents to overlook the subtle signs of drowsiness in their baby, and thus miss the window of opportunity to reinforce the baby's natural sleep rhythms.

But not to worry. We all can muddle through in our efforts to help our baby learn self-soothing skills, and most of us usually do, even though there may be some setbacks. Take heart! It might be three steps forward and one step back, but with patience and reasonable consistency the reward of a well-rested family is within reach.

The greater your resources to soothe your baby during the first few months, and the better you are able to become attuned to your baby's changing sleep needs, the more likely your baby will sleep well during the first four months. That, in turn, will help you *prevent* sleep problems from developing after four months.

Now, if you are like most parents, you do not have an ideal soothing support system, so there are likely to be moments during the first few months when your child might become more irritable and fussy and cry more because, despite your best efforts, she becomes overtired. Don't let these frustrating occasions get you down. Stick with the overall plan. Perseverance pays off in the long run, but if you give up, your infant will not learn the self-soothing skills essential to preventing later sleep problems from emerging.

If you have the misfortune to be dealing with a colicky infant, who appears to have less ability to soothe herself, your infant is likely to become mostly parent-soothed during the first few months. That is inevitable, and there is no reason to beat yourself up because of it. But after four months, even the colicky baby will more easily learn how to independently fall asleep and stay asleep. That is the time to start teaching self-soothing skills.

Parenting is the hardest work there is because there is no instruction manual that applies to all families. Not only that, but again and again, just when you think you've gotten the hang of it, your child changes and you have to start all over again. But if your baby sleeps well, you sleep well. Then not only will you be better able to figure out a plan that is a good fit for your family, you will be more adaptable to making changes in that plan as your baby changes.

Treatment of a sleep problem is more difficult when parents lack the resources that would have otherwise helped them teach self-soothing skills to their baby in the first few months. But sometimes there are parent issues or barriers that may make prevention and treatment of sleep problems more challenging. They make the hard work of parenting even harder. Some of these issues might be sensitive or highly personal matters that really could get in the way of your ability to do what is best for your child. Sometimes these barriers are only speed bumps that slow down the process of helping your child sleep better. However, if they are major roadblocks, consider professional counseling before working on your child's sleep problem. In such cases, you cannot help your baby until you help yourself.

What do I mean by speed bumps or roadblocks? Here are some examples.

Parents Lack Information or Tools

Your child does not come with a parenting manual. Starting in infancy or early childhood, parents may have unrealistic expectations or misunderstandings regarding age-appropriate sleep needs and sleep schedules. Or parents do not appreciate the benefits of healthy sleep and the harm caused by sleep deprivation in their children. Parents may be misguided or unaware regarding how to set limits, discipline, or socialize their children. Even if they have the right attitude, they may lack the proper techniques or tools and so become paralyzed or inconsistent.

Working Parents' Guilt, Exhaustion, or Absence

Parents may feel guilty because they are not available or do not want to be available to their child. So they give in to whatever their child wants. Or, selfishly, they feel that their child has to adapt to their work schedule and stay up late at night. A parent might truly believe that it is more important for the child to spend time late at night with her mother or father than it is for her to get more sleep from an earlier bedtime. Keeping a child up too late is more common with a parent who works outside the home, because he or she is not present to see the overtired child of late afternoon but instead sees only the child running on the fumes of a second wind. Sheer exhaustion from the demands of work may prevent the parent from being persistent and consistent. Too often, because of fatigue from work, the parent simply surrenders whenever the child cries. Sometimes the problem is neither guilt nor exhaustion but simply absence. Many modern parents do not do a lot of parenting. Because they spend so much time at work, they heavily rely on daycare or nannies. They are in denial or do not see the seriousness of the problem. Fathers especially, who are often less involved in child care than mothers, tend to say dismissively, "She'll outgrow it" or "It's not a big deal."

Bad Marriage

Three themes frequently occur here. The first is that one parent wants the child for support and love and thus becomes overly permissive in order to keep the child allied with him or her. This alliance maintains the parent's self-esteem. In the extreme version, one parent seeks the child's exclusive love as a means of expressing resentment or anger toward his or her spouse; in these cases, the child becomes a pawn in a struggle between mother and father. The second recurring theme is a control issue. A parent arrogantly asserts that he or she is right no matter what and knows best, end of story. There is no compromise in child raising. No shared philosophy. Just "my way or the highway." The third theme is lack of communication. The parents are unable to communicate effectively with each other to develop a practical plan that they can consistently implement. Thus they are constantly at loggerheads.

In a study of more than seven thousand children between 1 and 2 years of age, researchers compared those who frequently woke during the night with those who slept through the night. Among those who frequently woke during the night, the parents, usually mothers, were more likely (compared with the parents of infants who slept through the night) to *immediately go to their child when they heard a cry in order to prevent further crying*. These mothers were more likely to describe themselves as more irritable in general and "out of control." A sign of family tension was that these mothers were unable to confide in their husbands.

Parent Has Abandonment Issues

Because they had bad relations with their own parents, new parents might desperately want their child to like them. New parents might feel that their parents were not in tune with their feelings as a child, so they want to be very sensitive to and always address their child's feelings. They want to be their child's best friend. They do not want their child to feel hurt as they did when they were children. This leads to giving in to their child's every demand. A variation is that the parent does not want to break the child's spirit or damage her self-esteem. In these cases, parents are projecting onto their child, seeing their child less as a unique individual than as a "do-over" for unresolved issues from their own childhoods.

Parent Has Authority Issues

Some parents do not feel comfortable enforcing rules and communicating authority. This could be for a variety of reasons. Some are not comfortable with telling anyone what to do; they would rather ask for help. Others might have a "live and let live" philosophy and not want to enforce rules. Still others behave as if rules do not apply to them; because they act irresponsibly and cannot say no to themselves (with illicit drug use, for example), they cannot say no to their child. In the extreme version, a parent wants to be rebellious but cannot, and so he or she gets some gratification in seeing the child being rebellious.

Family Stress Issues

Parents facing money worries, job pressures and responsibilities, the illness of a loved one, or other sources of stress often do not have the energy to establish routines, plan events, or create schedules such as sleep times. In such cases, family life is chaotic, lurching from crisis to crisis. The parents are reactive instead of proactive; they respond emotionally instead of thoughtfully. These parents are not necessarily overindulgent; instead, they are overly inconsistent.

Parent Has Undiagnosed Anxiety Disorder, Depression, Attention Deficit Hyperactivity Disorder (ADHD), Bipolar Disorder, or Insomnia (pages 146 and 410)

When a person is sleep-deprived, the symptoms associated with these conditions can worsen. In this setting, education and coaching to help solve a sleep problem may fail because of the parent's significant unrecognized or untreated mental health issues. Adult

ADHD occurs equally in mothers and fathers. But problems regarding parenting are especially prominent if the mother is affected, because she is the one who is usually expected to organize schedules and routines such as regular bedtimes and naps.

Studies on night awakenings in infants sometimes focus on the role of *maternal depression*. One possibility is that children's sleep problems cause depression in the mother; it has been suggested (page 146) that by helping your child sleep better, you are less likely to become exhausted with sleep deprivation and/or frustrated with your child's sleep problems, and thus you are less likely to develop symptoms of depression. Your child's sleep patterns are always changing, so there are many opportunities, employing different strategies, to help her sleep better.

The alternative possibility is that maternal depression might cause sleep problems in the child. This is an extremely important consideration because, if true, the possible stability of maternal depression, which might worsen with sleep deprivation, might impair a mothers' ability to help her child sleep well throughout her entire childhood. Studies on this subject agree on some points and disagree on others. Therefore, it is not easy to give a short summary. So instead, I am going to present a few studies in detail for your understanding and motivation to seek help, if needed. Please skip the remainder of this section if this topic does not apply to you.

If maternal depression causes infant sleep problems, how does it occur? An extensive study, published in 2012, by Dr. Marsha Weinraub evaluated risk factors for nighttime sleep awakenings between 6 and 36 months of age. The study identified the following risk factors: being a boy, having a more difficult temperament, being breast-fed (being nursed to sleep), having a more *depressed mother,* and greater maternal sensitivity. Maternal sensitivity was measured by videotaping mother–child interactions in a semi-structured play activity. Maternal sensitivity means that, in Dr. Weinraub's words, "rather than allow infants to self-soothe and return to sleep on their own, parents who respond to awakenings with attempts to comfort or feed may interfere with their infant's growing ability to self-soothe and return to sleep independently. Parent responsiveness to infant night awakening may reinforce infants' signaling behavior following awakening and teach them to expect parental interventions. Alternatively, a lack of parental responsiveness can eventually . . . extinguish the signaling behaviors. Findings support this notion. *Feeding after awakening* [even when the child was not hungry] was the factor most strongly associated with infants not sleeping through the night at 5 months, and *parental presence until sleep onset* was the factor most strongly associated with sleep awakening at 17 and 29 months [emphasis added; also, pages 175, 194, and 223)]." The lead researcher in the study said, "The best advice is to put infants to bed at a regular time every night, allow them to fall asleep on their own [that is, put them down drowsy but awake] and *resist the urge to respond right away to awakenings* [emphasis added]." Contrary to what was seen in other studies, "infant-mother attachment measures were not related to these sleep awakenings . . . despite our attempt to use measures of attachment security and separation distress." These identical results of unnecessary attending to their child at night were found in another study of maternal depression.

A second study by Dr. Douglas Teti investigated the relationship between maternal depressive symptoms and their children's sleep issues. Because these researchers discovered the maternal behavior by which maternal depressive symptoms affect infant sleep, I wish to present this study in detail. The researchers documented what the mother was actually doing and not doing by placing multiple cameras in the home and child's bedroom:

> In the context of infant sleep, mothers who harbor *cognitions* [habitual thoughts and beliefs] that their infant will feel abandoned if they are not by the infant's side during the night or that their infant will go hungry if not fed (even when the infant is *not distressed*) may be more

likely to spend more time with their infants at bedtime and at night and in turn *awaken their infant more frequently* or *keep them awake longer* than mothers who do not harbor such *cognitions*. . . . Mothers reporting higher *depressive* symptoms [were much more likely to] not have a calming bedtime routine for their infant. Prior to the infants' bedtime, these mothers had the television on, allowed older children to play rough/make loud noises near the infant, appeared insensitive to the infant's needs (e.g., hunger), and *kept their infants awake after the infant appeared ready for sleep*. . . . Mothers with *elevated depressive symptoms* and *worries about infant nighttime needs* were more likely . . . to be hyper-responsive to *nondistressed* infant vocalizations (i.e., babbling or cooing that did not appear to function as a signal for parental assistance), to pick up and nurse the infants even when it appeared that the infants were *not* in need of nursing, to go to their soundly sleeping infants and move them from their cribs to the parents' bed to sleep (and in the process, *wake their infant up*), and to poorly structure bedtimes that in turn led to prolonged infant wakefulness. We suspect that mothers who *worry excessively* about their infants' well-being at night may be motivated to seek out and intervene with their infants, regardless of whether the infants require intervention or not, in order to alleviate *mothers' anxieties* about whether their infants are hungry, thirsty, uncomfortable, and so on. We suspect that mothers with elevated *depressive symptoms* may be motivated to spend time with their infant at night in order to satisfy mothers' emotional needs [emphasis added].

In a nutshell, both studies observed that among mothers with depressive symptoms, the mothers' behavior at nighttime was associated with infant night waking because they incorrectly believed (*dysfunctional cognition*) that they had to attend to their *non-distressed* infants and feed them even if they had just been fed.

Of course, if you think your baby is in distress (hungry, soiled, wet, cold, in pain), always respond promptly, but if you suspect your baby is not in distress, wait and watch a little, especially during the first three months. Other studies of parental response to nighttime infant crying (page 419) also suggest that prompt responses to distress vocalizations, of any intensity, during the first three months do not lead to later sleep problems. But after three months, perhaps delaying a response for a few seconds, for very mild distress vocalizations, might allow the child to self-soothe and return to sleep unassisted.

So during the first three months, if you suspect your baby is in distress or you are uncertain, always respond promptly. After three months, if you are uncertain or the distress is very mild, try to delay your response. At any age, but especially after 3 months, if you believe your child is making non-distress vocalizations, consider delaying your response.

In a third study regarding maternal depression, Dr. Johanna Petzoldt observed that "infant sleeping problems were related to maternal *depressive* (and comorbid *anxiety*) disorders" and she observed that preceding maternal anxiety (even before pregnancy) predicts both excessive infant crying and maternal postpartum depression. Perhaps the mother's insomnia associated with caring for an excessively crying or colicky baby and the stress from dealing with inconsolable crying might contribute to or cause maternal postpartum depression. But the trigger was preexisting or pre-pregnancy anxiety. As an anxious parent told me, "I was so worried that every time he made a sound at night, I rushed in to awaken him to make sure he was all right."

A criticism of some of these infant studies, and those described on page 146, is that because objective sleep data was not obtained documenting the night wakings, it may be that mental health issues in the mother are related not to objectively disturbed sleep in their child, but rather the maternal *perception* of infant sleep problems.

Another criticism is that common factors that might cause both maternal mental health issues and disturbed infant sleep, such as marital problems caused by issues involving the father, were not explored. Nevertheless, this research emphasizes a mother-driven path of influence whereby the mother's depressive symptoms (or anxiety or dysfunctional cognitions about infant sleep) cause maternal nighttime behavior that creates infant night waking (pages 232 and 408).

The other direction, or an infant-driven path of influence, is also possible (page 146). Here, infant night waking (for example, with a baby with colic) causes maternal night behavior that creates both Mother's depressive symptoms and Mother's dysfunctional cognitions about infant sleep behavior.

A third point of view is that the interaction between maternal depression and infant sleep is bidirectional. A study from Norway that included about one thousand children examined the infant-driven path, the mother-driven path, and a common-factor path. They concluded that the direction of effects between mothers' depressive symptoms and children's sleeping problems, at age 2.5 and 4 years, *went both ways;* "however the effect of the *child-driven* mechanism was significantly stronger than that of the mother-driven mechanism." The major sleep problem identified was "Co-sleeping in response to nocturnal awakenings."

> Mothers with depressive symptoms are more likely to have negative cognitions about setting limits for their children and increased doubts regarding parenting competence and to worry more often about their infant's sleep. These mothers more easily perceived themselves as insensitive, neglectful, or even abusive toward the child if they are not highly involved at bedtime or night time, and they even tend to more often interpret their children's crying as a sign of anxiety or distress.

Perhaps pre-pregnancy maternal anxiety is a trigger (mother-driven path) or infant colic is a trigger (baby-driven path) for initiating infant sleep issues, but as time passes, more interactions develop between maternal and infant issues so, later, more bidirectionality of effects is observed. I have tried to summarize what might be going on in "Big Picture" on page 234.

Dr. Liat Tikotzky also directly studied maternal sleep-related cognitions using a rating instrument describing fourteen hypothetical case descriptions of infants who have difficulty falling asleep and staying asleep. Parents were asked to rate on a 6-point scale (from highly agree to highly disagree) their agreement with assertions in two categories:

1. Distress (assertions that represent parental belief that infants experience distress or anxiety upon awakening and parents should therefore directly help or soothe them at night)
2. Limits (assertions that emphasize the importance of limiting parental involvement at night and focus on encouraging infants to learn self-soothing without or with minimal parental assistance)

She also performed assessments of parental soothing patterns at bedtime and during the night, using a bedtime scale from low involvement to high involvement:

1. In crib, by himself or herself, without caregiver's help
2. In crib with parent's passive presence (without talking, touching, etc.)
3. In crib with brief parental help for less than 2 minutes
4. In crib with parental extended help
5. While nursing, feeding, drinking, or outside the crib with caregiver's active help
6. Falling asleep in parent's bed

A similar scale was used for soothing during the night.
Objective sleep measures were obtained on the infants at 1, 6,

and 12 months. Her results showed that "maternal cognitions related to concerns about the infants' distress at night [were] associated with more disturbed sleep, as reflected by a higher number of objective and subjective night wakings, while maternal cognitions emphasizing the importance of *limiting* parental involvement were associated with more consolidated sleep." Further, "maternal prenatal cognitions . . . that are shaped even before the infant is born predicted the quality of the infant's sleep at later stages." Similarly, "mothers who put more emphasis on the infant's distress reported later greater parental involvement in soothing their infant to sleep at the age of 6 and 12 months. These findings support the hypothesis that parental soothing methods are not solely dependent on infant's characteristics. It appears that mothers bring their own perceptions into the interaction and those cognitions seem to shape their behavior toward the infant around bedtime." Just to be absolutely clear, "it would be wrong to conclude from these findings that parents should abstain from approaching their infant at night in order to facilitate good sleep patterns. Undoubtedly during the first months of life, infants need their parents for comfort and regulation, while gradually these functions shift from the caregiver to the infant . . . Parents emphasizing the importance of limiting parental involvement at night did not devaluate or disregard the interpretations underlying the need to soothe the infant. Moreover, in their actual soothing behavior, those parents who endorsed the limits interpretation were responsive to their infants and offered help although less intensively than parents who emphasized the distress interpretations and who relied more on active soothing."

Insomnia in mothers during pregnancy or in either parent postpartum may also be associated with adverse concerns. Objective measurements of mother's nighttime sleep during pregnancy at 16, 24, and 32 weeks showed that her short sleep durations were associated with objectively measured short nighttime sleep durations in her infant at three months of age. In a separate study, it was observed that insomnia in the mother is reduced when fathers are more involved in daytime and nighttime caregiving (when the baby is 3–6 months).

As you attempt to help your child sleep well, please be mindful to get sufficient sleep for yourself. After, all, our goal is a well-rested family.

Here is the bottom line. Ask yourself: Am I likely to be so concerned about my child at night that I might want to attend to her when she appears to be sleeping contentedly because I worry about her health or I feel that she needs my company? Do I have strong feelings of guilt, shame, or anger? Does my baby appear to be unusually fussy and hard to soothe to sleep or not able to sleep well, or is there stress in my marriage, perhaps because the father is not supportive in general and/or in baby care at night (page 410)? Under these circumstances, review the Step-by-Step Program in chapter 1, try some no-cry sleep solutions, and proceed slowly and gradually (page 240 and chapter 5) to help your baby sleep better, and discuss your overall situation with your husband, partner, or child's caregiver. Maybe consider engaging a community sleep consultant to help prevent sleep problems from developing or help solve existing sleep problems (page 329).

What about fathers? Becoming a father, in and of itself, does not cause depression in men. However, a separate study showed that "Men who enter the transition to parenthood with a tendency to interpret events negatively [*cognitive biases*] may respond to potential stressors, such as a fussy baby, with greater negative affect . . . [and] may be more likely to interpret such events in negative ways . . . [These] *cognitive biases* are associated with symptoms of *depression* and *anxiety* among fathers during the transition to parenthood [emphasis added]." In Australia, publicly funded Early Parenting Centers (EPC), also known as Sleep Schools, provide a residential program offering parenting support and education, commonly for sleep and settling issues with their children. The majority (84 percent) of fathers attending EPCs complained of "moderate to high fatigue," and the authors concluded that "distress among fathers may be experienced as psychological and physiological tension, agitation, and frustration rather than depressed mood. It is also possible that it is more socially acceptable for fathers to report symptoms of stress than depression." In another study, fathers of infants with sleep problems, at four months of age, had increased depressive symptoms, anger toward their child, poor personal sleep quantity and quality, and, at 6 months of age, increased depressive symptoms. A recent review by Tova Walsh noted that while some symptoms of maternal and paternal postpartum depression (PPD) ("decreased mood or loss of interest in activities") are similar, mothers are more likely to report sadness, and fathers are more likely to present with increased irritability and alcohol and substance use . . . Paternal PPD is associated with poorer child emotional and behavioral outcomes in childhood and adolescence." So fathers can be very helpful (page 163) or not so helpful (page 410).

The good news is that parents with depressive symptoms can be helped! Education about sleep helps parents: A 2014 paper titled "Preventing Early Infant Sleep and Crying Problems and Postnatal Depression: A Randomized Trial" showed that "Education about sleep and cry behavior at about 4 weeks caused caregivers to attend to infant night feeding less." And another paper concluded that prevention is successful when "Once the baby is 3 weeks old, healthy, and putting on weight normally, they can begin to delay feedings when baby wakes at night, in order to dissociate waking from feeding. This is done gradually, using [diaper] changing or handling to introduce a delay, and does not involve leaving babies to cry."

Big Picture: Maternal Anxiety and Infant Problems

A woman with anxiety symptoms or dysfunctional cognitions regarding how she will care for and respond to her baby at night (page 235) becomes pregnant. She worries about the pregnancy, her baby, and becoming a mother. During pregnancy, the anxiety leads to significant insomnia. After the baby is born, she worries about her child's weight gain and comfort level and/or interprets all infant vocalizations at night as distress. She may have a low tolerance for infant crying (page 417). She becomes too intrusive at night and fragments her child's sleep with unnecessary feeding and soothing. Her own insomnia during pregnancy and/or her own fragmented sleep postpartum depletes her reserves, and postpartum depression emerges. Her intensive involvement in putting her baby to sleep and/ or intrusiveness during the night results in her baby not learning self-soothing at bedtime or sleep onset. Subsequently, night waking as a sleep problem (signaling) during the night emerges in her baby, because after a normal nighttime arousal the baby has difficulty self-soothing, which is needed to return to sleep unassisted. The sleep-impaired baby becomes painfully tired near the end of the day, and after a few weeks excessive crying/colic emerges. For her own sense of comfort and to better calm her baby, the mother is more likely to choose to sleep with her baby in her bed, which further impairs the mother's sleep.

The baby's failure to learn self-soothing and subsequent impaired sleeping may create enduring sleep problems in both the child and the mother, worsening mental health symptoms in the mother and increasing family tension. When older, the direction of these effects goes both ways: from child to mother and from mother to child.

Older women with anxiety, knowing that their older husbands will be less involved in helping care for the baby, might be more likely to experience this sequence of events. Younger unmarried women with less support may also experience more anxiety. With symptoms of anxiety present, maternal smoking and drinking alcohol during pregnancy and postpartum might be viewed as a reflection of anxiety.

Variable #1 is maternal *depression* (or co-morbid anxiety *and* depression) before pregnancy, which worsens with increasing sleep deprivation during the pregnancy due to insomnia, and postpartum from caring for the baby at night.

Variable #2 is an infant's tendency toward *excessive fussing/crying,* which might be biologically associated with mother's mental health status and/or insomnia or smoking during pregnancy, or could be an independent factor. These children (about 20 percent) add more stress to the family and cause more sleep deprivation in the mother, which might contribute to or worsen preexisting maternal postpartum anxiety and/or depression.

Variable #3 is *low parental tolerance for infant crying* (page 417), which might interfere with a child having the opportunity to practice self-soothing.

Variable(s) #4-plus are other common variables affecting both mother and child, such as a nonsupportive or impaired father/husband/partner adversely affecting both the mother's mental health and the baby's ability to sleep well and self-soothe. Alternatively, any combination of these variables magnifies the stress in the mother and the challenges in parenting, causing a minority of children to continue to cry/fuss well beyond 2–4 months of age and/or continue to not sleep well during childhood. As a result, they are at a higher risk for future sleep problems and/or other problems driven by chronic sleepiness.

But there is a solution (page 240)! And it is simple, and it can be put in place even if there are adverse concerns in your family. Before presenting this treatment plan, let's first look at some specific adverse concerns affecting children's sleep.

Adverse Concerns Affecting Children's Sleep

Please do not be disheartened if some of the concerns I'm about to describe apply to you, because at the end, I will present a simple and straightforward plan to help you prevent or treat sleep problems despite any adversity. In addition to the parent issues and barriers previously discussed and the risk factors on page 105, there are specific concerns that might lead to sleep problems in your child. Because most of this information was published recently, 2018–2019, it might be surprising to you. Note that in the studies of mothers, fathers were not included. So it is possible that the fathers were directly contributing to or causing these issues in the mother.

BEFORE PREGNANCY

Expectant Mothers
Women with anxiety symptoms prior to pregnancy are more likely to have infants who experience excessive infant crying, and mothers with depressive symptoms prior to pregnancy are more likely to have infants with sleeping problems.

Medically assisted conception (assisted reproductive technology) is *not* associated with an increased risk of postpartum depressive symptoms.

Smoking before and during pregnancy reduces total sleep time in the infant and is a risk factor for SIDS.

Expectant Fathers
Smoking occurs more often if the mother smokes.

DURING PREGNANCY

Expectant Mothers

Depression during pregnancy in young mothers, age 19–24 years, has increased from 17 percent (1990–1992) to 25 percent (2012–2016). Depressed mothers during pregnancy describe feeling overwhelmed and having difficulty sleeping.

Poor quality sleep during pregnancy, independent of depression and anxiety symptoms, occurs in about 14 percent of women and at three years postpartum is associated with "demonstrated more disturbed mood including tension-anxiety, depression-dejection, anger-hostility, fatigue-inertia, and confusion-bewilderment." However, when significant symptoms of insomnia do occur, about 28 percent of the expectant mothers also had symptoms of depression. Additionally, insomnia during pregnancy is associated with increased risk of preterm birth.

Mothers who think that if they do not always respond promptly at night, their baby will feel abandoned, have babies at 1, 6 and 12 months with more night wakings.

Risk factors during pregnancy such as symptoms of insomnia, anxiety, depression, and attention deficit and hyperactivity disorder are related to sleep difficulties in infants at 3 months of age.

Smoking during pregnancy and postpartum increases the risk of infant colic.

Among pregnant women in the US, about 12 percent drink alcohol and 10 percent engage in binge drinking (four or more drinks in two hours).

Expectant Fathers

About 10 percent of expectant fathers experience significant depressive symptoms during pregnancy and the first postpartum year, which is about twice the rate in the general population. A father having depressive symptoms, independent of depressive symptoms in the mother, predicts excessive infant crying.

About 15 percent of expectant fathers had some symptoms of disturbed sleep. When significant symptoms of insomnia did occur, about 20 percent of the expectant fathers also had symptoms of depression.

A father's habitual or characteristic pattern of harboring negative thoughts about himself, the world, and the future is associated with depressive symptoms. Harboring thoughts of increased perception of threat and danger is associated with symptoms of anxiety. Expectant fathers with higher levels of thinking along both these lines report greater levels of distress.

Smoking during pregnancy and postpartum increases the risk of infant colic.

Alcohol use is described below.

AFTER PREGNANCY

Mothers

Risk factors for postpartum depression include younger maternal age, poverty, lack of social support, and single status. Postpartum depression doubles the risk of child behavior disturbances.

At 6 months, mothers who interpret their babies signaling at night as distress predict more maternal depressive symptoms and infant night wakings at 12 months.

Objective measurements of mothers' impaired sleep are associated with less observed positive parenting during the hour before the child's bedtime. Maternal disturbed sleep, independent of depression, is associated with more negative maternal perceptions of the mother–infant relationship.

Mothers of children with autism spectrum disorder did *not* have impaired sleep.

Sleep duration during the first three months postpartum is about one hour less per night compared with pre-pregnancy. During postpartum months four through six, sleep duration increases about thirty minutes per night but may not fully recover to pre-pregnancy levels even up to six years later.

Alcohol in breast milk, from one glass of wine or can of beer, may disrupt an infant's sleep if countermeasures are not taken.

Babies

Prematurely born infants (and small-for-gestational-age and low-birth-weight infants) had more night awakening at 18 months. Very premature infants (less than 28 weeks gestational age) have more regulatory problems (excessive crying and sleeping difficulties) at term.

Infants born to depressed mothers were matched with babies of mothers with no depression. Both groups underwent twenty-four-hour sleep studies performed on the second day and again at six months; altered sleep architecture was observed at both ages among those infants born to mothers with depression.

Sleep problems are more than twice as common in young children with autism spectrum disorder and other developmental delays.

When adverse circumstances cause naps to disappear prematurely, naps can be reestablished by maintaining daytime sleep schedules.

Fathers

Sleep duration decreases, compared to pre-pregnancy, but the amounts are much less than observed for mothers.

In Australia, fathers of unsettled babies (prolonged or inconsolable crying, frequent overnight waking, resistance to soothing, and feeding difficulties) whose wives sought residential early parenting services exhibited more fatigue, poor sleep quality, and risky alcohol use (episodic excessive drinking or daily alcohol use). Among these fathers, 20 percent had mental health problems, and risky alcohol use occurred in 82 percent; among the 80 percent without mental health problems, risky alcohol use occurred in 50 percent.

One in ten Australian fathers experienced mental health difficulties in the early parenting period. The most common attitudinal barriers to seeking help were (a) the need for control and self-reliance in managing one's own problems—"I like to be in charge of everything in my life"; (b) a tendency to downplay or minimize problems—"Problems like this are part of life; they're just something you have to deal with"; and (c) a sense of resignation that nothing will help—"I'd rather just suck it up than dwell on my problems." Fathers with the attitudinal barrier (a) regarding the need for control and self-reliance were more likely to have high levels of depression, anxiety, and stress symptoms.

If there are risk factors for unhealthy sleep in your child (page 105) or you are facing some of the previously discussed *parent issues* or adverse concerns discussed above—or perhaps you're experiencing a host of challenging events that, in combination, make it difficult to help your child sleep well—have hope. There is one simple sleep solution that may do wonders, and it does not involve ignoring your child at night: *Establish early bedtimes based on drowsy signs.*

Overcoming Adversity: You Do Not Have to Make Your Baby Cry to Have a Good Night's Sleep

Here is an edited parent's report describing a combination of circumstances that made sleeping through the night particularly challenging, but a go-slow, no-cry sleep solution (chapter 5) with an *earlier bedtime* (pages 65 and 300) *based on drowsy signs* produced a few minutes of extra sleep (page 55), which helped everyone sleep better!

> Go slowly: "Little by little . . . She is still very bonded and happy . . . She has never been let to 'cry it out,' and she has learned to sleep through the night."

We have a four-year-old son and after our daughter, Jane, was born, I fell into a pattern of nursing her to sleep. For the first few months she slept in a bedside sleeper. At 6 months, we moved, and stayed with my parents, and we ended up co-sleeping. Her pattern was that she usually awoke up four-plus times per night wanting to nurse and cries if I try any other method of soothing. In our new home, I tried to get her to sleep in a crib in her room, but she strongly disliked it. I started to try weaning at 12 months but she would not take much milk, so I continued nursing. She is now 15 months and continues to refuse to take a bottle. When a bottle is attempted, she cries until she vomits. She also has gastroesophageal reflux. We recently moved cross-country. Around 4:00 P.M., she'll play independently but it doesn't last long. Jane is very active around 5:00 P.M., less energetic around 6:30 P.M., and around 7:00 P.M. she will get rather suddenly clingy, fussy, even putting her head down on furniture while standing. After dinner, around 7:00 to 7:30, she will start to rub her eyes and become more irritable/sleepy. Bedtime is 7:00 to 7:30 and she's asleep around 8:00. She has never slept in her crib. My husband is unavailable most nights because of his work.

[Author's advice: Please read about drowsy signs, then move the dinner earlier and the bedtime to an earlier time based on those drowsy signs.]

I agree that we need to be more disciplined about feeding the kids earlier, but that means that my husband will never see them in the evening. The first attempt was a bedtime at 6:00 P.M. and she fell asleep at 6:50 P.M. and she awoke three or four times which was better than the four to eight times in the past. The second night, bedtime was 6:15 P.M. and because she started to cry, I nursed and rocked her until drowsy. She fell asleep a little earlier (6:45) and woke up only three times. Over the next week, she still woke up three or four times during the night, but there is no hard crying at all, just a few minutes of soft crying.

During the subsequent three weeks, I saw great progress with Jane's sleep. We put her to bed at 6:30 P.M., drowsy but awake, and she currently wakes up just one or maybe two times nightly, and the wakings are getting better with weaning the night nursing. I'm better rested and have more energy during the day and my husband is thrilled to have a wife who isn't always exhausted! And importantly, it's healthier for Jane to know how to self-soothe and get better sleep, too.

Four additional weeks later, I can report that I have stopped nursing Jane and Jane is sleeping through the night. I am glad that we did all of this gradually. *During all of this we did not let her cry.* Even now, I put her in the crib drowsy and stand next to the crib until she falls asleep. She isn't touching me but knows I'm there. After she falls asleep, I leave the room. Initially, she used to jolt awake at any sound of me trying to leave, and now I can pretty much walk out as soon as her eyes close.

My next step is to leave when she is drowsy in her crib. In another few weeks, we will try to have her go down without us in the room. It is little by little. She is still very bonded and happy, she likes her crib and doesn't see it as being away from me. *She has never been let to "cry it out."* And she has learned to sleep through the night. This process has been based on creating a loving, nurturing approach to help Jane learn how to self-soothe and sleep independently. Using this gentle and slow approach, I've had time to catch up on my own sleep, which gave me the energy to push ahead. I'd advise other parents to be gentle but firm and stick with limits that you've set around sleeping. I've learned that the key to helping babies sleep is allowing them the space to learn self-soothing, even if it's hard hearing them upset.

Therapist Failure

Sometimes a therapist has preconceived ideas that he or she attempts to shoehorn onto every family. Such therapists do not listen to parents and will often press them to try something experience has shown not to work for that particular family. Or the therapist gives good advice but fails to make clear to the parents that they must work every day to permanently prevent the problem from resurfacing. I see this time and time again in my patients. For example, after working hard to successfully correct a sleep problem caused by a bedtime that was too late, the parent asks me if he can now keep his child up later at night, since everyone is sleeping better!

Successful therapists such as Dr. Karen Pierce, a child psychiatrist, often start by asking a fundamental question: "There are many barriers to change. Is it the child, is it the parent, is it the couple, is it the larger family, or outside stress issues?" She emphasizes the importance of locating the particular barrier that prevents particular parents from solving problems. Identifying and dealing with the barrier allows the family to focus their energy on the solution to the child's sleep issue.

Dr. Robert Daniels, a child psychologist, often starts with questions such as: "What is the desired behavior you want from your child? What is the desired outcome? What is the endpoint of treatment? What would you like to see happen?" Both parents need to agree on what the goal is and how to achieve the goal before beginning a treatment plan. The failure to agree on a goal makes it difficult for parents to cooperate with each other to achieve success. Dr.

Daniels observes that most parents agree on the goal but not necessarily on the path to accomplish it.

Child psychologist Dr. Vicki Lavigne emphasizes that parents have to see the connection between what they do and the effect it will have on the behavior of the child. Parents have to be more focused on their behavior than worrying that their child has a problem or peculiar trait. For example, focusing on "He has a strong will" instead of your own behavior interferes with success.

Dr. John Bates, another child psychologist, encourages families to cast a wide net and seek support by talking to relatives and close friends, community mental health groups, parenting groups, or religious leaders, because resources and substantial support may be available but not known to new parents.

It is important for parents to try to figure out a way to separate their marriage issues from bedtime issues, compartmentalize other barriers, restructure their priorities, or seek professional counseling in order to heavily invest in soothing their newborn during the first few months. By gathering up all their resources for soothing during the first few months, parents are more likely to *prevent* sleep problems in the future.

Some parents may need professional help to establish reasonable, orderly home routines, to iron out conflicts between themselves, or to help an older child with a well-established sleep problem. To maintain healthy sleep for your young child, you need the courage to be firm without feeling guilt or fear that she will resent you or love you less. In fact, the best prescription I can offer for a loving home is a well-rested child and well-rested parents.

THE MOST IMPORTANT POINT

If some of these speed bumps or roadblocks occur in your family, then work extra hard with what resources you have available to teach self-soothing during the first four months in order to *prevent* sleep problems from ever arising in the first place.

Sleep Banking and Recovery from Insufficient Sleep

Sleep banking and caffeine (page 328) may be viewed as counter-measures to reduce the impairments caused by sleep loss. Sleep banking is extending time in bed for a few days, before an anticipated period of reduced sleep, in order to improve performance during the subsequent period of sleep restriction or sleep deprivation. This idea is similar to the concept of carbohydrate loading to improve athletic performance for endurance events; that is, storing energy for future use. However, another possible benefit is whether sleep banking can hasten the recovery of the impairments that developed during sleep deprivation after the sleep restriction period ends and regular sleep is now available. Two experiments in adults suggest that sleep banking accomplishes both goals. In both studies, sleep extension (more time in bed) for six or seven nights before a period of sleep restriction was shown to improve vigilance and sustained attention during a subsequent period of sleep restriction, and led to faster recovery when the period of sleep restriction ended. However, others have suggested that sleep banking in the sense of storing or banking sleep for future benefit does not occur and instead, the results that were observed occurred because the period of sleep extension actually simply reduced the habitual or baseline sleepiness of the subjects. Either way, if you are planning an extended holiday or crossing many time zones or anticipate a time when getting healthy sleep for your child might be more challenging, imposing an earlier bedtime for a week before the event might help keep everyone better rested and help everyone recover faster when you return home to your normal routines. How long does it take to actually recover from insufficient night sleep?

The largest study of sleep and performance studied, online, included thirty-one thousand adult participants over 18 years of age and examined three million nights of sleep. Insufficient sleep was defined as having less than six hours of time in bed along with a recovery period that extended over several days. "We find that, on average, it takes three nights to make up one insufficient night sleep and six nights to make up two insufficient nights of sleep in a row." However, during the next few nights of recovery sleep, there were no constraints regarding sleep duration, and it is possible that during the recovery period, some individuals had additional nights of insufficient sleep.

I asked one author, Dr. Zeiter, how fast recovery might occur if the individual actually obtained more than six hours on nights three through seven during the recovery period. "I think that, based on laboratory studies, one could assume that baseline performance could be obtained after two nights (following one night of sleep loss) and probably three or four nights after two nights of sleep loss. If by 'baseline' performance, we mean an average performance after average sleep, then it's probably one to two days of recovery per particularly bad day of sleep." In other words, if your child is chronically a little short on sleep, the return to this baseline state might take one or two days of recovery sleep to make up for one night of insufficient sleep. This only applies to an individual whose baseline reflects mild habitual sleep deprivation. "If by baseline performance we mean non-sleep-deprived performance, I think that most people would take a few weeks of good sleep" to more fully recover.

I think this fits nicely with my observation that well-rested children fully rebound quickly with a single reset (page 300) after an illness or holiday. In contrast, if young children who have been short on sleep due to long-term sleep problems embark on a sleep solution, it may take only a few nights to sleep better at night, but naps may not improve until several days or a few weeks later, once full recovery is achieved.

Summary and Action Plan for Exhausted Parents

1. *Teach self-soothing.* Learning self-soothing does not mean that your child will necessarily cry. Patience and perseverance will pay off.

Start early. It is never too late to start, but the earlier you start the easier it might be.
Many hands. Get Dad and others on board.
Put your child down drowsy but awake. Trial and error is needed to get it right.

2. *Soothing.* Find out what works for *your* baby. Don't compare babies. See page 178 for different ways to soothe your baby. To find out what works best for your baby, see page 516.

3. *Many naps.* After a brief interval of wakefulness, put your child down for a nap based on *drowsy signs* or clock time. This prevents a second wind. Sleep begets sleep!

Start early, right when you come home from the hospital, to put your child down, drowsy but awake, for a nap within one to two hours of waking up.

4. *Bedtime routines.* Consistency helps signal to your child, just like the yellow traffic light at the intersection, what will happen next (page 193).

5. *Leave the room* after you put your baby down to sleep.

6. *Breastfeeding versus formula, family bed versus crib.* These are decisions that should fit your family and not what someone else claims is best. The American Academy of Pediatrics

discourages the family bed because of sudden infant death syndrome.

7. *Earlier bedtime around 6 weeks old.* Once your baby is older, go ahead and experiment with an earlier bedtime.

8. *Protect naps around 3–4 months of age.* Establishing good naps and an early bedtime may be socially limiting, but it is liberating to have a well-rested child.

9. *No screens in the bedroom.* All screen-based media in the bedroom at bedtime will interfere with healthy sleep.

10. *Prevention versus treatment of sleep problems.* Expect no crying with successful prevention of sleep problems; crying may occur to treat sleep problems that you created or when you help a post-colic baby learn self-soothing.

11. *Parent issues or barriers that may make prevention or treatment of sleep problems more challenging.* When certain parent issues (page 219) are present, sleep problems are more likely to occur and persist. Recognition of these issues might lead to making a family plan of action, even before the baby is born, to help your baby sleep well, including, if necessary, seeking professional assistance.

What a Parent Can Do

Encourage your partner to help care for the baby daytime and nighttime.

Encourage self-soothing; the earlier, the better.

Put your child to sleep drowsy but awake, then leave the room.

Set an early bedtime based on drowsy signs; practice consistent bedtime routines, including massage; be emotionally available at bedtime.

Provide opportunities for naps based on drowsy signs.

Avoid irregularity of sleep schedules, including between weekdays and weekends.

Practice safe sleep recommendations.

No TV or digital screens in the child's room; limit screen time.

Seek help if your child is not sleeping well (from the child's primary care provider or a community sleep consultant—page 329) or for yourself or partner, especially if there are symptoms of anxiety or depression or significant risk factors (page 105), *parent issues*, or *adverse concerns*.

Chapter 5 Outline

SLEEP SOLUTIONS

Crying
Teach Self-Soothing
Extinction (or Unmodified Extinction)
 Extinction with a Cap
 Extinction with Parental Presence
 Graduated Extinction
Positive Routines Plus Faded Bedtime with Response Cost
Scheduled Awakenings
Pros and Cons of Different Methods
Check and Console
Sound Machines
Fading
Swings
Nap Drill
 Night Sleep Is Fine, Why Are Naps a Problem?
Control the Wake-Up Time
 When to Start the Day
 When the Wake-Up Time Is Too Early
Parent-Set Bedtimes
 Temporary 5:30 Bedtime
 Reset
 How to Choose an Earlier Bedtime
  Move the Bedtime Slightly Earlier
  Move the Bedtime Much Earlier
  The 5:30 P.M. Bedtime Rut!
 Regular Bedtimes
 Bedtime Routines
Sleep Log
Crib Tents, Gates, and Locking the Door
Sleep Rules and Silent Return to Sleep

Sleep Solutions

If you have not already done so, please go back and read chapter 1.

The previous chapter, Preventing Sleep Problems, could just as well have been titled How to Establish Healthy Sleep Habits. Parents teach healthy habits such as hand washing, toothbrushing, wearing helmets when riding bikes, and wearing seatbelts throughout their child's life. It's the same for healthy sleep habits. It's an ongoing process. This chapter, Sleep Solutions, may also be an ongoing process—not a onetime cure like a penicillin shot for strep throat—because of natural disruptions of sleep schedules. Because sleep schedules often may get derailed, think of helping your child return to a healthy sleep schedule more as an ongoing regimen of *care* and not as a onetime *cure*.

All parents want their child to sleep well so they themselves can have more calm private time and get more sleep. Some parents do not fully appreciate how powerfully the beneficial effects of sleep directly help their child (chapter 3) or, because of their own issues (including sleep deprivation), they find it difficult to make the lifestyle changes that are necessary to help their child sleep better (chapter 4). Because changing lifestyle habits is hard for everyone and even harder if you are sleep-deprived, I am presenting more facts in this chapter than you might think necessary. But

I believe that more information is empowering and will encourage and enable you to make changes. Also, because you may be struggling with your own sleep deprivation, some points are deliberately repeated here and elsewhere so the message will really sink in.

An important first step in actually doing something to achieve healthy sleep is knowing for certain that your child's sleep is impaired. For a moment, focus on the following five behaviors that might indicate your child is not getting healthy sleep. These are some of the target behaviors we want to reduce or eliminate.

IS MY CHILD GETTING HEALTHY SLEEP?

After 3-4 months of age, you can tell that your child is not getting healthy sleep if these are present:

1. Witching hour behavior
2. Sleep inertia and/or wakes up crying (chapter 2)
3. Fatigue signs or a second wind before naps (chapters 2 and 4)
4. Often easily falls asleep in the afternoon in a moving stroller in public or in a car
5. Difficulty getting out of bed and/or headaches in the morning

Children who often show these behaviors are *short on sleep* (SOS). Think of SOS behaviors as a distress signal: "Help me, I need sleep!"

Here are a few typical questions and answers:

Q: *Do I have to let my child cry to solve a sleep problem?*
A: "No-cry" sleep solutions (pages 240 and 332) will solve most sleep problems.

Q: *I don't believe in this kind of unnatural programming.*
A: Healthy sleep habits are learned, not innate. Unless you want your child to suffer the natural effects of chronic sleep fragmentation, you will have to help him learn how to sleep.

Q: *I've heard that if I nurse my baby to sleep, I'll create a night-waking problem.*

A: The issue isn't whether nursing to sleep is good or not, but rather whether nursing too frequently or nighttime nursing is part of a night-waking problem. Please include nursing, if you wish, in nap or bedtime rituals, but after you finish nursing, whether the child is asleep or awake, put him down, kiss his cheek, say good night, walk away, turn the lights off, and close the door.

Q: *I've heard that because my baby learns to associate my breast with falling asleep, he will be unable to return to sleep later in the night if my breast is not present.*

A: Nonsense! Almost all the mothers in my practice nurse their babies to sleep at bedtime, and at night, when the baby is hungry, either the mother nurses or the father bottle-feeds the child. Usually the babies are drowsy but not in a deep sleep when they are put down. I believe it is perfectly natural to nurse a baby to sleep, and by itself this act does not cause sleep disturbances. Older children can be very discriminating; they can learn to expect dessert after dinner, if that is the family custom, but not after breakfast. I think babies can also become very discriminating; they can learn to expect to be fed when they are hungry but not to be fed when they are not hungry in the middle of the night.

Q: *Once I let my child cry a long time and he vomited. Won't I be trading one problem for another?*

A: Consider other sleep strategies that involve less crying. However, if the vomiting always occurs, I think you will want to always go in to clean him promptly and then leave him again.

Q: *Won't my baby simply outgrow this habit?*

A: Believe it or not, 18-year-old college freshmen who don't sleep well had difficulties sleeping as infants, according to their mothers, as reported in one study. It seems that if the child doesn't have the early opportunity to practice falling asleep by himself, he'll never learn to fall asleep easily.

Q: *Even if he won't outgrow this habit, what's really wrong with my still going to him at night?*

A: Consider your own feelings. Good studies at Yale University show that all mothers eventually become anxious, develop angry feelings toward their child, and feel guilt about maintaining their child's poor sleep habits. These feelings may persist for years. If going to your child at night fragments his sleep, then eventually a *cumulative sleep deficit* will develop.

Sleep Solutions

CRYING

Chapter 1 explains why some sleep solutions are better for some families than others. There is not one single sleep solution that will work for all families.

Some parents wish to, and are able to, help their child sleep better by making small changes slowly (pages 240 and 309) and so avoid any crying. Subsequent unavoidable disruptions in sleep might be treated in the same fashion; or because everyone is now better rested and/or the child is older, the parents might opt for a quicker sleep solution that might involve some crying. Smooth sleep sailing ahead! However, especially if symptoms of anxiety or depression are present in either parent (page 408), this "relapse" into not sleeping well might be so disheartening that the parents choose to *not* try again to help their child sleep well. So the original solution does not stick. Sleepless storm clouds on the horizon! Professional counseling for *parent issues* or a *community sleep consultant* might be helpful to reestablish healthy sleep habits.

Some parents wish to, and are able to, help their child sleep better by making abrupt changes that might involve some crying. Because they quickly see how better-quality sleep in their child helps the entire family, when inevitable future disruptions of sleep occur, they are able to redo the original sleep solution or do a *"reset"* to restore healthy sleep. Smooth sleep seas ahead! The sleep solution sticks.

TEACH SELF-SOOTHING

Self-soothing skills are the foundation upon which any successful sleep solution rests (page 160). Understanding how to teach self-soothing skills and the related subjects (bedtime routines, early bedtimes, protecting naps, and parent issues) will give you a perspective on what you wish to accomplish with any sleep solution that you choose. Please review these subjects in chapter 4 and remember that sleep solutions will not work or will not work quickly if your child gets a second wind at night from not napping well or from a bedtime that is too late.

When treating a sleep problem, the improvement in sleeping is *sequential*, not *simultaneous*. First, improvement will be seen for night sleep, then for the midmorning nap, and lastly for the midday nap. Improvement in night sleep may take only a few days, but improvement in naps may take longer.

EXTINCTION (OR UNMODIFIED EXTINCTION)

Extinction, sometimes called unmodified extinction, means that after your child is put to bed, he is ignored, except for feedings, without time limit until morning to allow him to develop self-soothing skills. Of course, parents practicing extinction are mindful of and monitor issues of safety and illness. If you think your child might be ill, rush to him, feel his forehead for fever and take his temperature if needed, and look for signs of distress such as vomiting or difficulty breathing. But if when you arrive he smiles at you with a look of *Gotcha!* or appears well, turn around and leave without social interaction or soothing.

Going in to soothe sometimes and not going in at other times is called *intermittent reinforcement*. Intermittent reinforcement is a powerful way to teach your child to cry louder, longer, and more frequently at night, because he is sometimes rewarded by his effort to enjoy the pleasure of your company. This will occur even if your curtain calls involve minimal soothing such as only shushing or soft stroking. For your baby, even minimal social contact is a very powerful motivator. For extinction to work, there should consistently be no social contact except for the feeding that you have chosen.

After initial success, several days or weeks later, expect a *response burst:* a reappearance of crying or calling out for attention (page 315). Because it is now out of character, rush to your child to make sure he is healthy. Most likely he will stop crying and smile at you when you arrive. Maintain silence, kiss him, and leave. No soothing. Your child is testing to see whether he can return to the old style. This is frustrating for parents because they misinterpret it as a failure or a setback. No, it is to be expected. Stay the course.

Night sleep rhythms emerge around 6 weeks of age, so extinction might be used after 6 weeks to get night sleep in sync with sleep rhythms, but most commonly extinction is used after a few months of age. Nevertheless, it can work earlier: Parents' reports of success in helping babies, even with colic, sleep better starting at *3–4 weeks* are described in chapters 4 and 6.

For children over 3–4 months of age, when nap rhythms emerge, extinction might be used for only one hour at nap times.

Not responding to your child at night is most difficult for parents. It may not always be clear if your baby is hungry or not. Between 6–8 weeks and 4 months, some but not all babies might be hungry and need to be bottle-fed two or three times a night, but after 4 months only once or twice, and after 9 months not at all. The idea is to respond if you think your child is hungry or in distress but not at other times. This determination may be harder for a mother who is breastfeeding, because of uncertainty regarding her breast milk supply. When breastfeeding, if every suck is followed by a swallow, he is probably hungry. If you really think he is hungry, feed him. The middle-of-the night feeding is done lovingly but silently and without lots of social interaction. After the feeding, the child is put back in bed with a single kiss or brief hug, but the return to sleep is not associated with prolonged soothing. Then leave the room.

If your full-term child is several weeks old and needs to be fed at night, then the parents may choose to wait at least four hours after the last feeding, because babies this age can go without a feeding for four hours. For example, if your baby is fed at a 7:00 P.M. bedtime, do not attend to your child or go to feed before 11:00 P.M. Also, in the middle of the night (around 11:00 P.M. to midnight), your baby might vigorously suck during this first feeding and suck more leisurely a few hours later (for example, at 2:00 to 3:00 A.M.) and again appear to be hungry at 4:00 to 5:00 A.M. If this pattern occurs, always attend to your child for the strong feeding in the middle of the night and in the morning around 4:00 to 5:00 A.M. but ignore the feeding in between (2:00 to 3:00 A.M.). A common pattern is to feed only twice overnight.

Fathers may give a bottle of expressed breast milk or formula to help clarify whether the baby is hungry or not. Having Dad give a bottle at different times and watching how much and how fast your baby feeds might make it clear when he is really hungry. Whenever a bottle is given, watch your child's behavior and do not count ounces: when he really slows down in his sucking, end the feeding. Otherwise, the time spent trying to "top him off," with the misguided idea that he will sleep longer, is lost deep sleep for your child and for you.

When parents avoid unnecessary feedings at night and remove themselves as reinforcers of crying at bedtime or nighttime, crying decreases and then disappears. Giving your child less attention at night allows the sleep process to surface and lull him to sleep. Because night sleep and social smiling develop around 6 weeks of age, it is possible after this point that parents' attempts to soothe at night might be more socially stimulating than soothing. Too much middle-of-the-night soothing will interfere with the naturally evolving sleep wave, teaching the child to fight sleep in order to enjoy more parental contact.

As a practicing pediatrician, I have many families in my practice successfully use extinction to correct a sleep problem that evolved from a too-late bedtime, a disruption of routines, such as a long vacation, or unnecessary attention at night. As a sleep consultant, I had a rule that both parents participate, and many families chose extinction because they wanted to quickly get better sleep for the whole family. As a lecturer, I would ask the audience if anyone had used extinction and how it went. In all three instances, after three to four days it was over and done. Mothers hated to hear their child cry but loved the result: sleep for everyone. No regrets. Clear sailing. These experiences encouraged me to recommend extinction, or any other method a family might prefer.

Families who have talked to their child's health provider or read about helping their child sleep better and who are successful with extinction are families who are less likely to have anxiety regarding the process in the first place. But in some parenting books and academic articles, extinction is often described as effective but unacceptable because parents view the method as too harsh; they believe it will traumatize their child. Their view is: When a child is given less attention at night in order to help him sleep better (extinction or graduated extinction) and cries, then eventually stops crying and falls asleep, he has "given up" (page 331). Their interpretation is that crying is a form of communication that always expresses a need that must always be met in order to create "trust" between the parent and child. When the cry goes unanswered at night, the child "gives up" and the parent–child bond is weakened. The parent who disagrees with this "harms" the child because this parent is "selfish," putting the parent's "want" for sleep ahead of the child's "need" for parental attention. There is absolutely no evidence that this interpretation is correct and strong evidence from multiple studies that this interpretation is wrong (page 344).

Again, as a general pediatrician in private practice, I would see a wide range of parenting skills and challenges. But I think that researchers in academic centers are more likely to see more anxious families who are unable to solve their child's sleep problem because they're afraid that less attention at night to help their child sleep better might harm their child and/or there are stressful issues present as described in chapter 4. Generalizing from this selected population, extinction is promoted as an undesirable method, not because it is ineffective, but because these particular parents will not accept it. Other families just do it and get on with their lives.

> If your baby is hungry at night, feed him at night. If your baby is sleepy at night, let him sleep at night.

Extinction with a Cap

Some parents might wish to put a cap on the number of minutes of ignoring their child so they know they are not committing to endless crying. They fear that the crying will persist for hours. I recommend a cap of forty-five minutes. This cap may give you the peace of mind of knowing that you are not committing to ignoring crying forever and may enable you to have the confidence to try extinction. A much briefer cap might allow your child to learn to cry to the time limit and be rewarded by parental soothing. Crying for more than forty-five minutes typically occurs only when your child is extremely fatigued from not napping well or a bedtime is too late.

Extinction with Parental Presence

Some parents feel more comfortable using extinction if they remain in the room until their child falls asleep. Extinction with parental presence is based on the unproven assumption that sleep problems are due to separation anxiety. The parent remains in the room during the extinction procedure and can incorporate "fading out," whereby the parent gradually leaves the bedroom. This approach often takes at least seven nights to achieve results.

> Crying is hard, but sleeplessness is harder.

Q: *With extinction, how long will my child cry? (chapter 1)*
A: If, and only if, all the elements of self-soothing are in place (these elements, including enlisting many hands for help, putting your

baby down drowsy but awake, and allowing many naps, as discussed in chapter 4), the bedtime is not too late, and a child who is older than 4 months of age is napping well, the process usually takes only three to five nights, and dramatic improvement takes only one or two nights. In children who are short on sleep, there may be multiple bouts of crying of forty-five to fifty-five minutes the first night; the crying bouts on the second night are usually a little more or a little less. The reason there may be more crying on the second night, especially for older children, is that your child is trying harder to get your attention. The third night is much better (bouts of twenty to forty minutes), and by the fourth or fifth night there is no crying. Your baby will likely cry less at sleep onset if Dad is putting him down after soothing and Mom has left the house. This process might take longer for an older child and for a post-colic child. For children under 4 months of age without colic, there may be less crying.

Parents who do not see a rapid improvement usually do not have all the elements of self-soothing in place, and/or the bedtime is too late, and/or naps are not going well, and/or there is some other inconsistency in their approach to sleep.

In my research for *Healthy Sleep Habits, Happy Twins,* I found that many parents quickly became extremely sleep-deprived because of double-duty feeding at night and consequently did extinction when the twins were younger than 4 months old (counting from the due date). For twins who have an early bedtime and naps in place, extinction usually takes three to five nights. In general, the first night was associated with thirty to forty-five minutes of crying, the second night ten to thirty minutes, and the third night up to ten minutes. This suggests that *there is less crying associated with extinction when performed earlier than 4 months of age.*

I think there may be circumstances when a trial of extinction or extinction with a cap is warranted *at night* shortly after 6 weeks of age (counting from the due date), because night sleep is becoming organized around this time. I hesitate to list the exact circumstances, because my list could not cover all the possible variables that might go into making this decision. Briefly, when the parents are extremely stressed, the child's sleep is worsening or not improving despite the parents' heroic efforts, and other methods are not working or are considered by the parents to be unlikely to help, I think a five-night trial of extinction or extinction with a cap may be considered. Ideally, you try to maximize daytime sleep and minimize daytime crying by whatever soothing method works (for example, swings). And you might temporarily abandon attempts at putting your child down drowsy but awake. But it is necessary that you start the night sleep before your baby gets a second wind (put the baby to bed at 6:00 to 8:00 P.M., or earlier if needed). Practically, this might be started on a Saturday when both parents are available to work together as a team. Feed your baby at night whenever you think he is truly hungry, even more than twice if needed. If after the fifth night there is no clear improvement in night sleep, I would give it up, do whatever works to maximize night sleep, and consider trying again in a couple of weeks. Discuss your situation with your pediatrician, so that you can feel sure that your child is healthy and gaining weight well.

I know that this will help some babies shortly after 6 weeks to sleep better at night. When this fails, I do not know whether the lack of success resides in issues involving the baby (such as colic), the parents (such as inconsistency), or parent-child interactions (too many or unnecessary feedings). The most common reason for failure is a bedtime that is too late, so that your child develops a *second wind*.

Seeing Is Believing

I know that this will help some babies shortly after 6 weeks to sleep better at night. When this fails, I do not know whether the lack of success resides in issues involving the baby (such as colic), the parents (such as inconsistency), or parent-child interactions (too many or unnecessary feedings). The most common reason for failure is a bedtime that is too late, so that your child develops a second wind (page 43).

Seeing is believing, so here are some reports from parents who successfully used extinction.

We did extinction around 8 weeks for my first two children. The first was colicky, and I was at my wit's end. The second was one of those kids whose sleep was worsening. I was depressed, and my husband was the hero, sleeping with her in the living room so it didn't disturb me. Oh, and we had an 18-month-old at the time, too! By the third night, both babies were falling asleep, on their own, at a good time, and sleeping all night (with a couple of feeds).

I used extinction for my first two children at around 2 months. Both were still being swaddled at the time, and we kept them swaddled through extinction. They did not use pacifiers and did not suck fingers or thumb (though both started around 5 months). So it is entirely possible to do extinction with a swaddled baby (we started unswaddling them around 4 or 5 months with no problem at all).

My son, who was 11 weeks at the time, was extremely colicky. Having experienced colic in the past with my daughter (different type of colic, with more constant fussing and less crying), I felt that there might be the possibility of sleep training now rather than waiting until he was post-colic, around 4 months old. Not only was it for his sake, but in all honesty it was for us as a family also. We are so worn out and my poor little guy is so sleep-deprived. We started putting him down at 5:30 P.M. and did complete extinction. Within four or so days he started doing much longer stretches at night and better, not great, but definitely better sleep during the day as well. He still has days that seem more colicky than others, but our bedtime routine and early bedtime have made a world of difference for him.

I started sleep training my first at 10 weeks and my second at 12 weeks. My oldest was an extremely fussy baby who was insanely sleep-deprived, and waiting until he was 16 weeks old to sleep train him seemed impossible! While I was ready for him to sleep, I wasn't nearly as ready as I thought I was to hear all of the crying while training him! Regardless, he was ready, even if he didn't know it, because he needed sleep! We went from co-sleeping to putting him in his crib, so it was a significant difference for him. While he did cry, after the first couple of nights he fell asleep very quickly on his own in his crib. After the first two nights of sleep training, he made immense leaps and bounds. I found that it was more me who was not ready to sleep train, less the kids, but once I sucked it up (and had my husband hold me back from going in to check on them when they cry) they became happier kids, and I became a happier, less tense mom.

We just utilize the total extinction method for our 3-month-old (13 weeks) son. It took three or four days (the first two days of which were quite difficult) but has been unbelievably successful and a lifesaver for our family and our son. At least in our case, 3 months old was the right time for him. Essentially he would only sleep tightly swaddled in his car seat with a pacifier. We had to constantly reinsert his pacifier every fifteen minutes or he would cry and wake. It was exhausting for both us and him, as his sleep was terribly choppy. We tried graduated extinction at various times from 8 to 12 weeks—waiting ten, fifteen, or twenty minutes before going in to soothe—but he would always outlast us. Last week at 3 months old we decided to utilize total extinction, and while extremely difficult emotionally, it has been an unbelievable success. He is now going to sleep for naps and nighttime without any crying, and waking up cooing and smiling in his crib rather than crying.

We had success with my 4-month-old son (he's now 2 years old). We decided on extinction because it seemed to be likely to cause everyone, including my son, the least amount of stress. Our plan was to get him to a sleepy state and make sure all of his needs were met, and then put him down to bed awake. The first night, he cried for thirty-five minutes, and I cried, too. But then he slept seven hours! He woke once and went back to sleep for four more hours! I thought I'd died and gone to heaven. He was in a much better mood the next day, and his napping was much better as well. I began to wonder if this was really my son! The next night, he cried for twenty minutes and then slept for nine hours straight before waking. He was even more content and had even better naps the next day. I'll never forget how he had his first night without waking on Labor Day, a few days after starting the extinction method. I told everyone that it felt like a gift for all of my motherly labors. After a few days, he no longer cried when I put him down. My husband and I are such believers that babies/children (and parents!) need sleep to function well. We call what we did for him "sleep empowerment."

An important element for success is an *early bedtime* that prevents a second wind from developing. In general, using extinction past 4 months of age may be more difficult for the parents because everyone is more stressed from sleep deprivation and habits are more ingrained. But it still works quickly!

At 6 months of age, Stephen was strong, happy, and healthy in every respect but one—he didn't sleep well. He did all his daytime napping in the car, the stroller, or our arms. If we put him in his crib, he awoke immediately and cried until we picked him up. His nighttime pattern was different but equally exhausting. He went to sleep in his crib promptly at 8:00 P.M. but usually awoke within the first hour for a brief comforting, and two or three times between 11:00 P.M. and 5:00 A.M. for a feeding.

This routine was taking its toll. I was almost as tired as when Stephen was a newborn, and I had no emotional reserve for handling everyday problems. I was sharp with the rest of the family and got angry if my husband was even ten minutes late getting home from work. We needed to make a change. We had the weekend ahead of us, when my husband would be around for support, so we decided to start that night.

We put the baby to bed at 8:00 P.M., and he awoke for the first time around 9:30. We didn't go in to him, and he cried for twenty minutes before going back to sleep. He awoke again around 2:00 and 4:00 A.M. and cried about twenty minutes each time. When he cried at 6:00 A.M., I rushed into his room, anxious to hold him and be sure he was the same healthy, happy baby I had put down the night before.

Over the next few days it was amazing to see how quickly he fell into the schedule we had set up for him. He cried ten to fifteen minutes several times, but never again for an hour. Now he naps regularly and sleeps all night, occasionally crying for one or two minutes during the night as he puts himself back to sleep.

Letting my baby cry was one of the hardest things I've ever had to do. Now that the experience is behind us, however, I have no doubt at all that it was right. It gave me more confidence in my abilities to handle tough issues as a parent.

I read that you should always take your baby everywhere and "wear" your baby like the Native Americans did. I carried him around in a BabyBjörn carrier on walks and to do errands. By the time he was 10 months old, his nighttime routine was established. I would nurse him to sleep at 8:00 P.M., put him in his crib, and he would wake up at 10:00 P.M. and cry. I would change him and nurse him back to sleep, and carefully, oh so carefully, put him back in his crib, and repeat this process all night every two or so hours. Sometimes he would wake up when I put him back in bed and I would have to start all over again. As the night progressed, and he became more and more exhausted, he was more likely to wake up when I put him down, and it took longer to soothe him back to sleep. By 6:00 A.M. he was up for the day, napping occasionally and only briefly. Sometimes I couldn't even put him down long enough to eat dinner. I held him while I ate. One night I went to him when he cried and nursing did not soothe him. He could not stop crying no matter what I did. I realized at that moment that he didn't need me so much as he needed to sleep. We were all exhausted.

We had heard about "crying it out" before, and I thought it sounded cruel. But my husband wanted to do it, and it was clear that we had to change our methods, because although I was perfectly willing to deprive myself of sleep on his behalf, Ares was clearly suffering from sleep deprivation. Ares had all the symptoms of an overtired child. He was easily startled, and cried uncontrollably at sudden or loud noises. He was unable to go to sleep on his own, and unable to stay asleep once he did. The book explained that in going to Ares every time he cried at night, I was stimulating him and keeping him awake, not soothing him and reassuring him as I had thought. All that stuff I had read about "nighttime parenting" and "attachment parenting" was not only not helping, it was hurting Ares. We decided to try extinction.

The first night I put Ares to bed at 8:00 P.M. as usual, but when 10:00 came and he cried, I didn't go to him. It was one of the hardest things I have ever done, but I wanted to give it a try for his sake. He cried for forty-five minutes. I thought I would die. My nervous system went haywire. I cried, my whole body got hot, I was shaking and sweating, and my heart pounded. He's going to think I abandoned him, I thought. He will never trust me again. But once he stopped crying he slept all night long. Ares had never slept for more than four hours in a row. I thought for sure he had died. But he woke up the next morning happy and rested and then fell back to sleep a couple of hours later on his play rug, another first. Ares had never in his life fallen asleep without nursing.

We worked to make sure Ares got the sleep he needed. At night we developed a sleep ritual of bath time, reading to him, and nursing him at 6:00 P.M., and putting him down sleepy but awake. He took two naps a day, following a slightly abbreviated sleep ritual, and slept for two hours in the morning and one hour in the early afternoon. For some reason he didn't cry at nap time, he just went quietly to sleep. At night, however, for several weeks he still cried for forty-five minutes when I put him down. This was extremely difficult, even painful. But once he fell asleep he stayed asleep for twelve hours, which was incredible to me, and he was so much happier during the day that we stuck with it. In the daytime, he was so much calmer; he even seemed sleepier for the first few weeks. He almost never cried anymore, and his attention span was longer. Eventually Ares went to sleep without crying, and he still sleeps every night all night long, for at least twelve hours a night.

When I am doing a sleep consult, during the first two or three days mothers often call me, worried because there is still crying at night. Upon questioning, though, they might also describe a six-hour block of night sleep or a midmorning nap of two to three hours. When I ask if these events have ever occurred in the past, the answer is invariably "Never." Recognizing that a new, better sleep-ing event has occurred helps you accept the crying as a means to an end.

Here is an account that was published in a professional journal for psychologists, so please forgive the dry style of writing, which clearly describes that *extinction is not harmful.*

Case Report: The Elimination of Tantrum Behavior

Carl D. Williams

This paper reports the successful treatment of tyrantlike tantrum behavior in a male child by the removal of reinforcement. The subject child was approximately 21 months old. He had been seriously ill much of the first 18 months of his life. His health then improved considerably, and he gained weight and vigor. The child now demanded the special care and attention that had been given him over the many critical months. He enforced some of his wishes, especially at bedtime, by unleashing tantrum behavior to control the actions of his parents.

The parents and an aunt took turns in putting him to bed both at night and for the child's afternoon nap. If the parent left the bedroom after putting the child in his bed, the child would scream and fuss until the parent returned to the room. As a result, the parent was unable to leave the bedroom until after the child went to sleep. If the parent began to read while in the bedroom, the child would cry until the reading material was put down. The parents felt that the child enjoyed his control over them and that he fought off going to sleep as long as he could. In any event, a parent was spending from one-half to two hours each bedtime just waiting in the bedroom until the child went to sleep.

Following medical reassurance regarding the child's physical condition, it was decided to remove the reinforcement of this tyrantlike tantrum behavior. Consistent with the learning principle that, in general, behavior that is not reinforced will be extinguished, a parent or the aunt put the child to bed in a leisurely and relaxed fashion. After bedtime pleasantries, the parent left the bedroom and closed the door. The child screamed and raged, but the parent did not reenter the room. The duration of screaming and crying was measured from the time the door was closed.

The child continued screaming for forty-five minutes the first time he was put to bed. The child did not cry at all the second time he was put to bed. This is perhaps attributable to his fatigue from crying. By the tenth occasion, the child no longer whimpered, fussed, or cried when the parent left the room. Rather, he smiled as they left. The parents felt that he made happy sounds until he dropped off to sleep.

About a week later, the child screamed and fussed after the aunt put him to bed, probably reflecting spontaneous recovery of the tantrum behavior by returning to the child's bedroom and remaining there until he went to sleep. It was necessary to extinguish this behavior a second time.

No further tantrums at bedtime were reported during the next two years.

It should be emphasized that the treatment in this case did not involve aversive punishment. All that was done was to remove the reinforcement. Extinction of the tyrantlike tantrum behavior then occurred.

No unfortunate side- or after-effects of this treatment were observed. At three and three-quarters years of age, the child appears to be a friendly, expressive, outgoing child. (Emphasis added.)

My daughter Chelsea is almost 3 years old. Putting her to bed has always been an ordeal. At 18 months of age she started to climb out of her crib anywhere from seventy-five to a hundred times a night. The problem seemed to be solved with the advent of a "big bed." She now sleeps through the night. However, having her stay in bed and fall asleep is still an ordeal.

I have yelled and screamed. I have used gates and locks on her door to physically keep her in her room. I have used treats as an incentive for positive reinforcement of desired behavior. Unfortunately, the only consistent behavior has been my inconsistency.

If Chelsea knows that I will put a gate on her bedroom door if she leaves her room, even once, then she will gradually conform and stay in her room. But there is a catch! She eventually will start to challenge my inconsistent behavior. One night she will appear in the living room and say, "Mom, I need a hug and kiss good night." As a parent, do you deny your child such a loving request and lock her in her room? So you give her a hug and kiss and send her off to bed again. Then the next night she wants water, and before long she's out of bed three or four times a night for hugs and kisses, water, Band-Aids, scary noises—you name it! Within a week, saying good night and falling asleep takes an hour or more. Then we have to start over. Webster's dictionary defines the word consistent as "free from self-contradiction; in harmony with." I long for the night when I'm in harmony with Chelsea.

As this mother said, "Unfortunately, the only consistent behavior has been my inconsistency." In other words, when a behavioral approach fails with older children, it almost always is not a failure of the method but rather a failure of the parents' resolve to implement it consistently.

A father told me that it was painful for him and his wife to admit that what they had been doing was wrong and not good for their child. What were they doing? The child was several months of age, and they were going in about every two hours, every time the child cried a little. He said that it would have been much easier to blame or get angry with someone like me who said that too much attention at night was not good for their baby, and accuse me of giving bad advice, than it was to recognize that they were the ones responsible for her continued night wakings and irritability during the day. Another mother said that the reason some mothers and fathers have such strong emotional rejection of my advice is quite simple: parental guilt. Since they spend so little time with their child because they are both working, they feel bad and try to spend more time after work in the evening playing with their child. They cannot consider that the bedtime is too late for the child's health, so they conclude that my advice regarding early bedtimes must be incorrect. Some parents think that even if it is not incorrect, it must be harmful in the long run.

When parents stop reinforcing a child's night waking, the habit can be eliminated quickly. In fact, psychologists have shown that the more continuous or regular you are in reinforcing the night waking during the first few months, the more likely it will rapidly be reduced simply by stopping the reinforcing behavior. The advantages of ending the habit by not going to your baby at night are that the instructions are simple and easily remembered, and the whole process usually takes only a few days. But the seeming disadvantage is that a few nights of crying are unbearable for many parents. This procedure strikes many people as too harsh, too abrupt, or cruel. Those are personal value judgments, but bear in mind that this procedure is effective and safe. It works. But if you feel this way, consider "no-cry" sleep solutions (page 332), or simply move the bedtime a little earlier based on the onset of *drowsy signs*.

Please remember that providing minimal soothing in the middle of the night will sabotage your effort, and your child will cry longer and harder with the hope of receiving a major soothing intervention. Therefore, if you have decided to "rip the Band-Aid off" with extinction, then do not go to your child at all except for a feeding.

> Small soothing efforts such as kissing the forehead, rearranging the blankets, comforting, and patting appear trivial to parents, but they can interfere enormously with learning to fall asleep unassisted.

One parent described extinction as follows: "Extinction is intended to be a carefully monitored, intentional method of refraining from further stimulating overstimulated and overtired babies in order to allow them to fulfill their need for sleep."

Q: *I don't think I can do nothing when my baby cries for me at night.*

A: Letting your baby cry is not doing nothing. You are actively encouraging the development of independence, providing opportunities for him to learn how to sleep alone, and showing respect for his ability to change his behavior.

Q: *How long do I let my baby cry?*

A: To establish regular naps, no more than one hour, but to establish consolidated night sleep, there is no time limit at night if your child is not hungry or ill. If we place an arbitrary small limit on the duration of crying at night, we might train the child to cry to that predetermined time. When it is open-ended, the child learns to stop protesting and to fall asleep.

Q: *Why is it good for my child to cry? Why not delay sleep training until he is older and more reasonable?*

A: Crying is not the real issue. We are leaving the child alone to learn to sleep. We are leaving him alone to forget the expectation that he will be picked up. We *allow* him to cry; we are not *making* him cry in the sense that we are hurting him. When he is older and still not sleeping, it will be harder for him to learn how to sleep well. Plus, losing sleep is physically unhealthy, just as is too little iron or too few vitamins in his diet.

Q: *Isn't crying harmful?*

A: Not necessarily. In fact, studies have proven that *crying produces accelerated forgetting of a learned response*. So when a child cries, he may more quickly unlearn to expect to be picked up. When trying to stop an unhealthy habit, crying may have some benefit, because crying acts as an amnesic agent.

Graduated Extinction

Graduated extinction means that you let your baby fuss or cry for a predetermined brief period—say, five minutes. Then you pick up your baby, talk to him, feed him, and do whatever is necessary to calm him down. A progressive (graduated) checking schedule means that you leave your baby for five minutes the first time he cries; when he next cries, you leave him for ten minutes, and the next time for fifteen minutes. This sequence continues with an additional five minutes of ignoring before repeating the soothing process. The hope is that during one of these delays, your child learns to fall asleep unassisted because he is developing self-soothing skills. The major problem with a progressive checking schedule is that because you are likely to be sleep-deprived yourself and have to remember how long the new delay interval is, often the child outlasts the parents' resolve. An alternative is to keep the delay interval constant the first night, but progressively increase it on each subsequent night.

Your baby will likely cry less at sleep onset using this method if Dad is the one putting him down after soothing and Mom has left the house. This is for two reasons. First, your baby knows that Dad cannot nurse, so what is the point of crying? Second, moms are usually more sleep-deprived and therefore likely to be inconsistent with the schedule. Mom might go for a walk, get a cup of coffee, or hang out with friends until Dad calls to tell her that the baby is asleep.

Some mothers don't just leave at bedtime but spend the entire first night away at a friend's or at a hotel to get some much-needed rest and sleep. If affordable, one night of pampering self-maintenance at a spa hotel is a smart idea for the family and not selfish. Other mothers cannot bear the thought of being away from their baby, and that is fine, too.

Research has shown that graduated extinction takes about *four to nine nights*. Parents who do not see a rapid improvement usually do not have all the elements of self-soothing in place, and/or the bedtime is too late, and/or naps are not going well, and/or there is inconsistency in the approach to sleep. A common pitfall is to "just once" pick up your baby, bring him back to your bed, and nurse him back to sleep.

This method appears less harsh than extinction to many parents and works well for many children. However, graduated extinction may take longer than extinction, and if you are using a progressive checking schedule, it requires you to keep track of the delays. Because extinction is simpler and may succeed faster, when a natural sleep disruption inevitably occurs in the future, redoing extinction may be easier for the parents than redoing graduated extinction.

It is my impression that for extremely fussy/colicky babies and for babies much older than 4 months of age, because parents are so worn down from sleep deprivation and the child is way overtired, graduated extinction often fails or takes a long time because the child's crying outlasts the parents' resolve to be consistent. In these situations, extinction is more likely to succeed and produce results sooner.

My observations and sound scientific data show that if children are well rested during the day, if the bedtime is early enough to prevent a second wind, and if parents do not reinforce the crying by going in to comfort the child, then crying occurring with extinction lasts only *three to four nights,* after which the entire family enjoys the physical and psychological benefits of more sleep. My research shows that with extinction the average amount of crying is as follows:

In Children Younger than 4 Months

Night 1:   Crying lasts 30 to 45 minutes
Night 2:   Crying lasts 10 to 30 minutes
Night 3:   Crying lasts 0 to 10 minutes
Night 4:   No crying

In Children 4 Months of Age and Older

Night 1:   Crying lasts 45 to 55 minutes
Night 2:   A little more or a little less crying than night 1
Night 3:   Crying lasts 20 to 40 minutes
Night 4 or 5: No crying

If the bedtime (page 65) is too late or naps are not going well, there may be more crying on more nights.

Professor Sarah Honaker compared extinction with graduated extinction in a group of infants at about 5–6 months of age. In both groups, the first night of crying was about 43 minutes and *dramatically lessened after the first night,* similar to my observations. The highest first attempt success rate was for extinction, and the most common second attempt was a switch from graduated extinction to extinction. Both groups were highly satisfied with the interventions and reported that afterward, there was less difficulty falling asleep, fewer night wakings and feedings, and more consistent nighttime routines.

A group of 6-month-old children were continuously watched by nurses in the hospital during an extinction study, and they all exhibited two or more bouts of sustained distress with crying lasting five minutes or more before the study. By the *third night* of the study, there was no crying. Additionally, on the *third day,* compared to pre-study levels, there was no increase in cortisol levels in the babies; in fact, they appeared to be lower over the third and fourth day. However, the mothers' cortisol levels were significantly lower on the *third day.*

Among 7-month-old children, mothers were offered a choice between *graduated extinction* and fading. About 80 percent chose *graduated extinction*. Compared to a control group of infants, those children receiving either intervention slept better at 10 and 12 months of age and their mothers had fewer symptoms of depression. "Most mothers (80%) reported partner support with sleep strategies." Working as a team might be more important than choosing a particular sleep solution!

Also, a study, by Professor Michael Gradisar, of infants 6–16 months compared three groups: one using graduated extinction using a progressive checking schedule; a second gradually limiting the time in bed by delaying the infant's bedtime by fifteen minutes each night (bedtime *fading*); and a third, control group that only received a sleep information booklet. Objective data were gathered with ankle-worn movement detectors recording sleep data over a three-month study period. Infants in the graduated extinction group, compared with the other two groups, fell asleep faster, had fewer night wakings, less time awake after falling asleep, and longer total sleep time of *nineteen minutes*. Nineteen minutes of extra sleep every night can produce dramatic benefits over time (page 104). There were some small benefits in the bedtime fading group compared with the control group, but graduated extinction was clearly superior to bedtime fading.

Rapid improvement has also been reported in studies of bedtime routines (which involve no crying), especially when coupled with earlier bedtime. For example, a study of children age 8–18 months by Professor Jodi Mindell also showed *dramatic improvement over the first three nights* with the consistent implementation of a nightly bedtime routine including a bath, massage, and quiet activities (cuddling, singing lullabies), with lights out within thirty minutes of the bath. The only recommended change was the institution of a prescribed *bedtime routine*. The children fell asleep faster and had fewer night wakings.

An important point that bears restatement is that parents teach healthy habits such as nutrition, hand washing, toothbrushing,

wearing helmets when riding bikes, and wearing seatbelts throughout their child's life. It's the same for healthy sleep habits. It's an
ongoing process. Sleep solutions may also be an ongoing process—
not a onetime cure like a penicillin shot for strep throat—because of
natural disruptions of sleep schedules. Because sleep schedules
often may get derailed, think of helping your child return to a
healthy sleep schedule more as an ongoing regimen of *care* and not
as a onetime *cure*. Healthy sleep, like healthy food, provides lasting
benefits throughout childhood and beyond (chapter 3). Sometimes
parents do not appreciate that they must be mindful regarding
healthy sleep every day to permanently prevent the problem from
resurfacing. I suspect that this is the reason why some published
studies have shown only short-term benefits from a sleep intervention. Having the perspective of practicing pediatrics for forty years,
with frequent well-child visits, when families make a change to help
their child sleep well and continue to pay attention to their child's
sleep, benefits not only persist (page 141) but also increase as the
child develops cognitively and emotionally.

POSITIVE ROUTINES PLUS FADED BEDTIME WITH RESPONSE COST

With this method, parents minimize bedtime resistance by allowing
their child to go to sleep as late as the child wishes (the bedtime is
"faded"). The idea is that later bedtimes increase sleep pressure and
increase the child's ability to quickly fall asleep. By employing prolonged, calming, and pleasurable bedtime routines, the child's second wind is minimized or masked. If, upon being put to bed, the
child protests, he is immediately removed from the bed (*response
cost*); later, when the child is settled again, the soothing bedtime
routine is restarted. The process of falling asleep for the child is associated with parent soothing (positive routines), not with protest
crying or unpleasant associations, and he begins to associate his
bed with falling asleep. The association between being in bed and
falling asleep is called *stimulus control*. After the child is falling
asleep without protest, the bedtime is moved earlier.

In a study of 3-year-olds with difficulty falling asleep, night waking, or both, researchers used a faded bedtime without removing the child from the bed (no response cost), because it was thought that removing the child from the bed might reinforce his attempts to leave the bedroom; parents participated in two 90-minute group sessions of sleep education and sharing of experiences. Objective sleep measurements showed that there was a rapid and dramatic decrease in the time required to fall asleep (sleep onset latency), time awake after sleep onset (WASO), and number of bedtime tantrums. Objective data and parent diaries regarding number of awakenings and total sleep time did *not* show improvement, perhaps because the bedtime was *not* subsequently moved earlier. At a two-year follow-up, half of the families reported that they had again successfully used the procedure, but no objective sleep data were collected.

My experience with this method is that real-life issues with some parents make it difficult for them to remain calmly attentive to their overtired child late at night; they wish to hurry along the process to get their child asleep so they will have some time for themselves. This impatience interferes with their ability to remain calm late at night for prolonged soothing. Although this method and scheduled awakenings (described below) work in a structured research environment, parents may not find them acceptable or practical in the real world.

SCHEDULED AWAKENINGS

With this method, parents note the approximate times when their child wakes up at night and then wake him before those expected times, so that the child does not cry out. If needed, the child is fed and changed, and then he is soothed back to sleep. My observation is that most parents hate to wake a young child for scheduled awakenings because sleep is so precious for themselves and their child.

PROS AND CONS OF DIFFERENT METHODS

Research by Dr. Jodi Mindell has shown that extinction works much faster than scheduled awakenings, but that scheduled awakenings do work. A report by Dr. Timothy Morgenthaler examined many publications on the four sleep solutions above by looking at the designs of the study and the strengths of evidence. Each study was analyzed for its quality. For example, a prospective randomized study on a large number of children is superior to a retrospective nonrandomized study on a small number of children. Studies of superior quality support a "standard" recommendation of a sleep solution, indicating that there is very strong evidence to support the sleep solution's effectiveness, and studies of lesser quality support a "guideline" recommendation, indicating that the sleep solution may or may not be effective.

The only standard recommendation for effectiveness is extinction. "It should be noted that, although generally found to be effective, unmodified extinction [page 256] has limited parental acceptance. Some parents find extinction with parental presence, which involves a similar structure except that the parents remain in the child's room at bedtime during the extinction procedure, more acceptable." In other words, extinction has the strongest empirical support but seems too harsh to some parents.

The guideline recommendations include graduated extinction, positive routines plus faded bedtime with response cost, and scheduled awakening, but "studies suggest that [scheduled awakenings] may be less acceptable to parents and may have less utility in very young children."

While extinction may appear harsh, it is my impression that the total amount of crying with this method is less than with graduated extinction because success occurs faster. Some parents feel comfortable with either method, while other parents feel more uneasy about extinction.

Other research comparing extinction with graduated extinction

showed that parents using extinction reported less stress in parenting (page 332). This supports my observation that parents who are
less stressed about normal disruptions in sleep are more willing and
able to employ extinction repeatedly following changes of sleep
routines during special events such as birthdays, holidays, or illnesses. These repeat extinction events usually take only one night
and are called *resets*. If you can muster the courage to try extinction
once, when it is needed in the future you will be more able to do it
again, and the old sleep problems will be a thing of the past. In
contrast, because graduated extinction and some no-cry sleep solutions takes longer, those parents employing them, who are already
experiencing more stress regarding parenting, are less willing to repeat the procedure when changes of sleep routines cause the child to
become overtired, because the idea of adding more stress to an already stressful situation is unbearable. So the old sleep problems
return.

Another observation is that for older babies or children, where
there is less uncertainty regarding hunger at night, extinction is simpler to execute and parents can therefore be more consistent. In contrast, graduated extinction requires a detailed plan of action to be
modified gradually but consistently over several days or longer. I
think simpler is better.

CHECK AND CONSOLE

Responding to your child at night is less difficult than ignoring cries.
The process of *check and console* means that when your baby cries
at night, you immediately go to him and try to *minimally* soothe
him back to sleep by stroking, petting, making shushing sounds, or
gently rocking the crib or bassinet.

Check and console is different from graduated extinction. Graduated extinction involves a predetermined *delay* in your response
during which your baby may be crying hard. When you do go to
your baby, you do whatever is necessary to soothe him to a drowsy

but awake state or into a deep sleep even if you have to take him out of his crib. In contrast, with check and console, your response is *immediate,* so you are not ignoring crying. Because your response is *immediate,* your child is not fully awake or crying at full force, so *minimal* soothing is attempted. You quickly enter whenever your baby first cries to see that he is all right and gently soothe him in darkness, but you try *not* to pick him up. Instead, you rub his tummy, stroke his hair, or gently rock the crib. You do the least amount of rocking, singing, and, if necessary, nursing needed in order to soothe him back to a calm, sleepy state. This method appeals to those who practice attachment parenting (discussed in more detail below), because they believe that it provides *emotional security* to the child. When the child learns that his cries will not go unanswered, he learns to trust his mother, and in turn does *not feel abandoned*.

However, there is no evidence that babies are harmed when they are allowed to cry with extinction or graduated extinction. Furthermore, this method could teach some babies to cry more frequently and longer in order to receive more soothing. In addition, it is very hard to only partially soothe a crying baby at night. On the other hand, if your baby is well rested and does not have extreme fussiness/colic, this method might work well. The hope is that this minimal parental attention allows your baby to begin to learn some self-soothing skills. The method works best if it is Dad who is doing all the curtain calls. A common pitfall is to "just once" pick the baby up, bring him to your bed, and nurse him back to sleep.

Parents who do not see rapid improvement usually do not have all the elements of self-soothing in place, and/or the bedtime is too late, and/or naps are not going well, and/or the parents are inconsistent.

The check-and-console method is less likely to be successful in an infant 6 months of age or older because your soothing attempt is more likely to stimulate your baby and cause him to cry harder in the hope that you will pick him up and play with him.

Also, if your child is a post-colic child who became completely parent-soothed, or if the child is very sleep-deficient, then success might be elusive.

SOUND MACHINES

Continuous sounds help reduce the signal intensity of intermittent sounds. Tabletop fans or music may work well to partially drown out street noises. Sound machines should be on their lowest setting and farthest from the baby for safety.

FADING

A gradual approach to reducing the number of night wakings until the baby can return to sleep independently is called fading. Over a period of time, you gradually reduce your efforts at night so that your child takes over for himself and falls asleep or returns to sleep by himself. This is like teaching an older child how to ride a bike. You first provide balance and support or training wheels and then gradually withdraw assistance as the child gains confidence and skill. Here is an example of a fade sequence in an older child to eliminate night wakings.

Respond promptly; spend as much time as needed.

Father gives bottle or mother doesn't nurse.

Change from milk to juice.

Dilute juice to only water.

No bottle.

No picking up.

No singing, talking, verbal communication.

Minimal contact, patting, or hand-holding.

No eye contact; sober, unresponsive face.

No physical contact; sit next to child.

Move chair away from crib toward door, slowly over several days.

Reduce time with child.

Delay response.

At every stage of reduction of parental attention, expect the problem to get worse before improvement begins, because the child will put forth extra effort to cling to the old style.

Fading has also been called the chair method when done with an older child in a bed, because you are slowly moving the chair farther from your child until you are just outside the door.

In an English study of children about 3 years of age, psychiatrists examined children who displayed difficulty in going to bed, night waking, or both. Parents were counseled to keep a sleep diary for a week and establish goals for the child that included sleeping in his own bed, remaining in his bed throughout the night, and not disturbing his parents during the night. The treatment consisted of identifying the factors that reinforced the child's sleep problem and then gradually withdrawing them or temporarily substituting less potent rewards. It was a *fade* strategy, not a "cold turkey" approach. Here is an example of how parents in this study gradually reduced reinforcement:

1. The father reads a story to the child in bed for fifteen minutes.
2. The father reads a newspaper in the child's bedroom until the child falls asleep.
3. The child is placed back in bed with minimal interaction.
4. The father gradually withdraws from the bedroom before the child is asleep.

In another example:

1. The parents alternate, but respond to the child.
2. The parent gives no drinks but provides holding and comforting until the crying stops.

3. The parent only sits by the bedside until the child is asleep;
4. The parent provides less physical contact at bedtime.

In this study, 84 percent of the children improved. Not surprisingly, *the two factors that most likely predicted success were both parental: the absence of marital discord (page 220) and the attendance of both parents at the consultation sessions*. Also, when one problem such as resistance in going to sleep was reduced or resolved, other problems such as night waking rapidly disappeared. And although half of the mothers in this study had current psychiatric problems requiring treatment, this did *not* make failure more likely.

This study points out the importance of working with professionals who can provide guidance that is directed toward changing the child's behavior. Of course issues such as marital discord or maternal depression have to be considered and do affect treatment success, but the focus is on the child's behavior.

Another study from England included children who took at least an hour to go to bed, who woke at least three times a night or for more than twenty minutes at a time, or who went into their parents' bed. Treatment started with the parents recording the present sleep pattern in a sleep diary. A therapist worked with the parents to develop a program of treatment based on *fading* by gradually reducing or removing parental attention, adding positive reinforcement for the desired behavior, making bedtime earlier, and developing a bedtime ritual. Target behaviors were identified, and an individual treatment program was developed for each child. Also, mothers were evaluated for psychiatric problems. Mothers who showed psychiatric problems were more likely to terminate treatment, which again points out how stressful treatment can be. But for those families who completed four or five treatment sessions, 90 percent showed improvement. The authors concluded:

> The evidence that children's nighttime behavior could
> thus change so radically, often within a surprisingly

short time, suggests *that parental responses were extremely important in maintaining waking behavior. . . .*
A rapid achievement of improved sleep pattern with reduced parental attention would be unlikely if *anxiety in
the child or lack of parental attention were causing the
sleep difficulty. . . .* Parents needed help in analyzing goal
behavior into graded steps so they could achieve successes. Once some success was obtained, *the morale and
confidence of the parents rose,* and they were reinforced
in their determination to persist by the more peaceful
nights [emphasis added].

This improvement in the parents after a fade solution has also
been documented with extinction in several studies (page 344).

MAJOR POINT

**The rapid improvement of sleep patterns produced by reduced
parental attention tells us that neither lack of parental attention
nor anxiety in the child was causing the sleep difficulty.**

I have seen this over and over again: When you see even partial
improvement, you gain confidence and no longer feel guilty or rejecting when you are firm with your child. It is precisely this increased morale and confidence in parents who see some success
when they start with graduated extinction that emboldens them to
switch to extinction. In a 2017 survey by the Family Sleep Institute
(page 329), this was the most common switch (graduated extinction
to extinction) and occurred in 66 percent of those who made a
switch. In doing so, they are more able to redo extinction when a
natural sleep disruption occurs.

Often it appears that older children are listening to the treatment
plan in the office, because they often sleep better that very night, as
if they knew something was going to be different. I think they are
responding to the calm resolve and firm but gentle manner in their
parents, which tells them that things are going to change.

The apparent advantage of gradually weaning the child from prolonged, complex contact (fading) is its seeming gentleness. A disadvantage for many parents is that it takes several days or weeks, during which many brief crying spells may occur. The major reasons this approach usually succeeds only partially, or fails completely, are (1) unpredictable real-life events interfere with parents' best plans and schedules; (2) parents do not appreciate the enormous power of intermittent positive reinforcement to maintain a behavior ("I'll just nurse him this one time"); and (3) parents' resolve weakens from their own fatigue and sometimes from impatience.

As mentioned, it is common for parents to start with a gradual approach (fading or graduated extinction) and then, because of either frustration, exhaustion, or partial success, try extinction. The most important thing is to start early with any approach to see how it goes. Maybe just try a slightly earlier bedtime (page 240)!

SWINGS

Swings might be used to soothe a baby into a deep sleep. They may be the only way to get a nap for a baby with colic; they may be used by a parent with other children to have more time to be with them; or perhaps their use evolved out of simple habit. But regular use of swings for soothing may interfere with the ability of your child to learn self-soothing. After your child falls asleep, he may stay in the swing for an entire nap or be transferred to a crib for a nap. Eventually, all children will need to be transitioned to a crib and acquire some self-soothing skills. But the acquisition of self-soothing skills as you transfer from a swing to a crib might not be an all-or-none event, and there might be a messy month before your child gets better at self-soothing and accepts the crib without protest.

During the transition from sleeping in the swing to sleeping in the crib, parents should be mindful that other factors will help, such as putting the baby down drowsy but awake and instituting a bedtime that is early enough to prevent a second wind, especially around 6 weeks of age, when early bedtimes develop. Also helpful are brief intervals of wakefulness between naps before 3–4 months of age and synchronizing the soothing-to-sleep process with nap rhythms after 3–4 months of age, when nap rhythms emerge. After 6 months of age, when babies are more able to protest longer and louder, it will be necessary to ignore more protest crying.

To make the transition from swing sleep to crib sleep, your general plan is to allow your baby to fall asleep in the moving swing; once he is in a deep sleep, turn it off and leave him in it so he gets used to sleeping without the rocking. The next step is to transition him when in a deep sleep from the stationary swing to his crib. The next step is to not use the swing in the first place.

If your child is younger than 6 weeks of age and is not colicky, skip the swing and practice putting your baby down in the crib drowsy but awake after only one hour of wakefulness *in the morning* and maybe accept some low-level crying for several minutes in the crib. The reason for doing this in the morning and after only one hour of wakefulness is because he is best rested from night sleep and you avoid a second wind.

If your child is 6 weeks of age or older, also consider allowing some self-soothing skills to develop *at bedtime* by skipping the swing at bedtime and putting him down drowsy but awake, or by having the father do the soothing at bedtime. Here also, if there is some low-level fussiness when you place your baby in the crib, try to ignore it for several minutes to see if he will drift off to sleep. But if there is loud crying, pick him up and try again another day.

If loud crying frequently occurs when you try to transition your child from the swing to the crib, consider leaving him in the swing (moving or stationary) for a longer period of time. If you are successful in making the transition from the swing to the crib but initially the naps are shorter in the crib, temporarily move the bedtime earlier. Later, when the naps in the crib lengthen, the bedtime may be moved later.

Accept that this entire process will involve some trial and error and that there will be a trend toward success punctuated with frustrating setbacks. But if you stick to the age-appropriate plan and consider all sleep elements (bedtime, consolidated night sleep, and timing of naps), you will succeed.

NAP DRILL

Biological nap rhythms begin to develop between 3 and 4 months of age and are well established by 6 months of age. So beginning around 3–4 months of age, you want to try to harmonize the onset of soothing to a drowsy-but-awake state with the onset of the biological nap rhythm. The midmorning nap develops first. Initially naps tend to be regular but brief. The nap drill may be attempted anytime between 3 and 6 months when you think your baby is ready, and certainly anytime after 6 months of age. But the nap drill may fail in babies younger than 6 months because nap rhythms might be too weak. However, there is no harm in trying it for several days. Some young children, especially if they are post-colic, nap best in a very dark and quiet room, while others do not appear to be so sensitive. Experiment with different rooms in your home; one family living on a noisy street temporarily used a very large walk-in closet with the door open, because it was so dark and quiet. In addition to too much light or noise, the nap drill may fail at any age because the quality of night sleep is poor.

Here is the nap drill. Put your child down to sleep, after soothing, drowsy but awake around 9:00 A.M. or as close to this time as you can if he wakes up very early in the morning. There are three scenarios in which the nap is substantially less than one hour:

1. When you put him down, he might cry at this time and never fall asleep. Totally ignore him for one hour. This represents your attempt to get a midmorning nap. If he does not fall asleep, pick him up after one hour and actively play with him. This may be thought of as extinction with a one-hour cap.

Graduated extinction and check and console will not work for naps because the expected nap duration is not long.

2. When you put your baby down, he might fall asleep then or sometime during the hour of being alone, but after he falls asleep, the sleep duration is *less than thirty minutes*. Then you have two choices:

A. Try to extend the nap by quickly doing minimal and brief soothing such as feeding, rocking, shushing, patting, or stroking, and then leave him. If this fails to extend the nap and he cries, you might decide to end the nap opportunity or you might decide to ignore him for thirty minutes to see if he will return to sleep. If he has not fallen asleep after thirty minutes, pick him up and actively play with him.

B. Ignore him for an additional thirty minutes to see if he will return to sleep unassisted. If, at the end of that time, he is still awake, pick him up and actively play with him.

If your attempts to extend the nap or to ignore your baby for thirty additional minutes rarely work, then abandon them. Neither method is likely to work around or after 6 months of age.

3. When you put your baby down, he might fall asleep then or during the hour of being alone, but after he falls asleep, the sleep duration is *thirty minutes or longer* yet substantially less than one hour. In this case, you might try to extend the nap by quickly doing minimal soothing such as feeding, rocking, shushing, patting, or stroking. Because the longer the nap, the less successful you will be in extending it, you might decide to end the nap and pick your child up and have fun together. But do not ignore him for an additional thirty minutes to see if he will return to sleep unassisted.

For babies a little younger than 6 months of age, in all three scenarios, after you pick him up, enjoy his company and try to keep him up as long as possible for a midday nap. Your goal is to reach 12:00 to 1:00 P.M., but you might only get to 10:00 or 11:00 A.M. if there is no midmorning nap or the midmorning nap is brief. Alternatively, especially for babies substantially younger than 6 months of age, for the rest of the day you might do whatever you can to maximize sleep and minimize crying, but focus on maintaining brief intervals of wakefulness, putting the baby down drowsy but awake, getting Dad and others on board, and enabling good-quality night sleep. For these babies younger than 6 months of age, the midmorning nap usually falls in place several days after night sleep is going well.

The *midmorning* nap develops before the *midday* nap. Just as night sleep lays the foundation for the midmorning nap, the midmorning nap lays the foundation for the midday nap. So you probably want to work on the midmorning nap first and wait until it is well established before tackling the midday nap for infants less than 6 months.

If your baby is 6 months of age or older, because two major nap rhythms are well developed, definitely try for a midday nap as follows. Once a midmorning nap pattern is established, try putting your baby down drowsy but awake around 12:00 to 1:00 P.M., or earlier if needed, because the midmorning nap is regular but brief. Or you may wish to work on both naps at the same time. The three scenarios described above also constitute the nap drill for the midday nap.

Some babies take a third nap in the late afternoon, but this nap may be brief, and the time when it occurs is irregular. Other babies do not take this third nap. If you attempt a third nap and your baby cries, immediately pick him up. This is a no-cry nap, meaning that if he cries upon being put down or shortly thereafter, he is picked up immediately and you do not try to extend the nap by soothing or ignoring. In general, if this third nap starts too late in the afternoon or is too long, it will interfere with a reasonably early bedtime. A guideline is that if your child is allowed to sleep past 4:00 P.M. from a third nap, you may have difficulties with a bedtime that is in sync with his early night sleep rhythm.

As previously mentioned, establishing naps often works best when Dad puts the baby down for a nap and Mom leaves the house. By smell, babies know that Mom is gone, and they seem to protest less when Dad does the soothing to sleep. So consider starting the nap drill on a weekend, when Dad is available.

Night Sleep Is Fine; Why Are Naps a Problem?

There are three main determinants regarding your child's naps (and night sleep):

1. *What parents do*. Naps that take place while the parent is doing errands or socializing might be brief or have less restorative deep sleep.

2. *Innate traits in the child (page 85)*. For example, some children have a temperament trait called *regularity*. It appears that sleep rhythms are more regular for these children and more irregular for others. So some parents with an "irregular" child are naturally going to feel a bit frustrated because there is more variation in their child's sleep patterns compared with those of other, more "regular" children. Because temperament is mostly inherited, trying to mimic the sleep schedule that worked for a parent of a regular child to get more predictable sleep in your irregular child will not work. Also, the irregular child might need more regular and consistent parental efforts to keep on schedule. Another trait is *sensitivity*, which refers to the amount of external stimulation required for a child to respond. Some children are much more sensitive than others; they have a lower sensitivity threshold and are much more eas-

ily stimulated by light, noise, and vibrations. Also, there is *individual genetic variation* in the duration of naps. Some children take long naps during the first eighteen months, while others take short ones. Any or all three of these factors might affect naps more than night sleep.

3. *The child's environment.* Light, noise, and vibrations might affect naps but be absent at night.

Parents have more influence over night sleep than naps for three reasons:

1. Parents are tired themselves at the end of the day and really want their child to sleep, not only for the child's benefit but also so that the parents can have some private time for themselves. Parents are more able to have consistent bedtime routines.

2. The night sleep rhythm is a powerful and predictable wave within the child, developing at and after about 6 weeks of age.

3. It is more dark and quiet at night, and the child is home in the crib for night sleep.

Parents have less influence over naps for three reasons:

1. Parents are sometimes conflicted between naps and errands, scheduled events, visitors, and the needs of their other children during the day. There may be time pressure to do other things, so nap time routines may not be consistent. Daycare, nanny care, or grandparents may introduce more variables regarding naps. Digital distractions interfere with noticing subtle drowsy signs, so the timing of naps may be off. Dual-career parents may have a bedtime that is too late, or an oversolici-

tous nanny or night nurse might interfere with self-soothing at night, producing poor-quality night sleep that leads to problematic naps.

2. Nap rhythms develop around 3–4 months, and naps become more predictable and longer around 6 months of age. So between 6 weeks and 6 months, night sleep might be highly predictable . . . but not so for naps. Naps change over time; as your child gets older, he has fewer and then no naps. This lack of regularity and the transitions to fewer naps may make it difficult to catch the wave of emerging drowsiness. The congenital temperament features of sensitivity to environmental stimuli and regularity of nap rhythms create much nap variability among children of the same age. As previously mentioned, some children are born to take long naps and some are born to take short naps, adding to the variability among children of the same age.

3. It is more light and noisy during the day, and your child may be outside or moving about in a carrier or stroller during nap time.

When you're attempting to get naps in place around 9:00 A.M. and 12:00 to 2:00 P.M., it is important to *not let your baby nap at other times* or he will never get on this nap schedule.

CONTROL THE WAKE-UP TIME

If the bedtime is too late, there may be bedtime resistance or night wakings. Because of the late bedtime or fragmented night sleep, the wake-up time might also be late and mess up naps. A simple solution to help achieve an earlier bedtime is for the parents to wake the child early in the morning, say around 6:00 or 7:00. This helps shift the circadian night sleep rhythm to an earlier hour, especially if the child is exposed to bright sunlight after waking. In other words, the child's night sleep rhythm now starts earlier. This makes it easier for parents to establish an earlier bedtime. Published results have shown that this simple change may dramatically and swiftly reduce night wakings without the parents doing anything else differently. This strongly supports the idea that the time when your child falls asleep is especially important.

When to Start the Day

When you're using extinction, graduated extinction, check and console, or some other sleep solution, your child may often start the day around 6:00 A.M. This is approximate: 5:30 or 6:30 A.M. might be the time for now. A mistake is to start the day much earlier, at 4:00 or 4:30 A.M., because your child woke then and has difficulty returning to sleep. The reason starting the day too early is a problem is because your child will be sleepy around 8:00 A.M. and you will never be able to get naps in place around 9:00 A.M. and 12:00 to 1:00 P.M. Depending on your child's age, you might need to quietly feed him early in the morning, around 4:00 to 5:00 A.M., change him quickly, and then leave him, ignoring subsequent crying. Or you can try not going in at all if your child is not hungry.

When the Wake-Up Time Is Too Early

After a few months of age, when night and nap rhythms are in place, some very *well-rested* children wake up too early for the parents. They are ready to start the day around 5:00 or 5:30 A.M. I want to emphasize that I am now talking about *well-rested* babies who have an early bedtime, consolidated night sleep, and great naps. For these babies, I do not know how to make them sleep later in the morning. The logic of keeping them up later so that they will sleep in later appeals to many parents, but it rarely works during the first few months of life, when children need two or three naps per day. And keeping them up later often backfires because you create bedtime battles or night awakenings. But feel free to try it; move the bedtime later gradually. If bedtime battles emerge, abandon the effort. For older children who need only one nap, it sometimes works and sometimes does not work, and depending on your circumstances you might want to try this for several weeks, as long as bedtime battles do not emerge. Moving the bedtime later in well-rested older children who are not napping often works, but it may take several weeks to see the desired result. The reason it may take a long time to see improvement is because the slightly later bedtime is only slowly creating pressure to shift the wake-up time later.

In the long run, these *well-rested* babies eventually begin to sleep later on their own, but this may occur anytime between 4 and 12 months of age. Meanwhile, I urge parents to go to bed earlier themselves to better tolerate the early-morning wake-ups of their babies.

Sometimes a parent innocently helps create or perpetuate too-early wake-up times in the morning. Imagine a 3-year-old getting up around 5:00 A.M. and the parents turn on a video for him so they can get more sleep. After a while, the child might learn to fight the early-morning light sleep and force himself awake or refuse to return to sleep unassisted at earlier times (4:00 to 5:00 A.M.) in order to have the pleasure of watching the video. In my experience, when the parents stop the video and ignore the protests, eventually the child begins to sleep later. I am not sure whether highly pleasurable parental interaction early in the morning with younger children or babies might have a similar effect on the wake-up time. I have advised some parents whose babies used to get up around 5:00 to 5:30 A.M. but were now getting up earlier (these babies were completely well rested and had an early bedtime) to go to them around 5:30 but to try to not be highly stimulating. This means that you would change and feed your baby and be pleasant, but in a quiet way in dim light, instead of giving him your customary loud, bright, and enthusiastic greeting to start the day. The hope is that the baby does not fight the very early-morning light sleep to have the pleasure of playing with parents.

In *overtired* children, moving the bedtime later only makes matters worse. Overtired children, in contrast with well-rested children, are in a state of higher neurological arousal near the end of the day, so they may have more difficulty falling asleep or staying asleep either in the middle of the night or in the early morning during light sleep. This is especially true if they lack self-soothing skills. In fact, for many of these children, moving the bedtime earlier helps erase the sleep debt, and the child is better rested at 4:00 to 5:00 A.M., so he is able to return to sleep unassisted more easily and thus sleeps later! To help solve the problem of a too-early wake-up time in these children, all elements of healthy sleep have to be dealt with.

A common problem associated with these overtired children who get up too early is that they are at an age when they should be taking a single midday nap but are instead taking an early nap (because they got up too early). This causes them to not be tired between 12:00 and 2:00 P.M. (when they should be napping); instead, they take a late nap (between 2:00 and 3:00 P.M.), which interferes with an early bedtime, thus pushing the bedtime later and causing the wake-up time to be too early. To correct this vicious cycle, because your goal is to encourage the naps to be in harmony with nap rhythms, try hard to get a single midday nap. There will be a rough patch late in the morning because the wake-up time was too early. This overtired state around 10:00 A.M. to noon is fairly easy to deal with, because both parent and child are better rested in the morning from night sleep. In contrast, if you allow the single nap to occur before midday, you will have a much rougher patch between 4:00 and 5:00 P.M. because both parent and child are less well rested near the end of the day. The now earlier single nap will allow an earlier bedtime, which is likely to erase the too-early wake-up. Sleep begets sleep.

PARENT-SET BEDTIMES

Data show that children's bedtimes have become later since the 1970s. In children 6 months–5 years old, a statistically significant trend toward later bedtimes was reported by Dr. Igo Iglowstein in three birth cohorts: 1974–1978, 1979–1985, and 1986–1993. For example, for 2-year-olds in the first cohort, the bedtime was 7:08 P.M., and in the third cohort it was 8:30 P.M. This trend toward later bedtimes preceded the trend of having a *television* in the bedroom. For 10-year-olds and 14-year-olds, the bedtimes in the first and third cohort were 8:45 to 8:59 P.M. and 9:43 to 10:02 P.M., respectively; these differences were not statistically significantly different.

However, the *nineteen-minute difference* for 14-year-olds may be important! Different research, by Michelle Short, shows that teenagers with parent-set bedtimes on weekdays have earlier bedtimes, obtain more sleep, and experience improved daytime wakefulness and less fatigue during the day. The teens in her study went to bed twenty-three minutes earlier than teens without parent-set weekday bedtimes and obtained, on average, nineteen minutes of extra sleep. She concluded, "While the *19 extra minutes* of sleep per night . . . may seem small, the *cumulative effect* of this extra sleep was associated with improved daytime functioning and may have further reaching effects in terms of improved emotional regulation and reduced risk of psychopathology [emphasis added]." As discussed previously (page 102), small changes can make big differences when it comes to sleep!

As little as *nineteen extra minutes* of sleep may benefit your child.

Additionally, the children last studied by Dr. Iglowstein were born in 1993, and the trend toward using more screen-based electronic media in the bedroom at night has dramatically increased (page 681), contributing to even later bedtimes in children of all ages.

Temporary 5:30 Bedtime

A temporary 5:30 P.M. bedtime is useful to repay a sleep debt that accumulates because of brief naps, naps out of sync with biological nap rhythms, a too-late bedtime, or fragmented night sleep, or during the transition to fewer naps or no naps. How long does it take to see improvement with a 5:30 P.M. bedtime? It depends on many variables, such as whether there was an acute sleep disruption in a well-rested child or chronic sleep problems, the presence or absence of colic, your child's self-soothing skills, whether his night sleep is fragmented or consolidated, how well he naps, and the presence or absence of daycare. Older children with more sleep deprivation probably take longer to settle in. Do not always expect overnight improvement (but this can occur). Work on all the sleep issues at the same time, but do not expect a 5:30 P.M. bedtime to be a miracle cure if other sleep issues are ignored. It may take five to seven days or longer to be certain that a change was or was not helpful. Sometimes parents make a change to see if their child sleeps better, but do not allow several days to see whether there is improvement before they reverse course or make a different change. This results in too many changes occurring too quickly, and the parents get frustrated because none seems to help.

How do you know if a temporary 5:30 P.M. bedtime might be useful? The answer is based on how your baby looks between 4:00 and 5:00 P.M. If he appears slightly out of sorts, short-fused, frazzled, rough around the edges, clingy, whiny, or crisp, then his sleep tank is going dry and he needs a temporary 5:30 P.M. bedtime, or a slightly earlier bedtime in general. Sometimes these signs of sleep deprivation are masked by placing your child in front of a television or screen-based electronic media. If he appears socially animated, engaged, calm, focused, or independent, then he probably is fine with the current bedtime.

Some parents use the 5:30 P.M. bedtime for only one night after an acute sleep disruption. This is called a reset (discussed below).

Reset

If your child has been a good sleeper but develops cumulative sleepiness or sleep inertia, then repay the sleep debt quickly with a *reset* before major sleep problems develop. A reset is simply an extremely early bedtime that is strictly enforced for only one night to repay an accumulated sleep debt. Ignore all protests and excuses (extinction). Get him back in the good-sleep groove quickly. A reset might be done just a few times a year in some families, but in other families it may be necessary many times a year.

By temporarily getting more sleep at the front end, the hope is that your child will become better rested at night and a sleep debt will be repaid. This should enhance nap quality, and the subsequent improvement in naps will lead to a later bedtime—for example, 6:30 to 7:00 P.M. in young children. But after you see improvement, if the move to a later bedtime produces bedtime battles or night awakenings, try 6:00 P.M. Choosing an earlier bedtime to help your child sleep better may involve trial and error.

How to Choose an Earlier Bedtime

As previously discussed, early bedtimes (page 65) based on *drowsy signs* producing only a *few minutes* of additional sleep (page 102) will help prevent and treat sleep problems. If it is unrealistic to establish an early bedtime based on drowsy signs, a bedtime that is a little too late is still better than a bedtime that is very late.

Move the Bedtime Slightly Earlier

Parents coming home from work late or picking their child up from daycare want to play with him in the evening. This is understandably very important for them, and they fundamentally do not want to reduce the duration of this interaction. Such parents might try moving the bedtime earlier in small increments of fifteen to twenty minutes. If the sleep-deprived child does not show much improvement—evidenced in bedtime battles, long latency to sleep (time needed to fall asleep), night waking, daytime behavioral or developmental problems, and brief naps—then the bedtime is still too late. Do not become frustrated and declare the "treatment" a failure! Instead, after four or five nights incrementally move the bedtime an additional fifteen to twenty minutes earlier. Other families might feel more comfortable with smaller changes such as five to ten minutes earlier every few nights. Repeat this process until you reach a bedtime where the child calmly goes to bed. If you reach a point where he does not seem sleepy and calmly lies in bed but does not easily fall asleep, then simply reverse course and let him stay up an additional fifteen to twenty minutes. Still, the above plan may be impractical for some parents who return home late from work. How are they to get their child down to sleep at night? Your baby might need a 7:00 P.M. bedtime *based on drowsy signs,* but the best you can do is 8:00 P.M. This is still better than 9:00 P.M.! Simply try for the earliest possible bedtime. The reality, as with so much of parenting, is that you do the best you can. Life isn't perfect, so don't beat yourself up.

Have your child already bathed, fed, and dressed for sleep by the caretaker. Do minimal soothing to sleep and get the earliest bedtime you can for your child. Go to bed earlier yourself so you can enjoy morning time with your child. If you are not rushed, mornings may be filled with joy with your child: bathing, dressing, feeding, and playing together. Be rigidly strict with nap schedules, because the better rested he is from good-quality naps, the more likely he will be able to stay up comfortably later at night. On weekends, protect naps and an early bedtime so his sleep battery is recharged. I have dual-career parents in my practice who do not see their baby when they come home from work late but spend joyful time with him every morning and on weekends. Because everyone is always well rested, they accept this trade-off.

Move the Bedtime *Much* Earlier

Some parents are desperate to improve their child's sleep because they either are sleep-deprived themselves or recognize that their child is suffering from sleep deprivation—or both. These parents, eager for relief, choose a much earlier new bedtime, perhaps as much as *an hour or more* earlier (page 300). It may be that this much earlier bedtime is in sync with circadian rhythms and thus produces better-quality sleep and a better-rested child. But if the new bedtime is way too early, it may backfire, because although your child now might get up in the morning better rested, the wake-up time is too early, which makes for a napping problem. Although the parents might benefit in the short term by experiencing no bedtime battles or night waking in their child, the price they pay will be getting up earlier themselves or nap problems that will keep the child from showing any improvement during the day. The solution here is the same as above: By trial and error, find a sweet spot somewhere between the original too-late bedtime and the new too-early bedtime.

With either plan, remember that if you choose an earlier bedtime and your child falls asleep at this new earlier bedtime, then you have after-the-fact confirmation that the old later bedtime was too late. Choosing an earlier bedtime takes time, and the earlier bedtime should *vary* based on the child's mood and behavior around 4:00 to 5:00 P.M. In turn, the child's mood and behavior around that time might *vary* based on naps and outdoor exercise or play. If you do not see your child during the week in the late afternoon, be very attentive on weekends to observe his mood and behavior closely around 4:00 to 5:00 P.M. to determine the optimal bedtime. If he is in daycare and there is a big difference between nap duration in daycare and nap duration at home, then the bedtime has to vary in order to reflect this difference.

Of course, parents might not see the deterioration of mood and behavior at 4:00 to 5:00 P.M. because they are at work. Furthermore, upon arrival home, the joy and pleasure of parent–child interaction, with games, stories, and comforting, might mask the child's sleep-deprived state. These parents are skeptical that an earlier bedtime will help. Also, some parents fear that an earlier bedtime will always cause an earlier wake-up time, and this inhibits them from trying an earlier bedtime.

The early bedtime allows the child to wake up better rested. Thus, he takes better naps. *When naps improve, parents can move the bedtime a little later.* If he is now well rested but early-morning wake-ups still occur, consider moving the bedtime a little later. I've said this before, but it really bears repeating: A big part of finding the right bedtime for your child is trial and error. It can be a matter of hitting a moving target. But be cautious in pushing back the bed-time, because if you push it back too far, your child will once again start accumulating a sleep debt.

During the transition from three to two naps, or from two naps to one, some families temporarily move the bedtime earlier (5:30 P.M.) because of less day sleep. But again, this super-early bed-time might backfire and cause your child to wake up too early, with the result that he now has difficulty getting to his first 9:00 A.M. nap or his only midday nap because he is drowsy much earlier. This throws the entire day off kilter for naps, so that by 4:00 or 5:00 P.M. the child is exhausted and wants to fall asleep at 5:30 P.M. In this case, the early bedtime has created a problem—a too-early wake-up time. Yet when parents attempt to correct the problem by moving the bedtime later, the child gets a second wind, leading to bedtime battles. Many parents have described this dilemma to me as "being stuck in the 5:30 P.M. bedtime rut!"

The 5:30 Bedtime Rut
We have seen how well-meaning parents, attempting to secure sleep for themselves and their child, can wind up trapped in the 5:30 bed-time rut, seemingly with no way to get back out. For a *young child,* here is the solution to the 5:30 bedtime rut.

If your child is going from three naps to two, try to *keep him up for his first nap,* or else the rest of the day's naps will be off kilter. It is more tolerable to deal with early-morning fussing as you struggle to get to a 9:00 A.M. nap than it would be to let him nap around 7:30 or 8:00 A.M. and then have an off midday nap and a miserable late afternoon when his sleep tank goes dry.

Similarly, if your child is going from two naps to one, though you do have to temporarily maintain an early bedtime even when he wakes up too early, you can try to *push his single nap toward midday.* This will be difficult, and the going will be slow and rough in the late morning. But if you give in and allow a single nap early in the morning, you and your child will pay for it with a much more difficult fussy time in the late afternoon.

Often these nap transitions are messy because the child develops a second wind, so go slowly. It may take about a month, and during that time you may feel stuck with a too-early bedtime. But trust me: It will not last forever. The best way to transition smoothly is to ensure that your child is well rested at the outset. Then the nap transition will be easier for everyone. In contrast, children who are borderline short on sleep have much more difficulty when they drop a nap.

As stated earlier, by getting more sleep at the front end, the hope is that your child eventually becomes better rested at night or a sleep debt is repaid. This improved night sleep should enhance nap quality and eventually lead to a later bedtime, such as 6:30 to 7:00 P.M. in young children or later in older children. Sometimes parents find it frustratingly difficult to find the right bedtime. If the bedtime is too often just a little too late or a little too early, like Goldilocks tasting porridge, then the child may cycle in and out of good sleep.

For some *older, persistent children,* I have temporarily pushed the bedtime to a very late hour, and it caused them to sleep later. They receive lavish praise and token rewards (such as a small treat, stickers, or stars) for sleeping later. Then the bedtime is slowly and gradually moved to an earlier time, but the later wake-up time is preserved because the child continues to receive the praise and rewards. See also "Positive Routines Plus Faded Bedtime with Response Cost" (page 278).

Regular Bedtimes

Dr. John Bates and associates directly evaluated the interactions among family stress, family management, disrupted child sleep patterns (variability in amounts of sleep, variability in bedtime, and lateness of bedtime), and adjustment in preschool in children about 5 years old. Children with disrupted sleep did not adjust well in preschool. In the researchers' analysis, disrupted sleep directly caused the behavior problems. They did not find any evidence that family stress or family management problems caused both disrupted sleep and behavior problems. Dr. Bates concluded that "sleep irregularity accounted for variation in [behavioral] adjustment independently of variation in family stress and family management."

Research on 7-year-old children with irregular bedtimes or bedtimes later than 9:00 P.M. showed that they had more behavioral difficulties than children who had regular, earlier bedtimes. The effects of not having regular bedtimes appear to be reversible.

Bedtime Routines

Bedtime routines help children sleep better. My wife used to remind one of our sons about the "dolphin story" as part of his bedtime routine. She explained how a dolphin swims deep in the water and sleeps in the water but sometimes has to come up for air before returning to a deep sleep. Then she told our son to pretend that he was a dolphin at night and that it was perfectly all right to come up from sleep, but that he had to go back down by himself. It worked.

SLEEP LOG

The sleep log is a graph to help you see how your baby is sleeping—or not sleeping. Online sleep log graphs are available, or you can make your own. A sleep log is a series of bar graphs showing the times each day when your child was awake, asleep, quiet in bed or crib, and crying in bed or crib. A sleep log is superior to a diary because a detailed diary, in which parents keep a minute-by-minute daily record of all the times their child is awake and asleep, is so focused on the small details that it becomes hard for parents to see the forest for the trees. A sleep log shows the forest at a glance.

Here's how to make a sleep log. Each twenty-four-hour day is shown as a separate bar on a graph with the horizontal axis as the day of the week and the vertical axis the time of day. Each bar is color-coded for sleep times and wake times. Other times, such as crying times, feedings, periods in crib awake, periods in crib asleep, or periods asleep in a parent's arms, may also be included. Studying the sleep log allows you to pay closer attention to the timing of these events over several days and even weeks. The baseline data in these logs enable parents to compare interventions such as an earlier bedtime. Spotting trends such as less crying or longer naps is often easier when they are represented graphically. And if there is a setback amid success, the motivation to persist despite some crying or inconvenience is right there before your eyes.

For twins and triplets, instead of a single bar for each day on separate graphs for each child, put two or three bars, one for each child, next to each other for a given day on the same graph so you can see for any period of days whether one sibling's schedule can be slightly modified to help synchronize the entire group.

CRIB TENTS, GATES, AND LOCKING THE DOOR

One- or 2-year-olds who climb out of their bed may receive too much social interaction from parents and therefore continue the behavior because they are curious and social. To protect their sleep and prevent the development of sleep problems, consider buying a crib tent.

In 2012, the United States Consumer Product Safety Commission recalled all crib tents from a specific manufacturer because of the hazard of entrapment and strangulation. Since then, newer and allegedly safe crib tents, bed tents, and crib canopies have become available, and they might encourage your toddler to stay in the crib. A crib tent will usually prevent your child from getting out of the crib, and it allows you to remove yourself from his protest crying without fear that an injury might occur. Sometimes duct tape is needed to cover the zipper because your clever child otherwise figures out how to escape. Don't worry about some theoretical sense of failure if the child has to return to the crib with a crib tent. Many children fall in love with their crib tent as if it were their personal hideaway—they seem to view it like a personal tepee or fort. They do not appear sad or angry. The crib tent is useful for families who know that they are unable or unwilling to do the silent-return-to-sleep routine (page 309) when their child climbs out of the crib. For a minority of children, moving them to a bed solves the problem; they want to sleep in a bed and they will stay put to enjoy it. But in most young children, moving to a bed simply means it is now easier to go visit Mom and Dad.

Some parents feel that the crib tent "locks their child in the crib like an animal caged in the zoo" and prefer to place a gate at the door or lock the door instead. But if you stand at the door preventing your child from leaving the room, your child will fight sleep all the more because he is getting attention from you. Most families find the crib tent more acceptable and effective, but let's talk about gates and locking the door.

To me, this is absolutely the last thing a desperate family might want to try, and because it sounds so extreme, I want to share with you my observations in some detail. The reality is that not all marriages are made in heaven, not all jobs allow parents to spend much time with their children, not everyone can begin sleep training early and prevent sleep problems, and, to be perfectly honest, it is difficult and inconvenient to be consistent in handling sleep routines. Circumstances beyond your control, such as twins in a one-bedroom apartment, sick relatives who need your attention, or medical problems like frequent ear infections, conspire to rob children of healthy sleep. So what are we to do when all else fails and the entire family is stressed from sleep loss?

For younger children, around age 2, some parents place gates at the child's bedroom so he cannot leave his room, or, alternatively, safety gates are in place and the parent's bedroom is locked. Either way, the child is safe but receives no social stimulation from the parents at night. Usually everything begins to turn around within *one to two nights*. You may need earplugs in order to ignore the banging, crying, or yelling. You may or may not place the child back in his crib or bed after he falls asleep. Definitely praise him well when he eventually stays asleep in his own room.

For children about 3 years or older, perhaps you have already tried other sleep strategies, patient reasoning, threats, and criticisms. Perhaps you've even tried spanking, which of course never works by itself, but all methods have failed. Maybe the answer is a stiff door hook that, when locked, holds the door in a slightly open position but prevents opening or completely closing. The door is held locked in a slightly open position to protect the child's fingers from a crush injury. Completely closing and locking the door may be an overwhelming degree of separation for either you or the child.

Take your child with you to the store when you purchase the lock, and make your child watch or help you install the lock on the door. Often this installation of the lock alone will cause a change in your child's behavior. Your child is told that if he leaves the room, he will be put back in and the door will be locked. Almost all the time, the child picks up on his parents' serious demeanor and does not even attempt to leave the room in the first place. This is so important, I want to restate it: Many families desperate to get their well-rested child back never actually have to use the newly installed lock, because their child knows on the first night that this is the beginning of a new routine.

Buying and installing the lock establishes the unambiguous message that leaving the room after a certain time is unacceptable. The

child learns that you mean business. You avoid the repeated prolonged stresses of trying to physically separate from a child who is
clinging to you, or of trying to keep the door closed while your child
is in the room on the other side trying to pull it open.

If, however, the child tests the rules and leaves the room, and the
parents place him back into the room and lock the door, although
there may be loud and long protest crying, it is usually only for *one
night,* because the child is now highly motivated to prevent the door
being locked the next night.

Simply locking the door solves nothing, however, if your child is
going to bed too late, getting up too late or too early, not getting the
nap he needs, taking a nap too late in the afternoon, or having a
very irregular bedtime, or if you talk to your child through the
closed door. You will still have an overtired child. No quick fix,
whether a locked door, or, worse, drugs to make your child sleep,
will make an overtired child less tired.

SLEEP RULES AND SILENT RETURN TO SLEEP

It's quite natural for 2- and 3-year-olds to climb out of the crib or
bed to check out the interesting things they think their parents are
up to. Or maybe they just want to watch a late movie or have a bite
to eat. Of course, what they like to do most is to come visit with
their parents and perhaps get into their bed. This not only disrupts
their parents' sleep but also fragments the child's sleep.

Sleep Rules are a strategy I created that works well for children
over 2.5. The first step is to make a sleep rules poster and tape or pin
it to the wall in your child's bedroom. Just talking about what to do
without the poster is much less effective. The poster is essential because it serves as a constant reminder for your child. It encourages
behaviors compatible with sleep and discourages behaviors incompatible with sleep (such as singing, calling, and running around).
Decorate the poster with art, markers, and stickers, and let your
child help make it. The more colorful and dramatic it is, the more

motivational it will be. Insert your child's first name before the title so that John will listen carefully when a parent recites "John's Sleep Rules" every time he is put to sleep. At every bedtime and nap time, recite the rules and explain the consequences. Sleep Rules should be implemented for both naps and nighttime sleep in order to be consistent. At nap time, if the child follows the Sleep Rules for one hour but does not sleep, he is rewarded for a good-faith effort. For success, the bedtime must be early enough to prevent a second wind. You simply say, "John, remember your Sleep Rules. One, stay in bed; two, stay very quiet; three, close your eyes and keep them closed; and four, try to sleep."

_____'S SLEEP RULES

(insert your child's name)

1. Stay in bed.
2. Be quiet.
3. Keep your eyes closed.
4. Try to sleep.

In general, perfect consistency is the preserve of robots, not human beings. When it comes to parenting, if you are 80 percent consistent, then you should consider yourself as close to perfect as is humanly possible. But if you embark on Sleep Rules with silent return to sleep, try to be 100 percent consistent for five to seven days to convince your child that you are serious. Expect to see sequential improvement, first for night sleep and later for naps.

To indicate when the Sleep Rules are over in the morning, use a clock radio with very quiet classical music, a digital clock with a picture of the morning wake-up time, or a color-changing light that is set at the wake-up time you choose. If your child sleeps through this time, do not wake him. But explain to your child later that Sleep Rules are in place until he hears the music or sees the color change on the light or the digital clock looks like the picture. At that point, he can call out for you, and you will immediately go to him. Rewards and privileges are an important component of this plan.

Reward your child in the morning for compliance at night and immediately after a nap: a piece of candy, a cookie, wholesome snack foods, stickers, small toys, special events or trips, or more screen time (use a timer) in addition to hugs, kisses, and praise. After you recite the Sleep Rules at night, tell your child what the reward will be in the morning if he cooperates. If you use something like candy, place the treats in a glass jar above the refrigerator where they are visible to the child; this will enhance motivation. One mother rewarded cooperation by placing a piece of candy under a special doll after her child had gone to sleep; part of the motivation was the excitement of discovery in the morning when the child looked for her treat. Give an immediate reward in the morning and after a nap for compliance. In general, even if there is no problem around naps, for the sake of consistency, also give the reward after the nap. Also, use stickers or stars on a calendar so that three or four stickers equal a bigger reward. This way, there is both immediate and delayed gratification. After several weeks of smooth sleeping, instead of giving the child the treats immediately, they can be placed in a "treat bowl" to be given to the child after dinner. This delayed gratification helps the child to substitute heightened self-esteem for the treats. Later, forget the reward but continue with the hugs, kisses, and praise. Of course, this method is guaranteed to fail if the rewards are insufficiently motivational or if the rewards are stopped or inconsistently applied before new sleep habits are well established.

Let's take a moment to look more closely at the difference between rewards and bribes. I am sensitive to the fact that some people will claim that it is wrong to give something to a child to make a behavior occur—that it is like a bribe, which is given *before* the desired behavior. The simple answer is that we smile, hug, and praise our children *after* they perform in a socially desirable way. This is how a child learns to share toys and develop manners and desirable social habits. But our social rewards simply aren't powerful enough to change the behavior of a strong-willed 2- or 3-year-old who is dead-set on fighting sleep for the pleasure of your company. Opponents to giving rewards come up with theoretical objections, but the fact remains that when rewards are used in the context in which I am describing them, they work.

If your child is very young and you are not sure he understands the concept that actions have consequences, use the rewards alone and do not restrict privileges. But if your child is older and does understand, then *restrict privileges* for noncompliance: less light on in the bedroom, bedroom door is less open, less screen time, remove toys, and remove stuffed toys or other bed items. You might close the door in a progressive fashion every time he gets out of bed. You can put three or four white tape marks on the floor, and after each time he gets out of bed, the door is closed a little more until it is barely open. If he stays in the bed, the door is left open to the first tape mark. A similar progressive strategy could be used with brighter or dimmer night-lights.

After you recite the Sleep Rules and remind your child of the rewards he will receive in the morning for cooperation, tell him what privileges will be restricted for noncooperation. Remember, rewards are only half the story here. Think of what your child loves to do around the house and label it a privilege. Never restrict outdoor play and creative activities such as reading, painting, art, or building things. Rather, think of somewhat passive things, such as watching DVDs or television, playing videogames on the computer, or perhaps playing with some favorite dolls or trucks. Choose one activity to be the privilege. So, after you recite the Sleep Rules, you say, "John, remember to follow the Sleep Rules so that when you wake up you can choose a treat and play with your trucks." All the trucks are put in a box in the closet. If he follows the rules, after he wakes up you say, "Thank you for following the Sleep Rules. Here, choose a treat. And here are your trucks to play with." Or if he did not abide by the rules, say, "You did not follow the Sleep Rules, so no treat and no trucks to play with until you follow the rules." Alternatively, the restriction of privilege means that noncompliance causes one or a few trucks to be taken away each time and removed from play so that the child sees his truck supply dwindling. If he has a hundred trucks, remove ten at a time. The same number of trucks is taken from the locked closet each time and returned to him for compliance. If John decides he doesn't care about his trucks, then restrict some other privilege next time in addition to the trucks. Sequentially restrict additional privileges. Some families with older children do only the rewards but not the restriction of privileges, and the method fails.

> **Consider rewarding even partial cooperation: small rewards for some cooperation, bigger rewards for more cooperation. Rewards are best given in the morning after waking or immediately following a nap.**

Silent return to sleep means that if your child leaves his room, you gently pick him up and place him back in bed. Every time you determine that he is out of his crib or bed, or discover him in your bed, gently place him back in his bed. Put a bell on his doorknob so you know right away when he is leaving his room. The signal makes him aware of what he's doing, and it helps you to be consistent. If you hear the bell at night, by prior agreement one parent intercepts the child as he leaves his room. You are not sweet or stern; you are bland and silent.

> **Do not underestimate the enormous power of partial or intermittent reinforcement to ruin your efforts to overcome your baby's habit of getting out of the crib. If you are not *silent* and you discuss getting out of bed when it is occurring, your social behavior undercuts your words and reinforces getting out of the crib.**

Silence when you take your baby back to bed is important, because if you are sweet or stern while trying to explain why everyone needs sleep, the verbal attention will reinforce your child's desire to get out of bed to get more attention. Attending to the problem in this way will cause the problem to occur more often. Many parents do not understand that negative attention—even yelling or getting angry—is still attention, and it will encourage your child to continue the behavior.

> Be *silent* and unemotional; appear disinterested or mechanical. No social contact at night.

After you recite the Sleep Rules to your child, you might add: "I love you very much, but you need your sleep and I need my sleep, and if you leave your room, I am not going to start a conversation with you." Plan to not get much sleep the *first two nights,* as your child may try many, many times to get back to his old style. Parents might want to alternate nights so that at least someone gets some sleep. Do not take turns on the same night, because the child might think one parent will behave differently. When silent return to sleep is practiced consistently, children learn quickly that there's no benefit in getting out of bed, so they stay there and sleep through the night. In short, every time your child gets out of bed, he should encounter a silent, unemotional parent who gently picks him up and returns him to bed.

When your child refuses to comply with Sleep Rules, either at night or for one hour during the day when a nap should be taking place, employ the silent-return-to-sleep strategy. When you employ Sleep Rules and silent return to sleep, do not be surprised if your child's behavior gets worse for a short time. It's as if he is putting forth more effort to get back to the old way. But patience pays off. Many children become proud of their accomplishments and brag about how they are following their Sleep Rules. One very cute and bright girl ripped up three Sleep Rules posters before she got the message. Then she started to tell her friends, with great pride, that she now sleeps by the rules. Be optimistic!

> Problems may get *worse* before they get better during a retraining phase.

We know from many studies that when parents think they have finally solved a sleep problem, it may resurface sooner or later. This is known as a *response burst,* and it occurs either because the child is testing to see if the rules still apply or because the parents have slipped a little regarding consistency in enforcing the rules or maintaining a healthy sleep pattern. Parents have another name for it: "train wreck." Knowing that train wrecks occur is no reason for despair. On the contrary, it should give you confidence to stay the course and not give up in frustration by convincing yourself that you are back to square one. Don't be dismayed at these temporary if often striking setbacks. Stick to what worked, and usually the problem will subside for good.

Keeping track of progress with a sleep log will strengthen your resolve to continue even though you may be frustrated by many curtain calls. Once you have achieved success, feel free to occasionally skip naps and early bedtimes and enjoy special occasions maybe once or twice a month—but not once or twice a week. Do not be a slave to your child's sleep schedule. Well-rested children can tolerate occasional breaks in routine without going bonkers. However, even after you achieve success, there may be a few times a year when sleep gets seriously off track and you will want to use this method again as a reset with a super-early bedtime.

Now let us consider the fifth Sleep Rule, for older children in a bed.

SLEEP RULE #5
Do not leave your room until you hear the music (or hear the birds, or hear the alarm, or see the color change in the lamp).

This rule is for older children who like to get up too early, leave their room, and bother their brother, sister, or parents. Again, set a clock radio on a timer, or an alarm clock—placed under a pillow to muffle the loud noise—to the time it is okay for your child to leave his room. Or use a programmed light or bunny that changes color at a set time in the morning.

Some children who have never slept well and have just turned 3 might completely disregard all Sleep Rules and trash their room or simply stay up late playing in their room with the lights on. These children might need extra reinforcement. For example, they may have to be placed in a crib with a crib tent for a while, or the light-bulbs will have to be removed to keep the room dark, or a lock will need to be placed on the bedroom door. Whatever restriction you choose, compliance with Sleep Rules is rewarded by the removal of the crib tent, the return of the light, or no lock.

Expect Sleep Rules and the silent return to sleep to reduce or eliminate the getting-out-of-bed routine within *three to four days* for these older children. All you have to do is remove the previous nighttime social interaction (whether pleasant or unpleasant) as a reinforcer to your child's habit of getting out of his crib.

Here is a mother's story about her daughter, Zaylin. She was cared for at a nationally ranked academic pediatric center and was so severely impaired that her psychologists and psychiatrists thought she was autistic. Sleep Rules were used with positive and negative contingencies, Mom got Dad to put her to bed at night, and the bedtime hour was moved much earlier. Two years after her mother wrote her story, her bedtime is 7:00 P.M. and she continues to thrive academically, socially, and artistically!

My daughter Zaylin was born with complex birth defects requiring multiple surgeries and prolonged hospitalizations during her first few years. The consequence of this medical history, that resolved approximately one year ago, at age five, is that she had many behavioral problems not only at school but also in our home. We regularly got reports from her teachers for "acting out" and she had an IEP [Individualized Education Plan] as she struggled with academics in school. In addition, she was very mean and nasty to her brother and very defiant at bedtime. I sought out many therapists and advice in an effort to help her, but nothing seemed to work. Part of the stress for me was Zaylin's struggles and also, the difficulty for doctors to properly diagnose her problem. At first, she was diagnosed with autism. She was later diagnosed with developmental delay and PTSD (from her repeated and prolonged hospitalizations). After many tests and many therapists, none of these diagnoses seemed to fit my daughter.

We used Sleep Rules and she protested. I started by taking away her stuffed animals one by one. She loves them and has plenty of them on her bed. Then I offered her a cookie for breakfast. I would let her dad put her to sleep because I would baby her and he didn't. Her normal bedtime was 9:00 P.M. and we moved it to 6:00 P.M.

It was not until I got Zaylin on a better sleep schedule, at age 6 years, that I realized that her sleep deprivation was causing all of these behavioral issues. I was skeptical because of my past failed attempts. After one week of applying Dr. Weissbluth's advice, I saw some changes. It has been four months and my daughter is a new person! The sleep strategy allowed Zaylin to sleep longer through the night without any more bedtime battles and her improved behavior in school was noticed by her teachers, and, at home, she turned into an entirely new child, saving my daughter and our family.

Here are some typical questions and answers about this strategy.

Q: *My child is scared at night, and I don't want to leave him alone.*
A: Try to spend extra time soothing him to sleep, buy a dream catcher or guardian angel to protect him, or go around the room catching all the monsters and put them in a bag that you take out of the room. Maybe give him a bell that he can ring on one

occasion, and only one, at night when he is scared, to which you will respond promptly. This will give him a sense of security, knowing that you will come promptly once in the middle of the night. When you respond, consider using a timer, placed under a pillow to quiet it, for a measured amount of middle-of-the-night soothing. Controlling the duration of soothing creates expectations and a routine that both a parent and child will accept. If the duration of soothing is open-ended, sometimes the parent will have the ability to stay for a long time and sometime for a short time, and this irregularity might cause your child to learn to protest for more and more soothing. Tell your child that when the timer buzzes or the alarm goes off, you will kiss him and leave and not come back until morning. After a while, your child will learn to associate the sound of the timer with your departure and will return to sleep without protest, knowing not to expect any curtain calls. In fact, this could be a sixth Sleep Rule: "If you are scared, ring the bell and I will come, but I will come only once." Tell your child not to abuse ringing the bell. Ringing the bell on more than one occasion would violate this Sleep Rule and be a cause for some restriction of privileges that you should also make clear at bedtime. Alternatively, for older children, a pass system (page 320) might help your child sleep better.

Q: *Won't my child hurt himself when he climbs or falls out of his crib?*

A: This is a common worry and often used as an excuse to go to your child or buy a big-kid bed. But the truth is that serious injuries rarely occur when the child bumps on the floor as he lets himself down.

Q: *Can the plan fail?*

A: Yes, when both parents aren't committed, so that one partner passively or actively sabotages the program. One father in my practice loved to sneak a bottle of formula to his baby once or twice a night. This caused the baby to suffer excessive wetness and a severe, persistent, and painful diaper rash. Only in the course of trying to eradicate the rash did the father's behavior come to light. Failures also sometimes occur when the child is still chronically fatigued from too late a bedtime hour or nap deprivation.

Q: *What if he stays in his crib but cries?*
A: Letting your child cry when he protests going to sleep or staying in his crib is not the same as making your child cry as if you were hurting him. Leave him alone (extinction) or try graduated extinction.

One family instituted this five-step program when their daughter, Nicole, was 26 months old—after 26 months of poor sleeping. She had always had difficulty falling asleep and difficulty staying asleep. Nicole always wanted to, and did, get out of her bed and go into her parents' bed. After the birth of Daniel, her brother, her parents decided this had to stop.

Their record showed the following results:

Night 1: Between 8:13 and 9:45 P.M.—*69* return trips to bed. Slept until 8:30 A.M. with one brief awakening at 2:15 A.M.

Night 2: Between 8:20 and 10:30 P.M.—*145* return trips to bed. Slept until 7:20 A.M. with one brief awakening at 2:15 A.M.

Night 3: After 9:14 P.M. (bedtime)—*0* return trips to bed! Slept until 7:40 A.M., awakening once at 3:20 A.M.

That's it!

An important point to note is that almost all of Nicole's getting out of bed occurred within the first hour or two of the night. Many children follow this pattern, so don't expect that you will necessarily lose a complete night of sleep during this training period. I suggest that you sit near your child's room for an hour or so at bedtime for three or four nights when you do silent return to sleep.

After the third night of Nicole's program, the curtain calls at bedtime ceased. Furthermore, at naps her mother would now leave after fifteen or twenty minutes of reading, whereas before she had stayed in the room until Nicole fell asleep. The parents described Nicole as easier in many ways: less resistant in dressing, less argumentative, more charming, and better able to be by herself. It is possible that Nicole's bedtime, shown above, was too late and contributed to the development and maintenance of her poor sleeping.

PASS SYSTEM

In one study, 3- to 6-year-old children exhibiting bedtime resistance were given a card exchangeable for one parental visit or excused departure from the room after bedtime, with parents ignoring subsequent bids for attention. They left their rooms and called and cried out significantly less than control children who were not given a card. A variant of the pass system, discussed above, is placing a bell by the child's bed with the rule that the parents will respond promptly once, and only once, if the child rings the bell. Once the child learns that he can have his parents come to him at any time— but only once—he will use this power with restraint.

DAY CORRECTION OF BEDTIME PROBLEMS*

Another sleep strategy appropriate for 3-year-old or older children is called "Day Correction of Bedtime Problems." The idea here, developed by Dr. Edward Christophersen, a prominent child psychologist, is that because everyone is tired and less able to cope with the stress of bedtime battles or night-waking problems at the end of

---

* From *Beyond Discipline: Parenting That Lasts a Lifetime*, 2nd ed., by E. R. Christophersen (Shawnee Mission, KS: Overland Press, 1998), 127–128. Copyright 1998 by Edward R. Christophersen. Reprinted with permission.

the day, daytime behavior should be tackled first. The following instructions explain this strategy in detail. Under item number 3, "Relaxed," Dr. Christophersen says, "Perhaps the easiest way to teach self-quieting, during the day, is by allowing your child to self-quiet during naturally occurring times of frustration." (*Self-quieting* is Dr. Christophersen's term for what I call "self-soothing.") In a conversation with Dr. Christophersen, he clarified this statement by explaining that you do not always rush to help a child struggling with a puzzle or accomplishing some task. When there is something that is slightly bothering your child, it is sometimes better to leave him alone to learn to deal with it. Dr. Christophersen's observation is that some mothers need to be taught to disengage or to ignore some of their child's low-level distress. He does not mean you should ignore your child when he comes home from school crying or has had a very frightening experience! In one study, when children learned how to cope with frustration during the day, they were observed to settle themselves better at bedtime and later at night when they woke. I will let Dr. Christophersen speak for himself:

> There are three important components to getting a child to go to sleep at night. The child must be:
>
> 1. Tired
> 2. Quiet
> 3. Relaxed
>
> When these three components are in place, children who have adequate "self-quieting skills" will be able to go to sleep rather easily.
>
> 1. *Tired*. The easiest way to make sure that your child will be tired when he or she goes to bed is by getting him or her up at the same time every day and by getting him or her an adequate amount of exercise during the day—vigorous exercise that requires a good deal of energy. For an infant, include several long

periods of time when he or she is on the floor and can see what you are doing, but the infant must hold his or her head up in order to really see much. For almost any child, twenty minutes of good exercise each day, after a nap, is usually adequate.

2. *Quiet.* You can elect to either quiet down the entire house or quiet down your child's room. Quieting down your child's room by closing the door and keeping it closed is probably the easiest. . . . You might need to turn on the furnace or air-conditioning fan as a masking noise for the first few nights.

3. *Relaxed.* Children can relax only if they have learned self-quieting skills. Self-quieting skills refer to a child's ability to calm himself or herself, with no help from an adult, when the child is unhappy, angry, or frustrated. Whereas older children (at least age 6 years) can be taught relaxation procedures [see below], infants and toddlers need to practice self-quieting skills in order to know what works for them. Perhaps the easiest way to teach self-quieting during the day is by allowing your child to self-quiet during naturally occurring times of frustration.

Self-quieting behaviors. The baby who goes to sleep with help from one of his or her parents by nursing, rocking, or holding learns only adult transition skills and needs an adult present in order to fall asleep. The baby or toddler who goes to sleep alone cuddling a stuffed animal, holding his or her favorite blanket, or sucking his or her thumb learns valuable self-quieting skills that can be used for many years to come.

How they feel. Children who go to bed easily and sleep through the night uninterrupted get a good night's sleep. They will feel better during the day, just as the adults in their household will feel better during the day. It may take from several nights to one week to teach a child the skills he or she needs for going to sleep alone, but this is one behavior that the child will be able to use for the rest of his or her life.

These three components described here have the added advantage that they can be taught during the day, which removes many of the fears parents have about handling behavior problems at bedtime. Even parents who choose co-sleeping can allow their infant or toddler the opportunity to fall asleep on their own, with the parent joining the child at the parents' regular time for retiring. In this way, the infant or toddler gets the perceived advantages of co-sleeping and the known advantages of learning self-quieting skills.

REMOVE TELEVISION AND ALL OTHER SCREEN-BASED MEDIA FROM THE BEDROOM

Having a television or other electronic screen-based media in the bedroom is associated with a variety of sleep problems and short sleep durations. Removal of all electronic media by the parents at a parent-set lights-off time may be a powerful solution. I view this as an underappreciated public health problem that has quietly developed over the last thirty-five years. Data I collected around 1980 showed no strong correlation between more television viewing and less sleep, but at that time television was uncommon in children's bedrooms. Shortly thereafter the presence of a television in the bedroom became much more common. By 2005 it was 40 percent; even among children under 2 years old, 18 percent had a television in their bedroom! In 2013, more television viewing, computer use, mobile telephone use, and video gaming were associated with later bedtimes and less sleep in children. A 2018 review showed that screen-based media use at bedtime was associated with inadequate sleep duration, poor sleep quality, and excessive daytime sleepiness. Detrimental sleep outcomes were observed when media devices were present in the bedroom even when they were not used at bedtime!

The presence, and subsequent removal, of a TV in a child's bedroom might be thought of as a simple sleep solution. But, as described by Dr. Radesky, the TV in the bedroom might be a coping strategy employed by parents who have a child with regulatory problems (page 681). Additionally, the amount of TV actually watched by the child might be an example of differential susceptibility (page 85). That is, individuals might vary, in the degree to which TV viewing is pleasurable.

From a geneticist's point of view, chaotic family environment, a television in the bedroom, large amounts of television viewing, unhealthy sleep habits, and regulatory problems might be interrelated and under some genetic influence. From this perspective, the TV in the bedroom is a symptom of a much larger problem and simply removing the TV may *not* be easy to accomplish nor, upon doing so, lead to healthier sleep and improved regulation. Maybe, for some families, the presence of a TV in a child's bedroom is a red flag that signals that professional consultation is warranted.

RELAXATION TRAINING

Let's look at the two major areas of concern for older children: falling asleep and maintaining a healthy sleep schedule. In treating these sleep problems, we attempt to break the self-perpetuating sequence in which sleep disturbances cause hyperarousal, which further interferes with sleeping well. Working with a therapist, older children can learn to sleep better through relaxation training techniques similar to those used by adults. The attempt is to reduce the level of pre-sleep arousal, thereby permitting the sleep process to surface. Here are a few techniques:

1. *Progressive relaxation* is a method whereby you tense individual skeletal muscle groups, release the tension, and focus on the resulting feeling of relaxation.

2. *Biofeedback* involves focusing on a visual or auditory stimulus that changes in proportion to the tension within skeletal muscles. Both progressive relaxation and biofeedback techniques can help reduce muscle tension and thus make it easier to fall asleep.

3. *Self-suggestion* to produce relaxation involves repeating suggestions that your arms and legs feel heavy and warm.

4. *Paradoxical intention* is based on the idea that trying hard to spontaneously fall asleep might create a vicious circle, which can be broken by focusing on staying awake.

5. *Meditative relaxation* procedures vary, but simple instructions to focus on the physical sensation of breathing seem to help some people fall asleep.

STIMULUS CONTROL AND TEMPORAL CONTROL

Stimulus-control treatment tries to make the bedroom environment function as a cue for sleep. Spending lots of time in bed watching television, reading, or eating directly competes with sleeping, and therefore these activities must be discontinued. *Temporal control* means establishing a regular and healthy sleep schedule.

Richard R. Bootzin, a psychologist specializing in insomnia, incorporates the elements of stimulus control in the following instructions he developed:

Stimulus-Control Instructions

1. Lie down intending to go to sleep *only* when you are sleepy.

2. Do not use your bed for anything except sleep—that is, do not do homework, read, watch television, eat, or worry in bed.

3. If you find yourself unable to fall asleep, get up and go into another room. Although you should not watch the clock, you should get out of bed if you do not fall asleep within about ten minutes. Stay up as long as you wish, engaged in a focused activity (reading is best), but no screen-based media, and when

feeling sleepy return to the bedroom to sleep. Remember, the goal is to associate your bed with falling asleep *quickly*! If you are in bed for more than ten minutes without falling asleep and have not gotten up, you are not following this instruction. You want to avoid being in bed feeling upset or frustrated that you can't fall asleep.

4. If you still cannot fall asleep, repeat step 3. Do this as often as necessary throughout the night.

5. Set your alarm and get up at the same time every morning, irrespective of how much sleep you got during the night. This will help your body acquire a consistent sleep rhythm.

6. Do not nap during the day.

Dr. Rosalind Cartwright, a pioneer adult-sleep researcher, teaches a variation of Bootzin's stimulus control that has helped some older children fall asleep more easily.

1. Before bedtime, do something that is pleasurable for a limited amount of time, using a timer set for fifteen to twenty minutes. Do anything you want, but not in your bedroom.

2. Take the hottest lavender bubble bath you can tolerate for fifteen to twenty minutes. This is for relaxation, so don't read a book or listen to music while you're in the tub. The bath helps prevent the storm of thoughts and worries that strikes the brain like a meteor shower when the protective shield of activity, sports, or homework is down.

3. After the bubble bath, immediately get into bed. Don't start any other activities—no books, no music, no telephone calls. Close your eyes and try to sleep.

If these instructions do not provide help, consider encouraging your child to get involved in sports programs in order to increase the amount of physical exercise he gets during the day. If this fails and your child still can't sleep well and appears exhausted, too tired, and not interested in outside activities, ask yourself whether the cause might be a medical problem or depression.

Children do get depressed, and some crazy, risk-taking "accidents" in overtired teenagers are really deliberate suicide attempts. If this is a concern of yours, seek outside help immediately. Start with school social workers, your physician, or local suicide prevention centers.

COGNITIVE BEHAVIORAL THERAPY (CBT) AND PARENT–CHILD INTERACTION THERAPY (PCIT)

Severe nighttime fears and objectively measured sleep disruptions were reduced in children age 4–6 years with cognitive behavioral therapy. There were fewer night wakings and less wakeful time during the night. Co-sleeping with parents was also reduced. Among 7- to 13-year-old children, a separate study showed that CBT was effective: Children fell asleep faster, were less wakeful during the night, and had less separation anxiety. These benefits were maintained at the six-month follow-up. Another study, utilizing CBT for adolescents, age 12–19, with diagnosed insomnia and associated psychopathology symptoms produced improvements regarding insomnia and reduction in psychopathology that persisted at a twelve-month follow up. Therapists trained in CBT and behavioral sleep medicine are available in most sleep centers. In a study of children, 2–6 years, with developmental delays, Parent–Child Interaction Therapy significantly decreased sleep problems. Therapists trained in CBT and PCIT may be found online.

CAFFEINE

Caffeine and sleep banking (page 245) may be viewed as counter-measures to the effects of sleep loss. Caffeine is a stimulant that re-duces the consequences of sleep deprivation by increasing arousal, vigilance, and attention, but is ineffective in mitigating the degrada-tion of cognitive functions caused by severe sleep loss. As a stimu-lant, caffeine can cause a rapid heartbeat, increased blood pressure, nervousness, irritability, and impaired sleep (more difficulty falling asleep and reduced sleep duration). There appear to be genetic dif-ferences among individuals regarding the sleep disruption caused by caffeine. The American Academy of Pediatrics recommends that children under 12 years should not drink caffeinated beverages and for older children, no more than 100 milligrams of caffeine (about the amount in one cup of home-brewed coffee) a day.

MEDICATION

Dr. Judith Owens wrote in a review of medications used to help children sleep better that "in almost all cases, medication [including melatonin] is neither the first treatment choice nor the sole treat-ment strategy for children with insomnia. . . . Nonpharmacological treatments have been shown to have more long-lasting effects (i.e., persistent after medication has been discontinued)." More than thirty-five years ago, I incorrectly thought that an antihistamine that induces drowsiness might be used temporarily to help a child sleep so the exhausted parents could get more sleep and be better able to change their child's sleep routines. But instead, after only a few attempts, it became clear to me that the parents who desper-ately wanted medication were the same parents who were most un-willing to make the changes necessary to help their child sleep better. I have not prescribed medications for sleeping since then. Also, recent research has shown that antihistamines are ineffective for solving sleep problems.

WARNING

When your overtired child first starts to sleep better during a retraining period, he may appear, in the beginning, to be more tired than before! You are *unmasking* the underlying fatigue that had previously been present but was hidden by the turned-on, hyperalert state.

Community Sleep Consultants

Sleep consultants, locatable online, are available in most cities and give personalized face-to-face advice to help children sleep better. Often, consultants also perform services online. Their website will give information regarding fees, services, professional training, and educational background. Request a free initial encounter to see if there appears to be a good fit between you and the consultant's personality. Anyone can promote themselves as a sleep consultant because there are no state or national professional standards. However, some sleep consultants have received certification from online training programs. Anyone can create a training program because here, too, there are no state or professional standards. Investigating the training program founder's background, along with the program's course content, assessment methods, and recertification requirements might help in choosing a "certified" sleep consultant. A training program will help you find a consultant in your area. Training programs are available in many countries. One program that I am familiar with is the Family Sleep Institute: familysleepinstitute.com. (Full disclosure: I am an unpaid adviser to FSI with no financial interests or potential conflicts of interest.)

In 2020, the Family Sleep Institute conducted a survey of ninety-four consecutive sleep consultations performed by thirty-seven consultants in fifteen countries (46 percent of these consultations were in the US). The most common age of the child was 5 months (the range was 4 months to 5 years). Recommendations included safe sleep to prevent *SIDS*, putting the child to sleep independently, drowsy but awake, regular bedtimes, and age-appropriate sleep and night-feeding schedules.

At 12 months of age or younger, parents' concerns were night wakings (98 percent), napping (84 percent), nighttime eating at undesirable times (84 percent), and bedtime issues (71 percent). The success rates in resolving these concerns were 93, 82, 86, and 95 percent, respectively. Similar concerns and success rates were observed among children 13 months of age and older. Overall satisfaction rates with the consultation were high: Complete satisfaction, 89 percent; somewhat satisfied, 7 percent; neutral, 2 percent; and completely dissatisfied, 1 percent. Families that had a bedtime routine at initial contact were more likely to be satisfied. Increased parent satisfaction was associated with using extinction or graduated extinction at the end of the consultation.

Most families maintained their initial choice for a sleep solution throughout the consultation (thirteen for extinction, forty-five for graduated extinction, and twenty-three for fading or a version of check and console). For these families, "completely satisfied with the sleep training consultation" percentages were 100, 91, and 86, respectively. Other families changed from their initial choice for a sleep solution to a subsequent choice that involved attending to their child less at night.

Using extinction as an initial sleep solution was associated with increased likelihood that the child would be sleeping independently through the night, eating during the night at desirable times, and going to bed without bedtime issues at the end of the consultation. Using extinction, compared with other choices, at the end of the process was associated with increased satisfaction with the sleep-training consultation. Recommending extinction as an initial or subsequent sleep solution occurred almost exclusively in the US and Canada, and more experienced consultants were more likely to do so.

Choose a Sleep Solution

Happily, if a sleep problem exists, it usually can be corrected, even in older children. If your child is not sleeping well, the goal is to have parents impose upon him an age-appropriate, biologically healthy sleep schedule within the context of the family. This approach is no different from when parents choose a healthy selection of foods at meals. Parents' responsibility in teaching sleep habits is the same as teaching other health habits such as handwashing, toothbrushing, or wearing a helmet when riding a bike. But there is no one-size-fits-all approach to helping children sleep well, because all families are different (chapter 1).

There are many ways to help your child sleep. You should choose the solution that works best for you and your child. Some do not work well for the extremely fussy or colicky baby, some will be difficult to use because of limited resources for soothing, and some are appropriate only for older children. Also, one method may be more powerful in the hands of some families than in others.

In the past, I would often refer to ignoring all crying or extinction as the preferred solution to help your child sleep better, because I think this works best, after 2–4 months of age, for the 20 percent of babies who have extreme fussiness/colic. But effectiveness of a sleep method such as extinction does not mean it will be acceptable, especially for a parent who feels strongly that it is wrong for them.

I favored extinction because from my research and review of the literature, before writing a book for parents on infant colic in 1985 and the first edition of this book in 1987, it appeared that colicky infants represented the largest group of children with sleep problems or had more severe sleep problems. And it appeared, then, that colic was almost entirely a within-the-child or biologically based developmental issue. However, I did understand that this is probably the hardest sleep solution for parents and recommended that you should always first consider other sleep solutions that involve less crying, especially if your child does not have extreme fussiness/colic.

Today, research amply demonstrates interactive effects between babies and parents with regard to crying/fussing and not sleeping well. Also, there may be a real increase in the prevalence of anxiety among parents and/or a heightened appreciation of the effects of parental anxiety (or depression) in rearing a child. Finally, it appears that our busy lifestyle has pushed back the bedtimes of our children. So if anxiety or depression symptoms are present or you are just uncomfortable with extinction, simply first try to *move the bedtime a little earlier* (page 102) based on *drowsy signs* and consider other sleep solutions that do not involve crying. Later, you might feel more comfortable with a fade procedure or graduated extinction.

One way to think about different sleep solutions and help you choose one is to organize them into three groups:

1. "No-cry" sleep solutions
   Teach Self-Soothing
       Many hands, father care
       Drowsy but awake, soothing
       Many naps
   Move bedtime slightly earlier based on *drowsy signs*
   Fade Procedure
   Check and console
   Bedtime routines
   Motionless sleep
   Sleep log
   Sound machine, room-darkening curtains
   Positive routines plus faded bedtime with response cost
   Scheduled awakening
   Control the wake-up time

Relaxation training
Stimulus control
2. "Maybe-cry" sleep solutions
Move bedtime much earlier
Nap drill
Parent-set bedtimes, regular bedtimes, earlier bedtimes
Swings
Crib tent
Sleep Rules and silent return to sleep
Pass system
Day correction of bedtime problems
3. "Let-cry" sleep solutions
Extinction: with or without cap, with or without parent
   presence
Graduated extinction

Another way to think about choosing a sleep solution (see chapter 1):

1. If you practice limit setting and neither parent has anxiety or depression symptoms, choose extinction.
2. If you practice limit setting and one parent has anxiety or depression symptoms, choose graduated extinction.
3. If you practice limit setting and both parents have anxiety or depression symptoms, choose check and console or fading.
4. If you practice infant demand, choose fading.

For some parents, the major decision is whether to ever let their child cry (chapter 1). Some parents are strong believers in only one approach to soothing to sleep. They believe there should never be any crying and that by always holding their baby, frequently nursing their baby, and sleeping with their baby, they can prevent extreme fussiness/colic from occurring and prevent sleep problems. They characterize their approach as "gently to sleep" or "attachment parenting," a gentle, warm, child-centered style that enhances a sense of security because the baby is taught that the mother is always there. They are proud to "wear their baby" and proclaim themselves "twenty-four-hour parents." They characterize other approaches as "cry it out" or "detached parenting," a cold, rigid, parent-centered style that creates a sense of abandonment because the baby is taught that the mother is unresponsive. These parents say that when the baby stops crying and sleeps, he has "given up" trying to communicate with his mother and will grow up with feelings of insecurity (pages 255, 336, and 344). This stark contrast in parenting styles is supposed to produce differences in babies and differences in the bonding between the child and his parents.

However, there are some major problems with this way of thinking. First, there is no evidence that one style or another produces a specific outcome. Second, babies themselves contribute a lot to what will easily work or not work. Third, it's not just about the bond between babies and mothers; fathers, siblings, and real-life family issues help shape your ability to soothe, comfort, and put your baby to sleep. Fourth, there are methods in between always attending to night crying and never attending to night crying, such as those listed under "maybe-cry" above. "Attachment parenting" may or may not be your decision, but it may work well for babies who have common fussiness and develop an easy temperament. For these babies, everything you read in popular books about soothing and sleeping will likely work. Perhaps, for the majority of parents, the path to healthy sleep does not involve any crying. There is no reason to be judgmental and criticize other parents who are not so fortunate.

A minority of families become distressed or overwhelmed with the arrival of their baby because they lack sufficient resources to soothe the baby or the baby has extreme fussiness/colic, with the result being that the baby develops into an overtired 4-month-old with a difficult temperament. These parents may have started out with the crib and decided later to use the family bed for soothing and sleeping, and were still frustrated when, after four months, the baby still did not sleep well. Flexibility and sensitivity to your baby is important in choosing a sleep solution that fits your family.

Another important factor in choosing a sleep solution is sensitivity to your own personality and makeup (chapter 4). As mentioned previously, some parents feel more stressed, and for them graduated extinction is more acceptable than extinction. Some mothers have depressive symptoms and might find extinction too stressful, or they have anxiety symptoms that appear to be associated with infant colic.

Also, one study used a parenting scale to measure parental discipline style and discovered that certain maternal factors were associated with success in using extinction. The two main factors studied were laxness (the extent to which parents notice but do not discipline misbehavior) and verbosity (the extent to which parents respond to misbehavior with coaxing, begging, or lengthy explanations—not to be confused with appropriate parental reasoning, explanations, and conversations that are associated with greater compliance in toddlers and preschoolers).

For mothers who were less distressed with their roles as parents and "who made fewer lax and verbose disciplinary mistakes," there were better outcomes with extinction. These mothers were more compliant with the treatment protocol; that is, they more consistently followed the plan. So the recommendation or choice to use extinction might also be influenced by maternal discipline style. In this study, there were no maternal characteristics associated with graduated extinction. Graduated extinction, though, was easier to implement. As stated before, other research has shown that graduated extinction is more acceptable when parents report more stress in their marriage. Often, families start with graduated extinction and see some improvement in their child's sleeping, demeanor, and behavior and then shift to extinction. Both methods improve bedtime and nighttime sleep problems.

Another study followed a group of young women prior to, during, and after pregnancy. About 10 percent of the babies born had extreme fussiness/colic. Mothers who had anxiety before, during, or after the pregnancy were more likely to have a baby with extreme fussiness/colic. In this study, unlike others, there was no association between maternal depression and extreme fussiness/colic.

This study associating maternal anxiety before the pregnancy and extreme fussiness/colic and the previous study regarding discipline style and ability to use extinction highlights the interplay between maternal issues and baby issues. Sometimes this combination of maternal issues and baby issues is expressed as a fear of ever letting your baby cry.

WHY CAN'T I LET MY BABY CRY?

An important fact is that the meaning of crying changes with age. All babies cry some of the time and often, for no apparent reason (page 384). Also, as shown in studies by Dr. Emde, during the first few months your baby may have his eyes wide open and appear to be awake but actually be asleep; further, in this "indeterminate sleep," your baby may also smile, suck, or cry. Eyes open and crying while asleep! As Professor Barr wrote, "Crying is *at first* relatively undifferentiated ('expressive') whereas it *later* becomes more intentional ('communicative')." Of course, your baby may cry because he is hungry and needs food to survive. Your toddler may cry because he wants a second helping of dessert after dinner. Your child may cry when afraid. Your teenager may cry when feeling hopeless. You may cry from happiness at a wedding. Not all crying signifies pain. Unfortunately, when some parents talk about crying babies, the assumption is that *all* crying equals pain. This leads to the sometimes hidden thought, *If my baby cries, I am a bad parent.* Here are some reasons why some parents respond promptly to all cries no matter how quiet or mild:

1. *Unpleasant childhood memories.* These may surface and remind you of feelings of loneliness or being unwanted.

2. *Working parent's guilt.* You may feel guilty about being away from your child so much.

3. *We already tried and it didn't work.* Maybe your child was too young then; maybe you taught him, by your behavior, that if he cried for more than a certain amount of time you would go to him; maybe you unknowingly provided intermittent reinforcement by going to him at some times but not at others.

4. *I enjoy my baby's company too much at night.* This may be because you're not a good sleeper yourself.

5. *If I don't nurse my baby at night, he might lose weight.* This is usually not true.

6. *We're under a lot of stress.* In *My Child Won't Sleep,* Jo Douglas and Naomi Richman wrote: "If you are feeling stressed, your child may respond by not sleeping so well. If the stress is related to difficulties between you as parents, you may think that your young child will not notice, but the chances are that he will. His way of waking at night and coming into your bed can be a way of preventing you from talking to each other and sorting out your problems, and his presence can act as a useful contraceptive." Although this quote applies to older children, it's possible that maintaining the baby's night waking or having the baby sleep with you when he is younger also serves the purpose of avoiding marital problems.

7. *I feel that I am a bad parent if my baby cries.* You are not a bad parent if you are helping your baby learn healthy sleep habits.

What does it mean to be a "good parent"? Parents feed and protect their young and provide comfort and guidance. When your baby cries, you go to him. On the surface, it certainly seems reasonable to say that the cry of your baby communicates messages: "feed me," "change me," "pick me up," "hold me," "hug me," or "rock me." The question is, why is it that when a parent makes an immediate and complete response to these messages, some babies still cry? Alternatively, if crying is a form of necessary communication, why is it that many parents will deliver complete, loving, and sensitive care even when their babies do not cry? Perhaps crying as a signal system is not perfect: Some babies cry even when they don't need to, because their needs are being cared for, and other babies don't cry but still receive the care they need. Crying may be a fundamental part of what it means to be a baby: Birds fly, babies cry.

Some baby animals make sounds that always cause the mother to move closer to the baby animal; these have been called *proximity-promoting calls*. The obvious benefit for the baby animal is protection, nurturing, and not getting separated from the group. In infants, it is possible that crying originated as a similar signal that is no longer tightly linked to infant survival, but still occurs as a behavioral remnant of some distant past. For example, babies might have originally had gestations of more than nine months before our ancestors assumed an upright posture; now babies' brains at birth may be a few months biologically immature. The result is that during the first few months, some aspects of brain development may not be well attuned to the outside world, and this misalignment expresses itself as crying.

Thinking about how mothers relate to their babies during these early times and how they forge close relationships led to two popular concepts: infant bonding and attachment theory. Both focused almost exclusively on mothers and both claimed that future events would be strongly influenced by early experiences.

Infant bonding theories promoted the importance of early physical contact between baby and mother as a mechanism to a better adjustment later in life. The good news was that this concept caused the delivery of babies to become more comfortable, taking place in surroundings more like a hotel room than the cold, impersonal environment of a traditional delivery room. The bad news was that mothers who missed this experience because of complications around the delivery, and mothers who adopted older children, felt deprived and worried about their future relationship with their children. You see, infant bonding was thought to take place only during a critical period, very much like the imprinting of baby geese, who will follow any large, moving object they see at a specific time in their development. The fact is that there is no scientific evidence that a similar critical period exists for human babies, and there is no evidence that lack of "bonding" at a specific time right at birth affects subsequent behavior in either infant or mother.

Attachment theory not only considered the interaction between the mother and the child but claimed that if attachment didn't develop well, the infant would grow into an adult who had difficulty in peer relationships, romantic relationships, or parenthood. The good news was that mothers were encouraged to be affectionate, tactile, and warm without fear of spoiling their child. The bad news was that attention to children twenty-four hours a day was thought to be good. Today's "helicopter parents" are one result.

Popular distortions of attachment theory claimed that a "twenty-four-hour parent"—meaning one who attends to every cry day and night—would produce a more securely attached child than would a "selfish" parent who ignores a cry at night so she can get some sleep. Accumulated scientific data do not support these claims. In fact, published research on children between 7 and 27 months of age has shown that when parents are instructed not to attend to their children's protest crying at night (extinction), *measurements of infant security significantly improve and all the mothers become less anxious over time*. A similar study in sleep-disturbed infants also showed *no* evidence of detrimental effects on security.

In 2016, Professor Gradisar studied infants 6–16 months of age. "Do extinction-based techniques produce stress that leads to later problematic emotions and behavior, and thus insecure parent–child attachments?" Infants were randomized to receive graduated extinction, bedtime fading, or sleep education as a control group. Objective measurements of sleep showed improvements over a three-month study period for the treatment groups, especially graduated extinction. At the end of the three-month study, measurements of "Afternoon cortisol [a hormone related to stress] showed a large decline in the graduated extinction group, a moderate decline in the bedtime fading group, and a small decline in the control group." At the twelve-month follow-up, "Parents participated in the strange situation procedure to assess child–parent attachment . . . which were videotaped and blind scored according to gold standard criteria." They also completed a Child Behavior Checklist. "*No* significant differences were found between secure and insecure attachment styles between groups. There were *no* significant differences between groups for any emotional or behavioral problems on the Child Behavior Checklist. . . . *We do not interpret these data as the infant "giving up" but instead self-soothing* [emphasis added]." It's a simple but true statement that when the entire family gets more sleep, everyone feels better, even if the cries of one member of the family have to be ignored for a while to get there.

In discussing the myth of popular attachment theory, the famous child psychologist Michael Lewis emphasizes how the development of social skills and peer relation skills are encouraged and protected both by family members other than the mother and by people outside the family. Further, in his aptly titled book *Altering Fate: Why the Past Does Not Predict the Future,* he explains how this development depends more on current, ongoing relationships than on past experiences (page 363).

Extremely violent or catastrophic events aside, for ordinary families the power of past events has been extremely exaggerated, and the singular influence ascribed to the mother is unjustified. Strong proponents of the importance of early events have created in the minds of many mothers a *false* conclusion: "I am a bad mother if my child cries, because crying may cause permanent emotional damage."

The sad fact is that older theorists were unaware of the benefits of healthy sleep and how we are fundamentally different in sleep and wake modes. Child psychologists, child psychiatrists, and pediatricians did not know the benefits of healthy sleep until recently. Unfortunately, even today there are too many professionals who lack training regarding children's sleep.

The improvement in educating child health care professionals has been slow. A 2013 national survey of pediatric residency programs showed that half of all programs had only two hours of instruction on sleep and sleep disorders during their three years of training; the average number of hours was 4.4, but 23 percent of the programs provided no sleep education. In 1994, the mean number of hours was 4.8, and 46 percent of programs offered no education to pediatricians. So in nineteen years, the percent of pediatric residency programs that include instruction on sleep issues increased from 54 percent to 77 percent, but the average number of hours remained about the same, only about four to five hours. This partially explains why there is so much misunderstanding about the prevention and treatment of sleep issues in children and why, because they have not received much or any formal education in this area, pediatricians in practice so often incorrectly advise parents that their child is likely to "outgrow" the sleep problem.

When your baby was younger, he slept when he needed to. He controlled your relationship with him, in the sense that you met his needs whether you wanted to or not. You didn't let him go hungry simply because you didn't feel like feeding him just then. You didn't let him stay wet because you didn't feel like changing him. His needs determined your behavior.

But later on, a shift should occur so that *you* become in charge. For example, when your child is older, you may decide not to give him junk food simply because he asks for it. You will not risk his physical safety by letting him climb too high on a tree simply because he wants to. And you will not let him stay up late at night to play when he needs to sleep. What, then, are we to do when the child does not cooperate, crying because he does not *want* to go to sleep even though he *needs* to sleep?

"Let Them Cry": A Division of Popular Opinions

There is a long-standing disagreement among those who wrote for popular magazines or now online about what happens when children cry after being left alone at night to sleep. In September 1984, *McCall's* said: "Letting a baby 'cry it out' will not teach him the basic trust or confidence he needs to feel secure in his new world." *Parents* magazine, in November 1983, said: "It may give him the feeling that there's nobody out there who cares. The child may become a passive, ineffective person, or he may become angry or hostile."

However, the editor in chief of *Parents* wrote in the October 1985 issue, after the birth of her third child: "The trick was that after eight years of parenthood, my husband and I have discovered . . . [that] the first sound does not mean that the baby needs to be picked up immediately." Don't wait eight years to learn what she discovered a long time ago!

"Let Them Cry": An Agreement of Expert Opinions

While the popular press and the Internet may give all types of conflicting evidence from a variety of sources, expert opinion is solidly together. In fact, all evidence from an array of child health specialists concludes that ignoring "protest" crying at bedtime will not cause permanent emotional or psychological problems. In plain fact, the contrary is true. For example, while Dr. D. W. Winnicott, a British pediatrician and child psychiatrist, stressed the importance of mothers' attentive holding of their child, he also emphasized that the *capacity to be alone* is one of the most important signs of maturity in emotional development. In his view, parents can facilitate the development of the child's ability to soothe himself when left alone. Please don't confuse this with abandonment or, on the other hand, use this notion as an excuse for negligence.

Margaret S. Mahler, a prominent child psychoanalyst, identified the beginning of the separation-individuation process whereby the infant begins to differentiate from the mother at 4–5 months of age. This is the age when children naturally begin to develop some independence.

Dr. Alexander Thomas and Dr. Stella Chess, two American child psychiatrists, followed more than a hundred children from infancy through young adulthood. One item they examined was the regularity or irregularity of sleep and how parents responded. They wrote: "Removal of symptoms by a successful parent guidance procedure has had positive consequences for the child's functioning and has not resulted in the appearance of overt anxiety or new substitute symptoms. . . . The basic emphasis [of the] treatment technique is a change in the parents' behavior." So please don't fear when your child cries in protest at night, because he is being allowed to "practice" falling asleep, that this crying will cause emotional or psychological problems later. By itself, it will not.

Let me be very clear about this. During the periods of normally occurring day and night sleep times, emotional problems do *not* develop if parents ignore protest crying.

Drs. Thomas and Chess were sensitive to irregular sleep patterns in the infants in their study. Many of those infants also had frequent and prolonged bouts of loud crying. When I asked Dr. Thomas what advice he had given to the parents of those crying babies who did not sleep at night, he responded, "Close the door and walk away." Did this create or produce any problems? His answer: "No. None at all."

Always going to your crying child at night interferes with this natural learning and growth. Such behavior produces sleep fragmentation, destroys sleep continuity, and creates insomnia in your child.

One study examined infant crying at 1 year of age. It compared children over 6 months of age whose parents indiscriminately responded to every cry, day or night, to those children whose parents were trained to respond promptly to every intense, stressed, or demanding cry but to delay their response to quiet vocalizations or weak cries. The children in the first group, whose parents indiscriminately responded, cried much more than children in the second group. This study suggests that crying for attention can be learned or taught by at least 6 months of age. I suspect that this learning can occur even earlier, so I encourage parents to try to be discriminating in their responses to their baby's cries at night as early as possible. This is easier said than done for first-time mothers but much easier for second-time mothers.

Mothers who in general do not feel loving or empathetic toward their children, who are insensitive or emotionally unavailable to them, and who have a lack of warmth or affection are more likely to be referred to psychologists or psychiatrists. Consequently, these specialists sometimes take the attitude that *all* parents should be encouraged to *never* let their child cry, for fear of encouraging a cold parent–child relationship. Based on their observations of a small group of clinically referred families, they make this recommendation to all families. As a general-practice pediatrician, however, I don't share this view, because I see that the vast majority of parents are loving and sensitive to their child's needs. These parents should not fear letting their child cry at night to learn to sleep. Fading (page 283) is an alternative method and is effective even for mothers receiving psychiatric care.

DOES LETTING MY CHILD CRY TO HELP HIM SLEEP BETTER ACTUALLY HARM HIM INSTEAD?

Some parents worry, *I am afraid that letting my baby cry will cause permanent emotional harm.* There is no evidence that protest crying while your child is learning how to sleep better will cause any kind of emotional problems later in life. However, because many parents have this fear, I welcome the opportunity to directly address it.

The short answer is no—there is absolutely no scientific evidence to indicate harmful effects of crying to help a child sleep. However, some parents understandably have difficulty allowing their child to cry. For those parents, the following information should set your mind at ease on this point. If you are already secure in the knowledge that you can safely let your child cry in order to teach self-soothing skills, then you can skip this section.

One of the world's foremost researchers in sleep, William C. Dement, taught me at Stanford University Medical School in 1967 that we exist in three distinctly different biological domains: awake, REM sleep, and non-REM sleep. Although all three domains interact with one another, there are specific problems that can occur within each domain.

According to Dr. Dement, traditional medical science historically focused on only the first domain: wakefulness. His major point was that we are fundamentally different when we are asleep than when we are awake. The body's clock knows when we should be asleep and adjusts our brain, our temperature, and our hormone levels to the sleep mode. In sleep mode, we do not respond, think, or feel as we do when awake. If you do not believe this, ask any mother of a 6-week-old infant how she is when she is up at night soothing her baby!

There has been much misunderstanding about "insecurity" and "crying to sleep" because of a failure to make the distinction between (1) *the importance of sleeping well when we are in a biological sleep mode* and (2) *the importance of security of attachment when we are in a biological awake mode*. This failure is understandable, because most child psychologists, child psychiatrists, and pediatricians have not had the opportunity to do research or to receive training regarding the benefits of healthy sleep. They do not fully understand or appreciate the degree to which the sleeping brain is different from the awake brain. As previously mentioned (page 340), even today very little teaching regarding sleep (only about four to five hours) takes place during the standard three-year pediatric residency program. Sad to say, "expert" advice in books, on popular websites, and on podcasts often reflects this lack of knowledge.

Because there is a basic difference between the sleeping brain and the awake brain, different types of problems can develop. When the brain enters the biological domain of sleep, problems such as night terrors might appear. Night terrors and other sleep problems simply do not occur when the brain shifts to the awake domain.

Similarly, we are fundamentally different when we are awake. When our children are awake, we worry about problems such as temper tantrums, fighting, not sharing, or not eating well. Also, we sometimes wonder if we are making the appropriate emotional connection. Are our children getting enough love? Are they happy? Are they securely attached, or do they feel insecure? How we interact with our children while we feed them, bathe them, dress them, and play with them is very important. However, insecurity of attachment as a concept makes no sense when the brain shifts to the sleep domain. When your child's brain is in the sleep mode, he needs sleep and not more social interaction with parents. As stated before, during the periods of normally occurring day and night sleep, emotional problems do *not* develop if parents ignore protest crying.

Still, you might wonder about what goes on at the borderland between awake and asleep. Does crying harm your child when he is left alone to cross that border and fall asleep?

Dr. William Sears is a champion of attachment parenting, but he has never had the opportunity to do research on sleeping in children, and his fear of "crying it out" (extinction) as a method to help children sleep better appears to blind him to the real harm children suffer when they do not sleep well. On his website there is a list of publications that Dr. Sears falsely claims support his position. *Not a single item in his presentation deals with the question of whether using extinction to help a child sleep better harms the child* (see http://mainstreamparenting.wordpress.com/2008/06/25/of-sources -and-straw-houses-the-annotated-dr-sears-handout-on-cio). It is irresponsible for a professional such as Dr. Sears to claim that studies performed only on animals and severely abused or neglected children constitute evidence in support of his position. Dr. Sears is not a researcher, but among researchers, wildly inappropriate citations or selectively including only those citations that support your point of view is called intellectual dishonesty.

Contrary to Dr. Sears's view, scientific research published in twenty-one studies show that extinction to help an infant or child sleep better does *not* cause harm (page 339). In fact, the opposite is true: After extinction, there are improvements in the mother, the child, and the bond between them. Here are some of the studies:

> *Journal of Developmental and Behavioral Pediatrics* (1991): "Extinction is an effective, reasonably rapid, and durable treatment for infant sleep disturbance . . . mothers became less anxious as the study proceeded. . . . A measure of infant security was explicitly included in this study to test this hypothesis, and again, the results are clear. Infant security improved significantly over the course of the study . . . we can reject the hypothesis that exposure to extinction . . . will impair security."

> *Journal of Pediatric Psychology* (1992): "Measured and compared the behavior characteristics and security scores of infants (6–24 months) treated with extinction for sleep disturbances . . . There was no evidence of detrimental effects on the treated infants whose security, emotionality/tension, and likeability scores improved."

> *Attachment & Human Development* (2000): "Fifty families were observed at home during more than 20 hours, and infant crying behavior as well as maternal responses were recorded . . . the more frequently mothers ignored their infants crying bouts in the first nine-week period, the less frequently their infants cried in the following nine-week period." At fifteen months of age, there was *no* relation be-

tween crying at home and secure and insecure attachment classifications.

Sleep (2006): "A total of 13 studies [of behavioral management of sleep problems] have assessed a number of secondary treatment outcomes related to daytime functioning in the child (including behavior, mood, self-esteem, parent–child interactions). [I]nfants who participated in sleep interventions were found to be more secure, predictable, less irritable, and to cry and fuss less following treatment. . . . The results were remarkably consistent across studies. Following intervention for their child's sleep disturbance, parents exhibited rapid and dramatic improvements in their overall mental health status, reporting fewer symptoms of depression . . . an increased sense of parenting efficiency, enhanced marital satisfaction, and reduced parenting stress. The majority of these studies reported positive effects on daytime functioning; no adverse secondary effects were identified in any of these studies.

Early Child Development (2012): Cortisol levels after three days of "crying it out" on average showed *no increase* compared with before the sleep-training program began. Further, the cortisol level on the fourth day was less than the third day (personal communication). By the *third day* of the program, all infants settled to sleep independently without a bout of distress. Additionally, by the *third day,* the mothers' cortisol levels were significantly lower.

Pediatrics (2012): Behavioral sleep techniques have *no* harmful effect on measures of children's emotions, behaviors, psychosocial functioning, child–parent closeness, or attachment five years later.

Pediatrics (2016): "Both graduated extinction and bedtime fading provide significant sleep benefits above control, yet convey no adverse stress responses or long-term effects on parent–child attachment or child emotions and behavior. Our diurnal cortisol data indicate the active treatments did not result in chronically elevated levels over time. No significant differences in children's emotions and behaviors could be found between groups 12 months after intervention, with internalizing or externalizing behaviors comparable across groups. No significant differences were found in attachment styles between groups. For parental stress, mothers in both intervention groups reported less stress than mothers in the control group."

Journal of Child Psychology and Psychiatry (2020): *No* adverse impacts on leaving infants to cry it out in the first 6 months on infant–mother attachment and behavioural development at 18 months were found.

Journal of Developmental & Behavioral Pediatrics (2020): At 12 months of age, children whose mothers delayed their response to infant crying at 3-6 months, had an easier temperament, had fewer crying episodes, were less likely to cry at bedtime, had fewer night wakings, and had longer durations of sleep. "Cry out was *not* associated with observational measures of maternal sensitivity or infant–maternal attachment."

Dr. Johanna Petzoldt, a sleep researcher, psychologist, and mother, wrote that "attachment parenting" is very popular in Germany and "to my disappointment, it was often and fiercely misinterpreted as the one true parenting strategy . . . I fear that these opinions might put parents at risk for self-sacrifice and resulting mental problems . . . I would prefer parenting advice that is evidence-based, flexible, and balanced, so that every parent could choose their own path, without feeling guilty or intimidated."

My observations and sound scientific data show that if children are well rested during the day, the bedtime is early enough to prevent a second wind, and parents do not reinforce the crying by going in to comfort the child, then crying occurring with extinction lasts only a few days (page 257).

There are a few possible explanations for why there is so much misunderstanding and controversy regarding the subject of children, parents, and sleep. As mentioned previously, pediatricians between 1994 and 2013 spent only about four hours of their three-year training studying sleep, so they have at best only a cursory understanding of the benefits for the child and parents of sleeping well (chapter 3). Also, there is a trade-off in attachment parenting between less fussing/crying when younger and more night waking (signaling) when older (chapter 2), so it is not correct to state that one method of parenting is better than another. Finally, there may be more anxiety about parenting today than in previous generations. If true, this heightened anxiety creates not just fear but uncertainty, with parents worrying, *How do I start helping my child sleep better?*

I WANT TO START A SLEEP SOLUTION, BUT I AM NOT SURE HOW TO DO IT

There is no one-size-fits-all approach to implementing a sleep solution. Here are several factors to help you think about your particular situation.

Family

When a bedtime is way too late because of one or both parents' work schedule, sometimes a sleep solution depends on having someone other than the parent put the child to sleep earlier or having a parent come home earlier. For some families, neither option may be possible. In others, a parent might be able to come home a little earlier, but still not early enough for an improved bedtime. Even so, small improvements are better than none. Do what you can during the week, and then shift your focus to paying back the sleep debt on weekends, with good-quality naps and super-early bedtimes.

Sometimes a sleep solution should begin on a Saturday when both parents are available to support each other or care for other children. Parents should not start a sleep solution unless they are in complete agreement and can both commit to four to seven days. Teamwork and communication are the bedrock that will support your sleep solution success. As mentioned previously, humans are not robots and cannot realistically expect to achieve perfection. Nevertheless, during the first few days of implementing a new sleep plan, try hard to be 100 percent consistent. If you are inconsistent or cave after one or two days, you'll pay. You will have taught your child that crying is how to get more parental attention. If this happens, don't beat yourself up; try again a few days or weeks later. Often, after that time, families are more determined than ever to persevere, and this new resolve allows them to successfully execute the plan of action. I think this is worth restating, because some parents reading this are surely struggling with their own severe sleep deprivation and the guilt of previous failure to help their child sleep better. It's all right to take breaks when sleep solutions are not working, you feel overwhelmed, or you cannot take any more crying. Waving the white flag is fine when you get discouraged. You can retreat to swing sleep or naps in the stroller or car to regroup and get everyone better rested. Later, try again. Success often occurs on the second try.

It is smart, not selfish, for the mother to take breaks without guilt to recharge her battery, because she is the power source of most of the soothing effort.

Yet success does not rest on the mother alone. It often depends on whether the father remains calm, is willing to help solve the problem, and actively participates in the solution (page 163). If the father is not willing or able, then the mother might have to wait until he is away from home for an extended period, on a business trip or family visit, to fix a sleep problem. Alternatively, sometimes it's the father who sends the wife to a hotel for the first night of the solution because she is too sleep-deprived to tolerate any crying. Sometimes, though, a family feels stuck and has trouble making a start. If that describes your situation, try starting with a baby step.

Start with Small Steps and Simple Solutions

Sometimes a family is reluctant to begin a sleep solution because the mother is severely sleep-deprived and feels overwhelmed. Although she intellectually understands what to do, she is unable to execute because she is emotionally strung out. She is fearful that there will be more stress from her baby's crying, and she cannot handle any more stress. She is at her limit. Or she is in a sleep-deprived fog and cannot really see or believe in any viable sleep solution. In either case, try to get the father or others to take over; convince Mom to take a break. Fathers are usually less sleep-deprived than mothers, so dads need to step up in this situation and create a plan, if possible. Some dads need extra motivation, and being optimistic that he can succeed will go a long way toward giving him the confidence to try. Realistically, however, not all dads are always available or willing.

If the mother is doing the heavy lifting by herself, try small, simple, and acceptable steps first and later try to reach optimal sleep for the child. The simpler the solution, the more likely you will remember what to do and do it consistently. For example, a small step that is simple to remember might be a *slightly earlier bedtime*. A slightly earlier bedtime may jump-start healthy sleep (pages 102, 297, and 362). Another example might be letting someone else put your baby down drowsy but awake just once a day or once a week. The benefit is that when you see how improvement in your child's sleep causes improvement in his mood and performance, you will be emboldened to try more complex solutions and fine-tuning to improve sleep even though he might protest. Seeing is believing. Of course, a possible outcome is that no improvement might occur because the change in the bedtime is too small to be beneficial. But go ahead anyway and give it a try. What do you have to lose?

An optimal sleep plan for your child might be complex in order to accommodate many variables for your particular family, but it is not always practical to tackle the whole problem at once, and it may not be clear whether to go slowly or quickly.

Gradual versus Abrupt Changes

There is no hard-and-fast rule as to whether a sleep solution change should be implemented gradually (a check-and-console strategy or fading) or abruptly (extinction or graduated extinction). For some parents, gradual changes appear gentler and abrupt changes appear harsher. But gradual changes might take longer to see results. Often a family wishes to move gradually, but after seeing some improvement, they change course and make more dramatic changes. For example, they move quickly from fading to graduated extinction or extinction.

Parents who favor a more gradual approach (check and console or fading) over an abrupt approach (extinction) often complain of frequent relapses. The general reason a gradual approach tends to be less successful in the long run is that it takes longer and there are always natural disruptions of sleep, such as illnesses or vacations. The subsequent reestablishment of healthy sleep routines using a gradual approach becomes very stressful to the parents. Several days of a gradual approach often wear down parents, so they give up and revert to their old inconsistencies. Parents who have successfully used extinction know that they might have one, and only one, nasty reentry night of crying after they return home from several days on vacation or from a visit to a relative's house.

The truth is that some parents swing back and forth between firmness and permissiveness so often that they cannot make any cure stick. They confuse their wishful thinking with the child's actual behavior. This is why a sleep log can be an important tool to help document what you are really doing and how your child is really responding. After all, short-term "successes" might only reflect brief periods when your child crashes at night from chronic exhaustion. Or the actual improvement in sleep habits may be so marginal that the normal disruptions of vacations, trips, illnesses, or other irregularities constantly buffet the still-tired child and cause repeated relapses in which he wakes often during the night or fights going to sleep.

In contrast, parents who successfully carry out an abrupt retraining program—the cold-turkey approach—to improve sleep habits see immediate and dramatic improvement without any lasting ill effects. These children have fewer relapses and recover faster and more completely from natural disruptions of sleep routines. Seeing a cure really "stick" for a while gives you the confidence to keep tighter control over sleep patterns and to repeat the process again if needed.

Sometimes it appears more practical to gradually make a change in a daily sleep schedule, such as when there is a natural nap transition from two naps to one nap and the single midmorning nap is slowly pushed, over the course of a few weeks, toward midday. If you tried to do this abruptly, your child might get a second wind and take no nap! Other times it appears more practical to abruptly make a change, such as when there is a short nap around 6:00 P.M. and a way-too-late bedtime; in fact, this so-called nap should really be the bedtime. But here also, a family might fear that it is too much of a shock to his system to abruptly move the bedtime much earlier. Or perhaps they have difficulty themselves with such an early bedtime and want time to gradually make the adjustment. Here is a guideline: When you are keeping your child up later (for example, trying for a single midday nap by delaying the midmorning nap), do it gradually. When you want your child to have an earlier bedtime, if you wish, do it abruptly. But many families are reluctant to move the bedtime earlier.

Fear of an Early Bedtime

Parents often fear that an earlier bedtime will automatically produce an earlier wake-up time that is inconvenient for them. This usually does not occur because an earlier bedtime produces a better-sleeping child who is more able to self-soothe, even in the very early-morning hours. This is why sleep begets sleep. Also, a bedtime that is too late might occur because parents coming home late from work want to play with their child and think that the playtime is more important than sleep.

But an earlier bedtime directly benefits your child. And there are indirect benefits for the family as well: The stay-at-home mother doesn't have to deal with a witching hour in the late afternoon, and no witching hour means the father comes home from work to a calm, well-rested mother; both parents have relaxed private time in the evenings and overnight, which strengthens the marriage; the child is raised by well-rested parents.

How early is early? To repay a sleep debt as part of a sleep solution, a temporary super-early bedtime of 5:30 P.M. (under age 3) or 6:30 P.M. (for older children) might be needed for one or only a few nights. But if this super-early bedtime is kept in place too long, it may backfire and cause the now well-rested child to have a long latency to sleep or create a wake-up time that is way too early. So after a few days, when he is sleeping better, gradually move the bedtime back a little. Through trial and error, find that sweet spot for the new later bedtime hour that is not as late as the original too-late bedtime hour.

A 5:30 P.M. bedtime might also be used for only one night after a natural sleep disruption caused by an illness or family holiday. I call this a *reset*. Put your child to bed super early and ignore protest crying. One, but only one, night of protest might be the price you pay for a lovely family holiday. But this single super-early bedtime might be employed several times a year because of frequent grandparent visits or illnesses. Be firm.

So the bedtime is not a fixed clock time but is moved earlier when needed, then readjusted later again to keep your child well rested, which is the overall goal.

Competing Goals

One important goal is to synchronize soothing with the onset of the rising biological wave of sleepiness at nap times and bedtimes. So after your child reaches about 4 months of age, the advice is to keep him up until the time this wave is expected to occur, even if he is sleepy earlier. Keep him up to catch the wave!

Another important goal is to avoid a second wind by not keeping him up when he is short on sleep, because if he gets extremely short on sleep it will be harder for him to fall asleep and stay asleep. Put him down early before he gets keyed up!

These two goals may be in conflict, especially when your child is short on sleep. So to achieve the first goal, adopt a gradual approach and keep him up a little later each day or so to get closer to his natural sleep time. To do that, you might have to tolerate a little second wind and deal with it by distraction, entertainment, amusement, and longer soothing to sleep. Temporarily, the bedtime might be super early (5:30 P.M.) while you search for his best nap time and bedtime. Keeping track with a sleep log may help you discover his best sleep times by seeing the forest and not the trees. The big picture is most important, but when you are sleep-deprived, it may be hard to see.

Details and the Whole Picture

We often get caught up in the day-to-day details of our children's sleep and sometimes have to take a step back and look at the whole picture. For example, a parent might say, "Help! My son gets up too early, around 5:00 A.M." It is important to know how often this too-early wake-up time occurs. If the 5:00 A.M. wake-up time occurs 10 to 20 percent of the time, there may be circumstances in the family that render this too-early wake-up unavoidable. For instance, occasional late scheduled sports for an older sibling might cause the bedtime for the baby to be too late, which will cause him occasionally to wake too early in the morning. Perhaps the family will be able to hire a babysitter or have a relative or neighbor watch the baby when the older sibling has a late sports event. Or maybe they will have to accept this as an untreatable minor sleep problem and learn to live with it. On the other hand, if the 5:00 A.M. wake-up time occurs 80 to 90 percent of the time, the baby will eventually exhibit major adverse effects from cumulative sleepiness, and this should be viewed as definitely change-worthy.

Don't fret about naps or night sleep on a day-to-day or night-to-night basis. It will drive you crazy. That is missing the forest for the trees. When you're starting a sleep solution, be patient with your plan, and remember that it may take several days or several weeks before you see the benefits. Try something for at least several days before you conclude it is or it is not helpful. If you do not see improvement, step back and look at all the elements of healthy sleep (chapter 2), because focusing on only one sleep issue might have distracted you from noticing that other aspects of your child's sleep also need improvement. Improvement may be sequential (first night sleep, then the midmorning nap, and then the midday nap), not simultaneous. It may take weeks for naps to improve after night sleep has improved.

Relatives and Friends

There are individual variations in sleep patterns at any given age, even though there are general patterns that apply for every age. There is enormous variation among families regarding teamwork, number of rooms, the presence or absence of colic, and so forth. *Don't compare your child to other children;* just focus on your own child. For example, your child's naps might be shorter than your sister's child's naps, so your child should be going to bed a little earlier. What works for your relatives and friends may not work for you. Often a mother in my practice, who was successful in helping her child sleep well, might complain to me that her advice to a relative or friend went unheeded and wonder why their child's sleep deprivation was ongoing. Knowing that her husband had cooperated, I would ask whether the husband of her relative or friend was as supportive as her own husband, and the usual answer was no.

Regular sleep schedules in general help anchor healthy sleep. But *don't be a slave to a sleep schedule.* Exceptions to your sleep plan, such as skipping naps or staying up late for holidays or special occasions, are fine once or twice a month, but not much more often. Well-rested children tolerate these events and recover quickly. Early bedtimes or naps at home are *socially limiting.* But it is *liberating* to be out with a well-rested child who never fusses, and it is liberating for a couple to have relaxed private time in the evening when their child easily falls asleep early at night.

When starting a sleep solution, *be discreet* in confiding details of your plan to other people. You are in a vulnerable state because of your own sleep deprivation and therefore do not want to invite critical comments from relatives or friends who may not be supportive. Talk to your pediatrician, especially if your child has eczema or chronic snoring or mouth breathing during sleep, before embarking on any sleep-solution plan.

The Sleep Wheel: Sleep as a Twenty-Four-Hour Cycle

Imagine an upright wheel slowly rotating to make a complete revolution every twenty-four hours. It looks like a Ferris wheel, but I call it a Sleep Wheel. The Sleep Wheel illustrates how your child's sleep is not made up of independent, isolated parts but instead is composed of different but related parts.

The Sleep Wheel is driven by a giant engine, perhaps the largest motor you can imagine: the rotation of the earth on its axis. As the earth rotates, it creates alternating periods of light and darkness. You have no control over the speed of the Sleep Wheel. It turns round and round no matter what you do as a parent.

However, as a parent, you can build the spokes that radiate from the center to the rim and create the structural integrity of the wheel. The four spokes of the Sleep Wheel support the rim:

1. Start early.
2. Many hands (get Dad and others on board).
3. Put your child down while drowsy but still awake.
4. Many naps (no cumulative sleepiness, no second wind).

These spokes support the structure because they allow your baby to begin to learn self-soothing. If the spokes are strong, your child will have a smooth ride as the wheel turns round. If the spokes are weak, the rim will wobble in the wind. If some spokes are missing or there are no spokes at all, the rim will bend or collapse altogether.

Attached to the rim of a Ferris wheel are passenger cars, but attached to the Sleep Wheel are the six different parts of your child's twenty-four-hour sleep/wake cycle. Let's follow the Sleep Wheel through one complete revolution, beginning with the evening bedtime.

1. At 6 weeks of age (all ages are counted from the due date), an *early bedtime* develops. The failure to establish an early bedtime will result in a second wind that causes bedtime battles, difficulty in falling asleep, and difficulty staying asleep, such as night awakenings (fragmented night sleep) or waking up too early in the morning. If day sleep is deficient, a second wind will develop in the late afternoon or evening and make it difficult to easily fall asleep unattended (drowsy but awake) or stay asleep (consolidated sleep). You then might see bedtime battles and fragmented sleep (signaling).

2. *Consolidated night sleep* develops before or between 6 and 9 months of age, when babies no longer need to be fed at night. Feed your baby at night when hungry but do not respond to every sound. Responding to your baby at night for soothing when he is not hungry will create a night crying habit around or after 4–6 months of age. At that point, soothing becomes more socially stimulating. Fragmented night sleep is as harmful as brief night sleep and might cause your baby to wake up too early in the morning.

3. *Wake-up time* is not too early. If you go to your baby too early to start the day, he will not be able to nap well later because he starts the day too tired. Many young babies start the day between 5:30 and 6:30 A.M.

4. The *midmorning nap* is regular but initially brief and develops around 3–4 months of age. This nap should start around 9:00 A.M. If it starts much earlier than that because your child woke up tired (whether because the bedtime was too late, there was fragmented night sleep, or the morning wake-up time was too early), then the rest of the day's sleep will be thrown off schedule. On the other hand, if the nap starts too late, a second wind will make self-soothing for the midmorning nap difficult or impossible, or it may cause the nap to be way too brief. This nap may naturally become longer until 6 months of age, after which it will become shorter.

5. The *midday nap* is regular but initially brief and develops shortly after the midmorning nap. This nap starts around 12:00 to 2:00 P.M. If it starts too early because your child wakes up too tired from his midmorning nap (whether because the bedtime was too late, there was fragmented night sleep, wake-up time in the morning was too early, or a midmorning nap took place too early or too late), then the rest of the day's sleep will be thrown off schedule. On the other hand, if the nap starts too late, a second wind will make self-soothing difficult or impossible for the midday nap, or the midday nap might be too brief. This nap may naturally become longer until 6 months of age, after which it will become shorter.

6. *Late-afternoon nap(s)* tend(s) to be irregular and brief. They usually disappear by 9 months of age.

Good naps prevent a second wind in the evening and make it easier for your child to self-soothe for bedtime.

Whether you have a newborn or an older child of any age, your first task as a parent is to build the spokes of the Sleep Wheel. Then you start to assemble the six different parts of your child's twenty-four-hour sleep/wake cycle based on his age. There are two common pitfalls: that a parent is focused on one or more of the six parts but has not yet constructed the spokes, and that a parent is focused on only one (or two or three) of the six parts and ignores the others.

Each of the six parts affects the other five. If one is not developed at the appropriate age, the entire Sleep Wheel becomes unbalanced.

My Child Is Different; I Don't Believe You

Q: *Won't my child give up hope and trust that I love him and become insecure?*

A: No. Children do not become insecure; they learn self-soothing (page 344).

Q: *All children are different, and your suggestions to fix sleep problems will not work for my child.*

A: Some success occurs in *all* children when parents keep their children well rested during the day, establish a reasonably early bedtime that prevents a second wind, and consistently do not reinforce crying at night. All of these elements are necessary.

Q: *I think that you cherry-picked or faked the success stories in your book.*

A: Read at random a few of the more than seventeen hundred five-star parent reviews of the prior editions of this book online to see how quickly children can be helped to sleep better. Success is more elusive when the bedtime is too late, when the child does not sleep well during the day, and when there is too much parental attention during the night.

Q: *All children are different, and my child does not need to sleep when you suggest.*

A: The fundamental fact is that you can't fight circadian rhythms, and if you try to do so, it is your child who will pay the price. This is true for *all* children.

Q: *I think you are wrong that early bedtimes are such a big deal.*

A: During my forty years of general pediatric practice, I cared for many children from their first day to age 18–22. During a routine office visit, I might discuss a minor sleep issue such as a newly observed slightly longer time required for the child to fall asleep. In such a case, I would ask how the child appears between 4:00 and 5:00 P.M., and the mother might report, "He's fine. He's always sweet and charming, active and playful." Nevertheless, I would often suggest a slightly earlier bedtime for one to three nights as a trial. Usually, three days later the child would be falling asleep faster, the total night sleep duration would be slightly longer, and the mother's report would be, to her surprise, that her child was now even sweeter, calmer, more alert, and more patient between 4:00 and 5:00 P.M. than before. Skepticism about this scenario is a normal response.

When I would ask the mother if she'd ever thought her daughter would actually become sweeter with a slightly earlier bedtime, the answer would almost invariably come back as no. Still, the mother might protest that the earlier bedtime was inconvenient. My reply to this objection was to remind the mother that her child did in fact fall asleep at the earlier bedtime, with good results, which proves that her child needed the earlier bedtime and that the previous bedtime was too late. In this common scenario, the shift to an earlier bedtime might be as little as ten to twenty minutes! The fact that small changes like this may have profound consequences is discussed on page 102. Obviously, this slightly earlier bedtime will not help for major sleep problems caused by a bedtime that is way too late.

Q: *I think you are wrong that sleep is more important than classes.*

A: It is common for first-time parents to be anxious because of their inexperience. There is an enormous parenting-education industry trying to sell their goods and services to parents, and the industry deliberately preys on parents' worries and insecurities. The industry succeeds by implied fake promises: "Your child will be better (smarter, brighter, stronger, more successful) if you buy this product or take this class." Please stop eating the baloney sandwiches that they are trying to feed you.

Parents need to understand that much of what is being promoted to them is not based on any scientific evidence of benefit to their child. There is a long history of once popular but now thoroughly discredited parenting enterprises: "Patterning" as a treatment for children with developmental delays was sold by the Institutes for the Achievement of Human Potential (1955); therapy for autism, based on the false premise that autism is caused by "refrigerator mothers," was promoted by the Orthogenic School at the University of Chicago (1967); the now debunked "Mozart Effect" to raise your child's IQ (1997) was sold by CD purveyors; Baby Einstein DVD videos, advertised as educational for babies and sold by Disney, were recalled (2009); and probiotics, a $24 billion industry, were shown to not soothe babies' colic (2013). Yet even today, innumerable "educational" toys, videos, games, and computer-based activities are being marketed to naïve parents who only want the best for their children.

Just hanging out with or playing with your child, doing something together that you both enjoy, is easier said than done for many busy families who instead might purchase "educational toys" or enroll their child in a "class" with the expectation that their child will learn something now for a future benefit. Let's hear from seasoned experts who explain why this is misguided. Michael Lewis (page 336), University Distinguished Professor of Pediatrics and Psychiatry and director of the Institute for the Study of Child Development at Rutgers Robert Wood Johnson Medical School, wrote in 1997 in *Altering Fate: Why the Past*

Does Not Predict the Future, "The idea of progress . . . leads to the view that the child always is in the process of becoming and never just is. Consequently, parents play with their children to develop children's imagination or creativity in the future *rather than because it is fun for the children and enjoyable for them now.* Given the argument that it is difficult to demonstrate the antecedents of why children are the way they are now, as well as to predict the consequences of the child's status now for the child's future, *there is little reason to suggest to parents or teachers that they should do something for its good effects later.* They need to do what they do for children now, not because of their future but because it fits with our current value system. *Playing with children is good for them simply because playing is a good thing for children to do.* We know it is good because of the current patterns of covariation such as *smiling and attention* [emphasis added]." It is true that it is "difficult to demonstrate the antecedents of why children are the way now," but now we have genetic evidence that gives us strong clues to where the answer lies. Robert Plomin (page 85), Professor of Behavioral Genetics at the Institute of Psychiatry, Psychology and Neuroscience at King's College London, wrote in 2018, in *Blueprint: How DNA Makes Us Who We Are,* "Parents are not carpenters who construct a child. Although caring for children is crucial, parenting is *not a matter of shaping them to turn out a particular way.* Parents are not even gardeners [providing conditions for their children to thrive] if that implies nurturing and pruning plants to achieve a certain result. . . . Parents are neither carpenter nor gardeners in the sense that *parenting is not a means to an end. It is a relationship and, like our relationship with our partner and friends, our relationship with our children should be based on being with them, not changing them* [emphasis added]."

A contributing factor in today's rush to "improve my child" is that parents' challenges have increased in modern times. There are more mothers in the workforce and away from their children (contributing to so-called working mother's guilt); the global economy means that there are more people competing for fewer good jobs; parents want more educational activities for their children because there is more information available and more facts to be learned. And it is harder for parents to pay close attention to their children and harder for children to pay close attention to their parents and other children because of screen-based distractions. All these factors tend to inhibit early bedtimes or displace naps.

Simply ask yourself: What is the power of a nap that can turn a raving, ranting, and out-of-control toddler into a sweet and charming human being?

I know that I am ruffling some feathers to suggest that sleep may sometimes be more important than a scheduled activity. If you are skeptical that sleep is more important than another lesson, class, or sports activity, talk to a disinterested party such as your pediatrician, a child psychologist or child psychiatrist, or a specialist in early child development. Of course, you might get a different opinion from someone who will personally benefit, such as a coach, tutor, or preschool operator/owner. Even a mother who is using a drop-off class as a babysitter so she has more self-maintenance time might highly praise a class in order to feel better about not spending time with her child. So be careful whom you listen to and consider what is behind their recommendations. Again and again in this book, I show you what stands behind my recommendations: deep experience and solid scientific research.

My position is that sleep is of vital importance and well-rested children soak up knowledge like a dry sponge. Colors are more vivid, sounds are more interesting, smells and tastes are more exciting. Life and being with others are more enjoyable. Sleepy children experience a drabber, duller world, as through a glass darkly. Remember how it is for you when you get foggy or nod off at a class, concert, meeting, or party. Think of all that you have missed in your life because you were too sleepy or sleep-deprived. Is that how you want your child to grow up?

Of course, in real life it's often a matter of degree. We don't go through our days alternating between being fully alert and calm and being groggy and crabby. Most of us live in a gray zone somewhere in the middle of these extremes, occasionally moving more in one direction and then in the other. It's no different with your child, and part of your job as parent is to decide when it is more important to schedule an activity for your child and when you should focus on letting your child get the sleep he needs. My observation is that when parents routinely keep their child well rested, then that child is more able to deal with occasional sleep disruptions such as classes or family outings.

Marital disharmony or mental health problems in parents may express themselves in choices involving their children, such as classes versus extra sleep. Since these conflicts interfere with rapid success in correcting a sleep problem, these and similar challenges (page 219) should be explicitly dealt with first, if at all possible, because it is absurd to think that your child will get much benefit from some activity when he has a strong biological need for sleep.

REMEMBER
Different children require different approaches.

An easy, regular, common fussy baby may respond quickly to sleep-training strategies at around 6 weeks. A more irregular, extremely fussy/colicky child may respond well when 3–4 months of age.

How to Live with Your Choice

If you alone are doing the heavy lifting, keep it simple. There may be many variables and specific features about your family that you wish to change, but you are likely to be sleep-deprived yourself, so a single change in routine might be all that you can handle for now. For example, moving the bedtime earlier (pages 102, 297, and 362) is usually a powerful part of any sleep solution, so start with that. Complex solutions and fine-tuning might be left to a later time, when you get some help or you are less sleep-deprived.

If you have help and the ability to make a full-court press, work on all the age-appropriate sleep elements simultaneously.

Collect data. However, diary data are too detailed to be useful; instead, make a sleep log so you can see the forest and not just the trees. Look at the big picture to see if there is a pattern that explains why there are good sleep times and not-good sleep times.

Fathers are usually less sleep-deprived than mothers, so try to get the father to create a plan. Many fathers want to cooperate with helping their child sleep, but only in the sense that they will do what their wife tells them to do. They expect her to be the leader in all things related to child-rearing and view themselves as the helpful follower. This does not work for finding and successfully executing a sleep solution when the mother is very sleep-deprived. Assign Dad the responsibility of reading about sleep, collecting and analyzing data, and, with feedback from Mom if practicable, creating and executing a plan. Make it his job! Even if Mom isn't crazy about the plan, she should stand down for a few days to give it a chance . . . and to give herself time to recover energy, equilibrium, and insight. Remember: Allow a few days to go by before tweaking or abandoning the plan. Once you see some improvement, be patient; it may take several days or a few weeks to see the full benefit of your plan.

If you feel overwhelmed, take a break from your plan to give yourself time to regroup, and consider restarting it later. Success often occurs on the second try.

Don't compare children. There is individual variation in sleep patterns at any given age. Don't compare results. There is enormous variation among families regarding teamwork, number of bedrooms, the presence or absence of colic, and parent issues.

Exceptions to your sleep plan such as skipping naps or staying up late for holidays or special occasions are fine once or twice a month, but not much more often. Well-rested children tolerate these events and recover quickly.

Talk to your pediatrician if your child has eczema or chronic snoring or mouth breathing during sleep.

Choosing a sleep solution is a highly individualized process. While some parents might only wish to move the bedtime a little earlier, others might feel comfortable making several changes at the same time:

> "I learned to stay in the schedule in order to avoid fighting with circadian rhythms. I concluded that I won't win that fight, but my baby would lose!"

Summary and Action Plan for Exhausted Parents

Young children and infants cannot tell us how they feel, so parents need to be watchful. Is your child active, alert, vital, and wide awake, or is he fighting sleep and woozy?

MAJOR POINT
Junk food is bad for the body. Junk sleep is bad for the brain.

Obviously, sleeping is not an automatically regulated process like the control of body temperature. Sleeping is more like feeding. We do not expect children to grow well if all they eat is junk food. Children need a well-balanced diet in order to grow. If the food that is provided is insufficient or unbalanced, this unhealthy diet will interfere with the child's growth and development. The same is true for unhealthy sleep patterns.

The reality is that some sleep problems require multiple changes, but you might be able to make only some of the changes. Don't despair; make whatever changes you can. Still, if you are able, try to move the bedtime earlier, even just a little earlier. Anytime you make a change, allow at least four to five days before making another change to see whether you have helped your child. Be patient.

1. Keep a sleep log (page 305).
2. Identify the main sleep problem; review the chapter that fits your child's age.
3. Identify the elements of sleep that need improvement or correction for your child's sleep problem:
   Self-soothing (chapter 4)
   Sleep duration: night sleep and day sleep
   Naps
   Sleep consolidation
   Sleep schedule
   Sleep regularity
4. Determine what you can and cannot do (let-cry, maybe-cry, no-cry sleep solutions). Are there parent issues that need to be addressed (chapter 4)?

IMPORTANT POINTS

Sleeping well is a 24/7 process. It's not just about how we get our children to go to bed at night without crying. Solving sleep problems may be a very tough prescription and demands a consistent approach. There may or may not be increased crying in the beginning, but the payoff is that crying around sleep will be eliminated altogether in the end. Children benefit by becoming healthy sleepers and self-soothers who welcome each day with the resources of the well rested. Parents benefit by sleeping better themselves, which makes them better parents and partners.

What a Parent Can Do

Encourage your partner to help care for the baby daytime and nighttime.

Encourage self-soothing; the earlier, the better.

Put your child to sleep drowsy but awake, then leave the room.

Set an early bedtime based on drowsy signs; practice consistent bedtime routines, including massage; be emotionally available at bedtime.

Provide opportunities for naps based on drowsy signs.

Avoid irregularity of sleep schedules, including between weekdays and weekends.

Practice safe sleep recommendations.

No TV or digital screens in the child's room; limit screen time.

Seek help if your child is not sleeping well (from the child's primary care provider or a community sleep consultant) or for yourself or partner, especially if there are symptoms of anxiety or depression or significant *risk factors, parent issues,* or *adverse concerns.*

PART II

Establishing Healthy Sleep Habits from Infancy to Adolescence

Chapter 6 Outline

NEWBORN: THE FIRST WEEK

WEEKS 2-4: MORE FUSSINESS

FUSSINESS AND CRYING

Baby-Driven Path: The Role of the Baby
    Common Fussiness/Crying
        Fussiness
        Crying: All Babies Cry Some of the Time
        Some Crying Can't Be Attributed to an Obvious Cause
        Two to Three Hours of Crying per Day Is Average
        Many Babies Have Evening Crying Spells
        Crying Decreases at About 3 Months
    Extreme Fussiness/Colic
        Sleep
        Wakefulness
        Treatment
        Inconsolable versus Consolable
Parent-Driven Path: The Role of the Parent
    Mother: Anxiety and Depression
    Father: Depression, Partner Support, and Infant Care at Night
    Interaction between Baby and Parent
        Parental Tolerance for Infant Crying
    Interaction between Parents
Living with and Soothing a Colicky Baby
    How to Soothe a Colicky Baby

Healthy Sleep Habits in the First Month

If you have not already done so, please go back and read chapter 1.

A main goal at this age is to encourage the development of self-soothing skills.

Every newborn baby is unique. And the closer we look, the more differences we see. Some of these differences reflect genetic or inborn traits. Recent sleep research has focused on genes that control our biological clocks. For mothers of fraternal twins, the finding that sleep periods occur at different clock times will not be surprising. There are other differences present at birth that are not inherited but are caused by whether the baby was born at thirty-seven or forty-two weeks of gestation, or whether the mother smoked or drank large amounts of alcohol during her pregnancy. One area of research, based on animal studies, is how the mother's biological rhythms may help set or influence the rhythms of the fetus and the newborn baby: Based on the regularity or irregularity of the mother's sleep/wake patterns, activity/rest patterns, or eating patterns, there may be a kind of prenatal programming affecting the baby's own rhythms.

All of these differences—in smiling, sucking, sleeping, physical activity, and so on—combine to make a baby an individual. This chapter will describe the individual sleeping patterns in babies and how these patterns change as babies grow. Despite individual differences, there is some advice that applies to all babies:

Think and plan *how* you want to soothe your baby but, more important, *when* you soothe your baby.

- Babies quickly become overtired after only one or two hours of wakefulness, and some cannot comfortably stay up for even one hour! During the day, note the time when your baby wakes up and try to help her nap by soothing within the next one or two hours, before she becomes overtired. Try to keep the intervals of wakefulness brief.
- Babies less than 6 weeks old may fall asleep very late at night, and each bout of sleep may not be very long during the day or night. Try to soothe your baby to sleep during the day and at the end of the day before she becomes overtired. Always respond to your baby when you think she is hungry or in distress. Avoid the overtired state by keeping the intervals of wakefulness brief.
- By 6 weeks old, 80 percent of babies become more settled at night, sleep a little longer at night, and begin to become drowsy for night sleep at an earlier hour. If your baby shows signs of drowsiness earlier, try to soothe her to sleep at an earlier hour.
- By 6 weeks old, 20 percent of babies do not appear to become more settled at night, do not appear to sleep longer at night, and may not appear to become drowsy at an earlier hour. Nevertheless, try to soothe your baby to sleep at an earlier hour even if she does not show signs of drowsiness earlier. Spend extra time soothing: prolonged swinging, long luxurious baths, and never-ending car rides. Fathers should put forth extra effort to help out (page 163).

Newborn: The First Week

Night sleep: No established rhythms
Day sleep: No established rhythms
Bedtimes: No established rhythms

**Begin to teach self-soothing and bedtime routines (chapter 4)
and feed only when your baby is hungry at night.**

After your baby is born, you will experience the joy of becoming
a parent along with the exhaustion that follows labor and delivery
and perhaps the groggy aftereffects of anesthesia or pain medication. During the first few days, you don't have to worry about when
to feed your baby and put her to sleep because in hospitals without
total rooming-in, a feed/sleep schedule is imposed on baby care activities. The feed/sleep schedule is determined by general guidelines
to prevent low blood sugar as well as accounting for changes of
nursing shifts, visiting hours, and the need to measure vital signs.
You will receive instructions regarding when to feed your baby when
you are discharged but not when or how to put your baby to sleep.
Feelings of uncertainty or anxiety regarding feeding and sleeping
may surface as you prepare to go home. This is normal, because the
first-time parent is a rookie. Even the second-time parent is worried
about how to manage more than one child. Only the third-time parent is a true veteran!

**Your baby has no circadian rhythms or internal biological clocks
yet, so you can't set your baby to clock time.**

For most full-term babies, as soon as the parents arrive home,
they will need to disregard the clock and feed their baby whenever
she seems hungry, change her when she wets, and let her sleep when
she needs to sleep. Full-term babies sleep a lot during the first sev-

eral days; pre-term babies sleep even more, while post-term babies sleep less. For a few days, full-term babies eat very little and often lose weight. This is all very natural and should not alarm you. If your baby sleeps a lot, don't confuse sweetness with weakness.

> **Turn off your phone when nursing, when napping, and when with your husband. After a few weeks, if you are nursing, consider a once-a-day relief bottle (formula or expressed breast milk).**

Presumably this calm, quiet period during the first days is synchronized with the few days it takes for the mother's breast milk to come in. Babies sleep a lot, fifteen to eighteen hours a day, but usually in short stretches of two to four hours. These sleep periods do not follow a pattern related to day and night, so get your own rest whenever you are able.

Q: *I heard that I am supposed to put my baby to sleep when drowsy but awake. But every time I feed her, she quickly falls asleep. Am I supposed to wake her up and then put her down to sleep?*

A: Newborns usually fall asleep during a feeding, and it does not make sense to wake them simply in order to put them back to sleep. It goes against Mother Nature! But older babies, when they really slow down or finish sucking, may be almost but not quite asleep. When the breast or bottle is removed, older babies momentarily look around in a dazed fashion, just to check out that everything is okay, and then go into a deep, comfortable snooze.

Why, then, have you heard that you should not let your child fall asleep during soothing or feeding? The theory is that your child needs to learn self-soothing skills, and that she will not learn these skills if she comes to associate soothing or feeding with sleep. Consider two scenarios. In the first scenario, you keep the intervals of wakefulness brief, less than one to two hours, and you watch for signs of *drowsiness*. At the drowsy time, you soothe and feed your baby. She now may be drowsier and entering the sleep zone, but she is not completely asleep at the end of the soothing and feeding. That is when you put her down. Now she is able to self-soothe herself to deep slumber. This is easy because she was not overtired, and 80 percent of babies (those who display common fussiness/crying) can handle this well. But this scenario does not require you to wake your baby if she occasionally falls asleep during a feeding. There may be a lot of non-nutritive sucking after a feeding, so if your baby often falls into a deep sleep at the breast, slightly shorten the duration of the feeding plus sucking in order to put her in her crib drowsy but awake. As long as weight gain is fine, there is no harm in trying this.

In the second scenario, you allow your child to stay up too long and she becomes overtired. She has passed through the drowsy zone and is entering the fatigue zone. Now, when you soothe and feed your baby, you discover that she will not be easily placed in her crib or stay asleep unless she is already in a deep sleep at the end of the soothing and feeding. Soothing herself to sleep is difficult because she develops a second wind or she belongs to the 20 percent of babies (those afflicted with extreme fussiness/colic) who are often this way during the first few months. The problem is not your failure to "put her to sleep when drowsy but awake"; rather, the problem is allowing your baby to become overtired or being unlucky and having an extremely fussy/colicky baby.

WARNING!

The first week of life is like a honeymoon. Newborns "sleep like a baby" except when born post-term.

For all babies: It will become more and more difficult to soothe and put your baby to sleep in the evening hours at 6 weeks of age, counting from the due date.

For 80 percent of babies: They will settle down at night after 6 weeks.

> *For 20 percent of babies:* It will become more and more difficult
> to soothe and put your baby to sleep all the time starting at
> several days of age, counting from the due date. All these babies
> settle down at night around 3–4 months of age, some even at
> 2 months.

When your baby becomes more and more difficult to soothe and put to sleep, she appears to be completely out of your control, and your life will not be easy. Sleep training is described in detail in chapter 4 and does *not* mean simply letting your baby cry. Sleep training involves:

Teaching self-soothing
    Start early
    Many hands (enlist Dad and others)
    Put your baby down drowsy but awake
Many naps, with brief intervals of wakefulness
Bedtime routines and then leave the room

Weeks 2–4: More Fussiness

Night sleep: No established rhythms
Day sleep: No established rhythms
Bedtimes: No established rhythms

All babies are a little hard to "read" during the first few weeks. Most activities such as feeding, changing diapers, and soothing to sleep occur at irregular times. Do not expect your baby to adhere to a schedule, because her needs for food, cuddling, and sleeping are going to occur erratically and unpredictably. When your baby needs to be fed, feed her; when she needs to have her diaper changed, change her; and when she needs to sleep, allow her to sleep.

What do I mean by "allow her to sleep"? Try to provide a calm, quiet place for your baby if she sleeps better this way. Many babies are very portable at this age and seem to sleep well anywhere. You're lucky if your baby is like this, and you're even luckier if she is one of the few who have long night sleep periods. During weeks 2–4, most newborns don't sleep for long periods at night.

Studies have shown that for babies a few weeks old, the longest single sleep period may be only three to four hours, and it can occur at any time during the day or night. (This is known as day/night confusion, though the term is a bit misleading. It's not that your baby gets day and night mixed up; instead, your baby has not yet developed her internal timekeeping mechanisms that distinguish night from day.) Extremely fussy/colicky babies may not even have a single sleep period that is this long; premature babies may have longer sleep periods.

Parenting strategies such as changes in the amount of light or noise don't appear to greatly influence babies' sleep patterns at this stage. In fact, specific styles or methods of burping, changing, or feeding do not seem to really affect the baby at all. Try not to think of doing things *to* or *for* the baby. Instead, take time to enjoy doing things *with* your baby (page 363). Do the things that give you both pleasure: holding, cuddling, talking, singing, listening to music, walking, and bathing. This active love is sufficient stimulation for now; you don't have to worry about buying the right toy to stimulate your baby. Here are some concrete steps you can take to make it easier for everyone:

1. Take naps during the day when your baby is sleeping.
2. Turn off all phones in the house when your baby is sleeping.
3. Go out, without your baby, for breaks: a walk, a coffee date, or a movie.
4. Plan or arrange for a few hours of private time to take care of yourself.

5. Do whatever comes naturally to soothe your baby; don't worry about spoiling her or creating bad habits. But do try to ignore the very quiet vocalizations that normally occur during sleep and do not indicate hunger or distress.

6. Use swings, pacifiers, or anything else that safely provides rhythmic, rocking motions or engages the sucking reflex.

7. Look at the Step-by-Step Program to Prevent Sleep Problems (chapter 1); read about *parent issues* and *adverse concerns*. If you suspect that challenges lie ahead, sit down with your husband, wife, partner, or pediatrician for a frank talk. Perhaps this is the time to engage a community sleep consultant (page 329) to prevent sleep problems from developing.

If you find that your baby sleeps well everywhere and whenever she is tired, enjoy your freedom while you can. A time will come when you will be less able to visit friends, shop, or go to exercise classes, because your baby will need a more consistent soothing-to-sleep routine and a less stimulating sleep environment.

Q: *Why are breastfed babies fed more often at night than formula-fed babies?*

A: It may be that breast milk takes less time to digest, so the breastfed baby is hungrier sooner. It may be that the mother who has chosen to breastfeed is more sensitive or attuned to her baby and responds more frequently to the baby's sounds: both hungry sounds and sleep sounds. Maybe the breastfeeding mother is more committed to soothing or nurturing her baby, using her breasts as a pacifier even when her baby is just fussy and not hungry. Perhaps the breastfeeding mother responds more often because her breasts feel uncomfortably full. Or the mother who is breastfeeding is unsure whether her baby has gotten enough, because, unlike formula-feeding parents, she cannot see how much her baby has taken. Both breast milk and formula have the same number of calories per ounce even though formula appears to be thicker.

Q: *I've heard that my newborn should not sleep in the bassinet in my room because it will spoil her.*

A: Nonsense. Feeding and nursing are easier for both of you if your newborn is close. When your baby is older, both of you may sleep better if she is not in your room. Anyway, by then the number of night feedings is usually fewer. Please review the Safe Sleep Guidelines from the American Academy of Pediatrics (page 94).

Brief awakenings or complete arousals at night occur normally, at all ages (page 61). Quiet or brief vocalizations may accompany these arousals. Young infants, especially under 4 months of age, are fed at night, and some of these arousals might be misinterpreted as hunger. At any age, if parents attend to these normal arousals too frequently or provide too much intervention, the child may develop a night-crying or night-feeding habit. This becomes a sleep problem called *signaling,* and because it fragments both the child's and parents' sleep, the result is a sleep-deprived family. *Signaling* describes children who have difficulty or are unable or unwilling to return to sleep unassisted. Over time, the number of times the child wakes and signals tends to increase and the duration of wakefulness of each event also increases.

Q: *When will my child sleep through the night?*

A: After 6 weeks, infants tend to go to sleep earlier, around 6:00 to 8:00 P.M., and most need to be fed before they wake up to start the day. The need for night feedings disappears slowly over the next several months. After a few months, most babies do not need to be fed more than twice at night: in the middle of the night and early in the morning. Except for breastfed babies in a family bed, more than two night feedings after a few months will begin to create a night-waking habit. After 9 months, these night feedings are not needed. Sleeping through the night is discussed in detail in chapters 8 and 9.

A change occurs in all babies during these first few weeks, and you should prepare for it. When your baby is about to fall asleep or is just about to wake up, a sudden single jerk or massive twitch of her entire body may occur. As the drowsy baby drifts into a deeper sleep, the eyes sometimes appear to roll upward. This is normal behavior during sleep/wake transitions. Also, all babies become somewhat more alert, wakeful, and aroused as the brain develops. You may notice restless movements, such as shuddering, quivering, tremulousness, shaking or jerking, twisting or turning, and hiccups. There may be moments when your sweet little baby appears impatient, distressed, or agitated for no identifiable reason. This is all normal newborn behavior. These behaviors will soon disappear as the brain develops more inhibitory control, especially after 6 weeks of age.

During these spells of unexplainable restlessness or fussiness, your baby may swallow air and become gassy. Often she appears to be in pain. Sometimes she cries and you can't figure out why. The crying baby may be hungry or just fussy. This is confusing and frustrating to all parents.

All in all, at this point you may not have the baby you dreamed of having. She fusses or cries too much, sleeps too little, and spits up on you whenever you forget to cover your shoulder with a towel. This is known as reality, and the sooner parents learn to accept the baby they have, rather than stressing about some hypothetical perfect dream baby, the better everyone will be.

Fussiness and Crying

Baby-Driven Path: The Role of the Baby

COMMON FUSSINESS/CRYING

Fussiness
Fussiness is an unsettled or agitated state that often precedes crying if not attended to by parents with soothing efforts. A fussy child

appears to be in mild distress or mildly uncomfortable. But not all fussiness in children is created equal. How do you judge the degree of your child's fussiness? Measurements of fussiness are used by researchers and pediatricians to *arbitrarily* divide infants into groups with names like "common fussiness" or "extreme fussiness." But these measurements don't paint a complete picture, just as the measure of your weight in pounds does not say everything about your total health picture. That's why I advise parents not to worry about measurements and labels. Instead, keep in mind that your child will have a little, a medium amount, or a lot of unexplained fussiness and crying that is likely to first increase, then decrease after 6 weeks (counting from the due date), and then disappear more or less completely around 2–4 months of age.

But at 2–4 weeks, as fussiness and crying increase with attendant swallowed air (gassiness), you cannot predict how much fussiness and crying there will be in the future, so it is worthwhile to read this entire section to prepare yourself for possible challenges ahead.

Eighty percent of babies have common fussiness, and the parents of these babies are fortunate. These babies do not require a lot of parental soothing. They tend to be naturally self-soothing, mild, and calm; they fall asleep easily and sleep for long periods.

Breastfeeding these babies is relatively easy because the mothers tend to be better rested and the babies tend to be more regular in their habits. Feedings may be relatively short and infrequent because nursing is mainly for satisfying thirst and hunger. When these babies are fussy, methods of soothing other than breastfeeding often work. In fact, the popularity of many techniques or strategies for soothing babies is due to the fact that for these babies—the majority of babies—most everything for soothing works well!

Bottle-feeding these babies either formula or expressed breast milk with or without breastfeeding is a family decision that is usually easily made. Some considerations are to allow the father or other children the pleasure of feeding the baby, thus enabling the mother to get some needed extra sleep at night or to return to work by continuing to pump her breasts at work, or to make it easier for the parents to arrange an evening for an old-fashioned date.

Before your baby is born, you might decide that you want to sleep with your baby (see the discussion of SIDS on page 94) or that you want to use a crib or bassinet. For 80 percent of all babies, those with common fussiness, it doesn't matter which you choose; these babies are fairly adaptable and self-soothing. You might sleep with your baby both during naps and at night, or only at night. Or you might lie down with your baby when she first falls asleep, put her down in her crib, and then, at the first night feeding, bring her into bed with you. Or you might have a co-sleeper attached to your bed and use it for part or all of the night. You can easily put your baby to sleep within one to two hours of wakefulness, because drowsy cues are usually obvious in these babies. Any soothing-to-sleep method is likely to work, and the baby and parents usually sleep well. Parents are at a low risk for feeling distressed, and I think maternal depression and/or anxiety is not very likely. Some of these common fussy babies, however, will occasionally behave like the extremely fussy baby, and your plans might have to be altered. Only about 5 percent of these babies seem to develop into overtired 4-month-olds.

During the first four weeks after birth, your baby really is "sleeping like a baby." Elliot, my first son, described his own first son as having a look on his face like *I didn't do it* or seeming almost intoxicated during this time because he slept so much. Placing your baby in the crib is usually a piece of cake. During weeks 4–8, your baby will become more wakeful and alert and have more evening fussiness. Elliot said that his son now had a more quizzical look, like *Who are you?* and *Give me back my pacifier!*

Helping babies with common fussiness to sleep well using graduated extinction, extinction with a cap, or extinction may start early, even before 2 months of age, as described in chapter 4 (for soothing and crying) and in chapter 5 (for extinction).

Crying: All Babies Cry Some of the Time

Crying in infants was first intensively studied in 1945 by a group of dedicated researchers at the Mayo Clinic led by Dr. C. Anderson Aldrich. In their first study, they observed seventy-two newborn babies in a nursery. The researchers worked in shifts so that each baby was observed twenty-four hours a day. They recorded the onset of crying and how long it lasted. They tried to attribute a cause to the crying—wet or soiled diapers, hunger, cramped positions, chilling, and the like—if one was apparent. They found that most of the newborns cried between one and eleven minutes per hour for the duration of their stay in the nursery. The average daily total duration of crying was about *two hours* for these seventy-two babies. *All* of the infants cried for some time *every* day.

Continuous observations were also made for fifty of the original seventy-two babies staying in the nursery for eight days—the recommended stay at that time. Remember, these babies were being observed every minute during those eight days. Researchers found that the minimum amount of crying per day in this group was 48 minutes and the maximum amount was 243 minutes. *All* of the infants cried some of the time—at least forty-eight minutes per day. The average duration of crying was, as before, about *two hours* per day.

Some Crying Can't Be Attributed to an Obvious Cause

The researchers attempted to classify the causes of crying: hunger, vomiting, wet or soiled diapers, and unknown reasons. For example, if the baby was crying and sucking around feeding time, and was calmed by feeding, then the crying was attributed to hunger. They found that hunger appeared to cause 36 percent of all time spent crying. Wet diapers caused about 21 percent of crying time, and soiled diapers about 8 percent. Specifically interesting was that 35 percent of all time spent crying was due to "unknown reasons." The researchers were surprised that such a large part of crying—over one-third—could not be explained by any obvious causes.

Then they examined the number of separate crying spells. Each spell was counted once, regardless of its duration. They found that the number of crying spells for "unknown reasons" was greater than any other cause, including hunger. Their conclusion: Crying spells caused by hunger were slightly longer in duration, though less frequent, than those caused by "unknown reasons."

Thus, the findings of the Mayo study were that all babies cry during the newborn period and that much of this crying cannot be attributed to any obvious cause. The authors made some guesses about non-obvious causes: bright lights, peristaltic movements or contractions in the gut, loud noises, and loss of equilibrium. They added, almost as an afterthought, that perhaps the infants' crying expressed a need for fondling or rhythmic motion.

The authors continued the study at home on forty-two infants, using a detailed diary filled in by the mothers. These data covered about twenty-one days at home, after a nine- or ten-day stay in the nursery. The babies averaged four crying spells a day. *All* babies had some crying spells. Fifty-five percent of these spells were attributed to hunger. Crying associated with vomiting, stooling, urination, overheating, bathing, chilling, lights, or noises (the mothers making these attributions) were individually less common than crying for unknown reasons. Again, *unknown reasons (20 percent) seemed to be second only to hunger (25 percent) as a cause of crying.*

Two to Three Hours of Crying per Day Is Average

Dr. T. Berry Brazelton performed an important study on crying in 1962, utilizing diaries completed by parents to study crying in eighty infants. Fussy crying spells unrelated to hunger or to wet or soiled diapers occurred in virtually *all* the babies. Only twelve of the eighty fussed less than one and a half hours per day. About half cried for about two hours per day. This increased to an average of about three hours per day at age 6 weeks. Thereafter the amount of crying declined to about one hour per day by age 12 weeks.

Many Babies Have Evening Crying Spells

Dr. Brazelton also found that crying spells became much more focused or concentrated in the evening by the time the infants were
about 6 weeks of age, when the crying peaked. By this time, very
little crying occurred during the day. The spells of crying in the evening occurred around the same time every evening and began suddenly. The reason for this rapid shift in behavior from a calm/quiet
state to a crying state is not known. This was also observed in an
unpublished study by Dr. James A. Kleeman and Dr. John C. Cobb,
in which out of seventy-eight mothers questioned about their infants, sixty-eight reported "fussy periods," fifty of whom said that
the periods occurred in the later afternoon or evening, with the
fussiest hours coming between 7:00 and 9:00 P.M.

Crying Decreases at About 3 Months

Dr. Brazelton found that, on average, crying decreased to about one
hour per day by age 12 weeks. Another Harvard study verified Dr.
Brazelton's observations using tape recordings of infants crying in
their homes. This study observed the same time course: an increase
in crying at about 6 weeks, and a decrease by about 12 weeks. Although the amount of daily crying was less than that observed by
Dr. Brazelton, this may be because only ten infants were studied.
This means that the natural history of unexplained crying runs the
same time course as that of colicky behavior. In both cases, babies
calmed down at about 3 months of age.

You can see that, in at least five important particulars, what has
been called "colic" is just an extreme form of normal crying. Colic
may just be a lot of normal fussing/crying. In fact, even Dr. Brazelton suggested that those infants in his study who cried more than
the others were indistinguishable from infants with colic. I think
this is a very plausible suggestion. There is not a great gulf between
normal crying and colic. The idea that colic is an all-or-nothing
event (like pregnancy) is probably wrong. Colicky babies cry like

other babies, only more so. Or, if you prefer, most babies cry like colicky babies, only less so.

This is not to diminish the distress caused to parents because of their inability to deal with this crying. That difficulty cannot be overstated. Government data have shown that infant homicides increase after the second week and peak at the eighth week, and the researchers concluded that the "peak in risk in week eight might reflect the peak in the daily duration of crying among normal infants between weeks six and eight."

There are no clear cutoff points in measurements of irritability, fussing, or crying, whether by direct observation in hospital nurseries, voice-activated tape recordings in homes, or parent diaries. Thus, extreme fussiness/colic appears to represent an extreme amount of normally occurring, unexplained fussing/crying that is present in all healthy babies.

Because the spells of fussing or crying are universal, differing only in degree among infants; because the occurrence of spells peaks at 46 weeks after conception and seems to be independent of parenting practices; and because the behaviors exhibit behavioral state specificity (the babies are awake when the crying begins and fall asleep when the crying ends) and a day/night rhythm, it is reasonable to conclude that these behaviors reflect normal biological processes. One example is the normal biological process involving the development of sleep/wake control mechanisms: In all babies, the consolidation of night sleep develops during the second month (after the peak of crying occurs), and the periodic alternation of wake and sleep states during the day is well developed by 3–4 months of age (when colic ends).

> Because *all* babies fuss and cry, some a little and some a lot, it's best to think of colic as something a baby *does*, not something a baby *has*. It's a stage of life, not a medical problem.

EXTREME FUSSINESS/COLIC

In 1954, Drs. Morris Wessel and R. S. Illingworth published the first modern studies trying to define colic. Dr. Wessel, in America, defined a colicky infant as "one who is otherwise healthy and well fed, had paroxysms of irritability, fussing or crying lasting for a total of more than three hours a day and occurring on more than three days in any one week . . . and that the paroxysms continued to recur for more than three weeks." He told me that he added the criterion "more than three weeks" because many nannies left families after about three weeks of crying, and he thought that professional nannies, with their experience, knew that if babies cried for more than three weeks, then the crying was likely to continue. Because the mothers were now alone at night caring for their babies, they came to his office after three weeks, complaining that their children were always crying. About 26 percent of infants in his study had colic. Dr. Illingworth, in England, defined colic as "violent rhythmical, screaming attacks *which did not stop when the infants were picked up,* and for which no cause, such as underfeeding, could be found [emphasis added]." His observation of inconsolability has become the centerpiece of the current definition of *colic*. He also anticipated the terminology subsequently used to described *temperament* types and the association between temperament and extreme fussiness/colic: ". . . an important factor which governs the amount of cry is the personality. Some are placid *easy* babies who will accept anything . . . they are content [and rarely cry]. Others are determined *difficult* babies who almost from the moment of birth do not hesitate [to cry]." This was written many years before Drs. Thomas and Chess published their papers on "easy" and "difficult" *temperament* types and before anyone made an association between extreme fussiness/colic and temperament. His description of colic closely agreed with that of Dr. Wessel, and the data regarding the onset of colic and the disappearance of colic was virtually the same. Together, Drs. Wessel and Illingworth studied about 150 infants.

The *age of onset* of these behaviors is characteristic. Both Dr. Wessel and Dr. Illingworth found that the attacks were absent during the first few days after birth but were present in 80 percent of affected infants by 2 weeks and in about 100 percent by 4 weeks. Premature babies also start their attacks shortly after the expected due date, independent of their gestational age at birth. The *time of day* when these behaviors occur is another characteristic. During the first month, crying appears at any time of the day or night, but later it occurs predominantly in the evening hours. In 80 percent of infants, the attacks start between 5:00 and 8:00 P.M. and end by midnight. For 12 percent of infants, the attacks start between 7:00 and 10:00 P.M. and end by 2:00 A.M. In only 8 percent are the attacks distributed throughout the day and night. The *age of termination* of these spells is also characteristic. The attacks disappear by *2 months of age in 50 percent* of infants, by *3 months of age in 30 percent,* and by *4 months of age in 10 to 20 percent* of infants. The infant's *behavioral state* is associated with colicky behavior. Among colicky infants, 84 percent have crying spells that *begin when they are awake,* 8 percent have spells that start when they are asleep, and another 8 percent have spells under either condition. For 83 percent of infants, *when the crying spells end, they fall asleep.*

It is now known that persistent low-intensity fussing, rather than intense crying, characterizes infants diagnosed as having colic. In fact, to emphasize fussiness instead of crying, the title of a paper by Dr. Wessel was "Paroxysmal Fussing in Infants, Sometimes Called 'Colic.'" Fussing is not a well-defined behavior, and although not defined in Dr. Wessel's paper, it is usually described as an unsettled, agitated, wakeful state that would lead to crying if ignored by parents. Because sucking is soothing to infants, some parents misattribute the "fussing" state to hunger and vigorously attempt to feed their baby. These parents may misinterpret their infants as having a "growth spurt" at 6 weeks because they were "hungry" all the time, especially in the evening. That is, they want to suck much more at this time. They view their child as hungry, not fussy. Even if they spend more than three additional hours a day, more than three days a week, for more than three weeks feeding them at night to prevent crying, these parents do not think their baby is colicky because there is so little crying.

Over a thirty-four-month period, at newborn visits in my office, I routinely asked every new parent who joined my general pediatric practice whether their child fulfilled Dr. Wessel's exact diagnostic criteria for colic (paroxysms of irritability, fussiness, or crying lasting for more than three hours per day for more than three days per week, and lasting for more than three weeks in an otherwise healthy child). All families had been followed by me since the child's birth and received counseling regarding the normal development of crying or fussing. There were 118 extremely fussy/colicky infants out of 747 (16 percent). However, the vast majority of infants had *little or no crying*. Instead, they fulfilled Dr. Wessel's criteria for colic because they had long and frequent bouts of fussing, which did not lead to crying because of *intensive parental intervention*.

Studies also show that between 2 and 6 weeks there is an increase predominantly in fussing, not crying. Furthermore, fussing and sleeping, but notably not crying, were found to be stable individual characteristics from 6 weeks to 9 months of age. The amount of crying during the first 3 months does not predict crying behavior at 9 months. But in a study by Professor Olsen, sleeping *problems* ("The child has not established an age and developmentally appropriate pattern of falling asleep or maintaining sleep"), not short sleep durations, during the first two months are associated with excessive crying at 8–11 months.

One recent study showed that colic during the first few months that ends by 6 months is *not* associated with any adverse effects regarding child behavior, regulatory abilities, temperament, of family functioning at 2–3 years of age. Older literature showed different results—that is, colic is associated with a variety of unhealthy outcomes, such as emotional or behavioral problems in the child. However, the authors of the more recent study noted that the older studies might have included infants with persistent crying beyond 6 months. When infants with colic continue to cry substantially past 3–6 months of age, it may be due to a failure of the parents to help their child sleep well, and the persistent poor-quality sleep in the child or persistent parenting issues might lead to adverse long-term outcomes. Alternatively, there may be regulatory issues within the child that cause both the prolonged crying early in life and the later problems. The main message from the recent study strongly suggests that colic that ends within 6 months is *not* predictive of any long-term issues. However, a problem with this type of study is the definition of colic that they used (more than three hours a day of irritability, fussiness, or crying occurring on more than three days during a week). In this study, 35 percent of infants behaved this way. Dr. Wessel observed, in his original study, that 49 percent of infants behave this way. When you add Dr. Wessel's diagnostic criterion that this *behavior lasts for more than three weeks,* then only 26 percent of infants in Wessel's study and 16 percent of infants in my study behave this way. Selecting a smaller group of presumably more severely affected infants might reveal more adverse long-term outcomes that might not be detected when more mildly affected infants are included.

Also, as previously mentioned, crying, alone, is *not* a prediction of sleep problems. Two separate and well-designed studies agree with Dr. Ian St. James-Roberts that "high amounts of early crying do not make it highly probable that an infant will . . . have sleeping problems at nine months of age." In summary, early crying alone does not predict later crying and early crying alone does not predict later sleep problems. However, as discussed later (page 425), parenting style (either contributing to the crying or in reaction to the crying or both) does affect the likelihood that a child will be waking and crying at night when older.

What causes extreme fussiness/colic? A recent study performed brain imaging on infants during their first three days and recorded responses to olfactory stimuli (a rotten-cabbage-like odor, a banana-like odor, and a eucalyptus-like odor). Those infants who showed a strong reactivity to the cabbage-like odor were much more likely to develop excessive fussiness/crying at 5–6 weeks of age. Thus, the researchers said, "Shortly after birth, the central nervous system of babies developing infant colic has already greater reactivity to sensory stimuli than that of their noncolicky peers." Perhaps this heightened reactivity contributes to an impaired ability to self-soothe and sleep well.

Another study showed that colicky infants had higher levels of serotonin, a chemical found in the brain and in the gut. This supported the theory of my wife, Linda Weissbluth, that some features of colic might be caused by an imbalance between serotonin and melatonin, another chemical found in the brain and in the gut. Concentrations of serotonin are high and present in infants during the first month of life and decline after 3 months. Immediately after delivery, concentrations of serotonin are higher at night and lower during the day. Melatonin, flowing across the placenta from the mother, causes high concentrations immediately after birth, but they rapidly fall to extremely low levels within several days. Melatonin increases slightly between 1 and 3 months, and only after 3 months is there an abrupt increase in melatonin levels, with higher levels at night and lower levels during the day.

Serotonin and melatonin have opposite effects on the muscle around the gut—serotonin causes contraction, while melatonin causes relaxation. Linda Weissbluth's theory is that in some infants, high serotonin levels cause painful gastrointestinal cramps in the evening, when serotonin concentrations are at their highest. The high nighttime melatonin levels oppose the intestinal smooth muscle contraction caused by serotonin. On the other hand, melatonin and serotonin might be directly affecting the developing brain. For example, high levels of melatonin at night might cause night sleep to become longer.

Other hormones might be involved. In one study, extremely fussy/colicky infants had a blunted rhythm in cortisol production, while the control infants exhibited a clear and marked daily rhythm in cortisol that was not observed in the colicky infants. In addition, researchers in this study coded behavioral measures from video recordings made during the *day* and arrived at the same conclusion as have many other studies: The crying of these infants was not due to differences in handling by the mother, and the colic was not simply a maternal perception. While this supports a developmentally driven path regarding fussing and crying, more recent data, including video recordings made during the *night* (chapter 4), suggest that some parent behaviors also are important. Other studies have clearly shown that food hypersensitivity and gastroesophageal reflux are *not* linked to infantile colic.

Twenty percent of babies have extreme fussiness/colic, and the parents of these babies are unlucky. These babies require a lot of parental soothing. They tend not to be self-soothing, and they often appear intense, seem agitated, and have difficulty falling asleep and staying asleep.

Breastfeeding these babies is often difficult because the mothers tend to be exhausted or fatigued from sleep deprivation, and the babies tend to be irregular. Feedings may be long and frequent because in addition to satisfying thirst and hunger, much of the nursing is non-nutritive sucking to reduce fussiness. When these babies are extremely fussy, methods of soothing other than breastfeeding often do not work. Frustration or despair is common because many of the popular techniques or strategies for soothing babies fail, even though many other mothers (80 percent) swear by them.

Some considerations going through the mind of the mother of a colicky infant are whether something is wrong with her breast milk, whether her breast milk is sufficient, and whether her diet or the current formula is causing the extreme fussiness/colic. Because soothing at the breast often seems to work when other soothing methods fail, the mother does not want to give it up. But painfully dry or cracked skin around the nipple, from prolonged non-nutritive sucking, may make breastfeeding an ordeal. The discomfort and pain associated with breastfeeding, plus unrelenting exhaustion from sleep deprivation, may conspire to cause so much stress that the breast milk supply becomes insufficient. Mothers who have enormous support—a dedicated husband who spends a lot of time soothing, housekeeping help, or baby care help—can get through this difficult time much more easily than mothers who lack a support system. Mothers who have other children to care for, pressure to return to work, medical problems, baby blues, or postpartum depression may find the additional stresses associated with breast-feeding these extremely fussy/colicky babies to be overwhelming.

Bottle-feeding these babies either formula or expressed breast milk can be a benefit to some mothers, but it can also create more stress in others. The benefits of complete or partial bottle-feeding are that the mother might get more rest because others can feed her baby, and the parents are calmer—since bottle-feeding makes it easy to see how much the baby is swallowing, they can be certain their baby is not hungry. But in other mothers, giving bottles can create the feeling of having failed as a mother. Recognizing that bottles are not as soothing as the breast, these mothers feel guilty because they think they are causing their babies to fuss/cry more, and they worry that something in the formula may be causing the fussiness/crying.

If you want to breastfeed, a compromise position is to have someone else give a single bottle of expressed breast or formula once per twenty-four hours. This will not cause "nipple confusion" or interfere with lactation. It will give the mother a mini break, will allow her to get a little more sleep, and will allow the parents a night out.

Before your baby is born, you might decide that you want to sleep with her (please see page 94 regarding co-sleeping and SIDS) or that you want to use a crib or bassinet. But for the 20 percent of babies with extreme fussiness/colic, the plans that you made for sleeping with your baby or separate from her might have to be altered, because these babies tend to be difficult to soothe and have difficulty falling asleep and staying asleep. Watching for drowsy cues is usually frustrating in these babies because they are not obvious, and even if you keep the intervals of wakefulness less than one to two hours, it is still difficult to soothe them. When they finally do fall asleep, they do not stay asleep for long. As a result, parents are often sleep-deprived. Parents in this situation are at a high risk of feeling distressed, and I think that maternal depression is more likely to occur.

Because these babies are difficult to soothe, breastfeeding in the family bed may appear to be the best or only strategy that works. Although the mother's sleep may be fragmented by frequent feeding for both nutrition and soothing, this is probably the most powerful soothing method for these babies. During the first four weeks, these colicky babies are not really "sleeping like a baby." Placing a colicky baby in the crib is usually stressful. During weeks 4–8, the colicky baby may become even more wakeful and alert and have more evening fussiness, causing the parents to be at an even greater risk for distress. But about *50 percent* of these babies begin to settle down around *2 months* of age. About 27 percent of these infants, however, are at risk for becoming overtired 4-month-olds.

There is some research to suggest that parents who make the commitment to use the family bed from day one and stick with it will wind up with better-rested babies than those parents who initially wanted to use the crib but later brought their baby into their bed because it was the only way they could get any sleep. In the former group, proactive co-sleepers, sleep problems are less likely to develop as the children get older. But in the reactive group of co-sleepers, where the family bed was used only in response to soothing or sleeping difficulties, this short-term solution can create long-term sleep problems. What is happening is that parents, overwhelmed by the fussy/crying behavior, and with limited resources for soothing their baby, reluctantly use the family bed to gain relief, but the limited resources for soothing persist beyond the first months and may often cause sleep problems later in older children because those children have failed to learn self-soothing.

Sleep

I actually prefer the term *extreme fussiness/colic* instead of *colic* because fussiness is a bigger problem than crying. All babies have some fussing and crying, and for 80 percent of babies, I call this behavior common fussiness/crying. My idea is that extreme fussiness/colic is a sleep/wake disorder: The inability to sleep well or excessive wakefulness in about 20 percent of babies creates an agitated, uncomfortable state, especially in the evening or at night. I also suggest that post-colic sleep problems occur after 3–4 months of age because some parents experience difficulty in establishing age-appropriate sleep routines or fail to teach self-soothing after 3–4 months. A problem with associating colic with sleep is that we do not have an objective test for colic or a universally agreed-upon definition of it. Further, until recently we did not have objective measures of infant sleep. Let's look at the individual studies that suggest that infant colic and infant sleep are connected.

Dr. Jarkko Kirjavainen asked parents to keep a daily diary, and he performed sleep recordings in the lab at night between 9:00 P.M. and 7:00 A.M. At about 4.5 weeks, the total sleep time from the diary was significantly shorter in a colic group (12.7 versus 14.5 hours per day). The most dramatic decrease in sleep in the colicky babies occurred at night between 6:00 P.M. and 6:00 A.M. The diary data showed that by 6 months of age the extremely fussy/colicky infants slept slightly less than the non-colicky infants, but the group differences were small. Separate from the diary data, the first sleep lab recording was performed when the infants were about 9 weeks old. There were no differences in sleep characteristics between the groups in the night recordings. The second sleep lab recording was performed at about 30 weeks of age, and again, there were no differences in sleep characteristics between the infants formerly with and without extreme fussiness/colic.

Therefore, among infants with extreme fussiness/colic, parent diary data showed shorter total sleep times compared with the age-matched control group at 4.5 weeks, but by 9 weeks there were no group differences in sleep lab data obtained during the night. Also, this report suggests that over time, between the ages of 5 and 9 weeks, sleep duration increased among extremely fussy/colicky infants. Based on the sleep lab data and ignoring the parent diary data, the authors concluded that infantile colic was not associated with a sleep disorder. However, Dr. Kirjavainen told me that the lab data were questionable because all children slept poorly in the lab setting.

Dr. Ian St. James-Roberts used the term *persistent criers* to describe extremely fussy/colicky infants. At 6 weeks of age, the extremely fussy/colicky infants slept significantly less than non-colicky infants (12.5 versus 13.8 hours per day, which is similar to the 12.7 versus 14.5 hours per day at 4.5 weeks observed by Dr. Kirjavainen). There were no group differences regarding time spent awake or time spent feeding. Extremely fussy/colicky infants slept less throughout the twenty-four-hour diary record. The clearest group differences for sleep were during the day (in contrast to Dr. Kirjavainen, who found less sleep especially between 6:00 P.M. and 6:00 A.M.). In fact, there were no group differences regarding sleep at night. In addition, at night there were no group differences for fuss/cry behavior. The clearest group differences for fuss/cry behavior were in the daytime. The groups were similar in the timing and duration of the infant's longest sleep period. This analysis of sleep cycle maturation led to the conclusion that the "chief difference between them lies in amounts of daytime fuss/crying and sleeping, rather than in the diurnal organization of sleep and waking behavior." In addition, at 6 weeks of age, the less a baby slept, the greater the amounts of fussing/crying observed. Because the authors observed no deficit in calm wakefulness, only sleeping, they felt that there was a specific trade-off between fussing/crying and sleep. In other words, more fussing/crying behavior reduced sleep time only, not calm wakeful time. The researchers concluded that persistent crying is associated with a sleep deficit.

Another study of extremely fussy/colicky infants using sensors embedded within a mattress to continuously monitor body movements and respiratory patterns showed that at 7 and 13 weeks of age, they slept less than common fussy infants. The extremely fussy/colicky infants had more difficulty falling asleep, were more easily disturbed, and had less quiet, deep sleep.

A separate study, at about 8 weeks of age, noted that colicky infants slept significantly less (11.8 versus 14.0 hours per day). The colicky infants slept less during the day, evening, and night; however, the big difference in sleeping was during the nighttime. Again, crying more was associated with sleeping less. The authors concluded that extreme fussiness/colic might be associated with a disruption or delay in the establishment of the circadian rhythm of sleep/wake activity.

Here is a summary of the data:

SLEEP AND FUSSINESS

Age (Weeks)	Average Total Sleep Duration from Parents' Diaries	
	Extreme Fussiness/Colic	Common Fussiness/Crying
4.5	12.7	14.5
6	12.5	13.8
8	11.8	14.0

So at the 6-week-old peak of fussiness/crying (the average being about three hours, in the evening, in Dr. Brazelton's study), the difference in total sleep duration is about one hour, but during the two weeks before and after the peak, the difference is closer to two hours. Almost half of all babies will fuss or cry more than three hours a day on more than three days in a week around this time. Sometimes this is called the "modified" Wessel's criteria for colic, because it leaves out Dr. Wessel's additional requirement that the behavior continue for more than three weeks. If this definition is used around 6 weeks of age, the difference in sleeping durations above is not great, but if the definition includes Dr. Wessel's original criterion that fussing/crying behavior continue for more than three weeks, and ages before and after 6 weeks are included, the differences in sleep durations are much larger.

My study showed that at about 16 weeks of age, the average total sleep duration, based on parental reports, of forty-eight infants who previously exhibited extreme fussiness/colic (using Dr. Wessel's exact definition) was 13.9 plus or minus 2.2 hours—much less than those with common fussiness/crying.

In my general pediatric practice, where all parents receive anticipatory advice regarding sleep hygiene at every visit, parents of extremely fussy/colicky infants say that development of early bedtimes, self-soothing to fall asleep at night, longer night sleep periods, fewer night wakings, and regular, longer naps occur later in their babies compared with common fussy/crying infants. This suggests that while extreme fussiness/colic may be associated with a delay in maturation of sleep/wake control mechanisms at 4.5, 6, 7, 8, 13, and 16 weeks, the diary data show that by 6 months there are no differences in *duration of night sleep* between extreme fussiness/colic and common fussy/crying groups.

However, *night waking* has been reported to be more common following extreme fussiness/colic at 4, 8, and 12 months. This might be interpreted as a persistent impairment of the learned ability to return to sleep unassisted (a failure to learn self-soothing) during a naturally occurring nighttime arousal from sleep in a post-colic infant.

Colic is confusing to researchers as well as parents because there is no standard or universally accepted definition or diagnostic criteria.

In 2016, an updated version of diagnostic criteria for colic was published called the *Rome IV criteria*. "The committee decided to exclude Wessel's rule of threes [page 391] from the Rome IV criteria, as it was stated that a minimum of 3 hours per day was too arbitrary since no evidence exists that a child who cries 2 hours 50 minutes per day differs from one who cries 3 hours per day. . . . Another reason for abandoning Wessel's rule was the focus on crying amount instead of the . . . unsoothable character of the crying episodes. Moreover, the term 'paroxysmal' is left out, since evidence is lacking to support that infant colic differs in sound and starts more abrupt compared to normal crying bouts." The elements of Rome IV criteria are:

1. An infant who is younger than 5 months of age when the symptoms start and stop
2. Recurrent and prolonged periods of infant crying, fussing, or irritability reported by caregivers that occur without obvious cause and *cannot be prevented or resolved by caregivers* [emphasis added]
3. No evidence of infant failure to thrive, fever, or illness
4. Caregiver reports of infant crying or fussing for 3 or more hours per day during 3 or more days in 7 days

This definition actually retains the arbitrary cutoff of "3 or more hours" but shifts the focus to the notion of inconsolability (page 407).

Wakefulness
Parents of extremely fussy/colicky infants often report that daytime sleep periods are extremely irregular and brief. Also, some parents of extremely fussy/colicky infants describe a dramatic increase in daytime wakefulness and sometimes a temporary but complete cessation of napping when their infants approach their peak fussiness at age 6 weeks. I think that, before 3–4 months of age, the period of inconsolability in the evening hours, when the infant cannot sleep and cries, may reflect periods of high arousal similar to the circadian *forbidden zone*. In adults, the forbidden zone is a time period

(8:00 to 10:00 P.M.) during which sleep onset and prolonged, consolidated, and restorative sleep states do not easily occur. In this context, it might be more appropriate to describe colic not as a disorder of impaired sleep but as a disorder of excessive wakefulness in the evening. This view is supported by recent sleep lab investigations showing that, in infants, a circadian forbidden zone does exist between 5:00 and 8:00 P.M.

In summary, crying and fussing behavior is universal. Onset is around 1 week (or one week after the due date in a baby born prematurely). At 6 weeks, the behavior increases in duration and becomes focused in the evening hours. The behavior generally starts in a wakeful state and ends in a sleep state, and disappears around 2–4 months of age. Older studies failed to show substantial differences in daytime caretaking activities. All of this points to a biologically based or developmental basis for extreme fussiness/colic. In Wessel's report, about 49 percent of infants will behave this way for more than a total of three hours a day on more than three days in a week; 26 percent will behave this way for more than three weeks. In my study, 16 percent of infants fulfilled Wessel's exact criteria. So although the prevalence varies with the definition, about 20 percent is a common ballpark figure in many studies.

Additionally, in a 2013 review of a developmental explanation for crying during the first 4 months, Dr. St. James-Roberts explained that except for a very small group of infants allergic to cow's milk, there was no good evidence that colic represents a gastrointestinal problem. Also, in a 2013 review by Dr. R. Shamir, the conclusion was that colic reflects brain maturation.

If this is true, then treatment should revolve around helping families *cope* with the stress of having a fussy/crying/wakeful baby. If instead, colic is viewed as a medical problem that needs *treatment,* then desperate parents will grasp at unproven treatments or treatments proven to be ineffective.

Treatment

Probiotics (organisms such as certain bacteria or yeast thought to improve health), prebiotics (nondigestible fiber compounds), and synbiotics (nutritional supplements containing probiotics and prebiotics) were studied in a 2012 review by Dr. Mary Mugambi. She concluded that they "had no impact on the incidence of colic." In another study, the conclusion of a double-blind, placebo-controlled randomized trial of a popular probiotic was that the results "do not support a general recommendation for the use of probiotics to treat colic in infants."

When studies of manipulative therapies (chiropractic, osteopathic, and cranial manipulation) for infant colic have a "low risk of performance bias [that is, parents are blind to whether the child actually received the treatment], the results did not reach statistical significance," according to a 2012 review by Dr. Dawn Dobson. Dr. Paul Posadzki, in his 2013 review of osteopathic manipulative treatment, agreed that effectiveness remains unproven.

Although popular, evidence for simethicone for "gassiness" as effective treatment for colic is lacking in the review by Belinda Hall in 2012. Also, there was a lack of evidence for effectiveness for acupuncture in a study by Dr. Holgeir Skjeie in 2013.

None of these treatments are recommended by the group of experts who formulated the new (2016) Rome IV diagnostic criteria for infant *colic*.

Drugs commonly used for gastroesophageal reflux are often given to fussy or crying babies under the mistaken notion that the problem is acid reflux. A 2011 review by Dr. Pamela Douglas showed that these drugs do not improve symptoms in irritable infants.

If an infant has a medical problem causing painful crying, such as a urinary tract infection, then by definition the infant does not have excessive fussiness/colic, because the definition always includes the notion that the baby is gaining weight well and is otherwise healthy.

There are several reasons parents have the false impression that these so-called treatments work. One is that parents often begin a treatment near the 6-week peak of common fussiness/crying, and shortly thereafter the child becomes more settled. Another is that many individuals and companies profit by claiming that their treatments cure colic. A third is that one quick way for a pediatrician to shorten an office visit with a distraught sleep-deprived parent is to write a prescription or referral to a specialist. Please ask your pediatrician or child care provider whether he or she knows of any evidence that supports the recommendations.

The fundamental reason these treatments do not work for excessive fussiness/colic is that these children do not have a diagnosable medical problem. Excessive fussiness/colic is something some infants *do;* it is not a condition that they *have.* Think of *caring* for these infants and for yourself, not of searching for a *cure.*

MORE INFORMATION AND SUPPORT ARE AVAILABLE AT:

purplecrying.info

postpartum.net

whatwerewethinking.org.au (understanding baby's crying)

Caring involves getting help to take breaks without guilt and doing whatever you can to help prevent crying and fussing. Previous diagnostic criteria focused on the duration or amount of irritability, fussing, or crying and while the cutoff (more than three hours a day for more than three days in a week) was recognized to be arbitrary (like BMI measurements for obesity), it was often used to diagnose colic. As previously mentioned, new criteria were published in 2016 and deemphasized the amount of this behavior and focused instead on inconsolability. "Recurrent and prolonged periods of infant crying, fussing, or irritability reported by the caregivers that occur without obvious cause and *cannot be prevented or resolved by caregivers* [inconsolability]." Helping your baby sleep well during this difficult time has many benefits, such as preventing maternal depression (page 146). But some babies appear to be beyond help and are inconsolable.

Inconsolable Versus Consolable

Dr. Illingworth used inconsolability or unsoothability as part of his definition of colic. Is inconsolability or unsoothability a trait within the baby, a reflection of a parent's ability to soothe, or both? Let me share with you an observation I made in 1986. A mother with her colicky baby and her own mother came to my office. The mother had the baby on her lap; she was gently bouncing the baby up and down and patting the baby, but the baby was still crying loudly. The grandmother was reassuring and stroking the mother's hair. I asked the mother and grandmother if my nurse might take the baby outside the examining room so that we could talk without distraction for a few minutes, and they agreed. They passed the baby to my nurse, who then stepped out. Immediately, the baby stopped crying. My nurse, who was also a mother, was holding the baby chest-to-chest, with the baby's head resting on her right shoulder. The nurse's right cheek was gently pressed into the baby's right cheek, and the nurse gently rocked her body both from side to side and also with a slow and slightly rotational movement. It looked like my nurse was dancing with the baby in slow motion. The nurse was also whispering or shushing or humming directly into the child's right ear. Needless to say, we were all pleasantly surprised that the crying had abruptly stopped; in fact, we realized that the baby was now sound asleep. I clearly remember this event that happened more than thirty years ago, because it struck me that some mothers might have better soothing skills than other mothers and that the notion of inconsolability might, in part, reflect a mother's ability or inability to soothe. But at that time, I thought inconsolability was primarily a within-the-child trait, and in the absence of data I was strongly opposed to suggestions that mothers were responsible for or contributed to colic. Now we have data to consider a more nuanced view of the role of the mother, the father, and the couple as a unit.

Parent-Driven Path: The Role of the Parent

Mother: Anxiety and Depression

A 1965 study involving 103 mothers described a link between anxious mothers and colic. Dr. William Carey interviewed each mother within a few days after delivery. Forty of them expressed some anxiety. Dr. Carey compared their anxiety ratings with the presence or absence of colic in their children. He reported that only two of the colicky babies came from anxiety-free mothers, while eleven had mothers in the anxious category. This is a significant difference and supports Dr. Carey's conclusion that maternal anxiety appears at least partly responsible for, or contributory to, colic.

However, there are a couple of fairly significant flaws in the research. The first is with Dr. Carey's diagnosis of colic. He quotes and claims to have followed Wessel's definition; however, he reports that "colic began in the first month for five [infants], the second month for four and the third month for four." Wessel's data, and almost every other study of colic, report the onset of colic within two or three weeks after birth. This discrepancy causes one to apply a degree of skepticism to Dr. Carey's diagnoses. Also, Dr. Carey did both the interviewing of the mothers and the diagnosing of their babies. This means the study was not "blinded"; what a mother told Carey about her anxiety may have colored his view of whether or not her baby's crying ought to be considered colic. He recognized that maternal anxiety cannot be the only factor causing colic, because most anxious mothers did not have colicky babies and at least two non-anxious mothers did. Because of the weaknesses of this study, I did not find it a credible challenge to my strong belief that extreme fussiness/colic resulted from developmental issues.

Now, about fifty-five years later, we have better data . . . and much of it supports Dr. Carey. In 2014, Dr. Johanna Petzoldt showed that "infants of mothers with anxiety disorders *prior to pregnancy* were at higher risk for excessive crying [colic as exactly defined by Dr. Wessel] than infants of mothers without any anxiety disorder *prior to pregnancy*. . . . Maternal depressive disorders prior to pregnancy were not significantly associated with excessive crying." Additionally, she speculated that "maternal anxiety might lead to *intrusiveness* that possibly intensifies infant crying [emphasis added]." Intrusiveness, that is, regarding unnecessary night feedings and attention at night (page 219). In her 2018 review of all the literature, Dr. Petzoldt wrote that the best-supported path is that preceding maternal anxiety (even before pregnancy) predicts both subsequent excessive crying and maternal postpartum depression. When infant excessive crying and maternal depression are present simultaneously, "a vicious cycle of poor infant self-regulation [excessive crying] and hampered intuitive parenting [maternal depression] emerges." In a separate study, she showed that the strongest predictors for excessive infant crying, using Wessel's exact criteria, were maternal anxiety disorders and a fussy infant *temperament*; in contrast, infant sleeping problems were associated with maternal depressive disorders and not associated with a difficult infant temperament.

It should be noted that the mother's anxiety itself does not explain the observed typical onset (when awake) or cessation (when asleep) of colic or the 6-week peak. But perhaps if the anxiety is worse at night, it may contribute to the evening clustering of infant crying. Alternatively, the maternal *intrusiveness* at night fragments the child's sleep, and the sleep-deprived infant exhibits a prolonged witching hour or second wind at the end of the day or early evening called extreme fussiness/colic; she remains in this hyperaroused and painful *wakeful* state until she is exhausted and then crashes into *sleep*. Although anxiety and depression may occur together in an individual, in her original study, Dr. Petzoldt did not implicate maternal depression as a statistically significant factor but suggested that with a larger number of subjects, depression would likely also be found to be associated with colic.

Here is my interpretation. Anxious about her child's well-being at night, a mother might interfere with her baby's consolidated sleep or ability to learn self-soothing (page 219), causing her baby to have difficulties in falling asleep and staying asleep, which in turn causes the baby to fuss and cry more mostly at the end of the day when she is most sleep-deprived, causing the mother to become increasingly depleted from her own lack of sleep leading to her depressive symptoms (page 237).

Dr. Joseph Lonstein observed that elevated postpartum maternal anxiety "is particularly prevalent in women who experienced pregnancy complications, gave birth prematurely, delivered a low birthweight infant, or are caring for an infant with a birth defect." These births represent about 10 percent of all births in the United States, but "the actual rate [of postpartum maternal anxiety] may be greater than 20–25%." It may not be coincidental that colic also occurs in about 20 percent of babies.

Maternal depression or maternal "dysfunctional" cognitions (page 231) may be caused by a child who is not sleeping well (page 146) and may lead to unnecessary nighttime feedings or interventions that result in sleep fragmentation, causing a sleep-deprived baby to exhibit colic-like behavior. Alternatively, maternal depression independently might lead to nocturnal behaviors that disturb an infant's sleep, causing the sleep-deprived baby to become *colicky*. Thus, maternal depression may be a cause of colic, a consequence of colic, or both.

Father: Depression, Partner Support, and Infant Care at Night

I surveyed many families of twins to find out what factors were important for sleeping well. For the entire group, maternal age was perhaps the most important variable, in part because young mothers are usually married to young fathers. Here are some data for the *entire group*, which was a mixture of identical and fraternal twins and those who did and did not use assisted reproductive technology

(ART) such as in vitro fertilization. I compared families with younger mothers (at or under the median age for the group, which was 34 years) to families with mothers 35 years or older.

In the families with younger mothers, it was more common for both twins to sleep well, for the parents to start sleep training early (at 4 months or younger), and for there to be more success at breast-feeding. In addition, there was less baby blues or postpartum depression (BB/PPD), and the babies were less likely to have colic. These younger mothers were married to younger fathers (age 36 or younger). These younger fathers were more likely than older fathers to be involved in helping the twins sleep. I observed that when the younger fathers played an active role in caring for the twins and took an active part in sleep training them, the sleep training went more smoothly and was successful at an earlier point in the process. Among the entire group, almost 30 percent reported that at least one of their twins had colic based on Wessel's exact diagnostic criteria.

No other report showed such a high (30 percent) prevalence of colic. To better understand why colic was so common, I looked at different variables separately. I first divided the entire group by whether or not ART was utilized, because ART is associated with infertility, stressful fertility treatments and sometimes multiple unsuccessful attempts, and fraternal twins and older mothers. Within the group not using ART, a further division was made between identical twins (similar sleep rhythms would make sleep training easier) and fraternal twins. The oldest mother with identical twins was 37 years. Within the group using ART, a further division was made based on the age of the mothers, using 38 years of age as the cutoff. Here are the data:

VARIABLES ASSOCIATED WITH COLIC

	Both Twins Sleep Well	BB/PPD	Colic	Breast-feeding Only	Father's Involvement
No ART					
Group A: 37 years or younger, identical	60%	13%	9%	73%	92%
Group B: 38 years or older, fraternal	33%	20%	19%	33%	76%
ART, Fraternal					
Group C: 38 years or younger	28%	40%	32%	39%	88%
Group D: 39 years or older	22%	67%	40%	9%	70%

What puzzled me when I did this analysis in 2007 was that if colic was primarily a within-the-child characteristic, why would it be less common among younger mothers (a difference of 9 percent versus 19 percent or 32 percent versus 40 percent)? Younger mothers were more successful at breastfeeding (a difference of 73 percent versus 33 percent or 39 percent versus 9 percent), and their husbands were more involved in helping their babies sleep well (a difference of 92 percent versus 76 percent or 88 percent versus 70 percent).

From correspondence and conversations with all the mothers, it was clear to me that the stress of parenting increased with each group (from group A to group D). The dramatic trend of more colic from 9 percent to 40 percent may be a reflection of this increased stress of parenting. I understood how more colic might cause twins to sleep less well (from 60 percent to 22 percent) and mothers to have more BB/PPD (from 13 percent to 67 percent) and less ability to exclusively breastfeed (from 73 percent to 9 percent). In other words, colic might be causing these problems.

But mothers told me that fathers were highly involved or not involved at all in parenting *before the colic developed,* and the trend of fathers to be less involved in helping the child sleep well (from 92 percent to 70 percent) was a source of great stress for the marriage and for parenting in general. A common theme among older mothers, especially in group D, where 40 percent of the infants had colic, was that the lack of teamwork in the marriage between husband and wife continued to be an issue between father and mother after the babies were born.

I began to wonder whether the lack of involvement of the father in caring for the baby and his lack of teamwork in the marriage might be contributing to sleep deprivation in the baby and mother so that colicky behavior emerged. The important role of the father in helping children sleep well is discussed in on page 163.

Obviously, children's sleep issues reflect not only the mother's care for the baby but also the father's care and how well the parents cooperate or agree on parenting. An uninvolved, absent, abusive, or addicted husband or father may adversely affect a mother's mental health and a child's sleep. So studies that omit inclusion of the husband, father, or boyfriend may focus unwarranted blame on the mother or unwarranted attribution to the mother's mental health status. However, in the past, fathers were not usually mentioned in published scientific reports on maternal depression, maternal anxiety, or maternal mental health in association with children's sleep issues.

For example, in 2013, Dr. Jenny Radesky published a paper on a group of mothers, 89 percent of whom were married, that showed that "*inconsolable* infant crying may have a stronger association with postpartum depressive symptoms than infant colic." While this supports the notion that the baby's characteristics are the predominant factor (a baby-driven path), the father's role was not included in this study. Similarly, in Dr. Petzoldt's 2014 study regarding maternal anxiety disorders prior to pregnancy being associated with colic (which supports the notion that the mother plays a significant role—a mother-driven path), no mention is made about the role of fathers or boyfriends. In Dr. Petzoldt's study of mothers between 18 and 40 years old, those mothers who were younger and had only a tenth-grade education or less were more likely to have a colicky baby than older and more educated mothers. In her entire group, 61 percent were not married prior to the pregnancy, and among those reporting colic in their babies, 76 percent were not married prior to the pregnancy and 24 percent were married prior to their pregnancy. While marital status alone does not indicate the presence or absence of paternal support regarding parenting, it does appear that mothers who are younger, less educated, and single are more likely to have a colicky baby. Echoing the lack of teamwork described above in older mothers with colicky twins, Dr. Petzoldt told me, "When we looked at social support and partnership characteristics, we find that perceived [by the mothers] social support and tenderness in partnership reduce the risk for excessive crying. However, these results are only preliminary." It seems to me that if the fathers are not included in the study, one should be cautious about attributing problems associated with sleep or crying in the baby to the mother.

In 2010, Dr. Douglas Teti studied a group of families in which 93 percent of mothers were married. He documented that fathers' involvement with infants at bedtime and at night was much less than the mothers'. Also in 2007, Joanna Martin showed that infant sleep problems "were associated with serious psychological distress and poor general health" in fathers as well as mothers. However, "relationship happiness and partner support showed strong evidence of a protective effect . . . reducing the odds of serious psychological distress on average by almost half." She concluded, "Fathers should be actively engaged in the assessment and management of child sleep problems because their health is also at risk." In the same year, Dr. Harriet Hiscock found that behavioral strategies designed to improve babies' sleep also improved the mothers' well-being (fewer depressive symptoms and better maternal sleep quality) and that "most mothers (80 percent) reported partner support with sleep strategies." Another 2007 study by Dr. Hiscock showed that "preventive strategies for infant sleep problems need to begin early . . . to improve mother's health. . . . Infant sleep problems were associated with parental disagreement about sleep management." I learned early on that for a sleep consultation to be successful I needed the active support or passive cooperation of the father, and therefore I do not begin a consultation without both parents present. The importance of having the father present for a successful sleep consultation/intervention is discussed in chapter 5.

Sometimes a father is not able to be very helpful. A large population study of over four thousand children evaluated parental depressive symptoms at 20 weeks of pregnancy and excessive infant crying at 2 months after delivery. Independent of depressive symptoms of the mother, the fathers' depressive symptoms during pregnancy were associated with excessive infant crying. The researchers concluded that "because of the prospective design, we could rule out a child-to-parent effect, that is, that the excessive crying of the child contributed to the parental depressive symptoms. Therefore, the association we found provides evidence for a parent-to-child direction in the association between parental depressive symptoms and excessive crying." Another study of fathers showed that infant crying problems at 4 months were associated with increased anger toward their infant and doubt regarding their ability to parent their infant at bedtime; at 6 months, with increased depressive symptoms, anger, and less personal sleep. At 4 months, 10 percent of these fathers met criteria for postnatal depression.

Depressive symptom scores were significantly higher in fathers reporting an *unsettled infant,* that is, an infant with a sleep or crying problem. As previously mentioned, when fathers attend Early Parenting Centers in Australia for support, they complain more of *tension, agitation, and frustration* than depression (page 232). Fathers whose partners (mostly wives) were admitted to a residential Early Parenting Center for a brief structured psycho-educational treatment program were also studied. The most common reason their wives were admitted was for *unsettled infant behavior,* which included prolonged or inconsolable crying, frequent overnight waking, resistance to soothing, and feeding difficulties. These fathers reported more stress, irritability, fatigue, and sleepiness, and more than half (53 percent) reported possible misuse or risky alcohol use (episodic excessive drinking or daily alcohol use). Furthermore, the lead researcher told me that about 20 percent of the fathers had a history of mental health problems, and risky alcohol use in this group occurred in 82 percent of them; among the 80 percent of fathers with no history of mental health problems, risky alcohol use was 50 percent. Another study from the UK also noted that "Men largely described their 'stress' with reference to *exhaustion, poor concentration and irritability.* . . . Fathers experience psychological distress in the perinatal period but question the legitimacy of their experiences. Men may thus be reluctant to express their support needs or seek help amid concerns that to do so would detract from their partner's needs. Resources are needed that are tailored to men, *framed around fatherhood, rather than mental health or mental illness, and align men's self-care with their role as supporter and protector* [emphasis added]."

Obviously, a study of mothers and children that does not include the father, his mental health, and his risky habits might be incomplete.

Interaction between Baby and Parent

Parental Tolerance for Infant Crying

Professor Sadeh used "a two minute video clip of a 6-month-old baby playing on a carpet who then starts crying (after 10 seconds), with a gradual increase in crying intensity and visual distress signs. Prior to watching the video, a written cover story was presented to the participants: 'The following video is of a very demanding baby. His parents are trying to ignore some of his crying to allow him to calm down by himself [page 321]. Please look at the video and decide when you feel it is absolutely necessary to intervene.' The purpose of the cover story was to create a standardized description of the situation and to increase motivation to tolerate the crying and delay the response." Here are the results for three groups:

INTERVENTION DELAY (IN SECONDS, APPROXIMATELY)

Childless couple

Husband	60
Wife	50

Parents with child with no sleep problems

Father	50
Mother	45

Parents with child with sleep problems

Father	45
Mother	35

Parents with a child about 1 year old who had sleep problems "demonstrated shorter intervention delays in the crying clip and tended to attribute more distress to the crying infants compared to parents in both control groups. Additionally, women demonstrated lower tolerance for infant crying . . . compared to men. Our results suggest that parents of sleep-disturbed infants appear to have lower tolerance for infant crying, which may be a predisposition underlying their excessive involvement in soothing their infants to sleep which may lead to the development of sleep problems." I asked one of the researchers whether there was an association between maternal anxiety or depression and low tolerance for infant crying and the answer was no. So it is possible that parental tolerance for infant crying, anxiety and depressive symptoms, and "dysfunctional cognitions" (page 219) might coexist in a parent or any one of them individually might be an independent factor in the development of infant sleep problems. The reason that I show the actual number of seconds of delay before the intervention is because there is such a small difference between the two parent groups (only five to ten seconds). Maybe if the parents with a child with sleep problems could delay their responses just five to ten seconds more, their child would have more opportunity to develop self-soothing skills. However, "the associations between lower tolerance for infant crying and infant sleep problems are not indicative of causality. It could be hypothesized that infants who are more difficult (e.g. cry more, present sleep problems) might influence their parents' tolerance for crying." So the direction of effects might be bidirectional between parent and infant.

However, their next study, using the same video clip, does suggest that delaying the response *after three months* does promote better sleep. Professor Sadeh again measured the number of seconds of delay before intervention while watching the video; he called the ability to delay intervention "parental cry-tolerance (PCT)." In this study, however, they followed sixty-five couples from pregnancy through six months postpartum. The researchers measured PCT on pregnant women and later, recorded objective sleep measures on their child at 3 and 6 months postpartum. The PCT was also repeated at 6 months. Here are the results and interpretations:

1. Prompter responses during pregnancy predicted better infant sleep at 3 months. Prompter "Parental responsiveness in the early months promotes early infant sleep regulation"—that is, better sleep at 3 months.

2. More disrupted infant sleep at 3 months predicted prompter responses at 6 months. "Parents may become more sensitive to infant crying when they have to continuously take care of a night-waking infant" at 3 months. Subsequently, at 6 months, they respond more promptly to infant crying.

3. Prompter responses at 6 months is associated with poorer sleep at 6 months. Prompter responses for parental soothing of the infant at night at 6 months is associated with more night wakefulness (WASO) and more night wakings.

4. Fathers showed more delayed responses than mothers (page 163).

5. PCT decreased over time and parents became more similar regarding PCT to each other over time.

Before the age of 3 months, respond promptly to all distress crying. After the age of 3 months, briefly delaying parental response to very mild distress sounds (page 176) may lead to better infant sleep, but not before that. "During pregnancy, mothers place more emphasis on the importance of limiting parental night-time involvement to encourage self-soothing than they do at six months. Thus, it seems that after becoming a parent and accumulating experiences with a baby of their own, parents become more sensitive to infant signs of distress . . . This growing similarity [over six months] may be a result of shared experiences with their own child, including mutual discussions and reciprocal modeling of responses to their crying infant."

My view is that we should keep it simple! If your baby is hungry or soiled at night, promptly respond to her and feed or change her. If she quietly vocalizes at night, does *not* sound to be in distress, and you are not sure she is hungry, delay your response a little, maybe just thirty to sixty seconds, even before three months. But continuing to always respond promptly to *non-distress* vocalizations (page 176) after age 3–6 months will lead to sleep problems. Slightly delaying your response might help 80 percent of infants because you are giving them the opportunity to practice self-soothing. For 20 percent of infants with extreme fussiness/colic, probably always responding promptly at night, during the first few months, will head off some major crying storms. But remember, extreme fussiness/colic dissipates in 50 percent of children by 2 months of age. So you might be lucky and struggle for only two months. Or unlucky, because it can last for about four months.

Extreme fussiness/colic in babies, which appears to have a developmental component, along with the associated impairments in sleeping, may trigger depression in mothers and fathers. Furthermore, maternal anxiety or depression that is present before delivery might cause unnecessary feeding of or attending to babies at night. Because their sleep is fragmented, these babies become overtired and cry more. This in turn creates more sleep deprivation and emotional stress for the mother and father. The father may or may not be very involved in helping the child sleep (on his own or because the mother acts as a gatekeeper—either encouraging or inhibiting the father's involvement), be a partner in parenting in general, or be a team player in the marriage. So colicky behavior may have both a developmental and a parental component. Unresolved or unappreciated *parent issues* may be the root cause of crying/fussing and sleep problems in the baby.

Interaction between Parents

One study of about three thousand families examined:

1. General maternal social support (during pregnancy and post-partum)

2. The happiness of the mother–partner relationship (during pregnancy and postpartum)

3. Partner involvement in caring for the newborn

"The *postpartum maternal-rated happiness of her relationship with her partner* (in most cases the father of the baby) was the factor that was most protective for infant colic, even more protective than partner support with caring for the new baby and general social support for new mothers . . . This suggests that a happy mother–partner relationship can be a powerfully protective factor, *even if the mother is experiencing postpartum depression* [emphasis added]." In other words, lower risks of colic were mostly associated with the mother having a happier relationship with the father, and less so with the father being warm, loving, and affectionate to their baby (newborn care) or the mother having someone to turn to for suggestions about how to handle a personal problem (general maternal social support). This study also supports my earlier observation (for twins) that there is more colic among older mothers (who tend to be married to older men who, because they were less involved in parenting, caused stress in the marriage).

Another study focused on coparenting. Coparenting is the manner in which parents work together to raise their children. Coparenting quality may be evaluated by asking parents to report on how they see their partner as a coparent regarding *positive* features such as:

1. Agreement. ("My partner and I have the same goals for our child.")

2. Closeness. ("My relationship with my partner is stronger now than before we had a child.")

3. Support. ("My partner asks my opinion on issues related to parenting.")

4. Endorsement. ("I believe my partner is a good parent.")

5. Division of labor. ("My partner does carry his or her fair share of the parenting work.")

Or coparenting quality may be evaluated by asking parents how they see their partner as a coparent regarding *negative* features such as:

6. Exposure to conflict. ("How often in a typical week, when all three of you are together, do you yell at each other within earshot of the child?")

7. Undermining. ("My partner does not trust my abilities as a parent.")

Higher positive features indicate better quality of coparenting.

Evaluation of coparenting quality was performed when infants were 1, 3, 6, 9, and 12 months old. Additional evaluations were performed at these ages regarding parents' beliefs (page 219) about responding to infant night wakings ("My child will feel abandoned if I don't respond immediately"). The more strongly parents endorsed immediate responses to the infant night wakings, the higher the *negative* features of coparenting quality were rated. Additionally, a larger discrepancy in parents' beliefs about immediate response to infant night wakings (when the mother endorsed stronger beliefs to immediately respond than the father) predicted lower *positive* features of coparenting quality. "Results emphasize the importance of communication and concordance in nighttime parenting practices for aspects of parents' coparenting relationship."

Living with and Soothing a Colicky Baby

My son, now 4 months old, had colic. He lacked the ability to fall and stay asleep. He would startle at the slightest noise and required darkness in which to sleep. Sleep, by the way, was only obtained by a very specific rocking/holding motion day and night for three months straight. When you mention "colic" to people, they immediately give you advice on symptomatic GI treatment. When I tried to explain how he was, nobody understood. Nobody. When I told our son's pediatricians that he would stay awake for eighteen hours a day, they would just stare at me and make me take the Edinburgh Postnatal Depression Scale test once again. It was so very isolating. People would say, "You are spoiling him by holding him so much," "All babies are difficult; get used to it," "Just put him down and let him cry." The degree of isolation and amount of criticism while caring for such a difficult baby cannot be understated. There is no way to describe how it feels to watch your new baby be so miserable. There are no words to fully explain this experience. I have a small but firm support system, and this experience pushed us to our limits. I had to leave my hard-earned career because I could not imagine how daycare could put forth the effort of care our son required.

HOW TO SOOTHE A COLICKY BABY

I think ultimately parents have to experiment to find out what kind of soothing works best for their child at that par-

ticular time. I tried everything with my colicky child, who quickly became chronically overtired. We found that her preferred method of soothing changed as she learned to become a better sleeper over the course of one year. In the beginning, she seemed to like the "jiggle-sway." We would hold her and swing her side to side while simultaneously jiggling her. (I also think that I had an easier time using that method because I was frantic and nervous.) As time went on, she preferred to be held in a rocking chair with quick, jiggle-like rocking. Now she likes to sit in your lap with slow, long rocks while reading a story. Once she's ready for bed, she throws the book and starts to wiggle. You put her in her crib and she spends some time playing with her hair or pacifier and falls asleep. I also found that in the later stages of sleep training, Dad and Grandma had more success than me. Can't really explain it because we all use the same sleep routines. If I had to do it over again, I would have read Healthy Sleep Habits, Happy Child *before my daughter was born and not four months later. Then I would have understood that her extreme fussing was colic. I could have at least been armed with some tips and techniques to prevent or at least minimize the chronically overtired mess she became. I would also have made sure that I protected her naps and bedtime from day one. I also would have made sure that Dad was more involved and on the same page from day one.*

My first child was colicky, too, and we had to do an extreme amount of bouncing also. The rocking chair was absolutely useless! We had to swaddle him and walk around bouncing him. He also preferred the sideways, facing-out position. I definitely wonder if colicky babies need more motion—almost like they need some sort of distraction. I tried rocking with my second baby, non-colicky. But I quickly switched to walking and bouncing because that was what I was used to. I think she probably would have been fine with less motion, but I reverted to what I "knew" worked. With my third, we were able to rock in the rocking chair. She would just sit there in my arms and fall asleep. It was such a weird experience for me!

How Parenting Style Influences Crying (chapter 1)

Dr. St. James-Roberts showed that carrying a baby more during the day will reduce common fussiness/crying, but carrying a baby more during the day does not make extreme fussiness/colic go away (chapter 1). To clarify what it means to carry a child more to reduce fussiness and crying, he also studied different approaches to infant care in three groups of parents: London, United Kingdom, parents; Copenhagen, Denmark, parents; and a "proximal care" group of parents who planned to hold their infants 80 percent or more of the time between 8:00 A.M. and 8:00 P.M., breastfeed frequently, and respond rapidly to infant cries. Proximal care is also called infant-demand care or attachment parenting. Here are his results:

> Proximal care parents held infants for 15 to 16 hours per 24 hours and coslept with them through the night more often than other groups. London parents had 50% less physical contact with their infants than proximal care parents . . . [and] abandoned breastfeeding earlier than the other groups. . . . Copenhagen parents fell in between the other groups in measures of contact and care. *London infants cried 50% more overall than infants in both other groups at 2 and 5 weeks of age. However, bouts of unsoothable crying occurred in all 3 of the groups, and the groups did not differ in unsoothable bouts or in colicky crying at 5 weeks. Proximal care infants woke and cried at night most often at 12 weeks* [emphasis added].

My interpretation is that while the near-constant holding and co-sleeping reduced the overall crying of babies in the proximal care group, it also interfered with their development of self-soothing skills, so that by 12 weeks there was substantially more signaling at night, which may persist, as Dr. St. James-Roberts noted: "Most [proximal care] infants continue to wake their parents at night when 10 months of age." In another study, Dr. St. James-Roberts pointed out that while most infants who cry a lot at 5–6 weeks of age do sleep well at night at 12 weeks of age, "four randomized controlled trials have found that 'limit-setting' parenting prevents continuation of night waking and signaling beyond 3 months of age. In contrast . . . 'infant-demand' care . . . increase[s] the number of infants who continue to wake and signal in the night at 12 weeks of age." As he stated, "Rather than one being better, [different parenting styles] are associated with different benefits and costs."

When to Allow Babies with Colic to Learn Self-Soothing

If you suspect that your baby has extreme fussiness/colic, do everything you can to maximize sleep and minimize crying during the first weeks. Parents who are able to put forth heroic efforts to soothe their fussy baby may note that there is really minimal or no crying, only fussing. But their baby would cry in the absence of heroic soothing efforts. The attempt to help your colicky baby may be mildly or overwhelmingly stressful to parents. You are likely to be in survival mode. Success or failure in your attempt to help your colicky baby sleep better by learning self-soothing may be based on factors within your baby and on your and the other parent's soothing skills, mental health, and resources. The most important thing to remember is that you will be more successful in soothing your baby and surviving your baby's colic if you *get help in order to take breaks*. Also remember: This, too, shall pass.

Teamwork and constant communication between parents is the bedrock that permits a family to cope with and emerge from colic well rested. Starting early and tolerating some crying is common in some situations, and no adverse effects occur: Mothers of twins are much more willing to let a colicky baby cry to develop self-soothing skills because the reality of their situation is that they are not always available to soothe the crying twin. Mothers who have had a previous child are especially keen on having the colicky baby sleep so they can have some time with their older child, and mothers who had a previously colicky baby are more tolerant of letting their second baby cry as a means to the end of getting better sleep, because they are less likely to have a fear of crying it out or to worry about whether crying will hurt their child. I also think experienced mothers try hard to move the bedtime earlier after 6 weeks because they know that drowsy signs might not be very visible in their colicky baby. On the other hand, I think it is totally appropriate for some first-time mothers to have a go-slow approach and wait until colic passes.

All babies experience unexplained fussiness and crying in their first weeks of life, no matter what your ethnic group, no matter what birthing method brought your child into the world, no matter if your lifestyle is that of jet-setter or stay-at-home parent. All parents, too, tend to use the same techniques and strategies to successfully weather those first few months of life with their new baby, whether it's fair sailing for the most part or they feel storm-tossed by colicky waves of crying. Sleep problems arise after 3–4 months of age when some parents don't change their techniques for coping with crying and fussiness at bedtimes and nap times. That's when unhealthy sleep habits and their resulting problems begin.

Because colic winds down in 50 percent of babies at 2 months and 80 percent of babies at 3 months, you might try to help your baby sleep better before 4 months of age. Parents tell their stories of helping colicky babies sleep better at 8, 11, and 12 weeks in chapters 4 and 5. Here are some more reports from mothers of babies with extreme fussiness/colic (or perhaps sleep deprivation masquerading as colic) who helped their babies sleep better:

My baby was deemed colicky at 3 weeks old. I wasn't happy with that answer, and that is when I got the book Healthy

Sleep Habits, Happy Child. *This book changed my life. I really don't believe my child was colicky. I think she was just way overtired and completely strung out. She has always been a spirited baby and would never just fall asleep like typical babies. Ever since I started implementing Dr. Weissbluth's advice, she has become a totally different baby. Sometimes I wonder if a lack of sleep can cause colic or colic-like symptoms. I truly believe there are colicky babies, but sometimes I wonder if some are misdiagnosed.*

In retrospect, I think that my baby was colicky. He was terribly sensitive to light/noise—couldn't sleep anywhere but his quiet room by himself at 6 weeks, and would scream and scream to fall asleep even if I held him. Thankfully, my aunt had a colicky baby, and she recommended letting him cry. Starting at 4 weeks, I would just put him down in his room when he was tired [that is, drowsy but awake]. He would cry for five to ten minutes, and then sleep a full nap. If I had tried holding or rocking him, he would have screamed for a long, long time without sleeping. If it weren't for the fact that he got so much sleep (because I was willing to let him cry), he would have been full-blown colicky. As it was, he slept a lot! I am so grateful that I experimented with letting him cry to fall asleep. I can't even imagine how much screaming he would have done if I had insisted on holding him when he cried.

My maternity leave had ended, and I went back to work for the first full day. My 12-week-old daughter had "colic" (screamed for three to five hours every day) for the first 10 weeks, which I felt was 100 percent her being overtired. I did graduated extinction at 6 weeks to get her solid naps during the day, which helped her daytime crying/screaming immensely, but these naps were attained through use of a dark room, swaddle, and some quiet soothing.

We used extinction with a twenty-minute limit at 12 weeks. Our little guy would cry in our arms for two hours before he'd finally fall asleep. We'd take turns rocking him in our arms, swaying back and forth. When we finally decided to just try it, we were surprised at how little he cried before he fell asleep—eight minutes! The second day was equally easy, but then he quickly learned the twenty-minute time limit and would cry up to that point. We adjusted the bedtime from 6:30 to 5:30 [earlier bedtime] and removed the time limit [no cap]. First night, he cried for two hours. It was awful! But after four days, the crying stopped.

Our son was colicky and sleep was nonexistent in our house for three months. He refused to go in the swing or the bouncy seat, and hated the car even more (and still does!). If he did sleep, it was after being rocked for hours and he was put down in his crib in a dead sleep. At 12 weeks we did graduated extinction because he had no self-soothing skills. Our goal was four hours of sleep, and it worked. Within five nights, he was sleeping through the night! We were shocked to say the least. It was an absolute miracle and the best thing we ever did. Everyone in the house was much happier, and we started to really enjoy being parents. For the first 3 months he was definitely going to be an only child. ☺ *Your book* Your Fussy Baby *helped us tremendously!*

I have only one child, so my experience is limited to her. Based on our experience, at 6 weeks, all we were trying to do was survive. She was extremely fussy between 5 and 10 weeks. At the time, we felt that the best thing to do was soothe her and try to get the maximum sleep possible.

Things were "messy" in the sense that we used swing, holding, the crib, extensive soothing—whatever worked that day/night. We made repeated attempts at drowsy but awake, but it never worked before 3.5-4 months of age. Ultimately, we felt it was more important that she get some sleep in those earliest months, so we did what it took. From my perspective, parents of colicky children should be prepared to be somewhat flexible until about 4 months. You can attempt earlier bedtimes or some extinction, but if things are really disastrous, abandon the effort and try again later. We knew it was time around 3.5 months because we were soothing more and she was sleeping less—it was like we were annoying her! I would add that dealing with colic is incredibly taxing, physically and emotionally. In the first 4 months, we were lucky to get four to five hours of consolidated sleep in a day. Most days, it was two to three hours. Add to that dealing with a fussy child almost around the clock, and you have a recipe for frazzled and distressed parents. I can certainly understand why many parents struggle with a post-colic sleep plan, as it can be hard to be resolute when you are completely burned out.

My baby was colicky and never slept. He did not take naps at all for the first 3 months of his life. At 4 months he started taking naps only in the car or in the swing. I feel like he was in the swing more often than not. As soon as the swing was stopped, he would wake right up. At 4 months I decided to do extinction; graduated extinction only riled him up and extended the crying. So we did extinction with no problems at night. He always went right to sleep, no crying and no night-waking problems. He wakes two times a night to nurse. The problems were his naps. He did not know how to self-soothe. So I taught him, and he caught on rather quickly. After two weeks he was going down every two hours for

naps without much crying. At the beginning of this nap training there was a lot of crying. At first his naps were short,
forty-five minutes or so. After a few weeks the midmorning
nap lengthened to about an hour and a half, the midday nap
went from forty-five minutes to an hour, and the third nap
declined to about thirty-five minutes. I have been very happy
with this! My family and friends think I am out of my mind
because I schedule everything around his naps.

The hardest thing about dealing with colic was that we
didn't know when it would end. People kept telling us, "Don't
worry, it'll get better," but we had no idea whether that
would be in a week, a month, a year. The need for twenty-
four-hour intensive soothing efforts took a huge toll on me,
emotionally and physically, and on my relationship with my
husband. Almost a year later, I believe we are still dealing
with the fallout from our very intense and difficult first few
months. The turning point for us was when we discovered
Healthy Sleep Habits, Happy Child and began sleep training at 4.5 months. It was like suddenly we had our lives back.
We knew that he would be in bed at 5:30 P.M., and while he
would wake up to eat a few times during the night, he would
go right back to sleep. Once we had naps under control it
got even better. I believe that at a certain point, his natural
colicky tendencies were fading, but still being exacerbated
by his being horribly overtired. I will know for my next baby
(won't be for a while!) that healthy sleep habits begin on day
one, and that most babies don't just know when to sleep—
they need us to help them.

The moment my daughter, Amanda, arrived home from the
hospital, she exploded with a very bad case of colic. I took
her to the pediatrician's office several times, only to be told
there was "not a thing wrong, relax." I also received several

suggestions about nursing and a pat on the back. All of these suggestions irritated me, and I felt as though I was being perceived as an anxious, first-time mother.

After twelve weeks of crying and screaming, Amanda was evaluated by two child development specialists. I decided we should work with one until my daughter's crying and screaming settled down. We also saw a psychiatrist, who recommended medication and also suggested that we continue to be followed by the development specialists. In the meantime, our lives had become a nightmare. Amanda cried most of the day and always screamed in the evening. To our horror, this behavior had worked itself into the night hours, too.

By 5 months, we were referred to Dr. Weissbluth for what we hoped was a sleep disorder. I say "hoped," because we were at the point of seeing a pediatric neurologist and having an EEG done. I was very frightened for my daughter, and my husband and I were exhausted. I was eager for the consultation. My daughter had definitely been cursed with colic. Could this now be wired exhaustion from a sleep disorder caused by the treatment for colic—rocking, swinging, motion all the time? It was.

Amanda was old enough now to try "crying it out." It was the most difficult thing I've had to do as a new mother.

The first night, Amanda screamed, choked, and sobbed for thirty-two minutes. I remember feeling sick to my stomach.

The first two days weren't too terrible. However, the third and fourth were almost intolerable. Amanda would cry through her entire nap time. Then I would get her up to keep Dr. Weissbluth's time frame going. Her temperament after these episodes is known only to mothers who have been through the same ordeal! When she would scream for over an hour during nap time and in the evening, I felt cruel, insensitive, and guilty. Three things kept me going: my husband's support; Dr. Weissbluth's concern, encouragement, and compassion; and the fact that I knew it had to be done—Amanda had to learn to sleep.

It took Amanda about a week to catch on to the idea. The bags under her eyes faded, her sporadic screaming attacks stopped, and her personality was that of a predictable baby—a sweetheart when rested and a bear when past a nap time or her bedtime.

I would offer these suggestions to other mothers and fathers who have to take this measure in order to teach their babies to sleep. You, as parents, have to understand and believe intellectually that it is the right thing to do. Otherwise feelings of guilt will overpower you, and you will give in. You must have the support of your spouse, as it will be too much of a strain to bear alone.

You are doing what is best for your baby. It seems cruel and unacceptable, as a loving new mother, to let your baby cry. But it is a fact of parenting—many, many things will bring tears and protests in the years to come.

Enlist the support of a sympathetic friend as much as you feel the need to. I found close telephone contact a tremendous help. Some parents may not need this close interaction, but many of us do.

My son is now 5.5 months. He was extremely colicky and also had reflux. My son cried pretty much all day and evening. He would only sleep fully swaddled in a swing in our bedroom, and even then he probably averaged six to eight hours of fragmented sleep in a twenty-four-hour period. Needless to say, once the colic ended and his reflux turned into just being a "happy spitter," my husband and I were desperate to figure out how to get some sleep for all of us! After trying the gradual approach and graduated extinction with no success, we decided it was time for extinction. It was very hard to do, but luckily he didn't scream every night for as long as we had expected. I kept reminding myself that we weren't making him cry: we were allowing him to cry.

We decided that because our son had been premature, and so colicky and sick, we really needed to wait until he was closer to 5 or 6 months to start any kind of sleep training. So we did. My husband and I are both psychologists, and we both work with people who have been severely neglected or abused as children, so we are acutely aware of the importance of building a secure attachment in children. As such, we were also very nervous about trying any kind of cry-it-out method, fearing it might undermine our son's attachment to us. However, we were also desperate for sleep, and so was our son. I think the phrase that stuck out to me in Dr. Weissbluth's book (and that I still hang on to to this day) is that a sleepy brain is not an awake brain. When babies cry at night they are not lonely, afraid, and anxious or any of the other things they might be when they are awake; when babies cry at night, they are tired. So when our son was 6.5 months old we laid him down for the night at his usual time (7:00 P.M.) after his bath and bottle and left the room [extinction]. He cried for almost an hour and then fell asleep, and he didn't wake up until 5:30 the next morning. I couldn't believe it. The next night we did the same thing, and I was sure the night before had been a fluke, that there was no way he could sleep that well two nights in a row. He did. He cried for forty minutes and slept until 5:30 the next morning. He is now almost 3 years old, and we still put him to bed between 7:00 and 7:30 at night. He talks to himself happily in his crib for about thirty minutes and then sleeps until seven the next morning. He naps for anywhere from an hour and a half to two hours a day. If our premature, sick, colicky son can learn to be a good sleeper, any baby can. It was the most difficult thing we've had to do as parents, letting our son cry, but it also taught us an important lesson—that even as babies what our children want and what they need are not the same thing. Teaching our son to sleep gave me the confidence to trust my instincts as a mother and to weather the criticisms I receive from others for "letting my baby cry." We firmly believe that tolerating or accepting some crying is worth the payoff of teaching our children to sleep. Refusing to allow them to develop this skill constitutes a form of selfishness of the part of my husband and me. I hope our experience can give other families who are suffering the confidence to succeed.

For many reasons (living in a one-bedroom condo, et cetera), we did not sleep train our daughter until 10 months old. We thought things would improve once we moved into a larger townhouse when she was 9 months old and had her own room. To our surprise, her sleep got worse. What we thought would take a few days to adjust went on for weeks of disastrous sleep for all of us. One day I sat down and wrote up our typical daily routine. To my surprise, I realized that I was spending up to two hours total per day just soothing her to sleep. I told Dr. Weissbluth our story. Although he said she might fight us pretty hard at her age (10 months), he assured us that we could still sleep train her. He set us up with a weekend plan so my husband could help out. In just four nights we made it happen! Dr. Weissbluth followed up with me until we had reached success. Here's how it went:

First night: Cried intermittently for seventy-five minutes
Second night: Twenty-five minutes
Third night: Forty-five minutes
Fourth night: Fifteen minutes
Fifth night: Done!

She goes down without a fight and sleeps like a baby—or, shall I say, like a baby is supposed to sleep! We wished we'd done this sooner. The many sleepless nights really took a toll on our new marriage, our health, and being able to enjoy our new baby. I think many new parents get stuck in the fog and can't bear to hear their babies cry. While it does take a degree of courage, my husband and I were astounded by how quickly our baby learned to soothe herself to sleep. So to all the parents out there who are sleep-challenged, it doesn't get any easier the longer you wait. Educate yourself on the vital importance of sleep (not only for infants but adults, too). Start sleep training early, engage others to assist (Dad, partner, Grandma, best friend, et cetera), and you'll be healthier, happier, find newfound freedom, and enjoy quality sleep where everyone wins!

A Final Note on Extreme Fussiness/Colic

Using the modified Wessel's criteria for colic (discussed above), researchers have studied how often colic occurs in different populations, and how colic is associated with sleep duration, night awakenings (signaling), temperament, parenting styles, maternal and paternal depression and anxiety, and subsequent sleep or developmental problems. The results of some of these studies are sometimes contradictory because the children studied represent a heterogeneous population of moderate and severely affected infants. However, when using a more restrictive, exact Wessel's definition, researchers are looking at a much smaller (26 percent in Wessel's report; 16 percent in my study) and more homogeneous group of children with more extreme fussiness/colic, and they are more likely to discover associations between these babies and the issues above. The associations described in this chapter and subsequent chapters are mostly supported by multiple studies, and I have taken into account different definitions of colic.

Summary and Action Plan for Exhausted Parents

If you are too tired to read much and just want to do *something* to help your child sleep better, read chapter 1.

THE FIRST WEEK

Begin to teach your baby self-soothing: many hands (enlisting the help of the father and others), putting your baby down drowsy but awake and leaving the room, and many naps (chapter 4). At this age, there are no established biological rhythms for night sleep, day sleep, or bedtime, so you need to watch for drowsy signs. Develop bedtime routines and avoid unnecessary feedings or interventions at night.

All babies become fussy and have some uncategorizable crying a few days after they are born, or a few days after the expected date of delivery if they are born early. About 20 percent of babies will develop extreme fussiness/colic. The exact cause is not known. But the effect is crystal-clear. When babies fuss or cry, they do not sleep. When they do not sleep, mothers do not sleep. Mind-numbing fatigue from lack of sleep is your main enemy!

WEEKS 2–4

More fussing and crying will develop in all babies. Fussing occurs more than crying. Fussiness is a pre-cry state that will often change into crying if parents are unable to soothe their baby; some fussing leads to crying despite parents' soothing efforts. With increasing fussing and crying, your baby may sleep less. If you have not already begun, start to teach your child self-soothing, develop bedtime routines, and avoid unnecessary feedings or interventions at night. There are still no established biological rhythms for night sleep, day sleep, or bedtime, so you should continue to watch for drowsy signs.

As stated above, fussing and crying behavior can be expected to increase at this stage, and for about 80 percent of babies—the ones with common fussiness/crying—it peaks around 6 weeks of age and then decreases. About 20 percent of babies—those with extreme fussiness/colic—may not show a clear peak at 6 weeks, and for them the fussing and crying behavior lasts until about months 2–4. But at weeks 2–4, you do not know which path your baby will take, so to plan for the possible challenges ahead, arrange to get help from relatives, friends, and neighbors so that you can take breaks. Explore how parenting can be shared by both parents so that neither parent becomes totally exhausted.

If teaching self-soothing is not working, or if you think your child is developing extreme fussiness/colic, then temporarily abandon efforts to use drowsy but awake. You cannot spoil your 2- to 4-week-old baby, so do whatever you can to maximize sleep and minimize fussing and crying.

> Extreme fussiness/colic occurs in 20 percent of babies. It is not a medical condition requiring treatment. It is something babies *do*, not something they *have*. Remember: This, too, shall pass!

Babies behave this way because of factors within the baby and within the family. Give your baby the opportunity to learn self-soothing if possible, or get help so that you can take breaks from the constant soothing your baby might require. But also review the parent issues (chapter 4) that might make for a greater challenge to prevent fussing or crying.

What a Parent Can Do

Encourage your partner to help care for the baby daytime and nighttime.

Encourage self-soothing; the earlier, the better.

If there is no colic, put your child to sleep drowsy but awake, then leave the room.

If there is colic, focus on *care*, not *cure*. Develop coping strategies.

Set an early bedtime for all children around 6 weeks; practice consistent bedtime routines, including massage; be emotionally available at bedtime.

Feed when hungry but ignore nighttime *non-distress* vocalizations.

Provide opportunities for naps based on drowsy signs.

Avoid irregularity of sleep schedules, including between weekdays and weekends.

Practice safe sleep recommendations.

No TV or digital screens in your child's room; limit screen time.

Seek help if your child is not sleeping well (from the child's primary care provider or a community sleep consultant) or for yourself or your partner, especially if there are symptoms of anxiety or depression or significant *risk factors, parent issues*, or *adverse concerns*.

Chapter 7 Outline

WEEKS 5-6

Common Fussiness/Crying Peaks around 6 Weeks

WEEKS 7-8

Earlier Bedtime and Longer Periods of Night Sleep
Develop
Common Fussiness/Crying
Extreme Fussiness/Colic
   Helpful Tips for Parents
   Tips to Help Soothe Babies

SUMMARY AND ACTION PLAN FOR EXHAUSTED PARENTS

Healthy Sleep Habits in the Second Month

If you have not already done so, please go back and read chapter 1.

A main goal at this age is to encourage the development of self-soothing skills.

Weeks 5–6

Night sleep: More evening fussiness may be associated with less night sleep before 6 weeks; after 6 weeks, night sleep rhythms emerge.

Day sleep: Naps are brief and irregular; there may be many catnaps.

Bedtimes: Bedtimes are irregular and may occur late, between 9:00 and 11:00 P.M.

For babies with common fussiness/crying, getting Dad on board, recognizing and respecting drowsy signs, allowing only brief intervals of wakefulness during the day, and establishing bedtime routines might help your baby sleep better. Try these items even if your baby has extreme fussiness/colic. And if they do not help, do whatever works to maximize sleep and minimize crying: swings, strollers, car rides, or sleep at Mom's breast or on Dad's chest. Exhaustion is your main enemy, so get help in order to take breaks.

Remember that the division line between common fussiness/crying and extreme fussiness/colic is arbitrary, and these labels do not accurately describe all babies. At this age, it may or may not be clear to you that your baby has a little, a medium amount, or a lot of fussing/crying. And attaching a descriptive label to this behavior is less important than helping your baby sleep better and coping with the stress of sleep deprivation in the family.

Be experimental with different methods of soothing (page 178) and do not give up trying. Some methods that failed in the past might work now or in the future, or they might inconsistently help. For example, some but not all brief naps might be extended by re-swaddling, a quick feeding, or replacing a pacifier. Swaddling and pacifiers might help; they will not harm your baby and should not be viewed as a "crutch" that somehow interferes with learning self-soothing.

Try to meet your baby's needs. If your baby is hungry, feed him. If he's tired, put him down to sleep.

COMMON FUSSINESS/CRYING PEAKS AROUND 6 WEEKS

About 6 weeks of age (counting from the due date), around the time your baby produces his first social smiles, night sleep becomes more organized, and the longest single sleep period begins to occur with predictability and regularity in the evening hours. This long sleep period is about four to six hours. If your baby has extreme fussiness/colic, the longest sleep period might be less. This long sleep period may occur before or around midnight, and subsequent intervals of sleep may be much shorter. The maturation of the internal timing mechanism for night sleep rhythms takes time; please be patient.

Your baby will also start to settle down more and more. He will become more interested in objects such as mobiles and toys, he'll have more interest in playing games, and his repertoire of emotional expressions and social responses will dramatically increase. Yet many parents find this time particularly frustrating, especially in the evening, since many babies reach a peak of fussing/crying and wakefulness at about 6 weeks. Even extremely fussy/colicky babies may be at their worst at 6 weeks of age, as shown by Dr. T. Berry Brazelton, and some may not appear to settle down much after their peak.

In a recent review of twenty-eight different studies including almost nine thousand infants, the authors noted that the average minutes of crying and percent of infants with colic were greatest at 5–6 weeks of age, but the results were not statistically significant. Nevertheless, in this study, it is striking that colic ended in 99 percent of the infants by 9 *weeks of age,* not 3–4 months! They might have seen a more dramatic peak and a longer duration if they had studied more severely affected infants using Wessel's exact diagnostic criteria. Still, it seems totally appropriate to try to help your colicky baby sleep better after 2 months of age and not wait until 3–4 months.

THE 6-WEEK PEAK

At 6 weeks of age, *all* babies are most fussy, cry the most, and are most wakeful.

One mother told me about her son at 6 weeks: "He's a little excited about all the living going on."

Here is a vivid description of the 6-week peak:

Antonio was born two weeks early and without difficulty. I remember thinking several hours after his birth that he was going to be a very easy boy, since my pregnancy and delivery were both routine and relatively easy. Three days after we brought him home, however, I realized that my expecta-

tions might have been a little off. Over the next three weeks we started to notice a pattern of crying that started at about 5:00 P.M. and usually lasted for about six hours. In addition to that, Antonio awakened every two hours to be fed during the night and didn't take daytime naps! During these early weeks, the only way Antonio would sleep, night or day, was if either my husband or I held him. My husband thought we must be doing something wrong, and I was afraid he might be right, although I didn't admit it at the time.

When Antonio was about 3 weeks old, I brought him to see Dr. Weissbluth. We discussed his sleep patterns (or lack thereof), and he advised me that Antonio's evening fussiness would get worse until he was 6 weeks old, and then it would start to improve slowly and hopefully end at about 12 weeks. I was quite dismayed to also learn that since Antonio was born two weeks early, I had to count Antonio's age from his original due date, not his birth date. So instead of having only three more rough weeks, we would probably have at least five! That's an eternity when you're sleep-deprived! I really didn't know how we were going to make it through that rough period! I think the biggest worry we had was that Antonio's fussiness would never end. We knew in our minds that he had to get better, but the big question was when.

Then, at about 6 weeks after Antonio's original due date, I couldn't believe it, but I actually started to notice that his evening fussiness was decreasing! In addition, at the same time, his nighttime sleep started becoming a little longer, and he started falling asleep in his crib instead of having to sleep with me! The improvements were small, but at that point I was just ecstatic to have four solid hours of sleep at night! At about 10 weeks I called the doctor and received encouraging advice. He suggested that I start putting Antonio to bed earlier at night, as this might help him feel less tired and make him fall asleep more easily. At the time, Antonio was going to bed between 10:00 and 11:00 P.M. So I moved his bedtime to around 8:00 P.M. for a few nights, and I could not believe how well this worked! I then started putting him in his crib even earlier, as I noticed that he actually became tired at around 6:30 P.M. Antonio is now almost 5 months old, and he has been sleeping from 6:30 P.M. through the night to about 7:00 A.M. He has been doing this since he was 12 weeks old. He does wake up occasionally at 4:00 or 5:00 A.M. if he's hungry, but for the most part he sleeps extremely well at night, and is even starting to form regular daytime naps! Antonio is such a joy to be with, I actually might want to have a second baby. Yikes!

This report eloquently describes the fear faced by many parents at this time: that the fussing/crying will never end. During this time, your baby may irritate and exhaust you. He may give up napping altogether around 6 weeks of age and, to make matters worse, when awake may appear to be grumbling all day. You may feel battered at the end of each day; you may be at your wit's end. This, too, is natural. Being annoyed with your baby does not make you a bad parent. Just understand why you're annoyed. Remember that your baby's immature nervous system lacks inhibitory control: Your baby might have moments of tremulousness, quivering, or shaking of the arms or legs. The brain develops inhibitory capabilities as it matures, but this takes time; things will settle down after 6 weeks of age. This report also illustrates how an earlier bedtime, after 6 weeks of age, helps your baby sleep better.

A main goal after the 6-week peak is to ensure an early enough bedtime to prevent a second wind near the end of the day. Move bedtime earlier at 6 weeks of age.

Weeks 7–8

Night sleep: Becoming organized.

Day sleep: Naps are brief and irregular; there may be many catnaps.

Bedtime: Starting to be earlier.

EARLIER BEDTIMES AND LONGER PERIODS OF NIGHT SLEEP DEVELOP

The major biological changes starting now are a tendency for your baby to go to sleep earlier at night and for longer periods of uninterrupted night sleep.

Watch for *drowsy signs* developing earlier in the evening, and if you do not see them, experiment with different earlier bedtimes. A pitfall is to assume that any bedtime in the time frame of 6:00 to 8:00 P.M. will work for your baby. Your baby might be developing a second wind or fatigue signs at 8:00 P.M., but you do not notice because of digital distraction or the demands of another child or responsibilities like preparing dinner. Or maybe drowsy signs are emerging at 6:30 P.M., but you don't get home from work until 7:00 P.M. and drowsy signs are masked by excited playtime.

Your baby will now develop longer blocks of night sleep. The single longest sleep period is now four to six hours long and will occur in the evening hours. Often this occurs before midnight, and after midnight the blocks of sleep might be shorter. Feed your child only when necessary and try to avoid unnecessary feedings, which might create a night-feeding or night-waking habit.

The failure to establish an early bedtime after about 6 weeks of age means that your baby might accumulate a sleep deficit from a bedtime that is too late. If this occurs, it will appear that common fussiness/crying continues longer or worsens, but what is really going on is the emergence of sleep-deprivation-driven fussy behavior. Help your baby sleep better after 6 weeks of age by moving the bedtime earlier to prevent a second wind. Sometimes *parent issues* interfere with establishing an early bedtime, and this eventually causes an overtired family.

Every baby behaves a little differently during these first few weeks. Your baby most likely will fall somewhere in between the common fussy/crying baby and the extremely fussy/colic infant. And even if your baby has had mild fussing/crying, this may well be a period in which he becomes worse either because of the 6-week peak or because he begins to accumulate a sleep debt.

If social smiles are not already present, your baby will start to produce them shortly after 6 weeks of age (or 6 weeks after the expected date of delivery for preemies). Prepare yourself for changes resulting from your child's increased social maturation. The social smiles herald the onset of increased social awareness, and it may come to pass that your baby will now start to fight sleep in order to enjoy the pleasure of your company. This is natural!

During the day, when your baby appears slightly fidgety, ask yourself two questions. First, when did you last feed him? Second, how long has he been up? Sometimes you need to sleep him and not feed him. During the night, respond quickly to feed your baby when he is hungry, but when quiet, *non-distressed-sounding* vocalizations occur shortly after a feeding, try to delay your response to see if your child might return to sleep unassisted, or send Dad in promptly to check on your baby and do minimal soothing without feeding.

Here is an account of one mother's first weeks that describes how even colicky babies may be more settled after the 6-week peak:

> Today my baby girl, Sophia, is 8 weeks old. I celebrated by taking my first uninterrupted bath since her birth. Of course, she woke up just as I was toweling off, but I have learned to be grateful for small pleasures.
>
> Sophia doesn't sleep much, and when she's awake she's usually either crying or nursing. It's been a little better the

past week, but she still sleeps very little: six to eight hours at night and two to four hours during the day. And since I can't bear to hear her cry, that means she spends most of her time on my breast, where, mercifully, she can always be soothed. I can't hold her and play with her; she's always squirming to get at my breast. So, anyway, she's on my breast ten to twelve hours a day.

Lately she's good for a couple of ten- to twenty-minute play periods (on the floor on her back, me leaning over her, or on the changing table while I change her diaper).

When I talked with the doctor, he said it did seem my baby was colicky, and I took his book home to read. Finally, I found descriptions by other mothers of babies like mine! I was not alone. I came to understand how sleep problems, like those of my baby, appear to be hunger but really aren't. I also learned that there's nothing I can do for my baby that I'm not already doing, and so I might as well turn some of my energy around and start taking care of myself. Truly, I believe that in the case of a colicky baby, who in most cases cannot be treated for her condition, it is the mother who "needs treatment" or help, and to this end I suggest:

1. *Get out of the house an hour or two a day, minimum.*
2. *When out of the house, try to get some physical exercise to burn off the tension.*
3. *Don't feel guilty about doing anything that makes you feel good.*
4. *Socialize as much as possible outside the home.*
5. *Keep a diary or log of your baby's sleeping/feeding habits.*
6. *When the baby is asleep, get some sleep yourself, unless you're doing something for your own peace of mind.*

And things are getting better. Yesterday afternoon Sophia woke up from a three-hour nap, nursed calmly, and wasn't fussy for several hours afterward. She didn't behave in her old way, but I got to hold her and play with her for over an hour; then she stayed calm in the swing for a while.

And I got my first bath in eight weeks this morning.

If you are lucky enough to have a baby with common fussiness/crying, at 5–6 weeks, you may have already noticed his sleep patterns becoming somewhat regular. You can try to help your baby sleep better by putting him down drowsy but awake, or perhaps you want to lie down with him to sleep (page 94 regarding co-sleeping and SIDS) when he first appears tired, but in any case, you should put him down after no more than two hours of wakefulness. He may or may not drift into sleep easily. You do not need to let him cry at all, but some babies will fuss or cry in a mild fashion before falling asleep. If he quietly cries for five, ten, or twenty minutes, it will do him no harm, and he may drift off to sleep. If not, console him and try again at other times. Try to become sensitive to his need to sleep. The novelty of external noises, voices, lights, and vibrations will disrupt his sleep more and more, so try to have him in his crib or your bed when he needs to sleep. Go slowly and be flexible.

In summary, at or shortly after 6 weeks of age (counting from the due date), the brain matures predictably in three ways:

1. *Specific responsive social smiling.* When you smile at him, he returns your smile.

2. *Longer sleep periods (four to six hours) occurring predictably in the evening hours, usually before midnight.* This is part of the night sleep circadian rhythm.

3. *The brain wants to fall asleep earlier in the evening.* The biological time of evening drowsiness dictates an earlier bedtime,

about 6:00 to 8:00 P.M. It might be a little earlier or later for your child. This is part of the night sleep circadian rhythm.

One parent described the early bedtime this way: "The early bedtime is a non-negotiable component of healthy sleep training. If you want your child to sleep soundly and wake up well rested, you have to marry the idea of an early bedtime."

With two or more children, a common problem is that your older child distracts you early in the evening, so you miss signs of drowsiness in the baby and innocently keep him up too late. *Cumulative sleepiness* results and leads to major sleep problems. Also, sometimes it is hard to put an older child down at an earlier time than your baby, who needs a later bedtime because he has had a long midday nap. If so, begin the process of putting your older child to bed earlier when you have help, such as on a Saturday night, when Dad is home, so each child has one parent for soothing to sleep. Tell your first child, "Because you are a big boy, you do not need to nap like our baby. Our baby needs to nap, and that's why he can stay up a little later than you. Do you want to take naps?"

If you have only one bedroom and cannot sleep well because you find yourself awakened by or responding to every quiet sound your baby makes, consider *temporarily* giving your bedroom to your baby. Maybe you will have to camp out in your living room for a while until you or your baby sleeps better at night. If you have only one bedroom, *temporary* separation like this between parents and child is necessary for extinction, graduated extinction, and the check-and-console technique. If you have two bedrooms, consider *temporarily* moving him to his own room during this age range (page 94 regarding SIDS) to learn self-soothing.

After 6 weeks of age, you might want to try to help your baby sleep better at night. The ease with which you can accomplish this is related to whether your child is currently well rested or overtired. And this is related to whether he had common fussiness/crying or extreme fussiness/colic and whether you were able to successfully soothe him during the first 6 weeks. Please see chapters 4–6 for some parents' reports on helping their young babies, around 2 months of age and younger, get better sleep. For babies younger than 2 months of age, consider graduated extinction, extinction with a cap, or check and console. Extinction, even for extreme fussiness/colic, may also be considered and be successful at 2 months of age (chapter 5).

Alternatively, you may have no need or desire to try sleep training strategies. Your baby might be sleeping well at night, and there is no reason to rock the boat. Or you are enjoying the family bed and do not wish to change or allow your baby to cry. This is fine for now, but eventually you probably will want to consider some changes in sleep routines to accommodate your baby's need for an earlier bedtime. The sooner you attempt an earlier bedtime, the more quickly the family will become better rested. These changes do not necessarily mean that your baby will cry. Always consider both your child's ability to self-soothe and your resources for prolonged daytime and nighttime soothing. Do what works best for you and your baby.

If you are considering helping your baby sleep better, usually start at *bedtime* with an earlier bedtime and/or by putting your baby down drowsy but awake, because night sleep develops around or after 6 weeks of age and this natural sleep rhythm will help your attempts succeed. You are using the developing internal timing mechanism for night sleep as an aid to get better-quality sleep. At night, Mom might leave the house after feeding and let Dad do the soothing to sleep. In addition, or alternatively, try to help your baby sleep better for a nap in the *morning* by putting him down drowsy but awake and having Dad do the soothing. The reason you might see success here is that your baby is likely to be best rested from night sleep. In the morning, you might be even more successful if you try to put your child down drowsy but awake within only one hour after waking, to prevent a second wind. That is, you do the changing, feeding, a little playing, and soothing all within one hour.

Look at the clock when you think your baby wakes to start the day; this time may vary from day to day, but you should try to have him in his crib with lights out within one hour of that time. If the start-the-day hour is quite early, maybe this first "nap" is really a continuation of night sleep. Go for it anyway, and if you are successful with the drowsy-but-awake technique, celebrate your success even if this nap is frustratingly short.

Remember, early sleep training means starting to respect your baby's need to sleep by anticipating when he will need to sleep (within one to two hours of waking), introducing an earlier bedtime, learning to recognize drowsy signs, getting Dad on board, and developing a bedtime routine. Then your baby will not become overtired.

Encourage the development of self-soothing skills and bedtime routines as soon as possible.

Start helping your baby to sleep (chapter 5) at different ages, depending on the following circumstances:

- At a few weeks of age if you have to return to work or if you are totally exhausted and unable to function. This may work well for babies with common fussiness/crying.
- After 6 weeks of age for night sleep for babies with common fussiness/crying.
- Around 2–4 months of age at night for babies with extreme fussiness/colic. Success may be slow and difficult.

Again, if you have anxiety or depression symptoms, maybe only a gradual shift to an earlier bedtime (page 362) might be the best approach for now.

REMEMBER
Different children require different approaches.

Common challenges during the second month include:

- Sleep deprivation, excitement, and medical conditions push thinking about your child's sleep off your radar.
- Thinking that feeding directly causes sleeping makes you focus only on feeding, leading to unnecessary feeding at night.
- Unwarranted diagnosis of acid reflux is mistaken as the cause of not sleeping well.
- Distraction because an older child interferes with helping your baby learn self-soothing by causing you to miss drowsy signs in your baby, which results in a second wind.
- Extreme fussiness/colic interferes with learning self-soothing.

These common challenges may cause your child to become more parent-soothed than self-soothed. Don't necessarily worry now if your child is mostly or completely parent-soothed, but look forward or plan ahead to a time when your child is older and you can teach him self-soothing.

COMMON FUSSINESS/CRYING

Most babies with common fussiness/crying tend to be "easy" babies who are placid and easy to manage, quiet angels most nights. Sure, they may have a fussy period in the evening, but it's not too long, intense, or hard to deal with. They appear to sleep well anywhere and anytime during the day and quite regularly at night. In fact, the early development of regular, long night sleep periods—starting well before the age of 6 weeks—is a characteristic feature of "easy" babies. These kids are very portable, and parents bask in their sunny dispositions.

But shortly . . . dark clouds may gather. The baby starts to have some new grumbling or crabbiness that does not occur only in the evening. In fact, the quiet evenings might now be punctured by new, "painful" cries suggesting an illness. Or it might now take longer to put the baby to sleep. What has happened to your sound sleeper? Irregularities of sleep schedules, nap deprivation, and too late a bedtime are the chief culprits. Now is the time to become ever more sensitive to your child's need to sleep.

After your baby is about 6 weeks of age, the best strategy still is to try to synchronize your caretaking activities with his own rhythms. You should try to reestablish healthy sleep habits by removing the disruptive effects of external noises, lights, or vibrations. Although it may be inconvenient for you, try to have your baby back in his crib after no more than two hours of wakefulness. Consider this two-hour interval to be a rough guide to help organize the day into periods of naps and wakeful activities.

HINT
Be careful, but . . . no set schedules and no rigid rules.

Q: *How long can I keep my baby up?*
A: No more than two hours.

Two hours of wakefulness is about the maximum that most babies can endure without becoming overtired. Sometimes a baby may need to go to sleep after being up for only one hour or less. Often this brief wakeful period of just one hour occurs early in the morning. Try to soothe him to sleep *before* he becomes overtired—*before* he becomes slightly crabby, seems irritable, pulls his hair, or bats at his ears. Expect this type of behavior to develop within two hours of waking up if he is not put to sleep when he first shows signs of being tired. Look for *drowsy signs*. Please do not mistake this two-hour guide to mean that he should be up for two hours and then down for two hours. Rather, two hours is the time interval during which you should expect to put him to sleep.

When you have been out for a walk or running an errand with your baby, watch the clock and try to have him asleep within two hours after he wakes up. If upon returning home during this time interval you notice that he is becoming overtired, say to yourself, *I blew it this time; next time I'll return home sooner.* Also, by paying attention a little to clock time, you will discover how much wakefulness your baby can comfortably tolerate.

Expect your overtired child to protest when he is put down to sleep. This is natural, because he prefers the pleasure of your soothing comfort to being in a dark, quiet, boring room.

Keep in mind the distinction between a protest cry and a sad cry. You are leaving your baby alone to let him learn to soothe himself to sleep; you are not abandoning him.

Q: *How long should I let him cry?*

A: Not at all if you want to lie down with your child in your bed and soothe him to sleep or soothe him to sleep at your breast. Or you might start with ignoring the crying for five, ten, or twenty minutes. Try to decide whether your child is tired, basing your judgment on his behavior, the time of day, and the interval of wakefulness (how long he has been up). See chapters 4–6 for parents' reports about letting their child cry in this age range.

When you have decided your child is tired or overtired, consider putting him down to sleep—even if he doesn't want to sleep. Sometimes he'll fall asleep and sometimes he won't. When he doesn't, pick him up and soothe and comfort him. You may try again after several minutes to allow him to go to sleep on his own, or you may decide not to try again the next day or several days later. But remember, if your baby cries hard for three minutes, cries quietly for three minutes, and then sleeps for an hour, he would have lost that good hour-long nap if you had not left him alone for six minutes.

Also, when he needs to sleep but wants to play, then your playing with him is robbing him of sleep.

Keep a log or diary as you go through these trials to see if any trend or improvement occurs. Here's an account from Allyson's mother, who helped her baby make a dramatic—and permanent—improvement in her sleep habits at about 8 *weeks* of age:

Day 56: *Allyson woke up from an afternoon nap, and I thought she was ill—she was so calm! No jerky movements or agitated behavior, which I guess I'd assumed was just "normal" for her. About this time, though, she still cried a lot when not nursing, and she still had trouble falling asleep.*

On day 59, the mother decided to ignore some of the fussing/crying.

Day 59 (first day of extinction with a one-hour cap): *Let her fuss 1 hour—and she went to sleep for 3.25 hours (5:45 to 9:00 P.M.).*
      Day 60 (second day of extinction with a cap): *Allyson fussed all morning and wouldn't sleep, but I kept her in her crib from 10:15 A.M. to noon, staying with her most of the time. Got her up to nurse at noon. That night she woke up at 2:30 A.M.—for the first time in several weeks. I nursed her until 3:00 and then put her down. She fussed off and on until 4:00, when she went to sleep.*
      Day 63 (fifth day): *Breakthrough! She went to sleep for forty-five minutes in the morning and took a really long nap in the afternoon (12:45 to 5:00). But she woke in the middle of the night again (3:20 A.M.). She went back to sleep at 4:30 and slept until 8:30. She was happy in her crib—no screaming as I changed her diaper, which was new behavior!*

Review of this mother's records showed that up to day 59, the total sleep duration per twenty-four hours was about six to twelve hours. After day 63, the total sleep duration was longer—twelve to seventeen hours. The five-day training really helped her child sleep longer.

Day 64 (sixth day): *Two wonderful things happened. First, Allyson took a midmorning nap (10:45 A.M. to 1:30 P.M.), and when I put her down for the night, with her eyes wide open, she did not fuss at all. I quickly left the room and heard no crying. She slept from 8:35 P.M. to 5:05 A.M.*

Days 87–96: *Allyson is just about perfect. If she starts to fuss, I know she is hungry, wet, or tired. If she's tired, I simply put her in her crib and within two minutes she is asleep. It's a miracle!*

As this report and others in chapters 4–6 clearly demonstrate, parents can help their children sleep better at around *2 months of age* or younger, and it often works quickly, especially if the child has common fussiness/crying. Extinction for babies with extreme fussiness/colic may also succeed quickly at 2 months of age, as described in chapter 5. There is no compelling reason to wait until 3–4 months of age to help your child sleep better.

EXTREME FUSSINESS/COLIC

As previously discussed, 80 percent of babies exhibit common fussiness/crying, while 20 percent are extremely fussy or colicky. Colicky babies are difficult to manage for the first two to four months because they are intense, wakeful, stimulus-sensitive, and irregular when they do sleep—and they only sleep for brief periods. They have long periods of fussing and crying. And often a portion of their crying is inconsolable. Because of all this, many parents are reluctant to try to teach self-soothing at this time. These babies are hard to read. Most parents have difficulty telling whether they are hungry, fussy, or plain overtired. So leaving them alone to cry with the hope that they will sleep is potentially frustrating to everyone. The fear that the attempt will fail and that the crying will go on and on for hours and weeks inhibits many of these sleep-deprived parents.

458 MARC WEISSBLUTH, M.D.

So you might feel more comfortable waiting a little longer while you do whatever you can to maximize sleep and minimize crying. You might attempt an earlier bedtime after the 6-week peak. Try to get help so you can take breaks without any guilt. However, please note that some parents are successful with helping their babies with extreme fussiness/colic sleep better *before 4 months of age* (chapter 5). In Dr. R. S. Illingworth's review, colicky behavior ends in *50 percent* of afflicted babies by *2 months* of age, in an additional *30 percent* by *3 months* of age, and in an additional *10 percent* by *4 months* of age. So you might try to help your baby with extreme fussiness/colic sleep better with drowsy but awake, an earlier bedtime, and graduated extinction, extinction with a cap, or extinction for a four- to five-day trial and be successful before 4 months of age. If the trial fails, abandon it and try again when your child is older. Of course you will be frustrated, and maybe angry with me, but I know that a trial this short will not harm your baby.

The reason that it is commonly believed that colic ends by 3–4 months is because it is true that 80 to 90 percent of infants have outgrown it by then. But you might be in the more fortunate group of 50 percent of infants whose colic is winding down at 2 months! There is no harm in trying to help your child sleep better with a five-day trial, even if you try graduated extinction, extinction with a cap, or check and console.

These first few months are rugged for many mothers because their baby's sleep/wake patterns are unpredictable, there may be lots of fussing and crying, and the mothers may not have fully recovered from the stress or complications associated with labor and delivery. Information in chapter 6 and the following hints will help you get through these first few months.

Helpful Tips for Parents

Pamper yourself; remember, this is smart for the baby, not selfish for you. If you feel better, you will be better able to nurture your baby.

Forget errands, chores, housework.

Unplug the phone.

Ignore your baby's quiet *non-distress* vocalizations during sleep.

Nap when the baby sleeps.

Hire help for housework or breaks when your baby is most bothersome.

Plan pleasurable, brief outings without your baby (swimming, walking, and movies).

Tips to Help Soothe Babies

Definitely helpful in soothing:

Rhythmic rocking: in chair swing, arms, car rides.

Sucking: pacifier, thumb, wrist.

Gentle pressure: swaddling, massage.

Gentle sounds: lullabies, music, singing, humming.

Possibly helpful in soothing:

Lambskin rug.

Warm-water bottle placed on abdomen.

Recordings of heartbeat sound, womb sounds, vacuum cleaner, running water, sounds of nature.

Removal of stimulating toys from the crib or any bright night-lights.

Some babies nap best in a pitch-black and/or very quiet room. (One family in a noisy city even used a large walk-in closet with the door open for naps.)

Crying should not be thought of as a test for you. If your baby has extreme fussiness/colic, don't feel that you are necessarily creating a crying habit because of your prolonged, complex efforts to soothe him. Maybe your first test to help your baby sleep will come around 2 months of age, or perhaps it will occur later, at 3–4 months of age, when almost all colic subsides.

You can't treat colic with smiles, but there will be less crying in a home where there is a lot of social smiling. Practice smiling, smile broadly, open your eyes wide, regard your child as you nod, and say "Good boy" or "Good girl." Do all these especially when your baby calms down or smiles at you. Even if your child does not always respond to your smiles, this practice, like a rehearsal, will pay off big-time later.

Don't save your smiles until colic ends.

Summary and Action Plan for Exhausted Parents

If you are too tired to read much and just want to do *something* to help your child sleep better, read chapter 1.

WEEKS 5–6: FUSSINESS/CRYING PEAKS

A main goal at this age is to encourage the development of self-soothing skills.

At 6 weeks of age, all babies are most fussy, cry the most, and are most wakeful. At or after 6 weeks of age, the brain matures predictably in three ways:

1. *Specific responsive social smiling.* When you smile at him, he smiles back.

2. *Longer sleep periods (four to six hours) occurring predictably in the evening hours, usually before midnight.* This is part of the night sleep circadian rhythm.

3. *The brain wants to fall asleep earlier in the evening.* This, too, is part of the night sleep circadian rhythm. The biological

time of evening drowsiness dictates an earlier bedtime, about 6:00 to 8:00 P.M. It might be a little earlier or later for your child.

A main goal after the 6-week peak is to ensure an early enough bedtime to prevent a second wind near the end of the day.

Parent issues (chapter 4) may get in the way of an early bedtime. Encourage the development of self-soothing skills and bedtime routines as soon as possible:

- At a few weeks of age if you have to return to work or if you are totally exhausted and unable to function. This may work well for common fussiness/crying babies.
- After 6 weeks of age for night sleep for babies with common fussiness/crying.
- Around 2–4 months of age at night for babies with extreme fussiness/colic. Be patient: Success may be slow and difficult.

REMEMBER
Different children require different approaches.

Common challenges around 5–6 weeks (see above) may cause your child to become more parent-soothed than self-soothed.

WEEKS 7–8

For 80 percent of babies, those with common fussiness/crying, the worst is over, as long as you have established an earlier bedtime and taught your child some self-soothing skills. It's never too late, so if you have not yet begun, start now. "No-cry" or "maybe-cry" sleep solutions (chapter 5) may work quickly.

For those 20 percent of babies with extreme fussiness/colic, consider a five-day trial with an earlier bedtime, putting the baby down drowsy but awake, permitting only brief intervals of wakefulness during the day, plus maybe-cry or let-cry sleep solutions (chapter 5). If you see no benefit or would rather not try this now, then try it again in a few weeks or wait until your baby's extreme fussiness/colic naturally winds down at 3–4 months. Remember, though, that colic subsides in 50 percent of infants by 2 months, an additional 30 percent of infants by 3 months, and an additional 10 percent of infants by 4 months. Your child might be in the more fortunate group of 50 percent of infants whose colic is winding down at 2 months, so there is no harm in trying to help him sleep better with a five-day trial of the sleep solution of your choice at that time: also remember, however, that no-cry sleep solutions are less likely to work in babies with extreme fussiness/colic.

What a Parent Can Do

Encourage your partner to help care for the baby daytime and nighttime.

Encourage self-soothing; the earlier, the better.

If there is no colic, put your child to sleep drowsy but awake, then leave the room.

If there is colic, focus on *care,* not *cure.* Develop coping strategies.

Set an earlier bedtime for all children at 6 weeks of age.

Set an early bedtime based on drowsy signs; practice consistent bedtime routines, including massage; be emotionally available at bedtime.

Feed when hungry but ignore nighttime non-distress vocalizations.

Provide opportunities for naps based on drowsy signs.

Avoid irregularity of sleep schedules, including between weekdays and weekends.

Practice safe sleep recommendations.

No TV in the child's room; limit screen time.

Take breaks, because fussiness/crying will increase, especially in the evening.

Seek help if your child is not sleeping well (from the child's primary care provider or a community sleep consultant) or for yourself or partner, especially if there are symptoms of anxiety or depression or significant *risk factors* or *parent issues* or *adverse concerns*.

Chapter 8 Outline

MONTH 3: EXTREME FUSSINESS/COLIC WINDS DOWN

Naps
   The Midmorning Nap Develops between 9:00 and
      10:00 A.M.
   Timing of Naps
   Consistency in Soothing Styles for Naps

MONTH 4: PREVENT POST-COLIC SLEEP PROBLEMS

Baby-Driven Path: The Role of the Baby
   Night Waking, Sleep Duration, Sleep Problems: The Baby-
      Driven Path
Temperament
   Difficult Temperament
   Association between Temperament and Sleep
   Association between Temperament and Extreme
      Fussiness/Colic
Mother-Driven Path: The Role of the Mother
   Night Waking: The Mother-Driven Path
   Temperament: The Mother-Driven Path
Interaction between Baby and Mother
   Night Waking: Interaction between Baby and Mother (and
      Father)
Temperament: Interaction between Baby and Mother

DIFFERENT DECISIONS FOR DIFFERENT BABIES

Common Fussiness/Crying: Low Risk for Sleep Problems
   Developing
Extreme Fussiness/Colic: High Risk for Sleep Problems
   Developing

Healthy Sleep Habits in Months 3-4

A baby is an inestimable blessing and bother.

—Mark Twain

If you have not done so already, please go back and read chapter 1.

A main goal at this age is to encourage the development of self-soothing skills.

MONTH 3: EXTREME FUSSINESS/COLIC WINDS DOWN

Fifty-four percent of all babies with extreme fussiness/colic will be more settled at 2 months of age. By 3 months of age, 85 percent have improved, and by 4 months of age, 95 to 100 percent have. So between 2 and 4 months, your baby should begin to appear calmer in the early evening and to sleep better at night. When this typical time course occurs and there are no associated problems such as sleeping difficulties after colic ends, there are no adverse outcomes. For example, a recent study, from Australia, studied children at age 2–3 years who had colic as infants. "Infants with colic whose crying self-resolves do not experience adverse effects regarding child behavior, regulatory abilities, temperament or family functioning." In another study, 85 percent of infant colic *ended by three months,* and "once colic resolves, the residual effects on levels of maternal distress (anxiety and depression) are negligible." The researchers acknowledged that the fact that "most mothers in this study were married and financially secure, along with the relative universality of health care in Canada, suggests that the families in this study would have adequate resources to buffer the effects of their infants' colic." But those infants whose colic persisted beyond 3 months were considered to reflect a "persistent mother–infant distress syndrome."

Professor Antonia Smarius studied mothers who, unlike the Canadian mothers, might be less fortunate and experience a high "maternal burden of infant care" as determined by the answers to the following five questions:

1. All things considered, taking care of my baby is not so hard?
2. Taking care of my baby is quite a burden to me?
3. The care of my baby takes up so much of my energy that other family members are neglected?
4. My baby is not easy to take care of?
5. Taking care of my baby is too demanding for me?

Excessive infant crying (crying for three or more hours per day over the past week), at 13 weeks of age, "doubles the risk of behavioral, hyperactivity, and mood problems at age of 5–6 years, as reported by their mothers. Maternal burden of infant care partially mediates the association between excessive crying and behavioral and mood problems." I asked the lead author when the crying began and when it ended to see if this was a time course for typical colic, but she replied that no such data were collected. Also, no paternal data were collected. In addition to the retrospective maternal report of infant crying, "maternal perception of the child's emotion and behavior was measured rather than children's emotions and behaviors themselves"—that is, common method variance. So we do not know whether typical colic caused future problems. It is possible that mothers with a high "maternal burden of infant care" also had difficulty encouraging self-soothing in their babies with subsequent and persistent sleep problems and adverse outcomes.

If you have not done so already, now is the time to practice letting your child learn more self-soothing (chapters 4 and 5). Your child's transition from being parent-soothed to learning how to self-soothe may be easy in a well-rested baby or difficult in an overtired baby. I have examined many children who cry with such intensity and persistence at bedtime that their mothers are sure they're sick. During their crying, they may swallow air and become very gassy. If this happens, it is tempting to assume that their formula doesn't agree with them or that they have an intestinal disease—but only at bedtime or at night? These children are healthy but overtired. Not only do they cry hard and long when awake, they also cry loud and often during attempts to put them to sleep.

Your crying baby may be hungry, fussy, or *overtired*.

Let's consider the ways in which your child is changing. More smiles, coos, giggles, laughs, and squeals light up your life. Your child is now a more social creature. She is sleeping better at *night,* but *naps* may still be brief and irregular.

Become sensitive to her need to sleep and try to distinguish this need from her desire to play with you. If your child was previously or is currently primarily parent-soothed, she will naturally prefer the pleasure of your company to being left alone in a dark, quiet bedroom. Therefore, she may fight sleep to keep you around. This is in contrast with well-rested children with self-soothing skills, who usually go to sleep easily without protest.

In addition to your presence, which provides pleasurable stimulation, your baby's increasing curiosity about all the new and exciting parts of her expanding world may disrupt her sleep. How interesting it must be for an infant to observe the clouds in the sky, listen to the trees moving in the wind, hear the noise of barking dogs, or focus on the rhythms of adult chatter. When your baby needs to sleep, try to have her in an environment where she will sleep well. As she continues to grow, she will become more curious and social, and you will notice that she probably naps best in her crib.

Your child is becoming less portable. She cannot sleep equally well in any setting or situation, as she could when younger. Now you must become sensitive to the difference in quality between brief, interrupted daytime sleep and prolonged, consolidated naps. As your child's biological rhythms evolve for day sleep, your general goal is to *synchronize your soothing-to-sleep activities with her internal timing mechanism for sleep*. This is no different from being sensitive to her need to be fed or changed. Many children are overtired from not napping well or from going to sleep too late. They may not nap well because they're getting too much outside stimulation, too much handling, or too much irregular handling.

Sometimes at about 3 months of age, after the extreme fussiness/colic has dissipated, or in a baby who had common fussiness/crying, a child who had been sleeping well begins waking at night or crying at night and during the day. The parents also may note heightened activity with wild screaming spells. These children have accumulated a sleep debt (page 82) and decided that they would rather play with their parents than be placed in a dark, quiet, and boring room. Parents who do not recognize the new sleep debt might believe that this new night waking represents hunger due to a "growth spurt" or insufficient breast milk or an imaginary "sleep regression." But when these parents begin to focus on establishing a healthy night sleep schedule, when they put these babies in their cribs when the babies need to sleep, and when they shield their babies from overstimulation, the frequent night waking stops. If the children had developed irritability or fussiness, this disappears, too.

REMEMBER
The more rested a child is, the more she accepts sleep and expects to sleep.

NAPS

After she's been awake for no more than about two hours, plan to put your 3- or 4-month-old child somewhere semi-quiet or quiet to nap.

Q: *When I put my child to sleep after no more than two hours of wakefulness, how long should she sleep?*

A: At this point, the naps may be either short or long, without any particular pattern. This variability occurs because the part of the brain that establishes regular naps has not yet fully developed. By learning to recognize *drowsy signs*, you will be able to determine the best time to give your child the opportunity to nap. An awareness of *sleep inertia* will help you decide whether a particular nap was long enough. And sensitivity to the *witching hour* will help you determine whether naps on a particular day were long enough (chapters 2 and 4).

The two-hour limit on wakefulness is an approximation. Often there is a magic moment of tiredness when the baby will go to sleep easily. She is tired then but not overtired. If you go past this point in time, expect fatigue to set in. When your baby is up too long, she will tend to become overstimulated, overaroused, irritable, or peevish from a *second wind*. Please don't blame changes in weather—it's never too hot or too cold to sleep well.

Many parents misunderstand what overstimulation means. *A child becomes overstimulated when the duration of wakeful intervals is too long.* Overstimulation does not mean that you are too intense in your playfulness. It occurs once your baby has been awake for too long, regardless of what actions are taking place or not taking place. Your baby is a sponge; she soaks up input from the world around her whenever she is awake. And like a sponge, she will quickly reach an oversaturation point. That point is what we call overstimulation.

> Do not think of overstimulation as excessive intensity in play with your child; rather, think of it as too long a duration of the baby's normal period of wakefulness. It's not too much of a good thing; it's just being up too long.

The Midmorning Nap Develops between 9:00 and 10:00 A.M.
Watch the clock a little, but watch your baby more during the day, and expect her to need to sleep within two hours of wakefulness. Use whatever soothing method or wind-down routine works best to comfort and calm your baby. This may include a scheduled feeding, non-nutritive ("recreational") nursing, a session in a swing or a rocking chair, or a pacifier.

After a while you may notice, in the morning, a partial or a rough pattern of when your child's day sleep is best. Based on your child's behavior, the time of day, and how long she has been awake, you may reasonably conclude that she *needs* to sleep at any given time. However, she may *want* to play with you instead. Please try to distinguish between your child's needs and her wants. Have the confidence to be sensitive to her need to sleep, and lie down with her (see page 94 regarding co-sleeping and SIDS) or leave her alone a little to let her sleep. How long should you leave her alone? Maybe five, ten, or twenty minutes; there's no need for a rigid schedule. Simply test her once in a while to see whether she goes to sleep after five to twenty minutes of protest crying. When you put your baby down drowsy but awake and then leave the room (page 173), you are giving her the opportunity to develop *self-soothing skills,* to learn how to fall asleep unassisted. Some children learn this faster than others, so don't worry if your child seems always to cry up to your designated time. If this approach fails, pick her up, soothe her, comfort her, and then either try once more to get her to go to sleep or play with her for a while and try again later or the next day. Perhaps she was too young; wait a few weeks and try again. Never letting your child cry might reflect confusion in your mind between the healthy notion of allowing her to be alone sometimes and your fear that she will feel abandoned. But you are not abandoning your child by allowing her to learn self-soothing skills! You are protecting her. Always going to your child when she needs to sleep actually robs her of sleep.

Why focus on the midmorning nap? Simply because it develops before the midday nap. Try to teach self-soothing for the midmorning nap and then do whatever works to maximize sleep and minimize fussing/crying for the remainder of the day (being mindful to limit wakefulness to short intervals). Success or failure to achieve a regular midmorning nap depends on how well rested your child is when she wakes up to start the day; thus, a prerequisite for a good midmorning nap is good-quality night sleep.

This lack of rigid scheduling is appropriate for children a few months old, who are biologically immature. However, as the child gets older, extreme inconsistency will produce unhealthy sleep habits. Be flexible, but also become sensitive to your child's need to sleep. Remember, it's your responsibility as a parent to provide structure for your child: She cannot do it on her own. That doesn't mean imposing some arbitrary sleep regimen on her. It means being aware of the signals your child is sending about when she needs to sleep, and then acting on those signals in a firm but loving way to help her sleep better now and in the weeks, months, and years to come. Here's an account from the mother of a 3-month-old infant who successfully accomplished the midmorning nap and helped her baby sleep better at night:

It started at just 12 weeks. Katie was so fatigued she would cry for hours, screaming completely out of control, scratching her head, pulling her ears. Holding her didn't help, so it wasn't hard not to pick her up—she screamed anyway.

Instituting a new day schedule was easy. As soon as she started getting cranky, I rushed her to her crib to sleep. She would watch her mobile, and then sleep for hours at a time. The first week, she was so tired that she only stayed up thirty to fifty minutes at a time and slept three to four hours in between. The key for me was to get her down before she got really upset.

The afternoon was when she was awake the longest, and then it was hard getting her to sleep at night. The first few nights under our new regime were the worst. Positive reinforcement from my doctor was important then. I had to hear several times that this "cure" was the best thing to do.

The first night under our new strategy, my husband lay on the floor in her room (I guess to make sure she didn't choke) while I sat crying in our living room. Finally, after forty-five minutes, Katie was quiet! Hurray! Each night she cried less and less, and I handled it better and better. After a week, her hysteria was gone! Sure, she cried a little sometimes, but now she was on a schedule. She napped two or three times a day, two to four hours at a time, and slept twelve to fifteen hours a night. Sleeping promotes more sleep, and makes it easier to fall asleep. It's a catch-22.

Writing down the sleep patterns helped, too. For one week I kept track of every time I put her down and every time I picked her up from her nap. At the end of the week I noticed a distinct pattern. She fell into it herself!

Reports from other mothers with children at even younger ages can be found in chapters 4–7.

MAJOR POINTS

Letting your baby "cry it out" is not the only way your baby will learn to nap. Babies and children learn to nap well when parents focus on timing, motionless sleep (sleep in a crib or stationary stroller, as opposed to sleep while in a moving car or stroller), and consistency in soothing style.

As Katie's mother noticed, sleep begets sleep. This is a true statement. Even though it is not logical, it is biological!

Q: *My 3-month-old used to take very long midmorning naps, but now, at 4 months, they are shorter. What happened?*

A: Between 3 and 4 months, your child went to sleep later at night. She now goes to sleep earlier and wakes up better rested in the morning, so she no longer needs a very long midmorning nap.

Timing of Naps

Sleep periods for naps develop as the brain matures. This means that there are times during the day when your baby's brain will become drowsy and less alert. These "windows of opportunity" for sleep occur when the sleep process begins to overcome your baby. They are the best times for her to be soothed to sleep, both because it is easier to fall asleep at these times and because the restorative power of sleep is greatest when your baby's brain is in a drowsy state. Yes, of course your child is able to sleep at other times, but going to sleep is more difficult at such times, and the restorative power of sleep is much less. Unfortunately, your baby's brain may not be drowsy when you want her to sleep. You cannot control when she will become drowsy any more than you can control when she will become thirsty. As your infant's brain matures, these biologically determined periods of drowsiness will become more predictable and longer.

Here is a quick recap of the developmental time line for sleep.

After your baby is born, there is a quiet and calm honeymoon during which she is very sleepy, when your baby really will "sleep like a baby." This ends when she is a few days old (or a few days after her due date if she was born early). You may not even have a honeymoon if your baby was born several days late! After a few days of life, the sleepy brain wakes up, and during the first six weeks of life infants display increasing amounts of fussiness, crying, or agitated wakefulness, during which they swallow air and become gassy. At 6 weeks (or 6 weeks after the due date), the duration of these periods peaks, and they become more common in the evening hours. During these first weeks, the longest single sleep period is not very long and can occur at any time: This is day/night confusion. At about 6 weeks of age, something dramatic occurs naturally: Your baby begins to produce social smiles, and in most babies the evening fussiness begins to decrease. One mother asked me if she could "fast-forward to 6 weeks" and skip the hard part. Sorry! But from 6 weeks, a more predictable and longer midmorning nap will emerge.

REMEMBER
Night sleep periods will develop first, so you will notice longer sleeping at night before you will notice longer naps.

The onset of social smiles followed by a decrease in fussiness in the evening reflects maturational changes within your baby's brain. In addition, the brain becomes more able to inhibit the stimulating effects of sights, smells, sounds, and other sensations. Your baby is more able to console herself—she is becoming more capable of self-soothing. As a result of these biological changes, at 6 weeks of age your baby develops *night sleep organization*. This means that her longest single sleep period now occurs at night. This is the end of day/night confusion. This longest night sleep period may be only four to six hours, but it regularly occurs at night. You cannot control the exact time when this long sleep period will occur, but at least you now know that you will get a little more rest at night!

Night sleep usually develops without problems at 6 weeks of age because:

1. Darkness serves as a time cue.
2. We slow down our activities and become quieter at night.
3. We behave as if we expect our baby to sleep.

These three factors may be absent during the day, and so the major way to *prevent* sleep problems from developing now is to focus your efforts on *helping your baby nap during the day*.

There are three factors that will help your baby sleep well during the day: timing, motionless sleep, and consistency in soothing style. If you have experience already because you have more than one child, or if you have a child with common fussiness/crying, you may start your efforts early; if you have a colicky baby, you might have to start later.

Keep the intervals of wakefulness short. Look at the clock when your baby wakes up in the morning or after a nap. Within one to two hours after your baby wakes, begin a soothing process *before* she appears grumpy, crabby, or drowsy. Usually the total duration of wakefulness, including the time of soothing, should be *less than two hours*. This does not mean that you keep your baby awake for about two hours before trying to soothe her to sleep. The point is that young infants cannot comfortably tolerate long periods of wakefulness. In fact, some babies go to sleep after being awake for only *one* hour or less. You want to catch the approaching wave of *drowsiness* as it is rising, to enable your baby to have a long, smooth ride to deep, refreshing slumber.

MAJOR POINT
Perfect timing produces no crying.

If your timing is off and your child's sleep wave crashes into an overtired state, then the ride to slumber is bumpy and sleep itself brief. If your timing is off, your child will become overtired, and then there will be some crying. This you may safely ignore. Such crying is the consequence of your having accidentally allowed your child to become overtired.

Think of how your baby behaves when she becomes overly hungry. She twists, turns, and may dive-bomb at the breast for a few minutes before she settles down to suck well. Similarly, the overtired baby takes a few minutes to settle down to sleep. I repeat: Crying is the consequence of becoming overtired. At this particular time, your efforts to soothe—hugging, rocking, talking—may be stimulating and interfere with the natural surfacing of the sleep process. After all, your baby does not fall asleep immediately in the same way a light switch is turned off. Rather, the sleep process takes time. Remember, it is easier for her to fall asleep before she becomes grumpy, because when she becomes overtired—from nap deprivation or any other reason—her body produces stimulating hormones to fight the fatigue. This chemical stimulation interferes with sleeping well. This is why sleeping well during the day will improve night sleeping and why, conversely, *nap deprivation causes night waking.*

One mother told me that her child had been extremely fussy/colicky but that he began to slip into a better night-sleeping routine at 12 weeks of age and began taking longer naps during the day between 12 and 16 weeks of age. She was breastfeeding and used the family bed; her child went to sleep at about 10:00 P.M. around 12 weeks of age. Her 2-year-old son was not sleeping well at night, either, and distracted her, and this allowed the baby to become overtired. The predictable result: The baby's naps were a mess. He was "napping" between 5:00 and 6:00 P.M. and asleep for the night between 7:00 and 8:00 P.M. The mother recognized that her baby should be falling asleep for the night around 6:00 P.M., not napping then. Here was the solution that eventually corrected the overtired state:

Temporarily, her baby was put to sleep at a very early time, between 5:30 and 6:00 P.M. The plan was to help the child get more sleep at night and be asleep before a second wind developed. The mother was to soothe her baby at night and then either lie down with him or put him in his crib. She wanted to use the crib because the hour was so early and she had a 2-year-old to deal with. Because of the baby's age, because he had been extremely fussy/colicky, and because he had become accustomed to sleeping with his mother in her bed at the breast, we knew he would protest our plan. We decided that we would ignore his protest crying at the onset of sleep and would use the father to soothe him at night when he might cry but was not hungry. During the day, the mother would do whatever worked to maximize sleep and minimize crying to keep him as well rested as possible. The 2-year-old made this part of the plan a little difficult. But within eight days, there was substantially less crying at night, and longer and fewer naps were occurring during the day. Now that the baby was better rested, he was able to stay up a little later at night. However, he still needed to go to sleep between 6:00 and 6:30 P.M. Please get fathers on board (pages 163 and 513)!

EARLY BEDTIMES
A common complaint is "We don't get to eat dinner as a family." Or, "How can we play outside as a family after dinner?" My answer is that what is most important is a well-rested family.

Consistency in Soothing Styles for Naps
Parents often assume that there is a right and wrong way to soothe a baby to sleep. This is not the case. Falling asleep is simply learned behavior, a habit. The important thing is that the behavior is learned, not how it is learned. Your child will learn best if you are consistent in how you soothe her to sleep for naps. Below are two popular ways to soothe a baby to sleep. Either will work as long as you are consistent.

Method A: *At nap time your baby sometimes soothes herself to sleep unassisted.* After soothing your baby for several minutes, you *always* put her down to sleep *whether or not she is asleep.* You are practicing putting her down for a nap *drowsy but still awake.* The soothing is a winding down, a transition from active to quiet, from alert to drowsy. Soothing may include breast- or bottle-feeding. Contrary to popular belief, your child will not develop night sleep problems if you include breastfeeding as part of the soothing process. Also contrary to popular belief, it is not necessary that you always put her down fully awake. The key is that you consistently spend a relatively brief period of time soothing your baby to sleep for naps. Because she is not necessarily always asleep when you put her down, she eventually learns how to soothe herself to sleep without being held. In other words, you are always attempting to put your baby down for naps drowsy but awake, but sometimes she falls asleep during your soothing. If when the child is put down there are some vocalizations or low-level, quiet crying, some mothers will ignore it and other mothers, knowing from experience that with this child it will always escalate into hard crying, will resume soothing for a few more minutes. Also, if there is hard crying upon being put down, some mothers will ignore it for a while to see whether their child will soon fall asleep, while other mothers, again knowing from experience with their individual child that this always means there will not be a nap, will immediately pick up their baby for more pre-nap soothing or attempt the nap at some other time. Method A may be viewed positively (creating independence, learning self-soothing skills, acquiring the capacity to be alone) or negatively (creating insecurity, neglecting or abandoning your baby, selfishness in the mother). There is no benefit in being judgmental of yourself or others. Choose a method that is comfortable for you and be aware of how your behavior affects your child.

Method B: *Your baby always begins naps with your help.* You *always* hold and soothe your baby *until she is in a deep sleep state, no matter how long it takes.* You are not practicing putting her down for a nap drowsy but awake. You may lie down or sit down with your baby, nap with her, or perhaps put her down only after she is in a very deep sleep state. Your child learns to associate the process of falling asleep with the feel of your breast, your breathing and heart rhythm, and your body's scent. Contrary to popular belief, this association, in and of itself, does not automatically lead to a night-waking problem (signaling). A night-waking problem sometimes occurs when the mother indiscriminately responds to normal arousals, misinterprets them to reflect hunger, and, because of unnecessary feeding, inadvertently fragments the child's sleep. Perhaps this situation at night occurs more often in those mothers who choose method B for naps, but that is not because of the method itself but because of psychological factors that cause certain mothers to prefer method B over method A. Like method A, method B may be viewed positively (providing more security, being more natural) or negatively (creating dependence, spoiling). Method B is often what works best for babies with extreme fussiness/colic and is often a component of attachment parenting.

One method is not better than another; both method A and method B can help your child sleep well. There is no reason to be judgmental about soothing styles or brand other parents as "bad" simply because they do not agree with you. Different methods will seem more natural or more acceptable to different parents, and different methods work better for different children.

Be decisive; choose a soothing style and *be consistent*. Consistency helps your baby sleep better, because, as noted above, the process of falling asleep is a learned behavior. Please review chapter 4 to help you decide which method is best for you. Grandparents and babysitters should handle your baby just as you do. Sometimes grandparents are a major problem because they interfere with the baby's sleep schedule. They want to come over to play with their grandchild when it is convenient for them, or they see their role as being more permissive than the parents. This is a difficult problem without a simple answer, because, in addition to wanting your child to be well rested, you want to maintain family harmony. If the grandparents are the primary caregivers during the day, consistency may be difficult. Try to teach them how important sleep is for their grandchild.

Q: *When should I start to try to establish regular naps? When should I start to become consistent in how I soothe my baby before naps?*

A: Day sleep organization develops at 3–4 months of age. A regularly occurring midmorning nap appears first, followed by a regularly occurring midday nap a few or several weeks later. The age when you start nap training depends on your experience and your baby's degree of fussiness/crying.

Regardless of when you begin to start nap training, the sooner you develop a consistent approach, the easier it will be for the family. Please begin to be consistent around 6 weeks of age, when your child is clearly becoming more social and everyone is getting more rest at night. For babies born before their due date, these changes occur about 6 weeks after the due date, and that is when you should start.

I encourage fathers to become as involved as possible for naps— for example, on weekends. With either method A or B, sometimes the mother breastfeeds the baby and then passes the baby to the father to be soothed to sleep (chapter 4). As I said, either soothing method works well, but my observation is that for well-rested babies whose parents have consistently used method B and sometime later decide to switch to method A, the transition is made with very little or no crying. However, the children of parents who use method B *inconsistently* (because of real-life events that often interfere with prolonged soothing for naps) may never develop regular naps; they then become overtired, and when the parents switch to method A, the overtired child cries a lot. For some parents, then, it is simply easier to be consistent using method A.

If you have more than one child, it is very difficult to consistently use method B, even with full-time help, because an older child's time demands may make it impossible to devote sufficient time to getting your younger child into a deep sleep before putting her down. Therefore, it is more practical to use method A. In addition, because of your experience, you can begin helping your younger child sleep well as soon as you get home from the hospital. With two children, starting sleep training early for your newborn is especially important. Here, too, fathers need to help out more. As one basketball fan told me after the arrival of his second son, "Now I have to shift from one-on-one to zone defense!" Here is an account from a mother who started early with her second child using method A:

> As patients of Dr. Weissbluth, we were ready to commit ourselves to promoting good sleep habits in our children. When our first son, Hayden, was born, it was easier said than done. Being new parents and not knowing what the different cries meant, we would pick Hayden up at the slightest whimper. We were quick believers when at 4 months we were a bit more seasoned and decided not to rush in at the first cry. The cry lasted fifteen minutes, and then it was smooth sailing; he gradually went to bed earlier and earlier until we reached a 6:00 P.M. bedtime with a 6:30 A.M. wake-up, and then naps at 9:00 A.M. and 1:00 P.M. This pattern still holds true minus the first nap, and bedtime is at 6:30 P.M. at almost 3 years old. He is social, happy, sweet, and most of all well rested.
>
> With the birth of our second child, a girl, Lily, we were busy with Hayden, now a toddler, and were quite the ex-

perts on all the "signs" babies give out. We had a rule: If she was sleepy and not crying (even at a few days old), she was to be put in her bassinet. We still played with her and enjoyed her, but we were not walking around the house with her twenty-four hours a day. We also provided Lily with the same nighttime routine we give Hayden: dim the lights and give a massage, bath, bottle, book, and bed. This prompted Lily to develop a quicker sleep schedule, and we found by 2.5 months she was sleeping through the late-night feedings. By 3 months she was going to bed at 5:00 to 5:30 P.M. and sleeping until 6:30 A.M. Also at 3 months we began putting her down for her midmorning nap two hours after she woke up, and that began her nap schedule. Now Lily, almost one, wakes up at 6:30 A.M., takes her first nap at 8:15 A.M., takes her second nap at 12:30 P.M., and is in the bathtub by 5:00 P.M. and asleep by 5:30 P.M.

We are vigilant about not letting either child nap in the car, strollers, or for that matter miss naps or have delayed naps. Once our children are in their cribs for the night, we don't hear from them until the morning . . . no night waking or games! We greet them each morning with a smile on their faces.

We are committed to having well-rested children and will defend our decisions with any naysayer suggesting we don't get to be with our children at night or we are too strict with the daytime schedule. We find too often it is the parent who is putting the child on their schedule instead of vice versa.

Babies yearn for routines and respond unbelievably to them. Again, we feel that we have two of the happiest, sweetest children, and knowing that teaching them good sleep habits and, more important, the ability to fall asleep unassisted is the best gift you can ever give!

Your goal is to synchronize your caretaking with your baby's needs: feed her when she's hungry, change her when she's wet, play with her when she's awake, and help her sleep when she's tired. Because of the irregularity with which these events occur, it's hard for first-time parents to "read" their baby's needs, but experienced parents should trust their instincts and put their baby to sleep when she appears tired.

If you have an extremely fussy/colicky baby, one who is more irritable, wakeful, harder to soothe, and harder to read, you may find that only method B will help her sleep at nap time without crying. Later you will want to make a transition from method B to method A in the colicky baby so that learning self-soothing for naps will occur.

Here are some common nap mistakes:

Keeping the intervals of wakefulness too long
Using swings, cars, or strollers during naps too much with
    older children
Inconsistency in methods used to soothe your baby to sleep

Q: *Doesn't this mean I have to become a slave to my baby's nap schedule?*
A: Not at all. Simply respect her need to have good-quality naps. Try to distinguish between routine days and exceptional days. On routine days, try to partially organize your activities around the naps. On exceptional days, naps may be lost because of special events: for example, birthdays, holidays, and family vacations. Well-rested children tolerate not sleeping well if such episodes occur once or twice a month, but not if they are happening once or twice a week. A *reset* might be needed after a special event.

If you are suffering from the inconvenience of hanging around your house on routine days when you think your baby will need to nap, perhaps it will help to keep in mind that between 12 and 16 weeks (or maybe somewhat later in colicky babies) your child will start taking fewer and longer naps, and longer periods of wakefulness between naps will develop during the day. There will be no late-afternoon fussiness, and your baby will have longer periods of night sleep. So while it is socially *limiting* to plan ahead and protect naps, it is *liberating* to have a well-rested child who never fusses or cries during the day at home or in public. An early bedtime with consolidated night sleep is also liberating for parents, who can enjoy calm private time together early in the evening and overnight. Isn't all that worth a little temporary inconvenience?

Remember that healthy sleep depends on different but interrelated elements (chapter 2):

Sleep duration
Naps
Sleep consolidation
Sleep schedule, timing of sleep, bedtime
Sleep regularity

When all the pieces are considered, healthy sleep will be accomplished. It won't happen overnight, but it will happen, and sooner than you think, if not as soon as you may desire.

Month 4: Prevent Post-Colic Sleep Problems

A main goal at this age is to encourage the development of self-soothing skills for night sleep, the midmorning nap, and the midday nap.

If your baby has self-soothing skills and is sleeping well at night without bedtime or nighttime problems, and if naps are going well, consider skipping or skimming the following section and resume reading about naps on page 533.

How to prevent post-colic sleep problems? The discussion that immediately follows assumes that infant-driven influences are most important. Later I will give equal weight to the idea that mother-driven influences are most important. Finally, I will discuss how both infant- and mother-driven influences interact with each other. The reason I say "mother-driven" instead of "parent-driven" is because all research on these subject focuses on the mother, but obviously the role of the father, or lack thereof, may be equally or even more important in some families (chapter 4).

Baby-Driven Path: The Role of the Baby

What is meant by *infant-driven influences*? Studies by Dr. C. Anderson Aldrich have shown that all babies have some uncategorizable crying: that is, they cry for no apparent reason. From studies by Dr. Ian St. James-Roberts, we know that no matter what the parenting style, bouts of inconsolable crying can occur (chapter 2). Also, Dr. T. Berry Brazelton showed that fussing/crying behavior increases around 6 weeks (occurring mostly in the evening) and then decreases. These facts (universality, occurrence independent of parenting style, and predictable time course) strongly suggest that there is a developmental component underlying the behavior called extreme fussiness/colic during the first few months of life. Later this developmental feature may be expressed at 4 months of age as a difficult temperament. After 4 months of age, the developmental issue might cause the child to have sleep problems that persist despite the parents' efforts. With this developmental framework in mind, let's consider what we know about temperament and how we might prevent post-colic sleep problems.

After extreme fussiness/colic winds down around 4 months of age or sooner, your child may be overtired, not sleeping well, and difficult to manage. The observation that brief and interrupted sleep often follows extreme fussiness/colic might suggest that some genetic, or congenital but not genetic (for example, maternal smoking during pregnancy), or biological factors postpartum lead initially to extreme fussiness/colic. These factors may still present in the baby after the colicky period has passed. This is supported by the observation that despite successful drug therapy that eliminated or reduced colicky crying, brief sleep periods were still the norm at 4 months of age (chapter 6). In addition, some, but not all, post-colic infants continue to behave as if they had heightened activity levels and excessive sensitivity to environmental stimuli.

Night Waking, Sleep Duration, Sleep Problems: The Baby-Driven Path

I studied 141 infants between *4 and 8 months* of age from middle-class families and showed that the history of extreme fussiness/colic was associated with the parents' judgment that night waking was a current problem. The frequency of awakening was a problem in 76 percent of infants, the duration of awakenings a problem in 8 percent, and both frequency and duration a problem in 16 percent. The more often a child woke up, the longer were the durations of the night wakings. Other studies also reported more night waking at *8 and 12 months* and age *14–18 months* in post-colic children compared with babies who did not have colic. Also, among those post-colic infants, the total sleep duration was less (13.5 versus 14.3 hours). So post-colic infants tend to have, for several months, brief sleep durations and more frequent or longer night awakenings (signaling). These group differences in night waking and sleep durations between previously non-colicky and post-colic babies *decrease* as children become older.

There are studies suggesting that both infant irritability and sleep deficits are moderately stable individual characteristics during the first year of life and beyond. One study showed that children with extreme fussiness/colic had more sleep problems and the families exhibited more distress than a control group at age *3 years*. But the trend of decreasing group differences between colicky and non-colicky infants with age, at least on night waking and sleep as these were measured by parent diary reports or sleep lab recordings of colicky infants at 9 weeks of age, suggests that the biological differences *diminish* over time and/or parenting practices become more influential. Other studies suggest that *extreme fussiness/colic* alone does not predict future sleep problems.

However, it may be difficult for parents of post-colic infants after 4 months of age to eliminate frequent night wakings and lengthen sleep durations. Because of parental fatigue, parents may unintentionally become inconsistent and irregular in their responses to their infant. As a reminder, one mother wrote:

> Dealing with a fussy child almost around the clock, you have a recipe for frazzled and distressed parents. I can certainly understand why many parents struggle with a post-colic sleep plan, as it can be hard to be resolute when you are completely burned out.

I would like to emphasize that soothing a fussy or crying child is something both parents can do (chapter 4). Even if she is breastfeeding, it is not solely the mother's responsibility. Fathers can, and in my opinion should, help with their children. If a father can be at home to help the mother for a time after she arrives home from the hospital and again for a period when the baby is about 6 weeks old, then the mother will be able to adjust to the changes in her baby. One father called this "tag-team parenting" because whenever one parent became exhausted, the other one took over for car rides, walks, or trips in the stroller to let the other get some much-needed rest. Two exhausted parents don't make a good couple!

Treatments such as simethicone drops, probiotics, and chiropractic spinal manipulation have been proven to be completely ineffective (chapter 6). Gastroesophageal reflux disease is the newest popular diagnosis in fussy and crying babies, but research has shown it to be a coincidental finding and not the cause of irritability in babies. Although many remedies have been suggested for extreme fussiness/colic, including catnip or herbal tea, papaya juice, peppermint drops, recordings of heartbeat or womb sounds, hot-water bottles, or trying new baby formulas, three main maneuvers have been found to calm fussiness and crying. The three maneuvers are:

1. *Rhythmic motions:* rocking chairs, swings, cribs with springs attached to the casters, cradles, carriages, and strollers; walking, "taking ceiling tours," using your baby as a weight for biceps curl exercises, and taking car rides. However, avoid water beds, which are dangerous because they may cause suffocation (chapter 4). Other dangerous colic "treatments" include certain herbal remedies, which have caused poisoning; beanbag pillows, which have caused suffocation; and trampoline-like devices suspended in the crib, which have caused strangulation. Tryptophan was once used to help babies sleep well, but we now know that this is dangerous; similarly, melatonin should not be given to babies.

2. *Sucking:* at breast, bottle, fist, wrist, thumb, or pacifier.

3. *Swaddling:* wrapping the child in blankets; snuggling, cuddling, and nestling. After the first few weeks, however, this maneuver is often less effective.

You should avoid trying gimmick after gimmick; it will only make you feel more frustrated or helpless as the crying continues. You may also feel resentment or anger if your child, perhaps unlike your friend's child, doesn't seem to respond well to home remedies.

Feelings of anger toward your crying child are frightening—and normal. You can love your baby and hate her crying spells. All parents sometimes have contradictory feelings about their baby.

Take breaks when your baby is crying. This will enable you to better nurture your child; it's a smart strategy for baby care, not a selfish idea for parent care.

You may feel during the first few months that you are not influencing your extremely fussy/colicky child's behavior very much. And you are right, but consider this period to be a rehearsal. Your hugs, kisses, and lovingkindness are expressing the way you feel. Practice showering affection on your baby, even when she's crying. This loving attention is important for both of you.

However, unceasing attention showered on a fussing or crying baby, whether she is extremely fussy/colicky or just showing common fussiness during the first few months, *can* have complications if you continue this strategy of intervention for the older, post-colic child at bedtime and nap times. Thus, after the extreme fussiness/colic passes, if the older child is never left alone at sleep times, she is deprived of the opportunity to develop self-soothing skills. These children never learn to fall asleep unassisted. The resultant sleep fragmentation or deprivation in the child, driven by intermittent positive parental reinforcement, leads to fatigue-driven fussiness long after the biological factors that caused the extreme fussiness/*colic* have been resolved.

It cannot be overemphasized that, as stated by Dr. A. H. Parmelee, "parents are never truly prepared for the degree to which the babies' sleep/wake patterns will dominate and completely disrupt their daily activities."

Temperament

When the extreme crying and fussiness of your baby's first few months have passed and your child seems more settled, what next? After about 4 months of age, most parents have learned to differentiate between their child's *need* for consolidated sleep and the child's *preference* for soothing, pleasurable company at night. Most parents can learn to appreciate that prolonged, uninterrupted sleep is a health habit they can influence; they can quickly learn to stop reinforcing night wakings and irregular nap schedules that rob kids of needed rest. A process of "social weaning" from the pleasure of a parent's company at nap times and bedtimes is under way. As one young mother said, "I see—I should now forget the company she [the baby] wants."

But parents of post-colic babies still have a few challenges to face. That's because babies who have had extreme fussiness/colic appear more likely than other babies to develop shorter sleep durations and more frequent night wakings between 4 and 8 months of age. My research also has shown that parents of post-colic babies are more likely to view frequent (instead of prolonged) night wakings as a problem.

Additionally, around 4 months of age, a difficult temperament might occur. The term *temperament* refers to the behavioral style or the manner in which the child interacts with the environment. It does not describe the motivation of an action. The reason it is important to understand temperament in detail is that the behavior of a post-colic and/or sleep-deprived child is predictably stressful to parents, and recognizing how these children appear allows parents to better understand their behavior and to institute healthier sleep habits. All parents naturally make their own assessment of their babies' temperaments, but there is a standardized system for evaluating infant temperament, and although it is not absolutely objective, it has proved over the years to be very useful.

Dr. Alexander Thomas and his wife, Dr. Stella Chess, both pioneers in child development, described temperament differences among babies. In a study based on both his own careful observations and parent interviews, Dr. Thomas noted interrelations among four temperament characteristics: *mood, intensity, adaptability,* and *approach/withdrawal*. Infants who were moody, intense, slow to adapt, and withdrawing in Dr. Thomas's study were also rated as *irregular* in all bodily functions. Thus, they were diagnosed as having "difficult" temperaments because they were difficult for parents to manage! We don't know why these particular traits cluster together, but we do know that infants with "easy" temperaments have opposite characteristics. In Dr. Thomas's study, four additional temperament characteristics were described: *persistence, activity, distractibility,* and *threshold*. Threshold means how sensitive or insensitive the child appears to be to noises or changes in lighting. These four temperament characteristics were *not* part of either the easy or difficult temperament clusters.

The researchers who developed this system did not have extreme fussiness/colic anywhere in their minds. There is not even a specific crying dimension in their system. But the mood rating does include the notion of fussiness and crying, and the mood rating is highly correlated with the traits of intensity, adaptability, and approach/withdrawal (these four traits are used to define a "difficult" temperament), so the construct "difficult temperament" would be expected to be linked to extreme fussiness crying. Yet no one connected temperament, as rated on this scale, with extreme fussiness/colic until much later. However, as you will see, the connection proved to be striking. Below are the nine infant-temperament characteristics described by Drs. Thomas and Chess.

1. *Activity (general motion, energy)*. Does your baby squirm, bounce, or kick while lying awake in the crib? Does she move around when asleep? Does she kick or grab during diapering? Some infants always appear to be active, while others only appear active in specific circumstances, such as bathing. Activity levels in infants have nothing to do with "hyperactivity" in older children.

2. *Rhythmicity (regularity of bodily functions)*. Rhythmicity is a measure of how regular or predictable the infant appears. Is there a pattern in the time when she is hungry, how much she eats at each feeding, how often bowel movements occur, when she gets sleepy, when she wakes, when she appears most active, and when she gets fussy? Some babies are very regular at age 2 months, while others seem to be irregular throughout the first

year. As infants grow older, they tend to become more regular in their habits.

3. *Approach/withdrawal (first reaction)*. Approach/withdrawal is a temperament characteristic that defines the infant's initial reaction to something new. What does she do when meeting another child or a babysitter? Does she object to new procedures? Some infants reach out in new circumstances—accept, appear curious, approach—while others object, reject, turn away, appear shy, or withdraw.

4. *Adaptability (flexibility)*. Adaptability is measured by observing such activities as whether the infant accepts nail cutting without protest, accepts bathing without resistance, accepts changes in feeding schedule, accepts strangers within fifteen minutes, and accepts new foods. It is an attempt to measure the ease or difficulty with which a child can adjust to new circumstances or a change in routine.

5. *Intensity*. Intensity is the degree or amount of an infant's response, either pleasant or unpleasant. Think of it as the amount of emotional energy with which the child expresses her likes and dislikes. Intense infants react loudly, with much expression of likes and dislikes. During feeding they are vigorous in accepting or resisting food. They react strongly to abrupt exposure to bright lights; they greet a new toy with enthusiastic positive or negative expressions; they display much feeling during bathing, diapering, or dressing; and they react strongly to strangers or familiar people. One mother described her extremely fussy/colicky baby's intense all-or-nothing reactions: "Her mood changes quickly; she gives no warning—she can go from loud and happy to screaming." Intensity is measured separately from mood. Infants who are not intense are described as "mild."

6. *Mood*. If intensity is the degree of response, mood is the direction. It is measured in the same situations described previously. Negative mood is the presence of fussy/crying behavior or the absence of smiles, laughs, or coos. Positive mood is the absence of fussy/crying behavior or the presence of smiles, laughs, or coos. Most intense infants also tend to be more negative in mood, less adaptable, withdrawn (difficult temperament). Most mild infants also tend to be more positive in mood, more adaptable, and approaching (easy temperament).

7. *Persistence*. Persistence level, or attention span, is a measure of how long the infant engages in activity. Parents may value this trait under some circumstances but not under others. For instance, persistence is desirable when the child is trying to learn something new, like reaching for a rattle, but it is undesirable when the infant persists in throwing food on the floor. Unfortunately, some babies persist in their prolonged crying spells and their prolonged wakeful periods. One father described his persistently crying baby as follows: "We have a copper-top, alkaline-battery-powered baby, and we're powered by regular carbon batteries. He outlasts us every time."

8. *Distractibility*. Distractibility describes how easily the baby may be distracted by external events. Picking up the infant easily consoles a distractible infant's fatigue or hunger; soothing can stop fussing during a diaper change. New toys or unusual noises easily distract the infant. Distractibility and persistence are not related to each other, and neither trait is related to activity or threshold levels.

9. *Threshold (sensitivity)*. Threshold levels measure how much stimulus is required to produce a response in the infant in specific circumstances, such as loud noises, bright lights, and other situations previously discussed. While some infants are

very reactive or responsive to external or environmental changes, other infants barely react.

Difficult Temperament

As previously mentioned, while observing many children and analyzing many questionnaires, Drs. Thomas and Chess noticed that four, and only four, of these temperamental traits tended to cluster together: *intensity, adaptability, mood,* and *approach/withdrawal.* In particular, infants who were extreme or "intense" in their reactions also tended to be slowly adaptable, negative in mood, and withdrawn. This appeared to be a personality type.

According to their parents' descriptions and direct observation by the researchers, these infants seemed more difficult to manage than other infants. Consequently, a child whose temperament scores fall into this pattern is said to have a difficult temperament. One mother referred to her infant jokingly as a "mother-killer." Infants with the opposite temperamental traits are said to have easy temperaments. These are sometimes called "dream" babies. One father described his "easy" infant as a "low-maintenance baby." The difficult temperament and the easy temperament are only descriptions of a behavioral style. Temperament research usually does not ask why a child behaves in a particular way. There is no scientific basis for labeling a child with a difficult temperament as a "high-needs" child. In fact, there is no scientific support for labeling a child a "high-needs" child under any circumstances. Many so-called high-needs children are really very overtired children or children with a difficult temperament.

Of the original group of infants Thomas and Chess studied, about 10 percent fell into the difficult-temperament category. These infants also tended to be irregular in biological function such as sleep schedules and night awakenings. They were more likely to have behavioral problems—particularly sleep disturbances—when they grew older. One of the most interesting differences between difficult and easy babies is the way they cry when they are past the extreme fussiness period—that is, when they are 3–4 months old. Published research found that mothers listening to the taped cries of infants rated difficult (but who were not their own babies) described the crying as more irritable, grating, and arousing than the crying of easy infants. They said that the difficult-temperament group sounded spoiled and were crying because of frustration rather than hunger or wet diapers. An audio analysis of cries helped explain why this should be. The crying of the difficult-temperament infants was found to have more silent pauses between crying sounds than that of the easy babies. These silent pauses caused the listener to repeatedly think that the crying spell had ended. Also, at its most intense, the crying of difficult-temperament infants was actually pitched at a higher frequency. These two differences can make the crying seem much more frightening, piercing, and annoying.

What causes the difficult temperaments? Temperament is usually thought to be an expression of your nature. As we will see, nurture may also play a role.

Here's how child development specialist Laya Frischer described a post-colic baby:

> Jane is difficult and unpredictable, with less than average sleep and cuddling and more than average crying. Observations over five weeks have revealed an extremely sensitive infant. For a period of time, she could not even tolerate touches on her abdomen. Swaddling helps a little, and the rhythmic swing movement gives her some relief. If these things fail, the parents walk her around. Sometimes these efforts quiet her fussiness, but at other times it escalates to panic crying. Jane seems to have no capacity to console herself, and very little capacity to be consoled by usual methods of touch. The pacifier has been helpful, but not always successful. Jane does not have good state regulation. *She can be in a panic cry state when she seems to be asleep.*

Jane goes from sleep to distress in seconds. She becomes overtired and cannot sleep, which contributes to her irritability. She does not habituate easily to sensory stimulation of light and touch. Jane requires a very protective environment, which puts great stress on her parents, particularly her mother. Her cries are very hard to read; her parents feel she is unpredictable, and often uncommunicative [emphasis added].

Here is another example of sensitivity to environmental stimuli from my own experience. When my first son had colic, I had to keep the crib railing up and locked in place, because the clunk of the spring lock would always awaken him. That made it awkward for me to place him in his crib, but fortunately I was limber from college gymnastics. For my wife, it was an impossible situation until we got a sturdy stool for her to stand on—but it still hurt our backs!

Interestingly, two temperament characteristics (high activity and high sensitivity) are not part of the diagnostic criteria for babies who fall into the difficult-temperament category. But some post-colic infants are exquisitely sensitive to irregularities in their nap or night sleep schedule. Disruptions of regular routines due to painful ear infections or holidays and trips subsequently caused extreme resistance to falling asleep and frequent night waking, lasting up to several days after the disruptive event. These prolonged recovery periods might reflect easily disorganized internal biological rhythms caused by enduring congenital imbalances in arousal/inhibition or sleep/wake control mechanisms. Alternatively, parents who put their baby to sleep slightly too late, or who often cause their children to skip naps after 4 months of age, keep their post-colic infant close to the edge of overtiredness (page 516). What happens when some natural disruptive event occurs is that the child falls into the abyss of severe agitated wakefulness and irritability and is unable to easily get back into a regular sleep pattern.

Some post-colic kids are extremely active; they appear to have boundless energy. "She crawls like lightning" was how one mother described her baby. These babies are constantly on the move. They would rather crawl up Mom's chest to perch on her shoulder than sit quietly in her lap. But having reached the shoulder, they immediately want to get down and check out that dust ball or some equally exciting object off in the corner. They appear easily bored; they also seem very stimulus-sensitive, especially to mechanical noises such as those of a vacuum cleaner, hair dryer, or coffee grinder (which may have seemed to calm them down during colicky spells when they were younger). It's as if they have a heightened level of arousal, activity, and curiosity. When overtired, they are always crabby and socially demanding, needing Mommy's presence and wanting to be held all the time. They also are quick to fuss when Mom leaves the room for only a minute. But when they are well rested, it's a different story. They may remain very active but less frantic, and this suggests that whatever biological process may be contributing to high-activity behavior, lack of sleep is also part of the picture. When they've had enough sleep, these same babies appear to have boundless curiosity, actively seeking opportunities to learn.

Some pediatricians, in their attempt to shorten the discussion of colic in the office, simply tell parents not to worry, because nobody dies of colic; it will pass, and anyway, colicky babies turn out to be smarter kids. They suggest that these post-colic babies who are so alert, curious, and bright that they have difficulty controlling their impulses to explore or investigate the world are unusually intelligent. No data support the conclusion that post-colic kids in general are more intelligent, but there may be a small number who are so exceptionally bright that they gave birth to this myth. One study of infants published in 1964 connected increased crying (induced by snapping a rubber band on the sole of the foot at age 4–10 days) to increased intelligence at 3 years of age. Whether this artificially induced crying and its link with intelligence can be generalized to colicky crying is an open question.

Association between Temperament and Sleep

Recent research showed that the tendency for shorter sleep durations to be associated with more negative emotionality occurs only in children with a specific variant gene. In other words, not all children who have shorter sleep durations are at risk for developing the issues described below. Therefore, your child's behavior might give you a better clue to whether she needs more sleep than comparing her sleep duration with some table showing numerical averages. Similarly, please don't compare your child's sleep needs with other children's; remember, there is so much individual variation. Just ask any mother of fraternal twins!

Continuous recordings of sleep patterns during the *second day of life* were linked with temperament assessments at *8 months:* It was observed that infants with the most extreme values on all sleep variables were more likely to have difficult temperaments. Observations on such young babies tend to support a developmental or biological basis for this association as opposed to parenting. A separate study of children at 3, 6, and 11 months of age showed that increased night sleep is associated with an increased likelihood of approaching new and strange people and things.

In my study of sixty 4- to 5-month-old infants, the infants rated as difficult had average sleep times substantially less than the infants rated as easy (12.3 versus 15.6 hours). Although nine infant-temperament characteristics were measured, only five are used to establish the diagnosis of a difficult temperament. And four of these (mood, adaptability, rhythmicity, and approach/withdrawal) were individually highly associated with total sleep duration.

When this study was extended to include 105 infants, those infants with difficult temperaments slept 12.8 hours and those with easy temperaments slept 14.9 hours. This observation was subsequently confirmed in a Chinese American group with different parenting practices. It thus appears that infants who have a difficult temperament have briefer total sleep durations when assessed at 4–5 *months* of age regardless of differences in parenting practices. In addition to short sleep durations, a study of children between 6 and 36 months showed that more fragmented sleep is associated with a more difficult temperament. Also, as mentioned previously (page 143), a Canadian study showed that sleep difficulties starting around 5 months persist at age 6 years and that "sleep difficulties likely are part of the difficult temperament profile." Another study, of Swedish children, over the same age range, also noted stability over time of frequent night wakings and low quality of sleep. Here, too, this persistence was more common in children with a difficult temperament. While this might suggest a developmental link between sleep duration and/or sleep problems and difficult temperament, both short sleep durations or sleep problems and difficult temperament might have a common cause. It is also possible that despite differences in parenting practices, the difficult temperament at 4–5 months simply represents an overtired infant whose parents were unable to establish healthy sleep. The unhealthy sleep habits might persist.

Support for an association between sleep and temperament is also based on a study by Dr. Marcia Keener in which objective measures of sleep/wake organization, derived from time-lapse video recordings, were compared with parental perceptions of infant temperament at 6 *months* of age. Dr. Keener stated that "infants considered [temperamentally] easy have longer sleep periods and spend less time out of the crib for caretaking interventions during the night." Her analysis also led her to the conclusion that night waking is caused by environmental (parental) rather than biological factors. This observation of increased time out of the crib for temperamentally more difficult children at 6 months is similar to the observation that increased night waking occurs in formerly extremely fussy/colicky infants at 4, 8, and 12 months, and it is also similar to the observation that mothers with depressive symptoms unnecessarily attend to their babies by removing them from the crib more often than mothers without these symptoms.

Utilizing a computerized movement detector, it was observed that for *12-month-old* children, those with the temperament trait of increased rhythmicity went to sleep earlier and had longer sleep durations, and by *18 months* of age there was again the observation that both subjective and objective improved sleep measures were associated with easier-temperament assessments.

At several ages during the first year of life, using sleep diaries and objective measurements, more recent research by Dr. Karen Spruyt also confirmed that increased sleep is linked with an easy temperament.

Additionally, in a study of about one thousand Canadian families, temperament assessments were performed at age 5 and 17 months. "Maladaptive parental behaviors" were recorded at 29 and 41 months and included mother's presence until the child fell asleep, giving food/drink after child wakes in the night, and co-sleeping in the mother's bed after awakening at night. Analysis of the data "support the suggestion that difficult temperament is the original context within which sleep disturbances arise . . . when controlling for early sleep problems, difficult temperament remained predictive only of shorter total sleep time [at age 6 years]." Their findings further "suggest that sleep difficulties likely are part of the difficult temperament . . . [and maladaptive parental behaviors] develop *in reaction to* prior sleep problems [emphasis added]." Finally, a Swedish study of ten thousand children from birth to age 5 showed a tendency for frequent wakings and low-quality sleep to persist and to be associated with a difficult temperament at age 1 and 3 years.

Some of the above studies used different terms to describe temperament traits, but the theme is consistent. More sleep equals an easier temperament. But some share a problem called common method variance, which means that because the data obtained regarding sleep and temperament come from the same source, that is the mother, maybe the association between temperament and sleep is not real but instead reflects something about the mother.

However, a study of temperament and sleep was performed using both sleep diary reports from the mother and motion sensors on the child (actigraphs) to objectively measure sleep. At 30 months of age, actigraph reports showed that toddlers who were more physically active had *less* nighttime sleep, as was also observed in my study of 3-year-olds (page 514). Separately, those who were more soothable had *more* nighttime and daytime sleep. Soothability is the ease and speed with which a toddler is comforted after becoming agitated or upset. So objective sleep measurements are associated with temperament.

A careful analysis of forty-five longitudinal studies of sleep behavior in children 4–12 years found only twelve that were rated as "high quality." Examining these twelve studies, they looked at sixty-one possible determinants for sleep duration. Only three showed evidence for causing short sleep duration: difficult temperament, more screen time, and past history of short sleep duration. As previously discussed, short sleep durations are associated with a difficult temperament and more screen time and there may be a genetic component to more screen time (page 324), so all three items might be interrelated.

I believe that sleep modulates *temperament* so it is important to get a handle on your child's sleep early to influence temperament and thus mitigate the adverse sleep outcomes associated with a difficult temperament.

Association between Temperament and Extreme Fussiness/Colic

When parents performed a temperament assessment when their child was *2 weeks* of age and kept a twenty-four-hour behavior diary at *6 weeks* of age, it was observed that more difficult temperaments at 2 weeks predicted more crying and fussing at 6 weeks. At *4 weeks* of age, infants who were temperamentally more difficult in general, and more intense and less distractible (less consolable) in particular, cried more during their second month of life than other infants.

Another prospective study performed temperament assessments at the age of 3 and 12 *months*. At 3 *months,* the extremely fussy/colicky infants were more intense, more persistent, less distractible, and more negative in their mood. However, at 12 *months,* ratings on the temperament questionnaire showed no group differences between the formerly extremely fussy/colicky infants and the control group, but the general impression of the mothers of the colicky group was that they were more difficult.

Infants who had extreme fussiness/colic, using Dr. Wessel's exact criteria, are more likely to have a difficult temperament than non-colicky babies when the temperament assessment is performed at 4–5 *months* of age. Furthermore, this progression occurs even when extreme fussiness/colic is successfully treated with the no-longer-used drug dicyclomine hydrochloride. Similar results were observed in another study: While behavioral management significantly reduced evening fussing and crying, successful treatment had no effects on later temperament ratings—the infants were still described as difficult. This suggests the possibility that some developmental feature causing extreme fussiness/colic before 4 months was suppressed by the drug, but when the drug was stopped at 4 months, this developmental feature, no longer suppressed, expressed itself as short sleep durations, night wakings, and a difficult temperament.

Mother-Driven Path: The Role of the Mother

What is meant by *mother-driven influences*? Dr. Aldrich showed that all babies have some uncategorizable crying, or crying for no apparent reason. But in my study, I found that babies that fulfilled Wessel's exact criteria for colic did so because of lots of fussing *but not crying.* These mothers were my patients from the time they gave birth, and at each office visit I gave them information regarding fussing/crying, soothing, and sleeping. This strongly suggests that there is a mother-related component underlying the behavior called extreme fussiness/colic, because when mothers were armed with more information on how to soothe their babies, there was less crying.

Situations in which the mother might find parenting more challenging and thus be associated with extreme fussiness/colic in her baby include young single mothers, mothers with anxiety issues, older mothers of twins, mothers with baby blues or postpartum depression, and mothers who used assisted reproductive technology. These challenges might impair the mother's ability to calm a fussy baby and prevent crying. Later, when the baby is 4 months of age, the mother's influence may be expressed in an overtired infant who is difficult to manage. After 4 months, this child might have sleep problems that persist because of a failure to learn self-soothing or a continuation of parent issues that interfere with healthy sleep (chapter 4). With this mother-driven framework in mind, let's consider what we know about night waking and temperament and how we might prevent post-colic sleep problems.

Night Waking: The Mother-Driven Path

Previously, the infant-driven pathway emphasized developmental changes with the baby (page 486). An alternative view is that instead of or in addition to biological factors, parenting practices, such as unnecessary feedings at night, contribute to sleep fragmentation during the first few months (chapter 4). And these parenting practices may continue to cause fragmented night sleep even after the biologic factors subside around 3–4 months of age.

We know that different parenting styles influence crying and soothing, and we know, too, that differences in mothers' confidence in their role as a parent and differences in discipline style influence when and how babies learn self-soothing. Also suggestive of the important role of the mother is the fact that in industrial societies, attachment parenting practices reduce fussing and crying in some babies during the first few months, but later these same babies are more likely to be unable to sleep well during the night—possibly because they did not learn self-soothing skills (chapter 6).

Parents may become overindulgent and oversolicitous regarding night wakings and not appreciate that they are inadvertently depriving their child of the opportunity to learn how to fall asleep unassisted. Some mothers have difficulty separating from their child, especially at night, while other mothers have a tendency toward depression, which might be aggravated by the fatigue that results from struggling to cope with a colicky infant. In either case, simplistic suggestions to help the child sleep better often fail to motivate a change in parental behavior. If a child fails to learn to fall asleep unassisted, the result is sleep fragmentation or sleep deprivation driven by intermittent positive parental reinforcement. This causes fatigue-driven fussiness long after the colic has resolved, which ultimately creates an overtired family.

Support for this view comes from research on infants at 5 *months* of age who were followed to 56 *months* of age. Dr. Dieter Wolke showed that *crying alone* was not the problem, writing, "Long crying duration and having felt distressed about crying during the first five months were significant predictors of night waking problems at twenty months" but not at 56 months. In other words, the combined factors of long infant crying or fussing plus parental distress at 5 months of age make it more likely that a night-waking problem will develop. Even more significantly, crying with sleep problems at 5 months, rather than crying alone, predicts sleep problems when older. Sleep problems at 5 months remain the best predictor of sleep problems, especially night waking, at 20 months. Dr. Wolke concluded that post-colic "sleep problems are likely to be due to a failure of the parents to establish and maintain regular sleep schedules. . . . This conclusion does not blame parents for sleep difficulties. Rather, it recognizes why many parents adopt strategies to deal with night waking in the least conflictual manner by night feeding or co-sleeping. This may be especially true of parents who are dealing with a temperamentally more difficult infant." Thus long crying in and of itself at 5 months is less predictive of a future night-waking problem than the association of long crying plus parental distress or long crying plus sleep problems.

Although the night waking disappeared between 20 and 56 months in this study, children continued to not sleep well, with unhealthy consequences. In another study, Dr. Wolke examined sixty-four children, age 8–10 years, who as infants had "persistent crying," defined as fussing or crying more than three hours for three days or more each week. The author concluded that they were at risk for hyperactivity problems and academic difficulties. In addition, at 8–10 years of age, the previous persistent criers took a longer time to fall asleep, suggesting that "they were less effective in controlling their own behavioral state to fall asleep."

Therefore, it appears that the increased crying/fussing behavior in infancy is associated with less infant sleep and more signaling at night (fragmented sleep), but the crying/fussing alone does not directly cause later sleep problems. Although the post-colic child's family may be stressed, it appears that it is the failure to establish age-appropriate sleep hygiene that specifically leads to later disrupted sleep and behavioral problems (page 515).

Here is a story of a child who probably had extreme fussiness/colic, even though the parents wanted to call him sleep-deprived. Remember, these labels might be interchangeable and are far less important than your child's behavior. There was no quick sleep solution, but improvement did come slowly. Patience is always rewarded if you are reasonably consistent.

When Jackson was 4 months old, he had never been on any kind of sleep schedule. He seemed to cry all the time and would only sleep about four hours at a time (if we were lucky!). My husband and I would spend hours on end, holding, rocking, bouncing, singing, playing, and doing anything we could think to do to get him to stop crying. Our pediatrician said that he had colic and there was nothing we could do about it but to wait it out. Looking back on it all now, I am convinced that he didn't have colic at all, but was just plain sleep-deprived. At first we were hesitant to allow Jackson to cry without holding him. Given that we are both psychologists, we were scared that leaving him alone to cry would be emotionally scarring and would affect his attachment and self-esteem. But we were both sleep-deprived ourselves, stressed out, and desperate to try anything. Dr. Weissbluth's belief that to not allow him to learn to soothe himself to sleep was damaging in and of itself was what allowed us to finally take the plunge. The first time I put him to sleep in his crib for a nap, I left the room and he screamed bloody murder. I sat at the top of the stairs and just cried and cried. I was convinced I was the worst mother in the world. After twenty minutes (which felt like an eternity), he finally fell asleep and slept for two hours. Unfortunately, later naps did not prove to be so easy. There were times in which he screamed for the whole hour (and I cried for the whole hour) and we would get him and try again later. Jackson was a bit resistant to the whole idea, and even though we were very consistent, he always put up a good fight. Even now, at 9 months old, Jackson will still cry before most naps and bedtime. Sometimes it's thirty seconds, sometimes it's thirty minutes. He sleeps so much better and longer than he ever did. We calculated that before he was averaging ten hours of sleep per day, and after just a few weeks he was sleeping around seventeen hours a day. The best part of all was that he learned how to sleep through the night. Now he goes to bed most nights between 6:00 and 7:00 P.M., and he wakes up usually between 6:00 and 7:00 A.M. He takes two naps per day, one around 9:00 A.M. and the other in the early afternoon. My husband and I finally got the sleep we needed, and the stress level went down dramatically. We have our evenings together back, which we desperately needed. And Jackson's temperament is dramatically improved. I would still say he is a highly active baby, but would no longer say he is fussy. Before, I was certain we would never have an-

other child because it was just too much on us emotionally. But now we are planning to conceive again within the next year.

When you become your child's timekeeper and program her sleep schedules, she will be able to sleep day and night on a regular schedule. For most parents, this is a relatively easy adjustment to make. But for post-colic infants, expect to put forth a greater effort to get them to be regular and consistent. Your effort to keep the child well rested will be rewarded by a calmer, happier, easier-temperament child. Improvement in temperament with better sleep, as mentioned in the story above, is discussed a little later in this chapter. One family that was finally able to permanently "de-crab" their baby with better sleep explained, "The 'other' baby is back!"

Without your effort to maintain sleep schedules, your child will have a tendency to sleep irregularly and become unmanageably wild, screaming out of control with the slightest frustration and spending most of the day engaged in crazy, demanding, and impatient behaviors. The majority of post-colic infants do not fit this extreme picture, but they do require more parental control to establish healthy sleep schedules compared with non-colicky infants. Thus it appears that after about 3–4 months of age, poor sleep habits are learned, not developmentally driven (page 515).

For all post-colic infants over 4 months of age, my clinical observations are that frequent night wakings may be eliminated and sleep durations lengthened if, and only if, parents establish and maintain healthy sleep schedules for their child.

From the perspective of a mother-driven path, it appears that most post-colic sleep problems are not caused primarily by a biological disturbance of sleep/wake regulation; rather, the problem is the parents' failure to allow their baby to learn self-soothing between 2 and 4 months or to establish regular sleep patterns when the colic dissipates. Both obvious and subtle reasons can be cited as to why parents have difficulty in enforcing sleep schedules when colic ends.

Two or more months of crying sometimes adversely and permanently shapes parenting styles. An inconsolable infant triggers in some parents a perception that their baby's behavior is out of their control. They observe no obvious benefit to their young extremely fussy/colicky child when they try to be regular according to clock times or to be consistent in bedtime routines. Naturally, but falsely, they then assume that this handling will not help their post-colic child, either. Unfortunately, they do not observe the transition, at around 2–4 months, from colicky crying to fatigue-driven crying.

Alternatively, some parents may unintentionally and permanently become inconsistent and irregular in their responses to their infant simply because of their own fatigue. The constant, complex, and prolonged efforts they use to soothe or calm their extremely fussy/colicky baby are continued. But these ultimately lead to an overindulgent, oversolicitous approach to sleep scheduling when the colic has passed. Their nurturing at night, for example, becomes stimulating overattentiveness. In responding to their child's every cry, the parents inadvertently deprive her of the opportunity to learn how to fall asleep unassisted. The child then fails to learn the important skill of self-soothing, which she will need her entire life.

Effective behavioral therapy to establish healthy post-colic sleep patterns by teaching the child how to fall asleep and stay asleep may or may not be acceptable to you, depending on your ability to perceive and respond to the sleep needs of your infant (chapter 4).

Some parents, usually mothers, have extreme difficulty separating from their child, especially at night, as was discussed in chapter 4. They may have some difficulty themselves being alone at night because their husband's work requires frequent or prolonged absences, or because nights have always been lonely times for them as a result of anxiety or depression. They perceive every cry as a need for nurturing. These women are wonderful mothers, but they may be too good. The infant's every need is anticipated and met before it is experienced; in doing so, the mother unintentionally thwarts the development of her child's capacity to be alone. For example, she may block her infant's attempts to provide herself with a substitute (such as thumb sucking or use of a pacifier) for her physical presence.

These parents perpetuate brief and fragmented sleep patterns in their children. Their infants become, according to Dr. Thomas Ogden, a child psychiatrist, "addicted to the actual physical presence of the mother and [can]not sleep unless they are being held. These infants are unable to provide themselves an internal environment for sleep." Although the *child* has disturbed sleep, here the focus of the problem and the key to its solution lies with the *parent*.

WARNING

Persistent sleep problems in children have been linked to hyperactivity in children, psychiatric symptoms in adolescents, and depression in their mothers.

Extreme fussiness/colic is the most obvious example of extreme crying, but please remember that any painfully overtired infant or child might cry. In some nonindustrial societies and among parents practicing proximal care (attachment parenting), babies rarely cry, because they are always held close to the mother in a soft carrier, highlighting the role of the mother. However, even where there is constant holding and unrestricted breastfeeding throughout the day and night, babies still cry and fuss, which supports the notion of a baby-driven path. Here, too, the crying and fussing peak at about 6 weeks of age! Of course, the babies in nonindustrial cultures are less likely to have any tendency toward fussiness caused by overtiredness. These mothers do not drive cars, wear watches, text, check email, or keep many daily appointments to which they must drag their infants. Also, there is less environmental stimulation during the day, so the baby might sleep well outdoors when the mother is planting rice or cooking. Our lifestyles are different, and may cause our children to become overtired more often.

Temperament: The Mother-Driven Path

Early temperament research suggested to me that biological factors primarily or exclusively caused increased fuss/cry behavior during the first 3–4 months of age and subsequently led to difficult-temperament assessments. I recognized that colic-induced parental distress or fatigue occurred, but I thought that parenting behavior was a much less important factor. Now I have a slightly different view that includes parenting practices both in reaction to the baby and independently contributing to the baby's behavior. The mother's mental health may be a cause of, a reaction to, or both a cause of and a reaction to infant fussing/crying and sleeping issues. For example, Dr. Jordana Bayer found that mothers reporting infant sleep problems in their 4-month-olds "had poorer mental and physical health compared with those not reporting sleep problems. . . . [Those infants with sleep problems] were more likely to be 'exclusively breast fed and perceived by their mothers as temperamentally difficult.'" This topic and the contributing role of the father are also discussed in chapters 5 and 6.

To further confuse the contributions of nature and nurture, some researchers have suggested there is no connection between extreme fussiness/colic and a difficult temperament. According to Wessel, irritability, fussiness, or crying lasting more than three hours a day and occurring more than three days in a week occurs in 49 percent of babies. As described in chapter 7, these arbitrary criteria of more than three hours a day and more than three days a week are sometimes used to describe Wessel's "modified" criteria for colic. Using these modified criteria, some researchers have concluded that colic is not an early manifestation of a difficult temperament. However, Dr. Wessel defined colic as having the additional characteristic of lasting more than three weeks, and this led to the conclusion that about 26 percent of babies had colic. Looking at this smaller and more severely affected group, an opposite conclusion might be drawn: There is a strong association between extreme fussiness/colic before 4 months of age and difficult temperament at 4 months of age. So much depends on how researchers define *colic*. The newer definition focuses less on the amount of crying and more on whether the infant is or is not consolable during a crying spell (pages 391 and 407).

But even when Wessel's strict criteria are used, the reason that extreme fussiness/colic should be viewed perhaps as a risk factor but *not* as an inevitable path to a difficult temperament is that at 4 months of age about 40 percent of children with a difficult temperament did not have extreme fussiness/colic and about 73 percent of infants with excessive fussiness/colic do not develop a difficult temperament. So while there are developmental features contributing to fussing/crying behavior during the first 4 months and temperament at 4 months, these developmental features are not destiny (page 515). Parenting matters!

Also, the good news for parents is that extreme fussiness/colic does *not* appear to be an expression of a *permanently* difficult temperament. In one study of extremely fussy/colicky infants, subsequent measurements of temperament at 5 and 10 months did *not* show group differences between formerly extremely fussy/colicky and common fussy/crying infants. So by practicing healthy sleep habits when extreme fussiness winds down, you may increase the chances that your baby's temperament might dramatically improve. I will discuss how sleep modulates *temperament* below.

Interaction between Baby and Mother

Dr. Douglas Teti wrote, "There is general agreement that infant sleep patterns are complexly determined, and coregulated, with ongoing contributions from both infant and parent. . . . It is very likely that both mother- and infant-driven influences are at play in terms of linkages between maternal depressive symptoms and infant night waking."

Night Waking: Interaction between Baby and Mother (and Father)

Extreme fussiness/colic certainly does not necessarily cause the parents to have difficulty separating from their child. But it is more than a sufficient stimulus to cause some parents to regress toward the least adaptive level of adjustment: They respond and interact too often with their child at night. The result is severe, enduring sleep disturbance in the child. In this setting, simplistic suggestions to help the child sleep better often fail to motivate a change in how the parents approach the problem. Thus, while it is the wakeful child who may be brought for professional help, it may be the parent who has the unappreciated problem.

Night waking in the baby between 3 and 6 months is reduced when *fathers* are more involved during the daytime and nighttime. Here are the facts. In a study by Dr. Liat Tikotzky, of "the triadic links between infant sleep, maternal sleep, and paternal involvement in infant care," both the mothers' and infants' sleep were measured objectively with wrist-worn motion sensors. *Father's general involvement during the day* at 3 months was associated with better mother's sleep at 6 months. Previous studies "suggested that disturbed maternal sleep may contribute to the development of problematic infant sleep patterns. It could be that mothers who experience more nighttime alertness, vigilance, or wakefulness respond faster to the infants' signals at night and are more involved with active nighttime soothing, a behavior that may reinforce infant night wakings." So a father's involvement *at night* directly helps infants have fewer night wakings (page 163), and indirectly, by being *more involved during the day*, helping mothers sleep better, which in turn helps infants sleep better by reducing unnecessary maternal responses to night waking in the baby.

Temperament: Interaction between Baby and Mother

Temperament assessments, performed at an average age of 3.6 months, showed an association between problems of sleep/wake organization, difficult temperament, and extreme crying. Mothers of crying infants scored high on depression, anxiety, exhaustion, anger, adverse childhood memories, and marital distress (chapters 4 and 5). The authors concluded that factors related to parental care, while not *causing* persistent crying, did function to *maintain or worsen* the behavior. The persistence of parental factors may explain why at 1 year there is reported to be more difficulty in communication, more unresolved conflicts, more dissatisfaction, and greater lack of empathy in families with an extremely fussy/colicky infant, and after 4 years formerly extremely fussy/colicky children have been reported to be more negative in mood on temperament assessments.

The exact same sixty infants that I examined at 4–6 months of age were restudied at 3 years. Again, temperamentally easy children had longer sleep durations compared with children with more difficult temperaments. However, there was *no individual stability of temperament traits (except for adaptability) and no individual stability of sleep durations between the ages of 5 months and 3 years* (page 663). Thus, except for *adaptability,* temperament ratings and associated sleep patterns at age 5 months do not predict temperament or sleep patterns at 3 years. Another study, at 18.5 months, objectively measured night sleep durations and showed that children with more rhythmicity slept longer and had fewer wakings, and also that children who were more adaptable and less distractible slept longer. Sleep diary data from the mothers in this study again showed that only the temperament trait adaptability was associated with longer night sleep duration.

Infants who were ranked as having brief sleep periods and difficult temperaments at 5 months and who were ranked as sleeping longer at 3 years had easier temperaments. But for 5-month-olds with brief sleep durations and difficult temperaments who also had brief sleep durations at age 3 years, the difficult temperament persisted. Similarly, individual infants who were ranked as having long sleep periods and easy temperaments at 5 months and later, at 3 years, were ranked as sleeping for shorter durations had more difficult temperaments. But for those 5-month-olds with long sleep durations and easy temperaments who also had long sleep durations at age 3 years, the easy temperament persisted. Sleep modulates temperament!

Dr. John Bates agrees with my hypothesis that sleep modulates temperament and told me that "parenting responses to [sleep] issues would be involved in the continuity/discontinuity of temperament. . . . If parents make the effort to manage their kids' sleep schedules consistently, I would think that over the years they are going to see less difficult and unmanageable behavior."

It appears that both nature and nurture contribute to sleep, temperament, and fussing/crying. I believe that how babies sleep does influence the development of temperament *at 5 months* of age. And how babies sleep during the first few months is a combination of factors within the child and the parents' ability and skill at soothing. I also believe that *at 5 months* of age, the difficult temperament represents an overtired baby and the easy temperament represents a well-rested baby. However, temperament at 5 months of age is not like a fingerprint; it is *not* a permanent marker of your baby's personality.

Professor Isabel Morales-Muñoz (page 73) wrote me: "Concerning sleep duration and infant temperament, and as you suggest, this might be related indeed to the reciprocal influence between parents and children interaction. So in that case, maybe parental attitude toward the child (e.g. parenting strategies) might be a moderator factor of the associations between sleep duration and temperament. For instance, parents who report and experience that their children have longer sleep hours, would also sleep longer hours themselves and consequently might feel more relaxed and less tired during the day, and in that sense, they might interact more positively with their child, and this would indeed positively influence the infant temperament. I am currently on my first month of maternity leave, and I can honestly say that this might be indeed true. :) Those nights when my daughter has a better sleep (which means longer) I am much more relaxed, aware, and in a positive mood the following day, and this allows me to interact more positively with her, which might have some impact in her temperament."

Over time, temperament changes as babies develop and parents change how they soothe their children. Individual temperament measures become more stable during the second year of life or shortly after the second birthday. If you are reading this book before you have had your baby, be prepared to invest enormous efforts in soothing and consider yourself unlucky if your child is among the 20 percent of extremely fussy/colicky babies. However, if you have already had your baby and you are in the midst of suffering through four months of extreme fussiness/colic, reevaluate some of your decisions, if necessary, regarding how you soothe your baby and what is best for your baby and family. Be optimistic, because everything settles down at about 4 months. Everyone gets a second chance at about 4 months to help their child sleep better (page 514).

DIFFERENT DECISIONS FOR DIFFERENT BABIES

Research—both my own and others'—has shown that about 80 percent of babies develop common fussiness/crying and 20 percent develop extreme fussiness/colic. What happens to these babies over the first 4 months? At 4 months of age, some children are super-calm, regular, smiling all the time, and good sleepers, while other babies are the opposite. The good sleepers are described as having an "easy" temperament; the opposite have a "difficult" temperament. Some children are more in between and are described as having an "intermediate" temperament. Remember that the measurements of sleeping, crying/fussing, and temperament are graded or continuous, like your weight in pounds on a scale, and not discrete measurements, like positive or negative results on a pregnancy test. Also, the definitions of common fussiness/crying (or extreme fussiness/colic) and easy temperament (or difficult temperament) are arbitrary. So labels are far less important than your baby's actual behavior. The main message is to watch your baby and pay attention to your own behavior, because how you care for your baby influences your baby's sleeping, crying/fussing, and temperament.

For now, I wish to lead you through a numerical exercise involving a hypothetical group of *one hundred babies*. Skip or skim this numerical exercise if you already have strongly held convictions or if you find it not useful for you. The reason this exercise might be useful is because it might:

1. Help you set your expectations on what you will need to do with your baby, both during the first several weeks in terms of soothing and over the following several months to prevent sleep problems

2. Help you decide whether you will breastfeed or bottle-feed

3. Help you decide whether you will use a family bed, sleep with your baby (see the *SIDS* warning), use a co-sleeper, or use a crib

Out of a group of one hundred babies, during the first 3–4 months, 80 percent (eighty babies) will have common fussiness/crying and 20 percent (twenty babies) will have extreme fussiness/colic. My research has shown that these two groups of babies differ in how their temperaments develop.

Consider the *eighty* common fussy/crying babies at 5 months of age:

A. 49 percent, or *thirty-nine* babies, are temperamentally easy.
B. 46 percent, or *thirty-seven* babies, are temperamentally intermediate.
C. 5 percent, or *four* babies, are temperamentally difficult.

Consider the *twenty* extremely fussy/colicky babies at 5 months of age:

D. 14 percent, or *three* babies, are temperamentally easy.
E. 59 percent, or *twelve* babies, are temperamentally intermediate.
F. 27 percent, or *five* babies, are temperamentally difficult.

Another way to look at this is to note that out of our original hundred babies, at 5 months of age:

Among all forty-two temperamentally easy babies, thirty-nine, or 93 percent, had common fussiness/crying.

Among all forty-nine temperamentally intermediate babies, thirty-seven, or 76 percent, had common fussiness/crying.

Among all nine temperamentally difficult babies, four, or 44 percent, had common fussiness/crying.

A point of view that emphasizes a developmental perspective might argue that a baby with extreme fussiness/colic is five times more likely to develop a difficult temperament than a baby with common fussiness/crying (27 percent versus 5 percent). But obviously, the status of fussing/crying during the first few months is not destiny, because 73 percent of babies with extreme fussiness/colic do *not* develop a difficult temperament, and the role of the parent in modulating temperament is discussed above. It is informative to understand that at 5 months of age, most babies are neither easy nor difficult but somewhere in between.

Of the original hundred babies, the largest temperament group at age 5 months is "intermediate." Forty-nine babies (49 percent) are in this temperament category. Because temperament measurements form a gradation, and the temperament categories represent arbitrary cutoff points, it is possible that the thirty-seven babies in group B, who had common fussiness, tend toward being temperamentally easier than the twelve babies in group E, who had extreme fussiness/colic. I suspect that the parents of the twelve babies in group E had to put forth much more soothing effort into this intermediate temperament group than the parents of the thirty-seven babies in group B. So the biggest temperament group at 5 months of age is in between easy and difficult temperament. It is a mixed group, and within this group some babies may tend to be easier or more difficult but not extremely so in either direction. Enjoy your baby and try not to compare her with other babies who may have different temperaments.

Of the original hundred babies, the next largest temperament group at 5 months is "easy." Forty-two babies (42 percent) are in this temperament category. Of these, thirty-nine babies in group A were born mellow, self-soothing, and calm, and/or their parents were unusually skillful in soothing and/or had vast resources to help them soothe their babies. This was not the case with the three babies in group D. These babies had extreme fussiness/colic at birth. They were not born mellow, self-soothing, or calm. I think these lucky three babies had superhero parents who put forth enormous effort to soothe and probably also had lots of other resources to help them maintain this effort over a period of several months. For these families, it should be smooth sailing ahead regarding sleeping.

The smallest temperament group at 5 months is "difficult." Only nine babies of the original hundred are in this temperament category. The four babies in group C had common fussiness/crying, but they may have been almost, but not quite, extremely fussy/colicky. Alternatively, for these four common fussy babies, maybe something went wrong with the parents' ability to soothe or teach self-soothing. Why might parents be unable to effectively soothe their baby? As we have seen, reasons may include maternal anxiety and/or depression and/or "dysfunctional cognitions" and/or "low parental tolerance to infant crying" regarding infant sleep, an unsupportive husband, too many other children to care for, illness, financial problems, stress from an extended family, and marital problems between husband and wife (chapter 4). The five babies in group F may have over-whelmed all the resources that the parents could bring to bear on soothing their baby. This implies that factors within the baby were so powerful that no matter what the parents did, the baby's extreme fussiness/colic led to a difficult temperament at 5 months of age. It is also possible that the difficult temperament evolved because a combination of factors within the baby and problems within the parents or family conspired to create an overtired child. Preexisting problems such as marital discord, stress from an unsupportive hus-band/father/boyfriend, or maternal anxiety or depression only get worse when parents are trying to cope with an extremely fussy/col-icky baby. Parents' inability to soothe may grow out of, or be a re-sponse to, the fatigue, frustration, and exhaustion of trying, without much success, to soothe an extremely fussy/colicky baby. For these few families, it might be rough or very stormy seas ahead regarding sleeping.

As previously stated, the largest temperament group *at 5 months*, making up 49 percent of the total, is the intermediate temperament group. Some of these babies will closely but not quite resemble easy-temperament babies or difficult-temperament babies. Therefore, for almost half of all babies, advice regarding common fussiness/crying and extreme fussiness/colic (and their respective links to easy and difficult temperaments, and a correspondingly low and high risk of sleep problems) fits only approximately. So please read the entire following section and take out of it only that which applies to your baby.

The risk of developing sleep problems *after 4 months* of age probably looks something like this:

RISKS FOR SLEEP PROBLEMS AFTER 4 MONTHS

LOW RISK (42%)

39 percent of common fussy/crying babies who develop easy temperaments

3 percent of extremely fussy/colicky babies who develop easy temperaments

MEDIUM RISK (49%)

37 percent of common fussy/crying babies who develop intermediate temperaments

12 percent of extremely fussy/colicky babies who develop intermediate temperaments

HIGH RISK (9%)

4 percent of common fussy/crying babies who develop difficult temperaments

5 percent of extremely fussy/colicky babies who develop difficult temperaments

Different temperaments and perhaps different paths to these temperaments will lead to different sleep strategies for each child. It appears to me that the difficult temperament at 5 months mostly represents an extremely overtired baby, while the easy temperament represents an extremely well-rested baby. But keep in mind that biological factors within the baby, such as elevated serotonin levels or immature development of sleep/wake rhythms, may contribute to a baby's behavior during the first 4 months. It is equally necessary to remember that there is enormous variability regarding the resources with which parents are able to soothe their babies, as previously discussed (chapter 4), and there appear to be genetic differences regarding how a child might respond to short sleep durations. So it is important to look at the big picture: your baby, your ability to soothe, and the support structure and resources available to you. What will work for one family may not work for you. As Cindy Crawford says in the foreword, "The most important thing is a well-rested *family*." The goal is to develop a *caring* environment for the family, not a *cure* for extreme fussiness/colic.

Common Fussiness/Crying: Low Risk for Sleep Problems Developing

Breastfeeding becomes much easier around 4 months of age or sooner for babies exhibiting common fussiness/crying because everyone is better rested and life is more predictable. At several weeks of age, your baby will start to show drowsy signs earlier in the evening. Instead of becoming sleepy at 8:00 to 10:00 P.M., she will become sleepy at 6:00 to 8:00 P.M. Respect her need to sleep and *begin the soothing-to-sleep process at the earlier hour.* If you are using a crib, simply put her to sleep earlier. But if you are using a family bed, you have to make some choices. The first is to go to bed much earlier yourself, but this is not usually practical. The second would be to lie down with your baby in your bed and create a safe nest or use a co-sleeper where she will sleep, and then leave her after she has fallen asleep. One danger here is that she might roll off the bed and injure herself (page 93). The third is to transition her to a crib for the beginning of night sleep and until she wakes for her first night feeding, then bring her to your bed for the remainder of the night. Because these are well-rested 4-month-old babies, they are more adaptable and easy to transition to a crib. One strategy is to breastfeed at night and then pass your baby to her father, who soothes her in his arms and then puts her down in the crib. This breaks up the previous pattern of mother/breastfeeding/sleep in parents' bed. If your baby cries, soothe her without picking her up. But if this fails, pick her up and, after soothing, try again.

If you are bottle-feeding (formula or expressed breast milk) or breastfeeding and using a crib around 4 months of age, expect to feed your baby about four to six hours after her last evening bottle and again early in the morning around 4:00 to 5:00 until about 9 months of age. Some bottle-fed babies are fed only once, around 2:00 or 3:00 A.M. If you are breastfeeding and using a family bed, you might feed your baby many times throughout the night.

If you are using a crib, there is more social stimulation as you pick up your baby and more handling as you put the baby down to sleep again. Under these circumstances, after 4 months of age, feeding your baby more than twice at night is likely to create a night-waking or night-feeding habit. If you are breastfeeding, the obvious question is whether the awakenings at night, other than the two times mentioned, are due to hunger. If your breast milk supply has not kept pace with your baby's needs or has decreased, then your baby will wake more at night because of thirst or hunger. One clue suggesting inadequate breast milk is that you are thirsty throughout the day. If so, you are not drinking enough fluid. Or maybe there are some unusual stresses in your life, such as an important trip that you have to take. Are you worried about balancing child care and working, or worried about returning to work and continuing to breastfeed? Is your baby producing less urine? Has the volume of your expressed breast milk decreased? When offered a bottle of expressed breast milk or formula, does your baby now quickly take a much larger feeding? Does she now sleep better or longer after taking a bottle? If you think your child is hungry and you want to continue breastfeeding, contact a lactation consultant through your pediatrician or maternity hospital.

If you are using a family bed (page 93), feeding often throughout the night is not likely to create a night-waking habit. This is because your baby is partially asleep or barely awake when fed. Therefore, the risk of sleep fragmentation for both mother and baby from too much social stimulation is low. With early bedtimes in place, the family bed does not create any sleep problems, and in fact, the family bed may have been part of the soothing solution during the first few months.

After the development of an earlier bedtime, the next sleep change is the evolution of a regular midmorning nap around 9:00 to 10:00. This nap may initially be about forty minutes, but it will lengthen to one or two hours. The rest of the day may be snatches of brief and irregular sleep periods. After the midmorning nap develops, when the baby is a little older, the next regular nap occurs around noon to 2:00 P.M. This nap will also lengthen to become about one to two hours. There may be a third mini nap that is irregular and brief in the late afternoon.

These sleep rhythms are maturing for night sleep and day sleep. A common mistake is to approach the timing of naps and night sleep by strictly enforcing a "by the clock" (BTC) routine. A temperamentally very regular baby might appear to be sleeping BTC, but watching your baby's behavior for sleepy signs (page 167) is more important than watching the clock.

Consider our original group of one hundred babies. At 5 months, of the forty-nine babies in the intermediate temperament group, thirty-seven babies (about 76 percent) had common fussiness when younger. Also, at 5 months, of the forty-two babies in the easy-temperament group, thirty-nine babies (about 93 percent) had common fussiness when younger.

So out of the original *eighty babies* with common fussiness/crying before 4 months of age, the vast majority, seventy-six babies (thirty-nine babies with an easy temperament plus thirty-seven babies with intermediate temperament), or 95 percent, are at a low risk or medium risk at 4 months of age for developing sleep problems because:

Parents are not likely to be stressed.

The infant is likely to be well rested.

The infant is likely to be able to self-soothe.

At night, consolidated sleeping (long sleep duration) develops early.

During the day, regular and long naps naturally develop early, without parental scheduling.

If sleep problems exist, "no-cry" or "maybe-cry" solutions usually work.

Another way to look at this is that out of our original hundred babies, at 4–6 months of age, this low- or medium-risk group represents 91 percent of temperamentally easy and intermediate babies.

Extreme Fussiness/Colic: High Risk for Sleep Problems Developing
Out of the original *twenty babies* with extreme fussiness/colic before 4 months of age, the majority of babies (fifteen, or 75 percent) are at a low or medium risk for developing sleep problems, because they develop easy or intermediate temperaments. But five babies, or 25 percent, develop a difficult temperament and are at a high risk for developing sleep problems because:

Parents are likely to be stressed.
The infant is likely to be overtired.
The infant is likely to be only parent-soothed.
At night, fragmented sleep (night waking) persists.
During the day, irregular and brief naps persist.
If sleep problems exist, "let-cry" solutions might be necessary
    or unacceptable due to added parental stress (chapter 1).

Another way to look at this is that out of our original hundred babies, at 4–6 months of age, the high-risk group represents 9 percent of temperamentally difficult babies. These nine infants might represent two somewhat different groups of children. The first group with a difficult temperament comes from the large group (80 percent) of infants who previously had common fussiness/crying. Only about 4 percent of these children, or about four infants out of a hundred, fall into this category. I think they are less overtired than the second group of five infants who previously had extreme fussiness/colic.

For the first group of infants who had common fussiness/crying and now have a difficult temperament, there is relatively fast improvement when parents put forth great effort to help them sleep better. Such infants are more adaptable, and it is easier to change their sleep routines. No-cry or maybe-cry sleep strategies are likely to work well. Perhaps these parents simply failed to establish an early bedtime after 6 weeks of age or provide timely opportunities for naps after a few months of age, and their child developed cumulative sleepiness during the first 4 months. On the other hand, there may be parent issues (chapter 4) that contributed to the development of a difficult temperament, and these same issues, if they persist, may interfere with helping the child sleep better. Perhaps these babies reflect mainly a mother-driven path.

The second group with a difficult temperament comes from a small group (20 percent of all infants) who previously had extreme fussiness/colic. About five infants out of a hundred fall into this category. I think they are more overtired than the first group. When parents put forth great effort to help them sleep better, there is relatively slow improvement. They are less adaptable, and it is more difficult to change their sleep routines. No-cry or maybe-cry sleep strategies are not likely to work, and these parents might have to consider let-cry sleep strategies or if unacceptable, just start moving the bedtime a little earlier (page 240). Perhaps these babies reflect mainly a baby-driven path. This group represents the majority of children that are referred to me for a sleep consultation.

I believe this small percentage (9 percent) of all babies have the most severe and hard-to-solve sleep problems. There are two reasons for this. The first is that for five of the nine babies, the biological factors that led to extreme fussiness/colic in the first place might persist and frustrate the parents' best efforts to solve sleep problems. The second is that for four of the nine babies who started off with common fussiness/crying, something occurred that led to the children developing a difficult temperament, and whatever social, emotional, or family factors occurred during the first four months might persist thereafter (page 533).

However, this explanation is incomplete, because for the group of five babies with extreme fussiness/colic, maternal anxiety (or depression or "dysfunctional cognitions") may cause the behavior and/or maternal depression may result from this behavior; this suggests that baby–parent interaction is the main path. Also, for the group of four babies who had common fussiness/crying, the fact that measurements of fussiness and crying are graded or continuous means that they might have been close to but just did not quite meet the criteria for extreme fussiness/colic. So it might be an error to overly dwell on nonbiological factors such as the mother.

My idea that at 4–6 months of age there are *two groups* of overtired children who appear to have a difficult temperament is supported by research on an initial group of 1,019 Canadian mothers by Dr. Clifford. Many mothers dropped out of the study, but the 560 mothers who stayed were more likely to be married, have completed more formal education, have higher household incomes, be nonsmokers, breastfeed, and have "higher levels of social support." The researchers noted that at 3 months of age there were thirty-five children (6 percent of this selected population) who were crying enough to be called colicky. Of these thirty-five colicky infants, eighteen (51 percent) had been this way at 6 weeks of age (called "typical colic"), but seventeen (49 percent) had not (they were called "latent colic"). The researchers felt that typical colic and latent colic represented *two groups* of colicky infants. They went on to describe a third group (14 percent of all colicky infants) that continued to cry substantially past 3 months of age. This has been called "persistent mother–infant distress syndrome" by other researchers, who associate it with long-term adverse outcomes.

Interestingly, in Dr. William Carey's work with anxious mothers (chapter 6), he noted the time of onset of colic among thirteen babies: for five, or 38 percent, it was in the first month; for four, or 31 percent, it was in the second month; and for another four, or an additional 31 percent, it was in the third month. Maybe these three groups are similar to the three groups described above: typical colic, latent colic, and "mother–infant distress syndrome."

Maybe the typical colic infants were what I refer to as extreme fussiness/colic and reflect a mainly baby-driven pathway, while the

528   MARC WEISSBLUTH, M.D.

latent colic infants may have started out as common fussiness/cry-
ing and reflect a mainly mother-driven pathway, so after 6 weeks
these overtired infants (from sleep fragmentation or a late bedtime)
exhibited colicky behavior. In other words, comparing the above
study on 560 families with my analysis, I would say that at 4 months
of age there are about 9 percent of overtired children with difficult
temperaments, falling into two groups: the first, five out of nine
children (56 percent), were formerly extremely fussy/colicky babies
(similar to the 51 percent with typical colic); the second, four out of
nine (44 percent), had common fussiness/crying (similar to the 49
percent with "latent colic"). I believe that those families with limited resources for soothing or persistent parent issues (chapter 4) are
more likely to have babies who are at greater risk for the overtired/
fussy/crying state to persist. The term *mother–infant distress syndrome* (pages 467 and 527) is similar to the notion of mother–baby
interaction issues, discussed above. But this term and the general notion of a mother-driven path are objectionable because of the blame
they direct solely to the mother. Obviously, fathers, grandparents,
financial factors, and so forth can stress a family independent of the
mother's capabilities to nurture her child.

On the other hand, my research agrees with the typical time
course of colic originally described by Drs. Wessel and Illingworth
(page 391): Colic begins in 70 to 80 percent of infants by the second
week and 90 to 100 percent by the fourth week; colic disappears by
the end of the third month in 85 to 93 per cent of infants and about
100 per cent by the end of the fourth month. In Dr. Clifford's study,
about 85 per cent of colicky infants (typical colic plus latent colic)
had resolution of their colic by three months, and "once colic resolves, the residual effects on levels of maternal distress (anxiety
and depression) are negligible." She acknowledged that "most
mothers in this study were married and financially secure, along
with the relative universality of health care in Canada, [which] suggests that families in the study would have adequate resources to
buffer the effects of their infants' colic." So it appears that if colicky

fussiness/crying starts later, at 6 weeks, so-called latent colic, as long as it ends by 3 months there are no adverse outcomes. This idea is supported by a recent study from Australia on children at age 2–3 years who, as infants, previously had colic: "infants with colic whose crying self-resolves do not experience adverse effects regarding child behavior, regulatory abilities, temperament, or family functioning."

In contrast, there are published studies suggesting that infant colic is associated with long-term adverse outcomes, but they all contain flaws such as relying on retrospective reports of infant crying, lacking data regarding onset and disappearance of crying, lacking diagnostic criteria for colic, relying on mother's report for crying and mother's perception of later problems (common method variance), and preceding or concurrent associated problems such as sleeping difficulties or high "maternal burden of infant care" in a study by Dr. Smarius describing the opposite conditions experienced by the Canadian mothers in Dr. Clifford's study.

So by the fourth month, when extreme fussiness/colic is no longer present, take a deep breath, kick back, have a drink, and as long as there are no other worries, be confident that if your child is not sleeping so great now, soon she will be (page 533).

UNDERSTANDING YOUR BABY

Before 4 months: Was there extreme fussiness/colic or common fussiness/crying?

At 4–6 months: Is there a difficult or easy temperament?

After 4 months: Will there be a high or low risk for sleep problems?

UNDERSTANDING YOUR FAMILY

Consider the behavior of both parents and any parent issues.

Consider your resources for soothing.

Living with and soothing a baby who has extreme fussiness/colic is discussed in chapter 6. Here is some more information on how common fussiness/crying/easy temperament versus extreme fussiness/colic/difficult temperament may affect some parenting decisions.

HOW AND WHEN TO MOVE YOUR BABY OUT OF YOUR BED

If you decided that you wanted a family bed before your child was born (page 93), and if your child has common fussiness/crying, you might decide to continue the family bed for a long time. Then, when you move your baby out, the transition might be very easy if your baby now develops an easy temperament. But if your decision for a family bed was in reaction to extreme fussiness/colic and your child now has a difficult temperament, the transition might be very stressful for the entire family because your child may not have learned self-soothing.

Q: *I am breastfeeding and my child sleeps with us, but I want to move her out of our bed. How do I do this?*

A: There is no one right way to do this, but if your child has learned self-soothing, you can do this quickly at any age. However, if your child lacks self-soothing skills, you probably will do it gradually and slowly over several weeks or a few months. Make the move when both parents agree that it is the right time. Always be mindful of your baby's safety. Initially, respond promptly when your baby calls for you. Later, you might delay your response. A baby might be placed in a crib close to the side of your bed. Later, the crib is moved a few inches from your bed. Gradually the crib is moved farther away until it is in baby's room. An older child might sleep on a mattress on the floor in your room, with or without the parent. Later, the mattress is moved to the child's room, with or without the parent. Sometimes you might just want your child to be in her crib or bed but in your room. If you are going to use a separate room and your child is older, announce the planned move in advance, and make the room very attractive or let her help decorate her room. Alternatively, move your baby into the room or bed where the siblings are sleeping. Some parents will begin the night with the child in the parents' bed and then move the child to a crib after she has fallen asleep.

Q: *Do I have to wean my baby from breastfeeding before I move her out of our bed?*

A: I think the answer depends on your resources for soothing other than breastfeeding, especially the assistance of the father, plus your desire to continue or to discontinue breastfeeding. I see no reason why weaning from breastfeeding has to precede or accompany your moving the baby. But if non-nutritive breastfeeding is the only way your child will fall asleep, you probably will want to teach her some self-soothing before discontinuing completely the non-nutritive breastfeeding and moving her out of your bed.

BREASTFEEDING

Breastfeeding babies with extreme fussiness/colic/difficult temperament may be difficult because everyone is tired. As the biological need for an earlier bedtime develops, the best strategy is to temporarily try to put your baby to sleep earlier (page 300), but the main theme is to do whatever it takes to maximize sleep and minimize crying. The plan is to keep your child as well rested as possible in order to buy time for the development of more mature sleep/wake rhythms. Once these rhythms are developed, they may be used as an aid to help your child sleep better. For example, the breastfeeding mother of an infant with extreme fussiness/colic/difficult temperament might want to take the baby into her bed and nurse her to sleep at the earlier bedtime and then, once she is asleep, move her to a co-sleeper or crib or use a family bed (see the *SIDS* warning). However, real-life events, such as returning to work or caring for other family members, might not permit the luxury of always sleeping with your baby whenever she appears to be sleepy.

ATTACHMENT PARENTING

You may have wanted to practice attachment parenting before your baby was born (chapter 1). If your baby has common fussiness/crying/easy temperament and is at low risk for sleep problems, then it is more likely that caring for her will not be exhausting and both mother and baby will have opportunities for sleep, making attachment parenting attractive and easy to execute. The opposite scenario occurs with a baby with extreme fussiness/colic/difficult temperament and a high risk for sleep problems. With these babies, a proactive decision to practice attachment parenting or a decision made reactively to the child's behavior may succeed if there are enormous resources for soothing, but in their absence the result might be an extremely overtired family.

Can you change your lifestyle so that your child will receive the soothing to sleep at those times when your child needs to sleep? Can you avoid too much social stimulation from interfering with sleep even if it means ignoring your child's crying at those times when she needs to sleep? These are difficult questions that challenge about 20 percent of families during the first 2–4 months because of extreme fussiness/colic and about 9 percent of families at 4 months because of overtired child/difficult temperament. Successfully dealing with these challenges will prevent sleep problems in the future.

SLEEP MODULATES TEMPERAMENT

Understanding temperament allows you to more clearly identify specific features in your baby's personality. Sleeping better makes for an easier *temperament*, and healthier sleep is something that parents can accomplish.

I believe that the quality of your baby's sleep influences the development of temperament at 4–6 months of age. And how babies sleep during the first few months is a combination of factors within the child and the parents' ability and skill at soothing. It is also my belief that at 4–6 months of age, the difficult temperament represents an overtired baby and the easy temperament represents a well-rested baby. Remember: The temperament that your baby has at 4–6 months of age is *not* permanent. Temperament changes over time as babies develop and parents modify how they soothe their children.

Additionally, as described by parents in chapters 4–7, children's personalities may be severely and adversely affected when they are short of sleep, but the good news is that these changes are reversible!

NAPS

The Midday Nap

After the midmorning nap develops, a midday nap rhythm evolves that will have your baby sleeping best between 12:00 and 2:00 P.M. Some caveats are in order, however. The evolution of nap rhythms is not the same in all children, as mothers of fraternal twins can attest! Additionally, the window when naps are easily obtained varies among children in terms of being wide (for example, anytime between 12:00 and 2:00 P.M.) or narrow (for example, between 12:30 and 1:30 P.M.). There will be some trial and error to find the best times when your child's brain goes into nap mode, so be patient and do not compare your child with other children. Children who had common fussiness/crying and later an easy temperament might slip effortlessly and early into two long naps, while parents of children with extreme fussiness/colic who later have a difficult temperament might struggle longer with the challenge of establishing regular and predictable naps—and be frustrated because the naps are somewhat short! The foundation for the midday nap is the midmorning nap, just as the foundation for the midmorning nap is night sleep. Gradually, for all children, naps will become more predictable and longer. Attempts to extend naps by reswaddling, replacing a pacifier, or offering a quick feeding may help, especially for well-rested children.

A third, brief, late-afternoon nap is common, but this nap does not occur in all children, and among children who take this nap, some do not take it consistently.

Transition from Brief Intervals of Wakefulness to Clock Time

As nap rhythms mature, the naps will become more predictable and longer if and only if they are in sync with biological nap cycles. Although they will not occur at exactly the same clock time every day, you will be able to watch the clock a little more. If you have good timing, you might not see drowsy signs, because you are perfectly catching the sleep wave. Because drowsy signs might be absent and because the naps are now getting longer, you want to move away from the notion of brief intervals of wakefulness and focus more on the clock-time window when your child takes her nap best. (Naps are also discussed in chapters 2, 3, and 4.)

SLEEPING THROUGH THE NIGHT

What does the phrase *sleeping through the night* mean? You might be surprised that there is no standard or widely accepted definition. In 2010, Dr. Jacqueline Henderson studied three different definitions:

1. Sleeping uninterrupted from midnight to 5:00 A.M.
2. Sleeping eight hours uninterrupted between sleep onset and waking time in the morning, without regard to the clock time when the sleep occurred
3. Sleeping uninterrupted between 10:00 P.M., or earlier, and 6:00 A.M.

Sleeping uninterrupted means that there is no feeding or soothing.

Here are her data:

INFANTS SLEEPING THROUGH THE NIGHT

Age	Definition of *Sleeping through the Night*		
	12:00–5 A.M.	8 hours straight	10:00 P.M.–6:00 A.M.
3 months	58%	Less than 50%	Less than 40%
4 months	Almost 70%	58%	Less than 50%
5 months	More than 70%	About 60%	53%

So at 3 months of age, 58 percent of babies are able to sleep uninterrupted for five hours between midnight and 5:00 A.M. By 4 months of age, this number is almost 70 percent, and 58 percent of babies are able to sleep uninterrupted for eight hours. By 5 months of age, more than half of all babies (53 percent) sleep uninterrupted for eight hours or more when their parents are likely to sleep. So by any definition, more than half of all babies are sleeping through the night by age five months. The data about sleeping through the night describe a population of children. But what is most important for you is your own child's behavior and mood in the late afternoon and early evening, which can guide you toward a reasonably early bedtime and help you avoid unnecessary soothing and feeding in the middle of the night.

Dr. Henderson wrote, "The most rapid consolidation in infant sleep regulation occurs in the *first 4 months*. . . . [This] reflects the emergence of infant's self-regulation and self-soothing capacities [emphasis added]." A 2015 report showed that about 70 percent of 3-month-olds were described by parents to sleep continuously for five hours or more, but video evidence showed that about a quarter of them actually "resettle"—they wake and return to sleep unassisted (page 61). These reports support the idea of using the child's natural internal sleep regulation machinery as an aid to help your child sleep better during the *first 4 months*. Because this process of sleep regulation is developing during the first 4 months, there is no reason for most parents to delay and begin to think about helping their child sleep better only at 4 months of age. Starting earlier is easier.

As discussed in chapter 5, my research shows that with extinction in children *younger than 4 months,* the average amount of crying is as follows:

Night 1:	Crying lasts 30–45 minutes
Night 2:	Crying lasts 10–30 minutes
Night 3:	Crying lasts 0–10 minutes
Night 4:	No crying

In children *4 months of age* and older, the usual pattern is:

Night 1:	Crying lasts 45–55 minutes
Night 2:	A little more or a little less crying than night 1
Night 3:	Crying lasts 20–40 minutes
Night 4 or 5:	No crying

If the bedtime is too late or naps are not going well, the process might take longer or not work.

Therefore, because children may cry less and for fewer days when younger, parents should respect and take advantage of their baby's capabilities to sleep longer at night during the first 4 months of life and not wait until their child is older to help their baby sleep well. The earlier you start to teach self-soothing, the better. It is never too early to start—but it is also never too late to begin.

What We Know and What We Do Not Know

During the first four months, among infants and parents, there are:

A. Different amounts of infant *fussing/crying*
B. Different patterns of infant *sleeping*
C. Different ratings of infant *temperaments*
D. Different parental behaviors at bedtime and during the night

We do not know exactly to what degree these four items are independent or how they may be related to each other.

We do not know exactly how the mixture of within-the baby features and parenting behaviors affect these four items.

We do not know exactly how genetics plays a role in the interaction between babies and parents regarding these items.

But we do know some useful facts:

1. Biological development of adultlike sleep patterns for night sleep matures over the first few months.

2. During the first four months, we know what predicts future sleep problems.
   Yes: Failure to learn self-soothing
   No: Extreme fussing/crying alone
   No: Difficult temperament alone

3. Parents can help or hinder the development of the self-soothing skills needed for healthy sleep habits.

4. Parents can correct sleep problems, and the ill effects from unhealthy sleep are largely *reversible*.

5. Anxiety and depression in mothers and fathers may make promoting healthy sleep habits more difficult. Past-year preva-

lence means that during a twelve-month period, around 2002, 23 percent of women (and 20 percent of men) had an anxiety disorder and 14 percent of women (and 10 percent of men) had depression. But *31 percent* of adults experience an anxiety disorder at some time in their lives!

6. Children who do not sleep well when young are at a higher risk for adverse outcomes when older.

By the end of your child's fourth month, unexplained fussiness/crying should disappear and sleeping at night should be regular, consolidated, and not a problem (pages 525 and 535).

By the end of your child's fourth month, if your child's fussing/crying has not disappeared or if your child has difficulty falling asleep or staying asleep at night, and you do not see a sleep solution (chapter 5), *seek help*. Talk to your child's care provider, a professional counselor, or a community sleep consultant. A well-rested family is needed for the parents' mental health and the child's healthy development!

7. During the first four months and beyond, there are cultural differences regarding:

   A. Bedtimes
   B. Night sleep durations
   C. Sleeping arrangements

We do not know exactly how these three items affect children in different cultures.

Summary and Action Plan for Exhausted Parents

If you are too tired to read much and just want to do *something* to help your child sleep better, read chapter 1.

If you have symptoms of anxiety or depression, they might worsen because you have become short on sleep. Ask yourself: *Am I likely to be so concerned about my child at night that I might want to attend to her when she appears to be sleeping contentedly because I worry about her health?* Or: *I feel that she needs my company even when she is sleeping; does my baby appear to be unusually fussy and hard to soothe to sleep or not able to sleep well?* Or: *Is there stress in my marriage, perhaps because the father is not supportive during the day or in baby care at night?* Under these circumstances, review chapter 1, or if willing, have your husband read this, and try some no-cry sleep solutions and proceed slowly and gradually (chapter 5) with a slightly earlier bedtime (page 240) to help your baby sleep better. A little extra sleep at the front end may make a world of difference (page 102). Discuss your overall situation with your husband, partner, or child's caregiver. Maybe consider engaging a community sleep consultant to help prevent sleep problems from developing or find solutions (page 331).

MAJOR POINT

To help children sleep better, 91 percent of families never have to let their child cry, provided that they start helping their baby learn to sleep early. No-cry sleep solutions may be used successfully (pages 240 and 331).

During the first four months, colicky infants, by definition, exhibit more fuss/cry behavior. Extremely fussy/colicky infants sleep less than common fussy/crying infants at 4 months of age, but group differences disappear by 6–8 months. Also, by 6 months of age, researchers are more apt to describe parents contributing to sleep problems, especially night waking or signaling.

Infant crying alone does not predict the development of sleep problems. Rather, the combination of crying plus parental distress or crying plus sleep problems at 5 months predicts night waking at 20 months, but not at 56 months.

Assessments at 2 and 4 weeks of age showed that infant-temperament difficultness predicted increased crying/fussing at about 6 weeks of age. Infants with extreme fussiness/colic are more likely to have a difficult temperament when assessed at 4 months of age, but not at 12 months. A difficult temperament is associated, at many ages, with problems in sleeping, such as shorter sleep durations and night waking, but this association is not predictive of later sleep problems.

Despite successful treatment of colic, a difficult temperament and sleep problems may emerge after 4 months. This led to my original view that emphasized the baby-driven pathway. We now know that, at bedtime, the emotional availability of the mother and the quality of her bedtime behavior will influence the development of self-soothing skills in her child. We now know that maternal behavior during the night (unnecessary feeding and attending to the baby) causes sleep fragmentation, which in turn may contribute to or cause sleep problems such as night waking. We also know that a supportive and helpful partner directly helps the child sleep better and indirectly helps the child sleep better by helping the mother sleep better.

It is important for parents to help post-colic infants establish healthy sleep habits.

After extreme fussiness/colic winds down around 4 months of age or sooner, a child may be overtired, not sleeping well, and difficult to manage. But not all difficult-to-manage 4-month-olds have extreme fussiness/colic. I think there are two groups of children at 4–6 months of age, both of whom have difficult temperaments.

The first group with a difficult temperament comes from the large group (80 percent) of infants with common fussiness/crying. Only about 4 percent of the children with common fussiness/crying fall into this category. No-cry sleep strategies are likely to work well with these children.

The second group with a difficult temperament comes from a

small group (20 percent) of infants with extreme fussiness/colic. About 27 percent of children with a difficult temperament fall into this category. No-cry sleep strategies are not likely to work with these children, and parents might consider let-cry sleep strategies or simply move the bedtime earlier.

Difficult-temperament children in both groups have trouble falling asleep and staying asleep. At about 4 months, they might not have developed self-soothing skills, perhaps because parents invested constant soothing to prevent their child's fussiness from developing into crying; because anxious mothers caused sleep fragmentation; or because the inability to self-soothe is an integral component of colic. A successful intervention effort to help families cope with infant crying during colic will reduce parental distress. Continued age-appropriate sleep hygiene after colic ends is likely to prevent sleep problems persisting beyond 4 months of age. Unsuccessful intervention increases the likelihood that temperament issues, family stress, and sleep problems will persist beyond 4 months.

Intervention with extinction is effective, fast, and safe, but some parents are unable or unwilling to use this method. For these parents, graduated extinction or fading may offer a more palatable and still effective alternative (page 240 and chapter 4).

What a Parent Can Do

Encourage your partner to help care for the baby daytime and nighttime.

Encourage self-soothing; the earlier, the better.

If there is no colic, put your child to sleep drowsy but awake, then leave the room.

If there is colic, focus on *care*, not *cure*. Develop coping strategies.

Set an earlier bedtime for all children after 6 weeks of age.

Set an early bedtime based on drowsy signs; practice consistent bedtime routines, including massage; be emotionally available at bedtime.

Feed when hungry but ignore nighttime non-distress vocalizations.

Provide opportunities for naps based on drowsy signs.

Avoid irregularity of sleep schedules, including between weekdays and weekends.

Practice safe sleep recommendations.

No TV in the child's room; limit screen time.

Take breaks; try to get more sleep for yourself.

Now might be the time to change soothing and bedtime strategies, because extreme fussiness/colic is ending.

Appreciate the individuality of your child's temperament and sleep needs.

Seek help if your child is not sleeping well (from the child's primary care provider or a community sleep consultant) or for yourself or your partner, especially if there are symptoms of anxiety or depression or significant *risk factors, parent issues,* or *adverse concerns*.

Chapter 9 Outline

TOTAL SLEEP DURATION TRENDS OVER TIME

NIGHT SLEEP

Sleeping through the Night
Bedtime Hour Trends over Time
Bedtime
Night Wakings for Feeding
Bedtime Battles, Difficulty Falling Asleep
Night Wakings (Signaling), Difficulty Staying Asleep
Teething and Growing Pains
Common Night Sleep Issues
   Brief Sleep Durations
   Having More than One Child Creates Bedtime Problems
   Unable to Fall Asleep
   Will Not Sleep Anywhere Else
   Only One Bedroom

DAY SLEEP

Day Sleep Duration by Age
Number of Naps per Day by Age
Day Sleep Duration Trends over Time
Common Day Sleep Issues
   Nap Deprivation
   Fixing Nap Schedules

SLEEP RECOMMENDATIONS

Months 4–8
   Wake-Up Time in Morning
     When the Wake-Up Time Is Too Early
Morning Time Awake

Healthy Sleep Habits in Months 4–12

> *To White Noise*
> *You are the sound silence*
> *makes in its sleep, air made*
> *visible by smoke, deepest*
> *breath with no breathing*
> *O my digital ocean, O un-*
> *broken shush of mortality*
> *O my digital sister, thank*
> *you, thank you for keeping*
> *the children from climbing*
> *over the fence of sleep.*
>
> —Carrie Fountain

If you have not done so already, please go back and read chapter 1.

The main goals at this age are:

To encourage the development of self-soothing skills for night sleep, the midmorning nap, and the midday nap.

To synchronize the time when you put your child to sleep with the onset of your child's biological sleep rhythms.

Routines that comfort your baby, including rocking, lullabies, stroking, patting, and cuddling for bedtime (chapter 4), may also be used intact or modified for nap time. Maintain these routines so your child learns to associate certain behaviors occurring at certain times in a familiar place with the behavior called "falling asleep."

After 1 year of age, soft, silky, or furry-textured blankets, dolls, or stuffed animals in crib or a small soft blanket over the top of the head, like a scarf, may be comforting for your child.

Helpful Hints for Comforting Routines
　　Dim night-light
　　Nursing to sleep

Nurse to sleep? Isn't that contrary to the advice to always put your baby down drowsy but awake? There are many well-rested 4-month-old children with self-soothing skills who often fall asleep with nursing. Some of the parents of these children had practiced putting them down drowsy but awake when their children were younger so their baby could achieve self-soothing skills. If this is the case with your family, there is nothing wrong with nursing your baby to sleep. Most nursing mothers in my practice do this all the time. But if you have difficulty letting your child learn to fall asleep unassisted, if your child *always* falls asleep at the breast, and if your child has disturbed sleep, then nursing to sleep might be part of the sleep problem. It may reflect the kind of separation problems discussed in chapter 4.

Many mothers nurse their babies for soothing and comfort as well as feeding, and their babies may or may not fall asleep at the breast. In either case, the key is to place your baby in the crib when there is a *need* to sleep. I think that this intimacy between mother and infant is beautiful, and nursing to sleep, in itself, does not necessarily cause sleep problems.

Here are some common questions in this age range:

Q: *Do I roll my older child over to his favorite sleeping position when he wakes up during the night? Do I help him get down when he stands up and shakes the crib railings?*

A: No. I doubt that you like playing these games with your child at night. Think, too, about what you teach him when you go to him at night to roll him over to his favorite sleeping position or help him down. But if he rolls over only once at night or gets stuck in the railings of the crib, then help him go back to sleep.

Q: *Won't he hurt himself if he falls down in his crib? He can't get down by himself.*

A: No, he won't hurt himself. He may fall into an awkward heap . . . and sleep like a puppy.

Try to be reasonably regular: Watch the intervals of wakefulness in babies 4 months of age or younger, and when your baby is over 4 months, watch both him and the clock. However, try not to get locked into a fixed or unvarying bedtime or nap time hour; vary the times a little depending on the wake-up time, the duration of naps, when the second nap ended, and indoor versus outdoor activities. Often babies between 9 and 12 months need to go to bed earlier because of increased physical activity in the afternoon and the absence of a third nap. Remember, too late a bedtime causes disturbed sleep just as nap deprivation does.

When you are somewhat organized regarding sleep schedules, the child accepts and expects sleep. But don't feel you have to be so organized for feeding or other infant care practices! Probably the opposite is true for feeding. When parents are creative, free-spirited, and permissive regarding wholesome foods, feeding solid foods usually goes well. So respect the biological basis for regular sleep, and accept or reject popular practices for feeding wholesome solid food as you see fit. But sleeping and feeding are similar in that just as junk food is bad for the body, junk sleep is bad for the brain (chapters 2 and 3).

Our goal is to establish sleep habits, so we don't want to get sidetracked at this stage by worrying too much about crying. When your 2-year-old cries because he wants to play instead of having his diaper changed or your 1-year-old cries because he wants juice instead of milk, you don't let the crying prevent you from doing what is best for him. Establishing healthy sleep habits does not mean that there will always be a lot of crying, but there may be some in protest. If you find this to be unacceptable when your child is 4 months old or younger, then by all means consider waiting until he is older to help him sleep better. But also consider that it may be harder to achieve when older. And remember:

By the end of your child's fourth month, if your child's fussing/crying has not disappeared or if your child has difficulty falling asleep or staying asleep at night, and you do not see a sleep solution (chapter 5), *seek help.* Talk to your child's care provider, a professional counselor, or a community sleep consultant. A well-rested family is needed for the parents' mental health and the child's healthy development!

As discussed in chapter 5, my research shows that with extinction in children *younger than 4 months,* the average amount of crying is as follows:

Night 1:   Crying lasts 30–45 minutes
Night 2:   Crying lasts 10–30 minutes
Night 3:   Crying lasts 0–10 minutes
Night 4:   No crying

In children *4 months of age and older,* the usual pattern is:

Night 1:   Crying lasts 45–55 minutes
Night 2:   A little more or a little less crying than night 1
Night 3:   Crying lasts 20–40 minutes
Night 4 or 5: No crying

If the bedtime is too late or naps are not going well, the process might take longer or not work.

Therefore, because children may cry less and for fewer days when younger, parents should respect and take advantage of their baby's capabilities to sleep longer at night during the first four months of life and usually not wait until their child is older to help him sleep well at night. The earlier you start to teach self-soothing, the better. It is never too early, but it is also never too late to begin.

It will become more difficult to change your baby's sleep patterns after about 6 months of age because of the development of *self-agency*. Self-agency means that your child can express likes and dislikes with greater energy and persistence than previously. If your infant wants to reach a desired toy, he may persist longer in trying to get it into his grasp. Your infant might protest at being changed or being put down to sleep, and he can now express his protest more loudly and longer than when he was younger. This increased ability to express intentional behavior may be described as persistence, drive, or determination.

Self-agency becomes stronger over time. During the first few months, you could change the diaper whenever you wished, and there was no protest. Distraction was an effective method to help get the job done when he became squirmy. After 6 months, distraction is now less effective because your infant has a stronger sense of self-agency. Your baby thinks that he can do whatever he wants to do, whenever he wants to do it. This independence leads to persistence, which may be desirable ("My son is determined to walk") or undesirable ("He is so stubborn all the time"). We welcome some efforts, but willful opposition makes the daily ordinary chores of parenting much harder. Some infants are more strong-willed than others. This is their nature, and you cannot change this feature of their personality. Being strong-willed may have a negative ring to it, but maybe the trait of being persistent as an infant will turn into the desirable trait of ambition or grit as an adult.

Self-agency might lead your child to protest naps because he would rather play than sleep or stay up late for more soothing company with parents. If you allow him to not nap or to stay up late, then he will become fatigued. The adaptive response to fatigue is to fight it with stimulating hormones, which allow your baby to maintain more wakefulness. However, this heightened state of alertness or arousal creates an inability to easily fall asleep or stay asleep for subsequent naps or night sleep. Not only does a vicious cycle of sleep problems begin, but as a by-product, your child may develop emotional lability (swift, sharp changes in mood) or an impaired attention span.

Total Sleep Duration Trends over Time

A review by Lisa Matricciani found that "over the last 103 years, there have been consistent rapid declines in the sleep duration of children and adolescents." A study by Dr. Ivo Iglowstein showed that total sleep durations have decreased steadily from 1974 through 1979 and 1986. This trend was confirmed in studies by Dr. Anna Price and me for middle-class or middle-socioeconomic-status (SES) families.

AVERAGE TOTAL SLEEP DURATION, 1979–80 AND 2004

1979–80	2004
14.1 hours (4–11 months)	14.0 hours (4–6 months)
	13.6 hours (7–9 months)
	13.4 hours (10–12 months)

This trend was also noted for higher-SES families in the early part of the twentieth century by Dr. Josephine Foster and at the beginning of the twenty-first century by Dr. Avi Sadeh:

AVERAGE TOTAL SLEEP DURATION, 1927 AND 2006

1927	2006
14.0 hours (6–11 months)	13.3 hours (3–5 months)
	12.9 hours (6–8 months)
	12.8 hours (9–11 months)

We do not know why children are currently sleeping less than in the past. Here are three possible explanations:

1. Center-based daycare became more popular when mothers entered the workforce in large numbers between the 1970s and 1990s. Center-based daycare is associated with shorter naps according to two studies, one conducted by Dr. Price and the other by Dr. Janet Lam. In 2011, the Institute of Medicine published specific recommendations for center-based daycare with the expectation that they would be included in state regulations for licensing child care centers: (1) encourage practices that promote child self-regulation of sleep (putting infants to sleep drowsy but awake); (2) create an environment that ensures sleep, such as no screen media in sleeping rooms and low noise and light levels; and (3) encourage sleep-promoting behaviors and practices, such as calming nap time routines and avoiding stimulating children just before nap time. A 2014 review by Dr. Sara Neelon documented that only eleven states recommended both of the first two suggestions and no state recommended the third. Additionally, in my experience, the long drive home from the child care center, along with the natural desire of parents who did not see their child during the day to want to play with him in the evening, causes the bedtime to be too late. Even with an early bedtime, some families have to wake their child in the morning to get to the center on time.

2. Having a television in the child's bedroom became more popular after the 1980s. Dr. Judith Owens and others have documented that this is associated with less sleep and more sleep problems. Modern screen-based media use at night has only made matters worse (page 681).

3. More women are delaying the time when they have their first child. There was a sixfold increase in the rate of first births among women in the age range 35–39 years between 1973 and 2006, and a fourfold increase for the rate among women 40–44 years between 1985 and 2002. As previously discussed (chapter 6), helping children sleep well is more challenging for older mothers and fathers.

Night Sleep

SLEEPING THROUGH THE NIGHT

What does the phrase *sleeping through the night* mean? You might be surprised that there is no standard or widely accepted definition. In 2010, Dr. Jacqueline Henderson studied three different definitions. *Uninterrupted sleeping* means that there is no feeding or soothing.

1. Sleeping uninterrupted from midnight to 5:00 A.M.
2. Sleeping eight hours uninterrupted between sleep onset and waking time in the morning, without regard to the clock time when the sleep occurred
3. Sleeping uninterrupted between 10:00 P.M., or earlier, and 6:00 A.M.

Here are her data:

INFANTS SLEEPING THROUGH THE NIGHT

Age	Definition of *Sleeping through the Night*		
	12:00–5 A.M.	8 hours straight	10:00 P.M.– 6:00 A.M.
3 months	58%	Less than 50%	Less than 40%
4 months	Almost 70%	58%	Less than 50%
5 months	More than 70%	About 60%	53%
7 months	—	—	About 60%
8 months	About 80%	About 70%	—
11 months	—	About 80%	About 70%
12 months	87%	86%	73%

By 5 months of age, more than half of all babies (53 percent) sleep uninterrupted eight hours or more when their parents are likely to sleep. So by any definition, more than half of all babies are sleeping through the night by age 5 months.

Dr. Henderson wrote, "The most rapid consolidation in infant sleep regulation occurs in the first 4 months. . . . [This] reflects the emergence of infant's self-regulation and self-soothing capacities." This supports the idea of using your child's natural sleep regulation machinery as an aid to help your child sleep better during the *first 4 months*.

In her study, the average bedtime at 12 months was 8:30 P.M. Based on my research and experience, at 12 months, 8:30 P.M. is too late for many children (see below), especially those who are taking a single nap (17 percent of children) and those who have total nap duration of less than two hours (whether in one nap or two). A bedtime that is too late would likely produce a second wind that interferes with easily falling asleep and staying asleep. In my experience, all children who are napping well and have early bedtimes are sleeping uninterrupted through the night by 9 months or earlier. The data about sleeping through the night presented above describe a population of children. But what is most important for you is your own child's behavior and mood in the late afternoon and early evening, which can guide you toward a reasonably early bedtime and help you avoid unnecessary soothing and feeding in the middle of the night.

BEDTIME HOUR TRENDS OVER TIME

The shift in children's bedtimes toward later hours has run in tandem with advances in night illumination. On a historical scale, it is only fairly recently that more illumination at night has become available. The industrial production of candles began in the 1850s, the wide use of kerosene lamps in the 1860s, and the commercialization of lightbulbs in the 1880s. Shortly thereafter, physicians began to blame modern life and, more pointedly, late bedtimes for causing sleep problems.

The following quote from an editorial in the *British Medical Journal* in 1894 titled "Sleeplessness" is typical: "The subject of sleeplessness is once more under discussion. The hurry and excitement of modern life is quite correctly held to be responsible." Today, because keeping our children up at night is so common, we might give little thought to the consequences of late bedtimes. But that does not mean those consequences are nonexistent or benign. As discussed previously, threats to our children's health may go largely unnoticed for generations before slowly beginning to become known. It is the same with late bedtimes (page 148).

So how late are our children staying up?

Data collected by Dr. Iglowstein, Dr. Price, and me over many years show that the bedtime hour has shifted to later times. The cause of this shift is not known.

BEDTIME HOUR (P.M.) BY YEAR

Age	1974	1979	1979–80	1986	2004
6 months	7:18	7:41	8:00	8:16	8:00
			(4–11 months)		(4–9 months)
1 year	7:08	7:35	8:00	7:46	8:00
					(10–12 months)

After about 1980, the trend toward a later bedtime plateaued in young children, perhaps because increasingly later bedtimes would eventually be significantly disruptive to the child and the family. Although the wake-up times were a little later—for example, three minutes later in 1-year-olds—the later wake-up times failed to fully compensate for the later bedtimes. This means that children today are getting less night sleep than in the past. It is important to note that research has shown that just a *nineteen-minute* decrease in total sleep time may cause significant impairments (page 102).

In this discussion of a trend over the years of later bedtimes (and of trends over time for less night sleep, less day sleep, and less total sleep, to be discussed later), the general conclusions appear to be sound because they represent large numbers of children in many studies. Some caution is warranted regarding these conclusions, however, because at every specific age for every specific year, only the average value is reported, and the range in values around this average is often very wide. Therefore, small differences between reported values over a short period of time may occur by chance alone (for example, the difference between 7:08 and 7:35 P.M. bedtimes in 1-year-olds between 1974 and 1979). On the other hand, larger differences over a longer period of time and fairly consistent trend data in between from multiple sources suggest that the overall trend is real (for example, the difference between 7:08 and 8:00 P.M. bedtimes between 1974 and 2004).

Television and other electronic screen-based devices in the bedroom have recently become more popular. These intrusive objects cause later bedtimes, and they are associated with less sleep and more sleep problems (page 681).

BEDTIME

Remember, you are establishing an orderly home routine and enforcing a bedtime hour. You are not forcing your child to sleep. When your child starts to seem tired and needs to sleep, you try to begin his bedtime routine, whether he likes it or not. The bedtime routine (page 194) should be regular in terms of *what* you do: bathing, massage, reading a story, lullaby, rocking, or other soothing efforts. Approximately the same sequence each night, at approximately the same time, helps signal to the child that it is time for night sleep. Your child begins to associate the bedtime routine, which includes your leaving him, with falling asleep in the same way that you associate a yellow traffic light with slowing down before stopping on red. But don't be rigidly regular in terms of *when* you do it; there is enough normal irregularity in napping to produce some variability in bedtime. However, in much older children, extreme variability in bedtimes has been shown to be unhealthy.

Sometimes parent issues (chapter 4) interfere with a reasonably early bedtime or with consistency in bedtime routines and need to be directly addressed. A parent who keeps a baby up past his natural time to sleep may be using this playtime with the child to avoid unpleasant private time with the other parent.

Some parents make the mistake of always putting their baby down to sleep at exactly the same time every night. For a few months this may work well, but when naps are irregular or your child stops taking the third nap, parents should learn to be more flexible in the timing of soothing to sleep at night, especially in the direction toward an earlier bedtime!

Method A and method B for soothing to sleep (chapter 8) apply only to naps. At night, adopt whatever style seems comfortable to you. For example, at nap time you may wish to put your baby down drowsy but awake after soothing, and at night you may prefer to sleep with your baby (see the discussion of co-sleeping and *SIDS* prevention). No problem. It appears that different parts of the brain are responsible for day and night sleep, so simply be consistent in how you soothe to sleep for daytime naps and in how you soothe to sleep at night, even if the two routines are different. You are "training" different parts of the brain at different times.

If it is your desire to put your baby down for the night after soothing and he is *overtired,* then there may be some crying. During the day, limiting the amount of crying to one hour, in the hope of getting a nap at a time that will not mess up the rest of the schedule, is reasonable. But at night, if you chose to do extinction, the crying that occurs as you put your overtired child down should not be time-limited unless you decide to do extinction with a cap. If you go to him after a brief bout of crying or if you choose a short cap, you may train your child to cry to your predetermined time limit. If you do not check on your baby, he will eventually fall asleep. He may cry more the second night, but each subsequent night he will cry less. This assumes that the bedtime is early, naps are in place, and night sleep is not fragmented. Alternatively, you might use graduated extinction, check and console, or a fade procedure (chapter 5). If a sleep solution involves establishing an earlier bedtime and your child is taking long and late midday naps, a part of the solution will be to not allow him to sleep past 4:00 P.M., by awakening him if necessary.

This may be the first time you will ignore your child's protests, but it certainly will not be the last. As he becomes mobile, you will protect his physical safety by not allowing unreasonable risks involving playground equipment. At some future point, you will teach your child other health habits such as handwashing and toothbrushing. Later still, you're not going to risk brain damage by letting him ride his bike without a helmet. In each of these cases, you won't let protest crying discourage you from implementing healthy practices and safety rules. Starting early and being consistent are the keys to establishing good habits.

Now is the time to let your child learn to fall asleep at night by himself, to return to sleep at night by himself, and to learn that being alone at night in slumber is not scary, dangerous, or something to avoid. Keep everything calm and not too complicated as you go through a bedtime ritual. Fathers should be helping out at bedtime and nighttime, especially if the child is breastfed, because babies know dads cannot nurse them, and so any protest crying is likely to be less intense or shorter.

If you are using the extinction method, once your child is in bed, he is there to stay, no matter how long he cries. Please do not return with curtain calls. Little peeks, replacing pacifiers, or reswaddling may be relatively harmless for some babies when they are 4 months old or younger, but they will eventually sabotage your efforts to help your older child sleep well, because intermittent positive reinforcement has enormous teaching power.

HELPFUL SUGGESTION

When your child is crying and he is not hungry or ill, say to yourself: "My baby is crying because he loves me so much he wants my company, but he needs to sleep. I know the value of good sleep, and I love my baby so much that I am going to let him sleep."

NIGHT WAKINGS FOR FEEDING

Your child may wake at night to be fed four to six hours after his last feeding. Some children do not get up then. Others are actually hungry at this time, and you should promptly respond by feeding.

You may say, "But when my baby was younger, he slept through the night." Remember, in a child under 4 months, maybe the bedtime and the last feeding at bedtime were both much later. Now your baby is going to bed earlier, is fed earlier in the evening at bedtime, and may need a middle-of-the-night feeding; this is normal. This bedtime feeding, and an early-morning feeding, may be needed until your baby is about 9 months of age.

As you may recall, partial awakenings or light sleep stages, called arousals, occur every one to two hours when your child is asleep. Sometimes your child will quietly call out or cry during these arousals. Quiet, non-distressed vocalizations during arousals are normal and should be ignored. If your child is not sleeping with you in your bed, going in to him at the time of these partial awakenings will eventually lead to a night-waking or night-feeding habit. This is because picking up, holding, and feeding your baby will eventually cause him to force himself to a more alert state during these arousals for the pleasure of your company. He will learn to expect to be fed or played with at every arousal. He will learn to more loudly and persistently call out for your company.

However, if you are sleeping with your baby (page 93) and breastfeeding, you might promptly nurse at all of these arousals while you and the baby are still in a somewhat deeper sleep state, and then there is no real sleep fragmentation. No night-waking habit might develop.

Parents should not project their own emotions or misinterpret these naturally occurring arousals with vocalizations as signifying loneliness, fear of the dark, or fear of abandonment. This might be especially difficult for a mother with depression or anxiety issues (chapters 4 and 6), and if so, professional help for the mother might be needed.

If your baby wakes at night and behaves as if he is hungry, feed him. If your baby appears to want to play at night, stop going to him. At night, the question is "Does my baby *need* me or *want* me?"

As mentioned, a second waking for feeding may occur around 4:00 or 5:00 A.M. Some children do not get up at this time, but those children who do wake are wet, soiled, hungry, or thirsty, and a prompt response is appropriate. While you attend to your baby's needs, maintain silence and darkness so your child will return to sleep. A common mistake is to quietly play with your child, preventing the return to sleep. But the return to sleep around 4:00 or 5:00 A.M. is important, so that with a later wake-up time, at 6:00 to 7:00 A.M., your child will be able to comfortably stay up in the morning until the time of the first nap. Actually, many children do not need to be fed twice at night; they simply get up at 2:00 or 3:00 A.M. or not at all. A common mistake is to feed around midnight, at 2:00 A.M., and again around 4:00 or 5:00 A.M. If you feed your baby around midnight, please do not respond again at the 2:00 A.M. time; your baby is not hungry then. The general guideline after 4 months of age is to feed your baby overnight when hungry, but no more than two times.

BEDTIME BATTLES, DIFFICULTY FALLING ASLEEP

Past 6 weeks of age, biologically driven bedtimes tend to become earlier. If you are unable or unwilling to allow these early bedtimes, your child will become overtired, develop a second wind at bedtime, and have difficulty falling asleep drowsy but awake. He will protest at bedtime and fight falling asleep. Problems commonly occur (1) in the post-colic child who is dependent on the family bed and breast-feeding to sleep but now needs to sleep much earlier at night than the parents; (2) when parents use daycare with a long commute time to bring the child home, causing a late bedtime; or (3) when dual-career families have long commute times from work. In the first situation, the solution involves allowing your child to learn self-soothing. In the next two situations, solutions involve using others to help prepare the baby or child for bed (bathing, dressing for sleep, and feeding dinner) and, as early as possible, the parents beginning a *brief* bedtime routine. Although you will see your child less at night, you will have lovely morning time. To really enjoy the mornings, some parents will have to go to sleep earlier themselves! Other parents may be able to alter their work schedule to come home early on some days or do some of their work at home in the evenings after their child has gone to sleep. In one dual-career family, one parent was able to go to work extra early in order to come home earlier. Obviously, not all parents can come up with a complete solution, but a bedtime that is a little too late is preferable to one that is way too late. If a sleep debt accumulates during the week from a bedtime that is a little too late, try to focus on protecting naps and early bedtimes on weekends.

REMEMBER

If circumstances cause your baby to go to bed too late, do the best you can, but try for the earliest bedtime possible. A bedtime that is a little late is better than a bedtime that is very late.

One mother with an executive position said: "The reality of my job was that I would usually get home around 9:00 P.M. and try to put my child to bed around that time. Now I understand that she is looking drowsy around 7:00 P.M. I was able then to rearrange my schedule so that I could be at home to put my child to sleep around 8:00 P.M. She's sleeping so much better. It's not perfect, but it's my new reality."

NIGHT WAKINGS (SIGNALING), DIFFICULTY STAYING ASLEEP

Night waking normally occurs in all children; the real problem is failure to develop the ability to return to sleep unassisted after the awakening. All sleep problems eventually lead to night waking. The specific treatments (chapter 5) depend on the child's age and are discussed in the appropriate age chapter.

In this age range, 4–12 months, night wakings are typically the complete arousals from sleep associated with disturbed sleep in post-colic babies and are discussed in chapter 8. Other causes include severe eczema, chronic snoring associated with partial airway obstruction during sleep, general disorganization of sleep with chronic fatigue, or parental reinforcement of naturally occurring wakings.

Two separate groups of infants after 4 months of age seem especially prone to night waking. The first, larger group—about 20 percent of infants—includes those infants who had colic when they were younger. Not only do these infants wake more often, but their total sleep time is less. Although boys and girls in this group wake the same number of times, parents are more likely to state that it is their sons who have a night-waking problem. In fact, boys are handled in a more irregular way than girls when they wake at night. This was shown in studies using video footage taken in dim light in the children's own bedrooms at home. Even when the colic either has or had been successfully treated with a drug (which is no longer used for colic due to safety concerns) during the first few months, by 4 months of age the children still were reported frequently awakening at night.

One possibility is that biological disturbances in infants can cause an overaroused, too-wakeful, hyperalert, irregular state full of fussing and/or crying, especially in the late afternoon or early evening. In the past, the crying part of colic was thought to be the major problem, but as discussed in chapter 8, fussiness is now considered to be a more common behavior. In any case, though evening crying generally diminishes at about 2–4 months, the wakeful, non-sleeping state may continue and thus is more serious and harmful in the long run.

This is because parents, defeated in the short term by colic, prematurely give up the effort to teach self-soothing. They do not realize that after 2–4 months of age, regular and consistent attention to bedtimes and nap times really does help their older infant sleep better. The parents' failure to develop and maintain healthy sleep patterns in these older post-colic babies then leads to prolonged fussiness driven by chronic fatigue.

Another possibility is that maternal anxiety leads to fragmented infant night sleep caused by unnecessary feedings at night over the first few months. The fragmented night sleep causes the infant to become overtired, and he fusses and cries more than well-rested infants. Alternatively, the child continues to sleep in the parents' bed for comforting, and as a Norwegian study of over fifty thousand families showed, "bedsharing was an independent and graded predictor of nocturnal awakenings and short sleep durations" in children 6–18 months. "The longer the infant is bedsharing, the higher the risk of nightly awakenings." Even when biological factors settle down after 2–4 months, the persistent maternal nighttime behavior mediates night waking in her baby (page 438). Of course, this is not an either–or scenario: Both the child's nature and parental nurturing practices influence sleep.

The second group of children with frequent night wakings after 4 months includes the approximately 10 percent who snore or breathe through their mouths during sleep (page 714). This difficulty in breathing during sleep might be due to allergies or large adenoids or tonsils. These infants wake as frequently as do those with post-colic night waking, but their parents do not label this night waking as a problem. Probably the parents had not worried about night waking, because the infants had not suffered from colic. Those infants who snored also had shorter sleep durations than other infants. As in many sleep disturbances, when one element of healthy sleep is disrupted, other elements are disturbed. Please alert your child's health care provider if your child commonly snores or mouth-breathes during sleep.

Another cause of night waking in this age group is abnormal sleep schedules. Going to bed too late and getting up too late seems to set the stage for frequent night waking. This is especially common among mothers who like to sleep in late in the morning, and so keep their child up too late at night or do not rouse their child early enough in the morning. Sleeping out of phase with biological rhythms produces an overtired and hyperaroused child who has difficulty falling asleep and staying asleep. One child I cared for took two to two and a half hours of soothing, rocking, or holding before she would go to sleep, and then would usually wake three to four times each night, sometimes as often as ten times. This prolonged period to put a child to sleep might be called *increased latency to sleep*. It's also called a waste of parents' time, and because the off/ on twilight sleep for the child during the rocking, walking, and hugging is light sleep, it represents lost good-quality, restorative deep sleep. Correcting the sleep schedule quickly eliminated the night wakings and long latency to sleep, highlighting the importance of *when* sleep occurs and not just *how long* the sleep period lasts.

Night wakings that are not for feeding or changing diapers but involve parental interaction are called *signaling* and they might occur occasionally because of a bedtime that is too late or some noise outside your home woke your child. If these are uncommon events, rush in to check your child to make sure he is well and help him return to sleep with mild soothing.

My research showed that most parents are more bothered about how many times their child wakes at night and less so about the duration of each awakening. But actually, even though they are associated (the more frequent the number of wakings, the longer each one tends to last), perhaps parents should be more concerned about their duration. A long night wakeful period, whether you are present and trying to soothe your child or your child is quietly alone, but awake, is measured objectively with wrist-worn motion sensors and referred to as wake after sleep onset (WASO, page 91). The night waking is causing *sleep fragmentation*, and large amounts of WASO (whether due to many brief-duration night wakings or infrequent long-duration night wakings) *shortens the duration of night sleep*, both of which result in poor-quality sleep (chapter 2).

One study described earlier (page 60), focused on infants with night wakings that were each 20 minutes or longer, based on parents' reports, and over time major adverse outcomes were observed. A more objective study was recently published by Dr. Manuela Pisch, using wrist-worn motion sensors to measure infant sleep, including wake after sleep onset at 4, 6, 8, and 10 months. At each of those four evaluations, "eye-tracking was employed to examine developmental cognitive trajectories. Infants had to remember the location of a toy [on a screen] that had previously been linked to a sound and an eye-tracker recorded whether they were searching the correct location upon hearing the sound." This is a task to measure working memory. Working memory is short-term and contains a small amount of information that can be held in the mind and used in the execution of cognitive tasks such as remembering a phone number someone tells you. "Infants were grouped depending on whether they looked correctly at 4 month trials[. Those] with more than 50% of looking time to the correct side were labelled as 'correct' and those with less than 50% of looking time to the correct side were labelled as 'incorrect' . . . when infants initially began to remember the location and the toy they were expecting, they looked more to the correct side. For some infants, this was the case at 4 months, for others only at 8 months." After succeeding in this first step, infants shifted their search strategy to look at the whole screen because they expected the toy to appear elsewhere when it did not show up in the familiar location (a "more mature level of ability"). Those infants who performed better at the 4-month time (correct responders) "reached the mature level of ability by 6 months, whereas the [incorrect responders] reached it by 10 months."

Ready for the punch line? "*The group with an earlier maturation of memory performance spend less time awake during the night* (WASO) in the first months of life, [but] night and day sleep time as well as night waking frequency were *not* related to working memory performance . . . moreover, only the time spent awake during the night, but not the number of night awakenings were associated with working memory development, suggesting that *infants who settled back to sleep more easily after waking in the night are more likely to perform better in working memory tasks* [emphasis added]." The title of their paper says it all: "Infant Wake after Sleep Onset Serves as a Marker for Different Trajectories in Cognitive Development."

She discussed how the role of habitual sleep might be important for learning and development: "quality sleep enhances the general subsequent ability for the brain to store and memorise events at one point in time [or] habitual sleep has an effect on performance during the day by increasing attentiveness and focus which could lead to a better performance in the working memory task." So the duration of night wakings, whether recognized by parents or not, seems to be more harmful than the number of night wakings, and for working memory, more harmful than short night and day sleep durations.

Infants might continue their night waking for a long time. Another study showed that those children with night wakings at 8–12 months continued to have night wakings when reexamined at 18–24 months. This night-waking group slept less in total and spent more time awake during the night than the non-waking group. Further, they did not compensate by sleeping more during the day. "However, psychomotor development did not differ between infants with and without fragmented sleep at 8 or 24 months of age." Working memory was not studied in these infants.

Regarding attention span, in one study, "Sleep duration at the age of 3, 8, and 24 months was associated with inattentiveness at 5 years of age. Moreover, parent-reported sleep problems [short sleep duration, many night awakenings] at the age of 24 months were related to both inattentiveness and hyperactive symptoms at the age of 5 years. Finally, at the age of 5 years, parent-reported sleep problems and night awakenings were associated with concurrent symptoms of inattention and hyperactivity." Dr. Fallon Cook studied infants when they were 8–12 months old. About 25 percent had *only* mild-to-moderate sleep problems, 39 percent had combinations of sleep problems, crying problems, tantrums, or mood swings, and 36 percent had none of these issues ("settled" infants). Comparing these settled infants with those with *only* sleep problems, he noted that there was twice as much psychological distress in the mothers. When these children were restudied at age 5 and 11 years, the ones who had only sleep problems scored higher on scales for conduct disorder and hyperactivity at age 11. In a separate study, Dr. Fallon found that severe and persistent infant sleep difficulties across the first year were associated with increased diagnoses of emotional disorders (particularly anxiety and hyperactivity) at age 10 years. So night wakings and/or short sleep duration or other sleep problems don't just bother parents, but might also predict long-term problems for the child. Please remember, though, that most of the consequences of not sleeping well are *reversible* (page 578); further, the benefits from helping your child sleep better when young will also last a long time (page 142).

A general problem with some older studies, and my own research, is the reliance on the mothers' reports without objective measurements of the infants' sleep. Additionally, these, and many other studies, omit studying the bedtime (and the father), which might be important for the quality of sleep. Nevertheless, we now have objective measurements of night wakings and WASO. Night wakings between 4 and 12 months that occur frequently should not be accepted as a normal phase of development. The bottom line is: If your infant has a lot of awakenings at night, don't be a martyr and wait for him to outgrow it. Rather, view it as change-worthy behavior for your child's sake, and for yours too!

IMPORTANT POINT

The more tired your child, the harder it is for him to fall asleep, stay asleep, or both, because unhealthy sleep causes hyperarousal during the night and day.

Another consequence of increased arousal at bedtime is that *disturbed sleep* produces more wakeful, irritable, and active behaviors during the day. Also, these children often have increased physical activity when asleep. Although all babies can have movements involving the entire body or localized movements or twitches involving only one limb, these are brief motions lasting only a second or less. But chronically fatigued babies who are overly aroused move around more in a restless, squirmy, crawly fashion when sleeping. It seems that their motor is always running at a higher speed, awake or asleep. I will explain how you can reduce your child's idle speed by making sure he gets the sleep he needs.

What is *disturbed sleep*?

Abnormal sleep schedules (going to bed too late, sleeping in too late in the morning, napping at the wrong times)
Brief sleep durations (not enough sleep overall)
Sleep fragmentation (waking up too often)
Nap deprivation (no naps or brief naps)
Prolonged latency to sleep (taking a long time to fall asleep)
Prolonged wakefulness after sleep onset (page 71)
Lower proportion of total sleep occurring at night (page 71)
Too-active sleep (lots of tossing and turning)
Difficulty breathing during sleep

Disturbed sleep or night waking is *not* caused by:

Too much sugar in the diet
Hypoglycemia at night
Zinc deficiency
Pinworms
Gastroesophageal reflux

TEETHING AND GROWING PAINS

Teething, contrary to popular belief, does not cause night waking. If you ask parents what happens when teething occurs, the answer is everything! All illnesses, fevers, and ear infections that happen to occur around the time a tooth erupts are blamed on teething. Throughout medical history, doctors used the diagnosis "teething problems" as a smoke screen to hide their ignorance. In fact, at the turn of the twentieth century, 5 percent of deaths in children in England were misattributed to teething.

A proper study, by Dr. Arvi Tasanen, of problems caused by eruption of teeth was performed in Finland in 1968. Based on daily visits and the testing of 233 children between the ages of 4 and 30 months, he concluded that teething does not cause fevers, elevated white blood cell counts, or inflammation. Most important, teething did not cause night waking. Despite this study being published more than fifty years ago, many parents and professionals still believe in this myth. Two separate studies by Dr. Melissa Wake and Dr. Michael Macknin in 2000 also found no association between infant teething and sleep, wakefulness, or sleep disturbances. A 2016 review of over one thousand articles also found no evidence connecting teething with sleep issues. Night waking between the ages of 6 and 18 months is more likely due to nap deprivation, fragmented night sleep, or abnormal sleep schedules—not teething.

A warning: Allowing your child to hold a bottle of milk or juice while falling asleep, or resting the bottle on a pillow when putting your baby to bed, will cause "baby-bottle cavities." Protect your child's teeth. Hold your baby in your arms when you give a bottle.

Growing pains also do not cause night waking. One study examined 2,178 children between 6 and 19 years of age and found that 16 percent complained of severe pain localized deep in the arms or legs. Usually the pain was deep in the thighs, behind the knees, or in the calves. The pain usually occurred late in the afternoon or in the evenings. But when the growth rates of these affected children were compared with those of children without pain, there was no difference. In other words, growing pains do not occur during periods of rapid growth! Blaming night waking on growing pains is a handy excuse. But the rubbing, massaging, hot-water bottles, or other forms of parent soothing at night are really serving the emotional needs of the parent and/or child, not reducing organic pain.

Night waking may be caused by:

Fever
Painful ear infections
Atopic dermatitis (eczema) and breathing problems during
    sleep (chapter 12)

If you think your child is ill, call the doctor. If your child has a diaper rash or eczema that is moderate or severe, consider using thick layers of zinc oxide paste in the diaper region so that no rash will develop when you do not go to your baby at night to change diapers. Ordinary mineral oil will make removal of the paste easier in the morning.

> **Do not attempt to correct unhealthy sleep habits unless you see a clear period ahead of several days when you will be in control. Don't trust most relatives or babysitters to do as good a job as you can to correct unhealthy sleep habits. Also, if your child's sleep improves during a training period but suddenly he becomes worse, appears ill, or seems to be in pain, let your pediatrician examine him for the possibility of an ear or throat infection.**

COMMON NIGHT SLEEP ISSUES

Brief Sleep Durations

If your child is on an apparently normal sleep schedule and napping well, you might presume he is getting enough sleep because he doesn't look tired, and thus you might decide that no adjustments regarding sleep will be needed. But then, around 10, 11, or 12 months, your child starts waking at night. What's happening?

Many times, physical and mental activity increases at around 9 months. Your child is now moving around more, exploring more, becoming more active and independent. Also, there may have been a third nap that disappeared around 9 months, and afterward your child began to slowly acquire a sleep debt. The problem will often disappear when the bedtime is shifted to an earlier hour. Most families find that if they gradually shift the bedtime earlier in twenty-minute increments, they reach a time when night wakings melt away. Usually this change is easy for the baby, but sometimes it is hard for the parent who returns home late from work to accept that he or she will miss out on playtime with the baby due to the earlier bedtime. Just remember that small changes in sleep patterns often make big differences in sleep quality (page 102). Even a small change, as little as an additional *nineteen minutes* of sleep at the front end of the night, can cause a big change in your child's behavior during the day (page 298).

Having More than One Child Creates Bedtime Problems

Experienced mothers often try to help their babies learn self-soothing from the day they come home from the hospital (chapter 4) in order to create more time to be with their older child. Still, there may be conflicts between the social needs of your older child and the nap or early bedtime needs of your baby. When there are such conflicts, try to strike a balance. For example, perhaps Mom or Dad has to go to an older child's soccer practice on one day, interfering with the baby's optimal nap time, while on another day the older child might be late to some event because it's important for the baby to finish his nap.

Also, an older child, about age 3 years, might not nap and will need to go to sleep fairly early, especially if he has had a very active day. His younger sister, about age 6 months, might be taking three naps and be able to stay up later. If the mother is by herself, she cannot ignore her baby and fully attend to her 3-year-old's earlier bedtime routine. Perhaps the solution is to eliminate the third nap for the baby so she goes down earlier, before her older brother, while the 3-year-old is playing by himself. Sometimes when the older child protests that he has to go to bed earlier than the baby, the solution is to tell the older child that because the baby naps, she can stay up later, and if he wants to nap like the baby, then he, too, can stay up later.

Fraternal twins who have different sleeping schedules, causing different bedtimes, are challenging to parents. Sometimes there is no solution except to put them down at about the same time; if there is any crying associated with falling asleep, then temporarily separate them. More information on twins can be found in my book *Healthy Sleep Habits, Happy Twins*.

Unable to Fall Asleep

Young babies or children may have difficulty falling asleep except when they are in bed with their parents or in their arms. Most of these are children who had colic (chapter 6) or whose parents had used the family bed from the beginning. The "no-cry," "maybe-cry," and "let-cry" sleep solutions that may be helpful for these children are discussed in chapter 5.

If your child has a sleep problem that requires multiple changes but you are only able to make some of them, go ahead and do the best you can. Try to identify the major sleep issue and focus your attention on a solution that you feel comfortable with (chapter 4). Be consistent and patient. Anytime you make a change, allow at least four to five days before making another change, in order to see whether you have helped your child. Keeping a sleep log (page 305) is helpful to see objectively whether the change you made is helping, because you might be under such stress that you fail to see a little improvement in the beginning. For example, there may be protest crying at night that is unbearable for you, but the sleep log shows that for the very first time, your child took a substantially longer nap.

An important issue is worth repeating: If you have symptoms of anxiety or depression, they might worsen because you have become short on sleep. Ask yourself: *Am I likely to be so concerned about my child at night that I might want to attend to her when she appears to be sleeping contentedly because I worry about her health,*

*or I feel that she needs my company; does my baby appear to be
unusually fussy and hard to soothe to sleep or unable to sleep well?
Or: Is there stress in my marriage, perhaps because the father is not
supportive in baby care at night?* Under these circumstances, review
chapter 1, or if willing, have your husband read this, and try some
no-cry sleep solutions and proceed slowly and gradually (chapter
5)—say, trying a slightly earlier bedtime (page 240) to help your
baby sleep better. A little extra sleep at the front end may make a
world of difference (page 102). Discuss your overall situation with
your husband, partner, or child's caregiver. Maybe, consider engaging a community sleep consultant (page 329) to help prevent sleep
problems from developing or find solutions.

Remember: Sleeping well is a 24/7 process. It's not just about how
we get our children to go to bed at night without crying.

> **Solving sleep problems may be a very tough prescription and de-
> mands a consistent approach.**
>
> There may be increased crying in the beginning, but the upside is
> that crying around sleep will ultimately be eliminated altogether.

Will Not Sleep Anywhere Else

Maybe your baby sleeps well in your home but does not sleep well at
Grandma's. Try to play the same music only at sleep times at both
homes. Spray some fragrance or perfume around the crib or bed
only at sleep times at both homes. Try to use the same sleep schedules and nap time and bedtime routines at both homes. After 1 year
of age, buy something soft and safe for your baby to feel or clutch
and use it only at sleep times at both homes.

Only One Bedroom

When your baby becomes more curious and aware of the sounds
and movements of people around him, and you are using a crib, it
might be time to move your baby to his own room. But what do you
do if you don't have an additional bedroom? Some families have

their baby sleep at night in their bedroom, then use a sofa bed to convert their living room into the parents' bedroom at night. In this way, the baby can go to bed early in a dark and quiet room, and the parents know that their nighttime sounds will not wake him. Encouraging your child to practice self-soothing may be more important than having a separate room for sleeping (page 95).

REMEMBER

If you want to make a change, but you are totally exhausted and unsure which way to go, just move the bedtime *a few minutes earlier!*

Day Sleep

Please review the sections "Consistency in Soothing Styles for Naps" and "Different Decisions for Different Babies" in chapter 8.

DAY SLEEP DURATION BY AGE

In my nap survey of children born between 1984 and 1986, starting at 6 months of age, I divided them into five nap duration groups (see below; each group represented about 20 percent of the children). I found that children typically remained in their initial nap duration group until 21–24 months. In other words, for babies whose average nap duration was 3 hours at 6 months of age, by 9 months it was 2.9 hours and by 12 months it was 2.8 hours; most did not move to a different nap duration group with much shorter or longer naps. Stated another way, children with long naps at 6 months of age continue to take long naps until 21–24 months, and the same is true for children with short or intermediate nap durations. So while there is a large variation in nap duration among children, there is also a stable tendency for nap durations for an individual child. This individual stability of nap durations probably reflects a *genetic* influence over sleep. Also, for the vast majority of infants, nap durations were restricted to narrower time frames (shown below) as the children got older, despite variations in caretaking and social activities. This suggests that *biological* processes affect naps. Nevertheless, considering the actual minimum and maximum duration of naps, the wide total range of nap durations (shown below) suggests that *parents* do play an important role.

AVERAGE DAY SLEEP DURATION

Initial Nap Duration Group (Hours)	6 months	9 months	12 months
1–2.5	2.3	2.7	2.5
3	3.0	2.9	2.8
3.5	3.5	3.1	3.1
4	4.0	3.2	3.2
More than 4	4.8	3.6	3.3

Most children nap within a narrow range:

At 6 months: For 80 percent of children, the range is between 2.5 and 4.0 hours; 5 percent nap less than 2.5 hours and 15 percent more than 4.0 hours.

At 9 months: For 93 percent of children, the range is between 2.0 and 4.0 hours.

At 12 months: For 94 percent of children, the range is between 2.0 and 4.0 hours.

Some children nap far outside the narrow range that occurs for most children:

Minimum	1.0	1.0	1.5
Maximum	6.0	5.5	5.5

Average nap durations apply to groups only, of course, not individual children:

| **Average** | 3.5 | 3.1 | 3.0 |

As previously mentioned, post-colic children might be over-represented in the 20 percent of children in the shortest nap duration group (1 to 2.5 hours), but the good news is that this is the only group that did not show a decrease in nap duration between 6 and 9 months; in fact, their average nap duration *increased* from 2.3 to 2.7 hours, suggesting a slower maturation of day sleep rhythms. This increase of *twenty-four minutes* may seem small, but we know that small changes in sleep can have a huge impact (pages 102 and 298). Although some studies on large groups of children show no consistent relationship between the durations of daytime sleep and nighttime sleep, I think it is likely that most of the children who sleep near the minimum number of hours for naps have problems with night sleep and/or naps. This may also be true for some of the children who sleep near the maximum number of hours for naps, although I have encountered some very well-rested children, later determined to be highly intelligent, who had, at these young ages, very long naps.

You may have a well-rested child who does well with short naps, even though his fraternal twin wants long naps or your older child took long naps. Now that you appreciate how wide the nap duration range is, you can see how important it is to not compare your child's naps with other children's, because all children are a little different. No matter what the nap duration is for your child, all of these numbers are less important than your observation of whether or not your child is well rested.

NUMBER OF NAPS PER DAY BY AGE

In my nap survey of children born between 1984 and 1986, I asked how many naps were taken per day.

NAPS PER DAY BY AGE

Age (months)	Percentage of Children Taking 1, 2, or 3 Naps per Day		
	1/day	2/day	3/day
6	0%	84%	16%
9	4%	91%	5%
12	17%	82%	1%

By 9 months of age, the vast majority (91 percent) of children are taking two naps. As previously stated, these numbers are less important than how your child looks, but if your child is under 9 months of age and is taking only one nap or your child is over 9 months of age and taking three naps, his sleep schedule may be off and in need of adjustment.

DAY SLEEP DURATION TRENDS OVER TIME

In addition to the previously discussed trend of bedtimes becoming later, causing less night sleep, data are available from studies by Dr. Price and me that show a trend for less day sleep over time. The cause of this shift is unknown.

AVERAGE DAY SLEEP DURATION

1979–80

3.2 hours (4–11 months)

2004

3.0 hours (4–6 months)

2.8 hours (7–9 months)

2.6 hours (10–12 months)

COMMON DAY SLEEP ISSUES

Nap Deprivation

When parents have invested the effort to create an age-appropriate sleep schedule and their child is well rested, occasional disruptions due to illness, trips, parties, or holiday visits cause only minor disruptions of sleep. The well-rested child requires only a brief recovery period—for example, a single reset—before getting back on track. But when parents allow poor-quality sleep patterns to emerge and persist, then significant sleep deficits accumulate gradually. Now even minor disturbances might create long-lasting havoc.

In this age range, nap deprivation seems to be a major culprit in ruining healthy sleep patterns. It's only natural that you want to get out more and do more things with your child, who is now full of new social charms, cheerful, and crawling or maybe even walking . . . why not hang out together and enjoy the good weather at the park or beach? Children at this age are fearless, full of grace and self-confidence, and very explorative. Hanging out with parents and siblings is simply a lot of fun for everyone. The main message is to enjoy socializing out of the house but not so frequently that your child is often shortchanged on day sleep.

Willfulness (self-agency) might lead your child to protest naps because he would rather play than sleep. If you often allow him to skip his nap, then he will become fatigued. The natural adaptive response to fatigue is to fight it with stimulating hormones, which allow him to maintain more wakefulness. However, this heightened state of alertness or arousal creates an inability to easily fall asleep or stay asleep for subsequent naps and night sleep. Not only does a vicious circle of sleep problems begin, but your child may also develop emotional ups and downs or a reduced attention span as a by-product.

If naps slip and slide too much, a trend of increasing fatigue will clearly develop. First, the child becomes a little more crabby, irritable, or fussy, maybe only in the late afternoon or early evening. You might think it's normal for children this age to be easily frustrated or sometimes bored. Then he starts to get up at night for the first time ever, "for no reason." Later, maybe following a cold or a day-long visit with his grandparents, he starts fighting going to sleep at night, and you wonder why night sleep is suddenly a problem.

When you reestablish healthy, regular nap routines, the witching hour, bedtime battles, and night awakenings *disappear*. I have seen this over and over again. That's why I think nap deprivation and not a particular "stage" is the culprit behind disturbed night sleep.

> **Sleep deprivation may appear as boredom. If your child's motor is idling and he's not going anywhere, maybe he's short on sleep.**

Some parents, unsure of when their child naturally shifts to need-ing only one nap, try to get by with one nap before their child is ready. If this occurs, late afternoons full of activities can help smooth over rocky moments of heightened emotionality or grumpi-ness. Anyway, Mom or Dad returns from work shortly thereafter, so there is a loving play period early in the evening.

However, the fatigue from nap deprivation eventually leads to increased levels of arousal and alertness, and this causes difficulties in falling asleep, staying asleep, or both. These changes in the direc-tion of disturbed sleep and behavioral changes during the day may be very gradual, so initially it may appear that a single nap is all right. The effects of persistent sleep deficits are *cumulative*, though, and eventually your fatigued child starts to behave differently.

Sometimes, the changes in behavior can be striking. For example, two children in my practice, 5 and 6 months of age, had severe bob-bing, turning, and jerking of the head and facial wincing or grimac-ing. The parents of both children were physicians and were worried about neurological problems. So both children were hospitalized and evaluated for seizures or epilepsy, but all the test results were normal. Nap deprivation turned out to be the problem, as I had al-ways suspected, and both children *recovered completely* when they were better rested, though the movements transiently returned for each child during a temporary period of overtiredness.

Here is one parent's account of how shortening the interval of wakefulness helped her child sleep better during the day.

In November, our third daughter, Rebecca, was born. At that time I prided myself on how well I schlepped our new baby everywhere and how wonderfully she slept in and out of the car seat all day.

Our days were filled with errands and car pools; Rebecca would be nursing and napping on and off all day. What a cooperative baby, I used to think. But I was so exhausted by evening that I found the only way to survive was to sleep with her, waking up every hour or so to shift her so that she could nurse on the other side. I knew then that having her in bed with me wasn't such a terrific idea, but it was the only way for me to get any rest.

When Rebecca turned 5 months old, I placed her in her crib instead of going to sleep with her at my breast. As I anticipated, every few hours she began to cry, expecting me to be by her side. I would quickly run into her room and rock and nurse her back to sleep . . . until the next time she woke up.

And so our next pattern began. She would wake up every few hours, and I would faithfully run in and get her back to sleep. I was certain she would grow out of this bad habit . . . our other two had.

A few months passed. By now Rebecca was weaned to a bottle and I was sure things would change for the better. That didn't happen. In fact, things got worse. There were many nights when Rebecca would get up every hour on the hour. I tried letting her cry, fifteen minutes at a time, but it was much easier to just go in and give her a bottle.

When Rebecca was 1 year old, this pattern of frequent

waking continued. It was difficult leaving her with a babysitter on the occasional evening we went out. I knew that within an hour or so of our leaving she would be up crying for me. I actually felt sick leaving her.

When Rebecca was almost 13 months old we went to see Dr. Weissbluth. When we left his office I felt prepared for battle—armed with all the mental ammunition I needed to change Rebecca's nightly wakings. We started the program of shorter intervals of wakefulness the next day.

In a week's time, the change in Rebecca was phenomenal! She was always a happy baby, but when she began to sleep better, she became even more relaxed, more affectionate, and more fun to be with.

The change in her sleeping pattern has had an effect on everyone in the family. I don't yell and lose my patience with my older children quite as much, for I am better rested and I feel so much better physically and emotionally.

This has been one of the most rewarding and positive experiences that we have shared as parents. We are so proud of Rebecca and also pat ourselves on the backs for a job well done.

Shhh! Rebecca's sleeping!

As this mother wrote, "She was always a happy baby, but when she began to sleep better, she became *even more relaxed, more affectionate, and more fun to be with.*" Parents are usually skeptical that their charming and sweet baby can become even more so with healthier sleep. But it's true!

The treatment strategy to go back to two naps involves (1) shortening the interval of wakefulness *before* the first nap and reestablishing the midday nap by making sure the wakeful period after the midmorning nap is not too long; (2) making sure the midday nap does not start too late in the afternoon, in order to protect a reasonable evening bedtime; and (3) consistency in the nap time ritual.

Don't disrupt your efforts by allowing your child to stay up too late before bedtime. If you do, he is likely to become overtired and over-aroused, and will experience disturbed night sleep, which in turn means he will start the day short on sleep.

It's not uncommon for a child to sleep well at night but not nap well, especially in the afternoon. At night it is dark, everyone is more tired, and parents want to be regular with bedtimes because they want to enjoy each other's company or just go to sleep them-selves. During the day, it is light, everyone is more alert, and parents are more irregular because they want to run errands or enjoy recre-ational activities.

So during a training period, it's easier to establish good night sleep than naps, and easier to establish regular midmorning naps than midday naps. Don't expect improvement to occur equally at all times. Still, it's best to implement a twenty-four-hour sleep retrain-ing program, because if you focus only on one feature, such as bed-time, and ignore naps, you will be less likely to succeed.

In general, I recommend a twenty-four-hour sleep package to help restore healthy sleep habits. Here is an example of an excep-tion. A single mother has limited resources for soothing and is completely exhausted. The child does not sleep well day or night. The mother wants to continue breastfeeding, but now she wants to transition the baby from her bed to a crib. The first step might only be a *temporarily ultra-early bedtime* in the mother's bed to help the child get more sleep. Everything else stays the same. The advice is to do whatever is necessary to maximize sleep and minimize crying during the day. After the child is a little better rested, the second step might be to make the transition to the crib. This might involve crying, but because both child and mother are better rested, the crying may be very little and the mother is more able to cope. The third step is to work on naps. This will now be easier because ev-eryone is better rested. If, instead, this mother had an enormous support system to help her soothe the baby, she might try to do ev-erything at the same time. Her child might become better rested faster, and the greater stress in making all these changes abruptly would be shared by people other than the mother. Moving the bedtime earlier, as a stand-alone first step (page 240), might kick-start a sleep solution!

Some families have found it difficult to establish naps because their bedrooms are too bright or noisy during the day. One family I know was fortunate enough to have a large walk-in closet, which they furnished like a little bedroom and which was used only for naps. Other families have problems because they live in a one-bedroom apartment and it is difficult for anyone to sleep well when a child shares a bedroom with the parents. These parents sometimes relocate to the living room and turn the bedroom over to the child so that the entire family can stay well rested. If you do not want to have a family bed, expect it to become difficult for your child to sleep well in your room. Plan ahead, before the family becomes overtired.

> As long as your child retains the expectation that he can convince you to play during nap time, he won't nap well. If he thinks he can outlast you, he won't give up his protesting.

Fixing Nap Schedules

When the bedtime hour and sleep periods are not in synchrony with other biological rhythms, we don't get the full restorative benefit of sleep. Please refer to figures 5 and 6 (page 66) for age-appropriate times when children fall asleep or awaken.

At any age, abnormal sleep schedules can lead to night wakings and night terrors in older children. The schedule often gets shifted to a too-late bedtime hour because Mom or Dad (or both), returning late from work, wants to play with their baby. Or parents deliberately keep their baby up late in a misguided attempt to encourage a later awakening in the morning. Or perhaps they discovered that if they kept their baby up late, their child would eventually crash due to exhaustion, and in this way they avoided stressful bedtime battles. Or there may be parent issues (chapter 4) causing a late bedtime.

The strategy for bringing sleep schedules back to normal is based on developing an age-appropriate wake-up at 6:00 or 7:00 A.M.; a mid-morning nap around 9:00; a midday nap, usually around 12:00 to 1:00 P.M., but always starting before 3:00 P.M.; an early bedtime, 6:00 to 8:00 P.M.; and consolidated night sleep. This package of advice ensures good sleep quality, and it is quality, not just quantity, that really matters.

MAJOR POINT

The major fear that inhibits parents from establishing an earlier bedtime is that this will cause their child to get up earlier to start the day. In fact, the opposite will occur. An earlier bedtime will allow your child to sleep later, just as a too-late bedtime will eventually cause a too-early wake-up time. Remember, sleep begets sleep. This is not logical, but it *is* biological.

Q: *Why do you recommend 6:00 to 8:00 P.M. as an appropriate bedtime?*

A: Survey data from my earlier research showed that the vast majority of children between the ages of 4 and 12 months went to sleep between 7:00 and 9:00 P.M., and so I used to recommend those hours. However, as I have helped families correct sleep problems over the past forty years, it has become clearer that children who go to bed earlier tend to not develop sleep problems in the first place. In addition, children in this age range who did have sleep problems almost always benefited from an earlier bedtime. I think we have simply grown accustomed to having overtired children in the evening hours, and because it is so common, we have assumed that fussiness or irritability near the end of the day is normal. Imagine what a "normal" bedtime was before candles, kerosene lamps, electric lights, radio, television, videos, commuting, smartphones, or dual-income families traveling from work to daycare to home.

A reasonably early bedtime means that your child wakes up well rested and is better able to nap. So think of an early bedtime and consolidated night sleep as prerequisites for good naps. Naps can be established or reestablished by the nap drill and controlling the wake-up time (chapter 5), and by focusing on consistency in soothing style for naps (chapter 8).

It's up to *you* to enforce an age-appropriate nap and bedtime schedule. Your child initially may not cooperate by falling asleep immediately. Don't give up.

Studies have shown that when sleep disturbances are associated with abnormal sleep schedules, control of the wake-up time (page 294) may be sufficient to establish a healthy twenty-four-hour sleep rhythm. In other words, *you* set the clock in the morning!

Nap patterns are as varied as children themselves, family sizes, and parental lifestyles. One 5-month-old always woke briefly at 6:00 A.M. and then promptly returned to sleep until 10:00 A.M. A long midday nap occurred from noon to 3:00 P.M. and a brief nap from 5:00 to 5:45 P.M. Between 7:30 and 8:00 P.M. the child went to sleep for the night, until about 6:00 the following morning. This child was well rested, and the midday nap coincided with his older brother's single nap. For the time being, this pattern met both children's sleep needs. By 6–7 months, this child developed the more common pattern of a midmorning nap and a midday nap.

However, other children whose naps are not in sync with biological rhythms begin to accumulate a sleep deficit that grows, often slowly, over time. Eventually, daytime mood or behavior problems develop, as do sleep disturbances at night.

Please review "Choose a Sleep Solution" in chapter 5.

A temporary disturbance or mild variation in sleep schedules, nap patterns, amount of sleep, or early awakenings may not be worth changing. But if chronic or severe problems cause your child to become tired, then try to help him become more rested. Watch your child's behavior, not some inflexible schedule.

SLEEP RECOMMENDATIONS

Recall Lisa Matricciani's point from her 2013 review of the literature: Published recommendations for children's sleep are not based on empirical evidence, and "*sleep timing* [the time when sleep occurs] may be even more important than *sleep duration* [emphasis added]."

The take-home message is that what is common regarding bedtimes and naps among your relatives, friends, and neighbors might not be what is right for your child. See chapters 2 and 10 for more information on sleep recommendations.

> Commonly occurring sleep patterns among your relatives, friends, and neighbors might not fit your child. Ignore what they recommend and what you read about bedtimes, naps, and total sleep needs and instead *watch your child.* Don't be surprised if he needs an earlier bedtime and/or takes longer naps than other children.
>
> *When* your child sleeps might be more important than *how long* he sleeps.

MONTHS 4–8

Midday nap from 12:00 to 2:00 P.M.; a variable late-afternoon nap around 3:00–5:00 P.M. develops.

As months 3 and 4 blend into months 5–8, your child's behavior slowly changes toward increased sociability, which permits more playfulness and gamelike interactions between you and your infant. Your child may roll over, sit, imitate your voice with babbling, or respond quickly to your quiet sounds. This increased social interaction certainly makes having a baby more fun.

Infants really do enjoy their parents' company; they thrive in response to your laughter and smiles. However, your baby is not like an empty vessel you can fill with love, warmth, hugs, kisses, and soothing until it is full, thus leading to satisfaction, blissful content-ment, or undemanding repose. The more you entertain him, the more he will want to be amused. So it is natural and reasonable to expect your baby to protest when you stop playing with him. In fact, the more you play with your child, the more he will come to expect that this is the natural order of things. Nothing is wrong with this, except that there are times when you have to dress your baby or leave him to amuse himself for a while, and he will probably resist the partial restraint needed for dressing or the curtailment of fun and games. When this happens, please remember that leaving your baby alone protesting for more fun with you while you get dressed is not the same thing as abandonment! Similarly, leaving your baby alone protesting for more fun when he needs to sleep is not neglect. You have become sensitive to your child's need to sleep, and he is now old enough for you to recognize and respect his internal timing mechanism for naps. Our goal is to synchronize caretaking activi-ties with your child's needs to be fed, to be kept warm, to be played with, and to sleep.

After 4 months of age, an infant's sleep becomes more like an adult's. Younger infants enter sleep with a period of REM sleep, but around 4 months, like adults, they begin to enter sleep with a non-REM sleep period. Sleep cycling, from deep to light non-REM sleep with interruptions of REM sleep, also matures into adultlike pat-terns around 4 months of age.

As discussed previously, the five major elements of healthy sleep are (1) sleep duration (night and day), (2) naps, (3) sleep consolidation, (4) sleep schedule, and (5) sleep regularity. Now let's look at figure 7. This circle graph is a navigational aid for parents to help them understand sleep/wake rhythms. Although I designed this graph, I did not create it any more than a mapmaker creates the shape or location of an island. As your child gets older, the times when he will become sleepy become more pre-dictable. Another way of saying this is that the biological sleep/wake rhythms mature. This allows you to change your strategy for keeping your child well rested. Previously, the focus was on *brief intervals of wakefulness* to avoid the overtired state; now you can begin to use *clock time* as an aid to help your child sleep well. Some parents call this sleeping "by the clock," or BTC. Stated simply, you are using your child's natural sleep rhythms to help him fall asleep.

Data for the circular graph in figure 7 were derived from my research in the late 1970s on children living in northern Indiana and Illinois. The ranges for the wake-up time are about 6:00 to 8:00 A.M.; the first nap takes place about 9:00 to 10:00 A.M., and the second nap about 12:00 to 2:00 P.M. The range for the bedtime includes 8:00 P.M., but this time is too late for children who have brief naps and/or no third nap.

You want your child to sleep well by synchronizing parent-set naps and bedtimes with the sleep schedule set by your child's developing internal timing mechanism. Let's start in the morning and go around the clock.

Wake-Up Time in the Morning

Some babies tend to wake up early, 5:00 or 6:00 A.M., and return to sleep after a brief feeding or diaper change. This is a true continuation of night sleep and not a nap. Other babies wake up later and start the day then. Most children will wake to start the day about 7:00 A.M., but there is a wide range (between 6:00 and 8:00). In general, it is not a good idea to go to your child to start the day before 6:00 A.M., even if he is crying, because if you do, he will begin to force himself to wake up earlier and earlier in order to enjoy your company. The natural wake-up time seems to be an independent, neurological alarm clock in these young infants that is somewhat independent of the part of the brain that puts them to sleep or keeps them asleep. In fact, despite what is commonly believed, you usually *cannot* change the wake-up time by keeping your baby up later, feeding solids before bedtime, or waking your baby for a feeding before you go to sleep. The last seems insensitive, anyway. How

Figure 7: Healthy Sleep Schedule for Infants 4 to 8 Months Old

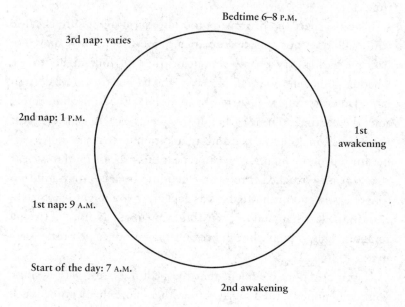

Bedtime 6–8 P.M.

3rd nap: varies

2nd nap: 1 P.M.

1st awakening

1st nap: 9 A.M.

Start of the day: 7 A.M.

2nd awakening

would you feel if someone woke you from a deep sleep and started to feed you when you weren't hungry?

When your child is well rested and has no disturbed sleep, an early wake-up hour may be inconvenient but not necessarily changeable. If your child is near his first birthday, you might consider some of the items discussed in the next chapter on older children.

When the Wake-Up Time Is Too Early

Make sure that the bedroom is dark and quiet in the morning. Window-darkening shades and a white-noise machine or noise from a humidifier will help reduce the startling effect of street noises. Keep a sleep log to help find the best bedtime.

The most common cause for waking up too early before 4 months of age is *extreme fussiness/colic*; after 4 months, it is a too-late bed-time.

If you suspect the bedtime is too late but are not sure because your child does not appear dramatically overtired, slowly move the bedtime earlier. Try twenty minutes earlier for four nights to see whether your child will fall asleep at the earlier time and sleep in later. Do everything you currently are doing at bedtime, but simply start the bedtime routine earlier. If this seems to help a little, repeat the process, making the bedtime an additional twenty minutes earlier for four more nights. You can repeat this process until it is clear that you have reached a too-early bedtime because your child no longer easily and promptly falls asleep. Now you might want to return to the last step and let your child stay up an additional twenty minutes. This gradual shift in bedtime may produce no protest crying.

If you are more confident that the bedtime is too late because your child appears tired much earlier, then move the bedtime much earlier right away; a slightly earlier bedtime might not help and only frustrate you. The abrupt shift may or may not produce protest crying. Review the no-cry, maybe-cry, and let-cry sleep solutions in chapter 5. It will probably be necessary to ignore your child until 6:00 to 7:00 A.M. For younger children, the option of bringing them to your bed for soothing may produce extra Z's in the morning, but after 6 months this is more likely to be stimulating than soothing.

Sometimes, after 4 months, a child is already going to bed very early, around 5:30 or 6:00 P.M., and this causes the entire schedule to shift: Too early a wake-up time causes too-early or poorly timed naps and a very tired child in the late afternoon who goes to sleep easily very early in the evening (page 303). For young children, it may help to simultaneously move their bedtime a little later, maybe twenty to thirty minutes every four nights, and ignore them until about 6:00 A.M. If you move the bedtime abruptly too late, your child might become so overtired that instead of the wake-up time becoming later, he simply wakes up more overtired.

Finding the bedtime that is just right for your child might require some back-and-forth adjustments; make one change and then wait four days to see whether it helps. And *be patient*.

Morning Time Awake

Morning wakeful time will last about two hours for 4- to 5-month-olds or about three hours for 8-month-olds. Some easy babies or babies born early may be able to stay up for only one hour at 4 months of age. In that case, plan a wind-down or nap time routine of up to thirty minutes. You decide what you want to do: bath, bottle, breastfeeding, lullaby, massage—but limit it, because spending hours holding your baby produces only a light or twilight sleep state, which is poor-quality sleep. Begin this routine as *drowsy* signs emerge or just before they are expected, about half an hour or less *before* the end of your baby's wakeful period, not after it's over. At the end of your predetermined nap time routine, whether your baby is asleep or awake, lie down with him (see the discussion of co-sleeping and the *SIDS* warning) or put him in his crib. As one mother commented to me, "I cannot tell you what a liberating experience it was to be able to put my baby down in her crib before she fell asleep in my arms." Your baby may now cry a little, a lot, or not at all.

The temperamentally easy child cries very little, and the routine is repeated for a midday nap. The temperamentally more difficult child, who may have also been an extremely fussy/colicky infant, might now cry a lot. The preemie also may cry a lot, and if so, the following approach might be delayed until 4 months after the expected date of delivery.

Nap #1: Midmorning

There are "windows" of clock time for naps. When your child is awake, watch your baby *and the clock* to determine the time when it is easiest for your child to take an age-appropriate nap. The nap windows of "sleep propensity" open and close, and they represent times during which it is easiest to fall asleep and stay asleep.

This midmorning nap develops first, usually between 12 and 16 weeks of age, counting from the due date. It occurs about 9:00 A.M. and may last an hour or two. Sometimes you can stretch your child's morning wakeful period by a few minutes each day to get to this time, or you might wake him up at 7:00 A.M. in order for him to be able to take this nap. This violation of the rule "Never wake a sleeping baby" is to help maintain an age-appropriate sleep schedule for the benefit of the baby. The rule mainly applies to waking babies for our social convenience, but to their detriment. Try to anticipate your child's best nap time. If he takes this nap too early or too late, then it may be difficult for him to take the second nap on time.

Consider a sleep period to be a restorative nap if it is about an hour or longer. Forty to forty-five minutes is sometimes enough, but most babies in this age range sleep at least a solid hour. Sleep periods shorter than thirty minutes should not count as good-quality naps.

If you are using method A for naps (page 478) or have a temperamentally easy baby, after putting your baby down for this nap, leave him completely alone for no more than one hour to allow him to (1) learn to fall asleep unassisted and (2) return to sleep unassisted until he has slept about an hour in an uninterrupted fashion. Easy babies may cry very little or not at all; the temperamentally more difficult child may cry a lot. Remember, you are responding sensitively to his need to sleep by not providing too much attention. You are decisive in establishing a routine because you are upholding his right to sleep. Be calm and firm and consistent, because *consistency helps your baby learn rapidly.*

He will pick up on your calm, firm attitude and will learn quickly not to expect the pleasure of your company at nap time. You are not abandoning your child in his moment of need; you are giving him all the attention he needs when he is awake. Now he needs to be alone to sleep. Please review, if needed, the prevention of nap problems (chapter 4) and treatment for them (chapter 5), and why consistency in soothing for naps may be helpful (chapter 8).

Q: *How long do I let my baby cry?*

A: No more than one hour.

Q: *What do I do if the nap is short? When I put my child down to sleep, he cries a long time, but for less than an hour, and then falls asleep, but he doesn't sleep very long. Do I let him cry again? Sometimes he doesn't cry when I put him down for a nap, but he still doesn't sleep very long. Do I let him cry after the brief nap to see if he will sleep longer?*

A: If the nap is substantially less than thirty minutes, you might try to leave him alone for an additional thirty to sixty minutes, even if he cries, to see whether he will return to sleep unassisted. If the nap is substantially more than thirty minutes, it is less likely that he will return to sleep unassisted, so you might want to leave him alone for an additional thirty minutes or go to him immediately and not let him cry anymore. In general, the shorter the nap and the less restorative it appears, the longer you should leave him alone to see if he will return to sleep unassisted. Alternatively, you might want to try to lengthen the nap by rushing to your child at the first sound of awakening from a brief nap (less than an hour) and attempting to soothe him back to sleep for a continuation of the nap. However, especially over 6 months of age, this might be counterproductive and simply stimulate your child to fight sleep more for the pleasure of your company.

Q: *After one hour of crying, what do I do?*

A: Go to your baby and soothe him. Now you have two choices. Your baby might remain wakeful, and you might decide that this was so stressful for you or him that you want to go outside for a walk, relax, and try again the next day to get a midmorning nap. Or after all this crying your baby might be falling asleep in your arms when you pick him up; if you feel that he will now be able to fall asleep, put him back down to see if he will nap. But do not let him cry anymore if this new attempt fails.

Q: *What's wrong if I quickly check my baby when he first cries, and I give him a pacifier or roll him back over? He always immediately stops crying and returns to sleep.*

A: Checking on your baby like this when he should be napping may not interfere with naps or night sleep in some infants between 4 and 6 months. But please be careful, because eventually all babies learn to turn these brief visits into prolonged playtimes. This learning process may develop more slowly if it is the father who does the checking and provides minimal intervention.

Q: *My child had extreme fussiness/colic. Now he is about 5 months old. How do I get him on a 9:00 A.M. and 1:00 P.M. nap schedule?*

A: Make sure he is sleeping well at night. Control the wake-up time; try to start the day around 6:00 to 7:00 A.M. by not going to him before 6:00 A.M. or by waking him up at 7:00 A.M. if he is still sleeping. Try intense but brief stimulation outdoors. Expose him to wind, rustling leaves, moving clouds, street noises, voices, barking dogs, sand in the playground, motion in the jogger or soft sling on your chest, swings, splashing in a swimming pool, and so forth. Try to stretch his wakeful period to about 9:00 a.m., but be mindful not to allow him to become so frantically over-tired that he will not be able to subsequently sleep well. He will get a little geared up, and initially he might get close to but not make it to 9:00 A.M. Tone it down a little as you get close to 9:00 A.M. Plan for a much longer and relaxing soothing-to-sleep routine before his midmorning nap, because he will be a little overtired. Consider including a bath for relaxation, not for hygiene. Bathing might be stimulating, but more often it is calm fun for babies. Around 9:00 A.M., lie down to sleep with him (see the co-sleeping and *SIDS* warning) or put him down to sleep. If he has a decent nap of close to one hour, repeat the same steps for his 1:00 P.M. nap. If he does not nap in the morning, get out of the house and try to not let him sleep until about 11:00 A.M.

Try the same soothing-to-sleep routine around 11:00 A.M. This means no car rides at 10:00 A.M.

Parents of post-colic babies or babies with a more difficult temperament might want to begin to practice method A (page 478) at this time. Many of these parents have been using method B (your baby always begins naps in deep sleep with your help). Ideally, you have been very consistent with method B up until now, because the better rested your baby is when you make the transition from method B to method A, the easier it will be.

> **WARNING**
>
> It may be very difficult to establish regular naps at 4–5 months of age in some babies because their biological nap rhythms are maturing very slowly. Some babies don't evolve into a schedule of regular long naps until 5–6 months of age, especially if they had extreme fussiness/colic when younger or if their parents were inconsistent or irregular about naps during the first 4 months.

Focus on the Midmorning Nap

For the difficult-temperament or post-colic baby, establishing the midmorning nap may be the toughest parenting maneuver that you have attempted so far. By focusing on the midmorning nap, we try to help a post-colic baby learn self-soothing skills. It's best to begin establishing an age-appropriate nap schedule with the midmorning nap because it is the first one to develop; it is the nap that should be the easiest to obtain, because your baby is most rested from the night sleep, and parents usually can be more consistent in the early morning, when scheduling conflicts are less likely to develop compared with the afternoon. After your child's day starts, look at the clock. *Within one hour of waking*, you will want to clean him, feed him, and then begin to soothe him using method A. If there is bright morning light during this hour, open up all your shades, because exposure to morning light might help establish sleep rhythms. If there is no bright natural light, make the room as bright as you can with room lights. Darken the room as you begin your soothing to sleep. After several minutes of soothing, which may include feeding, put your baby down to sleep. Remember, the soothing also occurs within the one-hour period of wakefulness. This ultra-short period of wakefulness is designed to prevent the overtired state from developing. Another reason it is important to establish the midmorning nap by keeping the interval of wakefulness very short is that the midmorning nap might represent a continuation of night sleep. The midmorning nap contains more REM sleep than the midday nap, and large amounts of REM sleep are a characteristic feature of a baby's night sleep. Eventually, this midmorning nap will be gradually and slowly delayed until about 9:00 A.M.

Q: *What if my child wants to go to sleep but is unable to do so?*
A: Here is a report from a mother who observed that her child was "so sleep-deprived he could not go to sleep. . . . Though he seemed to want to go to sleep, he appeared unable to get there."

I'll never forget the night and early morning at about 3 months of age when Eric was so sleep-deprived he could not go to sleep. I tried everything—nursing, rocking, walking, bouncing, and singing. Eventually he did fall asleep while I pushed him around the house in the stroller listening to his favorite CD, only to wake up the second I tried to move him into his crib. The hours stretched on and Eric became more and more tired, overstimulated, and agitated. He began trying to pick the flowers off my pajamas. Though he seemed to want to go to sleep, he appeared unable to get there. I felt I didn't have any choice but to put him in his crib, awake and crying. After about twenty minutes of crying, he fell asleep.

He did best with his first midmorning nap, crying only one or two minutes, if at all, before going to sleep. The evenings remained the most difficult. The longest crying episode was twenty-one minutes. My husband and I would sit in the den holding hands, listening to the baby monitor, and engaging in self-doubt: "Does he need us? Are we bad parents for let-ting him cry?" We kept reminding ourselves that Eric was learning a valuable skill that would serve him (and us!) well for life. After about three days, we felt he had achieved suc-cess. He has been a terrific sleeper ever since. Now, at age 11 months, he sleeps from 7:00 P.M. to 7:00 A.M. and naps twice for an hour or two. Everyone who meets him says he is happy, joyful, and alert.

This story describes the hyperaroused state caused by lack of sleep that interferes with sleeping well. It becomes a vicious circle. To prevent or correct this problem, consider rereading the parent reports about successfully helping babies with extreme fussiness/colic at ages as young as 8 weeks in chapter 5 and babies with common fussiness/crying at ages as young as 3–4 weeks in chapters 4 and 6.

If there is crying when you put your child down for a nap and you cannot leave him for one hour, ignore the crying for between five and twenty minutes. You be the judge of how much crying you think is appropriate, but watch the clock, because three minutes of hard crying might feel to you like three hours. The reason you might not let your difficult-temperament or post-colic baby cry for an hour, as you might with an easy-temperament baby, is that he has increased difficulty falling asleep unassisted. Parents of these babies are usu-ally extra stressed as well. I would, however, like to point out that some babies scream their brains out for two minutes, moan and whimper for three minutes, and then go to sleep for a great nap! You might lose the chance for a long nap if you do not let your child blow off steam for a minute or two. As before, when you feel there has been enough crying, rescue your child and try again the next day—or maybe put him back down if you think he will now go to sleep. For the remainder of the day, try to keep each interval of wakefulness to no more than two hours, or do whatever works to maximize sleeping and minimize crying.

An alternative to putting children in their crib for naps is to sleep with them in your bed (see the co-sleeping and *SIDS* warning). This may work well for first-time mothers who do not have other children to care for. However, as your child becomes older, he becomes more aware of his environment while awake, drowsy, and asleep. So you might have to use a co-sleeper next to your bed to ensure that your child is not stimulated by your body movements, coughing, or snoring.

Midmorning Nap Problems

Midmorning Nap Is Absent, Too Short, Too Long, or at the Wrong Time

The midmorning nap develops at 3–4 months of age in 80 percent of all children and a few months later in the 20 percent of children who had colic.

Sometimes the midmorning nap does not develop because the bedtime is way too late and your baby sleeps in too late in the morning to take a nap around 9:00 A.M., or he wakes up too early to make it until 9:00.

Sometimes the midmorning nap is short because that is all the sleep your child needs at that time—that is, your child is a short napper. As discussed earlier, about 20 percent of children between 6 and 21 months always have short naps in the morning and afternoon, no matter what parents do. These children may be well rested. In contrast, midmorning naps for other children between 6 and 9 months of age may be short, and the child may take many such short naps—or, as one mother called them, "snaps"—throughout the day. These children often appear tired even though the bedtime is early. However, as long as the bedtime is early, by 9–12 months most of these children are taking fewer and longer naps and no longer appear tired. I think that most of these short or irregular nappers are those who had colic when younger, and their biological nap rhythms need a longer time to mature, so their naps are actually longer at 9 months than at 6 months.

The most common cause of an absent or a too-short midmorning nap may be an interval of wakefulness that is too long between the wake-up time and the beginning of the nap. For the child under 4 months of age, sometimes starting the midmorning nap after only one hour of wakefulness allows the child to be soothed back to sleep before he becomes overtired. In an older child, starting the nap at the wrong time, either too early or too late, may either shorten the nap or make it less restorative; then it messes up the rest of the day. Use the midmorning nap rhythm as an aid to help your child sleep. If needed, stretch the interval of wakefulness, using approximately 9:00 A.M. as your target time. You might only get to 8:30 or 8:45 A.M. because your child is becoming overtired. It's a balancing act: You want to start the nap when the biological nap time begins, but you also want to avoid the overtired state. You are willing to allow the child to become a little overtired but not to become so wigged out that he has great difficulty falling asleep (page 355).

Sometimes an older brother or sister has a scheduled activity that interferes with the midmorning nap. Some options are to try to get relatives or a neighbor to watch your younger child at home while you drive your older child to the activity, or try to carpool to reduce the number of days per week your younger child misses out on a good midmorning nap. Often the younger child might fall asleep in the car seat during the drive; then the parent can allow the child to continue to nap in the car seat in the parked car. Transferring your child to the crib usually awakens him and ends the nap. It looks awkward to us, but many young children appear to sleep well in the cozy car seat.

Sometimes the wake-up time is too late because the bedtime is too late and your child cannot fall asleep at 9:00 or 10:00 A.M. for a nap. Controlling the wake-up time (page 294) simply means waking your child around 7:00 A.M. in order to get a good-quality nap to begin around 9:00 A.M. To avoid an overtired child, the bedtime will also have to be moved earlier. Parents may not like this solution, perhaps because they like to play with their child late at night or they like to sleep later in the morning.

If the midmorning nap is too long or too late in the morning, it may interfere with your child's ability to fall asleep easily around 12:00 to 2:00 P.M. for the second nap, and the result is an overtired child by late afternoon. The reason the midmorning nap is too long or too late is usually because the bedtime is too late. Limiting the midmorning nap to one to two hours by waking your child is necessary because it is important to protect the second nap. But many parents reject this suggestion because sleep is so precious! So it becomes essential to move the bedtime earlier, which will cause your child to wake in the morning better rested, and this will then automatically shorten the midmorning nap.

NAP HINTS

Before the midmorning or midday nap, go outside to briefly but intensely stimulate your child with physical activity at the park or in the sandbox; expose your child to light, wind, clouds, voices, music, traffic sounds; go for rides in the jogger or stroller. Then tone it down as you get near nap time. Now spend an extra-long time soothing; if your child finds baths soothing, include one in the nap time routine. Make the room dark and quiet.

Midmorning Time Awake

Expect your baby to be ready for another nap after two to three hours of wakefulness, depending on the length of the midmorning nap and whether your child is closer to 4 months or 12 months. In general, avoid long excursions, which might lead to mini snoozes in the car or park. Although I've been emphasizing sleep rhythms, remember that there are also wake rhythms—times during the day when the body clock automatically switches to a wakeful mode, just as it switches to sleep mode at night and at nap times. Wakefulness turns on as sleep turns off. The development of wakefulness is an active process; it is not just the turning off of sleep. During a wakeful mode, it is hard to fall asleep or stay asleep. Very tired children will sleep during the wakeful mode, but sleep quality during a wakeful mode—the ability of the sleep period to restore alertness and a sense of well-being—is lower compared with the same amount of sleep occurring during a sleep mode; that is, the sleep is less restorative. The result is similar to jet lag syndrome. It is equally important to sleep during the biological sleep mode and *not* sleep during the wakeful mode. If your child did not take a midmorning nap, do not allow him to take a snooze in the car or stroller at a time when he should be awake, because if your baby naps when he should be awake, it will throw the remaining sleep/wake schedule for the day off kilter.

For adults, there is a dramatic wakeful mode associated with a period of physical relaxation between about 6:00 and 9:00 P.M. Even if you are drowsy or sleep-deprived, it is hard to fall asleep during this time. This distinct zone of decreased sleepiness or increased arousal during the early-evening hours has been called the "forbidden zone" for sleep. This wakeful period has been recognized by the television industry, which calls it "prime time." This is the time when most adults do not and cannot sleep. Recent research also shows that there is also a forbidden zone for sleep in infants (page 403).

MAJOR POINT

It is as important to *not* let children sleep when they are in a biological wakeful mode as it is to help them sleep when they are in a biological sleep mode.

Usually if a nap doesn't occur, it is best to keep your baby awake and go to the next sleep period, whether it is another nap or nighttime sleep. Probably this next sleep period will take place a little earlier because of the missed nap. Try to strike a balance between not letting your child become extremely overtired by keeping him up, and at the same time preserving or protecting the age-appropriate sleep pattern.

Nap #2: Midday, Early Afternoon

The second nap usually occurs between noon and 2:00 P.M., most commonly around 1:00 P.M., but in any case it should usually begin before 3:00 P.M. in order to not interfere with an early bedtime. The nap should last about an hour or two. Please remember, this is an *outline* of a reasonable, age-appropriate, healthy sleep pattern, *not a set of rigid rules*. In order to describe sleep patterns, we have to use clock time and the number of hours of sleep, but it is more important to watch your baby than to watch the clock. There is nothing absolute about napping at 1:00 P.M. or any other time in this sleep schedule. You'll have to make some adjustments to fit your own lifestyle and family arrangements. There will be special occasions when your child does not get the sleep he needs. But he will recover from these exceptions faster if you have a regular pattern on most days. The problem with some families is that they never establish a regular pattern, so the child is always somewhat overtired, and exceptional days of missed naps create more extreme overtired behavior. The return to baseline in these children, which is slightly overtired behavior, is slow and stressful for families.

The midday nap commonly continues until the third birthday, but after age 3 it begins to drop out.

Midday Nap Problems

Midday Nap Is Absent, Too Short, Too Long, or at the Wrong Time

The most common problem with this second nap is that the interval of wakefulness following the first nap is too long. Maybe you lost track of time or traffic delayed your return home. Being up too long causes your baby to become overtired, and he has difficulty either falling asleep or staying asleep. If you are using method A (page 478), please leave your baby completely alone for one hour after soothing to see if he will fall asleep.

If the duration of crying and sleeping associated with the midday nap puts you way past 2:00 or 3:00 P.M., forget this nap and try to get your child to nap in the late afternoon if he is substantially younger than 9 months and has usually been taking a third, midday nap. If there is no midday nap and no third midday nap, prepare for a rocky afternoon and a long soothing period as you put your child to sleep super early that night, around 5:30 P.M. Even though your child might appear very sleepy at 4:00 to 5:00 P.M., going to sleep this early is likely to backfire with a too-early wake-up the next day.

Bad timing is a common cause of problems associated with the midday nap. If it is too early, way before noon, because of a too-short midmorning nap, the midday nap will not be as restorative and your child might be overtired by late afternoon. One mother said her son was a "french fry" by the end of the day because he was crispy. Under 9 months of age, this might lead to a late or long third nap that causes the bedtime to become too late. If the midday nap starts too late, way after 2:00 P.M., or if it lasts past 3:00 P.M., it may interfere with an early bedtime.

Sometimes the midday nap conflicts with scheduled activities, such as preschool for the child or scheduled activities for older brothers and sisters. Try to minimize these conflicts regarding the older children by using babysitters or car pools, or by skipping some (but not all) of the classes for your infant. An earlier bedtime might be essential when the midday nap is shortened or skipped.

Center-based daycare may be associated with poor-quality naps because of bad timing for soothing to sleep, not enough help for long soothing, too much light or noise from the environment, or crying from other children. Sometimes there are no alternatives available to the family in their choice of daycare, and although it is especially hard on these families, an earlier bedtime will help these children.

If the midmorning or midday nap is sometimes way too short or skipped, try to keep the child up and go to the next scheduled sleep time, but move it a little earlier. Protect the sleep schedule.

Nap #3: Late Afternoon

About 16 percent of children are still taking a third nap at 6 months; the frequency of this nap drops to 5 percent at 9 months and to 1 percent at 12 months. Therefore, after 6 months of age, more than 84 percent of children have no third nap, and their longest wakeful period occurs in the afternoon. This is the time to go on longer excursions, errands, or shopping trips. Scheduled events such as baby exercise classes and outings to the park may be fun during this longer wakeful period. In contrast, the morning wakeful period between the two major naps might not be very long.

If the late-afternoon nap does occur, the time when it starts may vary between 3:00 and 4:00 P.M. Also, the duration of this nap may vary, but it is usually very brief, maybe thirty to forty minutes. Some children take it daily and others take it occasionally. The presence of a third nap after 6–9 months is often associated with a bedtime that is too late, which in turn causes issues with the two major naps and may contribute to the bedtime battles that eventually emerge around 9–12 months of age, when there is increasing self-agency. If so, eliminate the third nap in order to accomplish an earlier bedtime. The earlier bedtime then abolishes the tiredness that had made the third nap appear necessary. Early bedtimes are especially difficult in families where both parents work outside the home, but the benefits for the entire family outweigh the difficulties (chapter 3). Try to overcome these difficulties as best you can.

Late-Afternoon Nap Problems

Sometimes, around 9–12 months of age, a child falls asleep around 4:30 to 5:30 P.M. and wakes around 7:30 or 8:00 P.M., then is kept up playing with parents for a few hours until 10:00 P.M., and finally goes back to sleep but may not sleep well at night. The parents think the child is taking a third nap at 4:30 to 5:30 P.M. But in reality the child needs a very early bedtime, maybe around 6:00 P.M., and no playing between 7:30 and 10:00 P.M. Eventually, the lost evening sleep during the wakeful evening play period produces a cumulative sleep debt.

REAL LIFE
Special events often result in skipped or shortened naps for children. Do not become a slave to your child's nap schedule. But the more you protect the sleep routine for regular days, the less disruptive those special days will be.

Q: *How long should my child nap?*

A: Ask yourself this question: Does your child appear tired or sleepy during the day? If your baby is tired in the late afternoon or early in the evening, this *might* indicate insufficient naps. A possible solution is simply to put your child to bed earlier at night. Keeping a baby up too late produces fatigue and sleep deprivation, and will ultimately lead the child to resist falling asleep or to wake at night. This may be a problem, especially when a working parent or parents arrive home late, feeling guilty about being away from the family so long.

To Sum Up: Months 4-8

In this age range, most babies accept naps without protest and fall asleep at night without difficulty. These easy babies may still wake once or twice in the middle of the night. I consider this behavior normal, natural, and not something that needs to be changed—as long as it's for a brief feeding and not prolonged playtime.

Choose the one or two times when you'll go to feed your baby and change diapers, and don't go at any other time. Please review the earlier discussion on arousals (page 61) if you are puzzled as to why babies sometimes get up or make sounds frequently throughout the night. If you have an intercom or baby monitor that allows you to hear all the quiet cries or sounds that occur during the arousals, turn it off. All you are accomplishing by listening to your child's awakenings is messing up your own sleep. A mother's sleeping brain is so sensitive to her baby's crying that any loud, urgent call will wake her. You do not need an amplification system to ruin your sleep over every little quiet sound your baby makes!

Most mothers will partially synchronize feedings to sleep patterns so that their child is fed around the time he gets up in the morning, around the time of (either before or after) the two naps, around bedtime, and one or twice at night under 9 months of age. In other words, bottle-feedings or breastfeedings now occur four times during the day. Frequent sips, snacks, or little feedings throughout the day are not necessary for nutrition, but the overtired child might appear to be "hungry" like this because sucking is soothing.

Gradually your child will begin to associate certain behaviors on your part, certain times of the day, his crib, and his sensation of tiredness with the process of falling asleep for naps. If you started early to teach your child self-soothing (chapter 4), falling asleep for naps usually involves no crying. If your child had extreme fussiness/colic or did not learn self-soothing early, learning to fall asleep for naps might involve maybe-cry or let-cry sleep solutions (chapter 5).

Stranger wariness or stranger anxiety may be present in some babies by about 6–9 months of age, and with this new behavior, some mothers note some separation anxiety—that is, the child shows distress when the mother leaves. I do not think this type of separation anxiety directly makes it more difficult for a child to fall asleep unassisted. I have observed that babies with separation anxiety learn to sleep well as rapidly as any other babies when their mothers leave them alone at sleep times. The problem is that some mothers also suffer from the thought of separation and will not leave their children alone enough at sleep times to allow healthy sleep habits to develop. Self-agency, described above, also develops around 6 months of age and may lead to major bedtime battles or signaling at night if your child is short on sleep.

A major problem in implementing an age-appropriate sleep schedule for naps and early bedtimes is that it is *inconvenient*. Many parents resent the fact that their babies are now less portable. It is inconvenient for parents to change their lifestyle to be at home twice a day on most days so that their baby can nap. But when parents initially suffer through the process of establishing a good sleep schedule and their child is well rested, occasional irregularities and special occasions that disrupt sleep usually produce only minor and transient disturbed sleep. The recovery time is *brief* (page 602), and the child responds to a prompt reestablishment of the routine.

Bluntly put, when parents are unwilling to alter their lifestyle so that regular naps are never well maintained or the bedtime is usually a little too late, the child always pays a price. The child's mood and learning suffer, and recovery time following outings or illness is much *longer*. These parents often unsuccessfully try many "helpful hints" to help their child sleep better. I'm not sure any or all of these hints can ever substitute for maintaining regular sleep schedules. Parents in my practice who have utilized regular sleep schedules have rarely, if ever, found these hints to be useful after 4 months of age.

Bureau of "Helpful" Hints of Dubious Value to Soothe Your Baby to Sleep

Lambskins

Heartbeat sounds

Womb sounds

Elevating head of crib

Maintaining motion sleep in swings

Changing formulas or eliminating iron supplement

Changing diet of nursing mother

Feeding solids only at bedtime

> You are harming your child when you allow unhealthy sleep
> patterns to evolve or persist—sleep deprivation is as unhealthy as
> feeding your child a nutritionally deficient diet.

Babies seem to respond quickly at this age to a somewhat scheduled, structured approach to sleep. If you can learn to detach yourself from your baby's protests and not respond reflexively by rushing in to him at the slightest whimper, he will learn to fall asleep by himself. As one mother said of her child, "She now goes down like warm butter on toast!"

COMMON DAY SLEEP ISSUES IN MONTH 9

Needs Two Naps but Can Get Only One

The bedtime might be too late and/or the wake-up time too early, causing your child to be very tired in the morning. This morning sleepiness causes him to take a mega-nap in the morning that interferes with his ability to take a midday nap. As a result, he is not well rested in the late afternoon or early evening. Or scheduled morning activities might conflict with a nap around 9:00 to 10:00 A.M., resulting in a very late midmorning nap around 10:30 or 11:00 A.M. Even if this is a brief nap, it may recharge your child's battery and interfere with a long midday nap.

The solution for needing two naps but only getting one is a bedtime that is twenty or thirty minutes earlier. More sleep at the front end allows young children, who need two naps, to wake up better rested, which means they are better able to take two naps. In older children who appear to need two naps but are really old enough for just one, more night sleep with an earlier bedtime erases the apparent need for two naps.

Needs to Nap but Refuses to Nap

When I studied naps in children, about 10 percent of children gave up naps early because of some stressful event that *disorganized home routines,* such as the death of a parent, divorce, moving to a new home, or the birth of twin siblings. Simply having a new sibling did not cause a change in napping. Also, there were three children who stopped napping for about a year during a period of marital discord or problems with caretakers. After resolution of the conflicts, all three children resumed napping and continued to nap for years. Additionally, there were many other children whose families experienced deaths (including SIDS), divorces, or moves but without associated napping problems. It appears that when parents and caretakers maintain nap routines despite potentially disruptive stressful events, most children continue to nap.

Holidays, trips, illnesses, or other changes in routine might cause your child to give up napping and be very tired during the day. Another common cause of no napping occurs when the child drops the midmorning nap but the parents do not make the bedtime a little earlier. Over many weeks or months, your child develops cumulative sleepiness (page 82) until he hits a wall and becomes way overtired. In this state, it is difficult for him to nap because his body is geared up to fight the fatigue. When you try to reestablish the nap, he just plays in his crib, cries, or does a combination of both.

Try a temporarily super-early bedtime to help him wake up better rested. In other words, for four or five nights, put him to sleep when he is drowsy at 5:00 or 5:30 P.M. This might backfire and cause him to wake up too early. If this happens, for those four or five mornings ignore him until 6:00 A.M. Often the temporary super-early bedtime will help erase his sleep debt so he is more able to relax and take a nap. To help reestablish the nap habit, you might want to have intense morning stimulation and an extra-long and soothing nap time ritual. Leaving him alone in his crib for no more than one hour, even if he cries, often will allow the nap to occur because he is tired and not receiving any stimulation from his parents (page 289). Or you might have to lie down with him in your bed to help induce sleep. If this is successful, then you would very slowly and gradually transition him back to his crib. Once the nap has been reestablished, the bedtime can be made a little later. Children who slip in and out of good sleeping patterns are usually going to bed slightly too late every day. They don't have major problems, but they are always on the edge of becoming overtired and they easily and quickly become very overtired whenever there is a disruption of sleep routines.

Here is a report of how a temporarily super-early bedtime helped create long and regular naps and a change in personality:

When our pastor asked us if our 8-month-old son, Henrik, was a "serious, sullen" boy, I knew we had a problem. Just one month before, my friend had sent us a note saying how Henrik was the happiest baby she'd ever seen. She could elicit a belly laugh from him with just a sideways glance. Now our pastor, an experienced grandfather, was pulling out all the stops—goofy faces and exaggerated sneezing— and Henrik wouldn't crack a smile. But it wasn't because he was suddenly sullen or serious; he was exhausted.

What I had hoped was just a napless phase that he'd outgrow was catching up to him and choking his vibrant personality. We needed help. While Henrik was sleeping better at night, his daytime naps were becoming history. Over the past two months, his decent, if erratic, nap schedule had faded into two brief naps and then disappeared altogether.

Getting my son to fall asleep was never an issue; nursing or rocking soothed him easily. The problem was getting him to stay asleep once I set him down. As soon as I'd set him in his crib, his back would arch and he'd be choked up before he touched the mattress. "Nap time" had come to mean Henrik crying in his crib until my nerves couldn't take it anymore, or him sleeping soundly on me.

I knew he needed to learn to soothe himself to sleep, but

crying it out just didn't seem to work. The longer I'd let him cry, the more he would work himself up. I knew sleeping on me wasn't a good solution, but when I'd see the dark circles under his eyes and hear his voice husky from crying—and especially when he got his first cold—I just couldn't let him cry anymore. He needed sleep. So I'd get comfortable with him on the sofa and hope a good movie was on cable.

We set off for our consultation with Dr. Weissbluth. After studying our son's erratic sleep patterns, he recommended an earlier bedtime and regular wake-up times for my son. Dr. Weissbluth explained that Henrik was going to bed too late and wasn't getting enough sleep at night. (Henrik usually fell asleep between 8:00 and 9:00 P.M. and woke up around 7:00 A.M.) This lack of sleep and a consistent schedule—as odd as it may seem—is what was keeping him from being able to cry himself to sleep during the day. He was too over-tired to sleep! Dr. Weissbluth suggested a 7:00 P.M. bedtime and a 7:00 A.M. wake-up for the long-term goal, but said that we'd probably be looking at a 5:30 P.M. bedtime until Henrik's napping got better.

Once Henrik was up in the morning, we were to stimulate him through walks, outings, and vigorous play. After that, a soothing period would precede his attempt at a 9:00 A.M. nap. I was to continue putting Henrik to sleep in my normal way (nursing and rocking) and then set him down in his crib. I was then to leave him alone for one hour either to sleep, cry, or a combination of the two.

Then, after his midmorning nap, we were to repeat the process for his attempt at a 1:00 P.M. nap (or earlier if no midmorning nap was taken). And then we'd go about our afternoon until it was time for the evening soothing. He asked us to chart our sleep data so we could clearly see Henrik's progress.

When we got home, we played and played, and then I soothed Henrik to sleep. When I set him down for his afternoon nap, he cried. I said a quick prayer, told him I loved him, walked out, and closed the door on my wailing son.

As I walked down the stairs, I breathed in slowly, reminded myself that I was doing this for my son's well-being, and hit the pause button on my emotions. I spent fifty-nine minutes emailing friends with one ear to the monitor to see if and when he'd stop crying. Didn't work today, I was telling myself on the way back up the stairs. But by the time I got to his door, I realized he was quiet. He fell asleep after fifty-nine and a half minutes of crying. If I had gone up one minute sooner, I would've cheated him out of this accomplishment. We were on our way.

The midday nap was the first to get back on track. It took about a week for him to be able to go down at all without crying, and he was still only sleeping for a half hour at a time. But he was sleeping—and on a schedule! I used to think that because Henrik was an erratic sleeper, a sleep schedule wouldn't work for him. Now I know that Henrik was an erratic sleeper because he lacked that schedule. While the idea of a schedule sounds limiting, establishing a schedule was the most freeing thing for our family. We are now able to make accurate plans instead of having to wait around and guess when our son would be ready to go.

The midmorning nap was more of a challenge. For two weeks he cried through his entire midmorning nap. It was difficult to put him down each day knowing he would cry, but his success in the afternoons, along with the giant hug I'd receive when I came to get my teary son, gave me the strength to keep going. Then one day he cried himself to sleep after just twenty minutes, and from then on he would stay sleeping after we put him down. It took two weeks for Henrik to get back to two naps a day, but he did it.

Despite Henrik's sleeping for only thirty to forty-five min-

utes at a time, Dr. Weissbluth told us we should get him as soon as he woke up. He suggested we keep the 5:30 bed-time, which would naturally help lengthen his naps. Our days are now virtually tear-free.

My son is thriving on his new schedule. He's back to his giggly, healthy, and well-rested self. Instead of being the sullen boy in church, he's now the chipper angel who sings out loud with joy—with or without the rest of the congre-gation.

As mentioned earlier, self-agency becomes more apparent at 9 months of age. *Strong-willed, willful, independent-minded, stub-born, headstrong, uncooperative.* Sound familiar? These are the words parents often use to describe their toddlers. You may observe that your young child is simply less cooperative. A psychologist might use the term *noncompliance* to describe this lack of coopera-tion, but the psychologist would also point out that these behaviors go hand in hand with the normal, healthy evolution of the child's autonomy or sense of independence. All infants can now express what they do and do not want, what they like or do not like, with greater energy and persistence than previously. Parents discover that their child is not as easily distracted as before. Get used to it, be-cause self-agency only becomes stronger with time! But don't forget that your child is also exhibiting positive qualities of drive and de-termination, qualities that, along with self-sufficiency, will stand him in good stead as he grows.

Usually, experts tell us, the times when you should expect the most difficulties, or "oppositional behaviors," are at transitions: for example, stopping play for dressing, mealtimes, and bedtimes. Since this is the beginning of the "stage" of autonomy (and noncompli-ance), some experts claim that it is natural for this independence/stubbornness to cause either resistance in going to sleep or night waking. I think this "stage" theory is an incorrect interpretation of fighting sleep, but self-agency and separation anxiety do develop around this age and are often used by parents to justify not helping their child sleep; they tell themselves, incorrectly, that all children have trouble sleeping during these stages.

Children in this age range also often develop behaviors described as social hesitation, shyness, or fear of strangers. A child also might cry or appear distressed when his mother leaves him alone in one room while she goes to another room or when she leaves the child with a babysitter. Psychologists call this behavior stranger wariness, stranger anxiety, or separation anxiety. So if a child develops increased resistance in going to sleep at night at this stage, some experts might say that separation anxiety, or fear of being away from the mother, is the cause. I think this is an incorrect interpretation also.

In my general pediatric practice, I have seen many children with intense self-agency and dramatic separation anxiety who have absolutely no problems with sleeping. Additionally, the vast majority of children with sleeping issues do not have big problems with self-agency or separation anxiety. When some children with significant challenges regarding self-agency or separation anxiety plus sleep problems see child psychiatrists or child psychologists, these professionals tend to misattribute the sleep problems to self-agency or separation anxiety. In part, as previously discussed, this is because there is little attention given to sleep during their professional training. But my experience and research show that the direction of effects is often likely the opposite: When overtired children become better rested, they then become more cooperative and less fearful.

Nap #3 Disappears

As mentioned above, the major sleep change that occurs before or around 9 months is the disappearance of the third nap. If the late afternoon nap persists, it often causes the bedtime to become too late. Also, children do not need to be fed at night after 9 months; children who are bottle-fed during the night are likely to develop a night-waking or night-feeding habit. If your baby goes right back to sleep after a feeding, then do not necessarily stop the feedings. But if he decides to play with you and does not easily and quickly return to sleep after the feeding, then stop going to him at night. Again, if you are breastfeeding in the family bed (see the co-sleeping and SIDS warning, page 94), no night-waking habit might develop. Additional changes in sleep routines are coming soon; the midmorning nap is going to disappear.

COMMON DAY SLEEP ISSUES IN MONTHS 10-12

Nap #1 Begins to Disappear

Beginning around 9 months of age, a small number of babies (4 percent) are now taking only one midday nap. This increases to 17 percent by the first birthday. The vast majority of children between 6 and 12 months are taking two naps. When your child drifts toward a single nap, which is always the midday nap, often the bedtime has to be twenty or thirty minutes earlier because children in this age range tend to get more tired near the end of the day. Sometimes it is the midday nap that starts to disappear because the midmorning nap is too long. In this case, move the bedtime much earlier; you can also wake your child after an hour or an hour and a half into the midmorning nap in order to protect the midday nap.

You may think your baby needs only one nap now, but most babies in this age range still need two. One clue that two naps are still needed is that some parents notice that their babysitter can have their child take two good naps, but they themselves can only get him to take one, if that. The child is obviously more rested after the sitter leaves, and the parents wonder how the sitter does it. Well, children are very discriminating at this age. They know that the sitter, following parents' instructions, has a no-nonsense approach and will put them to sleep on a fairly regular schedule. But they figure that with Mom or Dad, enough protesting may gain them more playtime together. After all, sometimes it works. And so long as your child retains the expectation that you will come to him and take him out of his boring, quiet room, he will fight naps.

Summary and Action Plan for Exhausted Parents

If you are too tired to read much and just want to do *something* to help your child sleep better, read chapter 1.

Now that your baby is older, the times when he will become sleepy are more predictable. Another way of saying this is that your baby's biological sleep/wake rhythms are more mature. This allows you to change your strategy to keep him well rested. Previously the focus was on *brief intervals of wakefulness* to avoid the overtired state; now you can begin to use *clock time* more as an aid to help your child sleep well.

REMEMBER
Timing is important, but watch your baby more than the clock.

Let's start in the morning and go around the clock.

Starting the day: Most children will wake to start the day about 7:00 A.M., but there is a wide range (between 6:00 and 8:00).

First nap: The first nap occurs about 9:00 A.M. and may last about an hour or two. Sometimes you will stretch your child to get to this time, or you may wake your child at 7:00 A.M. in order for him to be able to take this nap. Previously you focused on maintaining short intervals of wakefulness, but now you try to anticipate your child's predictable best nap time. If your child takes this first nap too early or too late, then it is difficult for him to take the second nap on time. The midmorning nap begins to disappear between 9 and 12 months, but 84 percent of children at 12 months are still taking this nap.

Second nap: The second nap occurs around 1:00 P.M. and may last about an hour or two. The most common problem at this nap time is too long an interval of wakefulness after the first nap. This causes your child to become overtired. The window for this second nap is between noon and 2:00 P.M., but you may notice that your child's own window, during which it is easiest for him to fall asleep, is much narrower. The midday nap commonly continues to about 3–4 years of age.

Third nap: The third nap may or may not occur. If it does occur, it may vary between 3:00 and 4:00 P.M. Also, the duration of this nap may vary, but it is usually very brief. Usually this nap disappears by about 9 months.

Bedtime: Because of the variability of the third nap, the bedtime may also vary. Most children are asleep between 6:00 and 8:00 P.M. The most common problem at bedtime is keeping your child up too late. If your child is put to sleep after his sleep wave has crested, he will have more difficulty falling asleep and staying asleep. If you keep your child up past the time when he is drowsy—for example, because you return home from work and want to play with him—then you are depriving him of sleep. Please try to avoid making your child overtired in this way, just as you would never deliberately make him go hungry by withholding food.

First night waking: This may occur four to six hours after your child's last feeding. Some children do not get up at this time. Feeding your child differently or giving cereal will not help him sleep better. There is a shifting from deep sleep to light sleep throughout the night. Partial awakenings or light sleep stages called arousals occur every one to two hours when your child is asleep, and sometimes he will make quiet, non-distressed sounds or loudly call out or cry during these arousals. Loud crying during these arousals usually signifies an overtired child. If your baby is not sleeping with you in your bed, going to him at the time of these partial awakenings will eventually lead to a night-waking or night-feeding habit, causing fragmented sleep. This is because the social stimulation that occurs when you pick up your baby, hold him, and feed him will eventually cause him to force himself to a more alert state during these arousals. Consequently, he will learn to expect to be fed or to enjoy the pleasure of playtime with his parents at every arousal. However, if you are sleeping with your baby and breastfeeding, you might promptly nurse at all of these arousals while your baby is still in a somewhat deep sleep state, and then no night-waking habit might develop. The most common problem regarding these naturally occurring arousals is to project psychological problems onto our children, such as saying that they must be lonely or afraid. *Just because the parents may be experiencing these emotions does not mean the child shares them!* However, four to six hours after the last feeding, many children are actually hungry, and you should promptly respond by feeding.

Second night waking: This may occur around 4:00 or 5:00 A.M. Some children do not get up at this time. Most children who do are wet, soiled, or hungry, and a prompt response is appropriate. Maintain silence and darkness, because your child should return to sleep. A common mistake is to play with your child and prevent the return to sleep. The return to sleep is important so that your child will wake up well rested and be able to comfortably stay up to the time of his first nap. Although this pattern of getting up once in the middle of the night and/or in the early morning is common, some children will simply get up once around 2:00 or 3:00 A.M. or not get up at all. Some night wakings for feeding are very common during the first 8–9 months.

Sleeping through the night: This may be defined in different ways, but if the bedtime is too late or if unnecessary feedings or attending to your child cause fragmented sleep, then he will continue to wake up at night.

There are trends over time for the bedtime hour to become later and for children to sleep less during the night and, for some children, to sleep less during the day. Pay attention to your own child's mood and behavior to determine what's best. Ignore advice from others or what you read. There is enormous variation at specific ages for bedtimes and sleep durations for night sleep and day sleep. Don't compare your child's sleep with other children's sleep.

There are three dramatic turning points in sleep maturation for young children:

1. At 6 weeks of age, night sleep becomes organized.
2. At 4 months of age, day sleep is developing and night sleep is becoming adultlike in terms of sleep cycles.
3. At 9 months of age, the third nap is eliminated, naps may be longer for post-colic babies, and there is no need to feed babies at night.

These turning points are so highly predictable and independent of parenting practices that we know they reflect maturation of the brain. Anticipating these changes and allowing them to occur naturally will set the stage for preventing all common sleep disturbances.

It cannot be emphasized enough that the major sleep problems in babies 4–12 months old develop and persist because parents:

• Reinforce bad sleep habits by unnecessarily feeding or attending to their baby at night

- Interfere with an important learning process in their child, namely, learning how to soothe himself to sleep unassisted
- Do not respect the child's biological nap and bedtime rhythms

The failure of children to fall asleep and stay asleep by themselves is the direct result of parents' behavior. Don't underestimate your child's competence and ability to learn healthy and unhealthy sleep habits during these early months!

What a Parent Can Do

Encourage your partner to help care for the baby daytime and nighttime.

Encourage self-soothing; the earlier, the better.

Put to sleep drowsy but awake, then leave the room.

Set an early bedtime based on drowsy signs; practice consistent bedtime routines, including massage; be emotionally available at bedtime.

Feed when hungry but ignore nighttime non-distress vocalizations.

Provide opportunities for naps based on drowsy signs and clock times, because naps are becoming more regular.

If a third nap was present but now has disappeared, move the bedtime slightly earlier.

When the morning nap disappears, consider moving the bedtime slightly earlier.

Avoid irregularity of sleep schedules, including between weekdays and weekends.

Practice safe sleep recommendations.

No TV in your child's room; limit screen time.

Take breaks; try to get more sleep for yourself.

Appreciate the individuality of your child's temperament and sleep needs.

Now is the time to change soothing and bedtime strategies, because extreme fussiness/colic is ending.

If fussiness/crying continues past 4–6 months, seek help.

Seek help if your child is not sleeping well (from your child's primary care provider or a community sleep consultant) or for yourself or partner, especially if there are symptoms of anxiety or depression or significant *risk factors, parent issues,* or *adverse concerns.*

Chapter 10 Outline

TOTAL SLEEP DURATION TRENDS OVER TIME

NIGHT SLEEP

Sleeping through the Night

Bedtime Hour Trends over Time

Bedtime

Bedtime Battles and Night Waking (Signaling)

Common Night Sleep Issues

Fears

Getting Out of the Crib or Bed

A Regular Bed and the Arrival of a New Baby

DAY SLEEP

Day Sleep Duration by Age

Individual Stability of Naps

Number of Naps per Day by Age

Day Sleep Duration Trends over Time

Trends over Time: Percentage of Children Taking Naps
and Number of Naps per Week

Common Day Sleep Problems

Routines and Schedules

Refusal to Take a Nap

Getting Up Too Early

SLEEP RECOMMENDATIONS

MONTHS 12–15

Night Sleep

Healthy Sleep Habits in Early Childhood: Age 1–7

If you have not done so already, please go back and read chapter 1.

Studying what constitutes a healthy diet has a long history, and today everyone appreciates that healthy food, for us and our children, is an essential part of staying healthy. Perhaps the reason that sleep gets far less attention today is because in the past, research regarding the link between sleep and health in children was not performed; sleep problems in our children were less of an issue . . . because they slept more! Let's look at how sleep in our children has changed over time.

Total Sleep Duration Trends over Time

A study by Dr. Ivo Iglowstein showed that total sleep durations decreased from 1974 to 1979 and from there to 1986. For example, "at two years of age, the decrease between 1974 and 1986 was from an average 14.2 hours to 13.5 hours for total sleep duration." Also, a review by Lisa Matricciani found that "over the last 103 years, there has been consistent rapid declines in the sleep duration of children and adolescents."

This trend was confirmed by studies by Dr. Anna Price and me for middle-class or middle-socioeconomic-status (SES) families:

AVERAGE TOTAL SLEEP DURATION

Age (Years)	1979–80	2004–08
1	13.8 hours	13.4 hours (2004)
2	12.8 hours	—
3	12.4 hours	11.7 hours (2006)
4	11.9	—
5	11.4	11.1 (2008)

As noted previously (pages 102 and 298), cumulatively small differences in sleep—for example, among the 5-year-olds, a decrease from 11.4 to 11.1 hours (*nineteen minutes*)—may have major consequences.

This same trend was noted for higher-SES families by Dr. Josephine Foster in the early part of the twentieth century and by Dr. Avi Sadeh at the beginning of the twenty-first century:

AVERAGE TOTAL SLEEP DURATION

Age	1927	2006
12–17 months	13.6 hours	12.8 hours
18–23 months	13.4 hours	12.5 hours
2–3 years	12.8 hours	11.9 hours
	(24–29 months)	(24–36 months)

The trend toward less sleep has also been documented in other countries. For example, in Spain, the mean sleep duration has decreased as follows:

AVERAGE TOTAL SLEEP DURATION

Age	1987	2011
2–5 years	10.7 hours	10.3 hours
6–9 years	9.9 hours	9.5 hours
10–14 years	9.3 hours	8.9 hours

Again, even though the absolute differences are small (twenty to thirty minutes), *small differences in sleep can have major consequences.*

Night Sleep

SLEEPING THROUGH THE NIGHT

What does the phrase *sleeping through the night* mean? This is discussed in detail in chapter 9. In my experience, all children who are napping well and have early bedtimes are sleeping uninterrupted through the night by *9 months or earlier.*

Don't hide behind excuses; there will always be one handy (page 134)!

BEDTIME HOUR TRENDS OVER TIME

I want to illustrate the enormous variability in children's sleeping, both in the past and currently. The age of your child is most important; older children stay up later and sleep less. But at every specific age, there is a wide range for the bedtime hour and for the duration of night sleep, day sleep, and total sleep. I present the average numbers to help you understand the main points. But, for clarity, I have deliberately excluded the very wide ranges that accompany each average number in order to show how *most* children were sleeping in the past. This guideline may or may not inform you how your child should sleep today.

It may be reassuring that your child's early bedtime was commonplace in the past, when parenting may have been less complicated. Skip all the number stuff if you wish; what counts is your child's mood and behavior—so watch your child!

As discussed in chapter 9, it is only recently, over the long history of parenting, that children have been able to stay up late at night. Data collected by Dr. Iglowstein, Dr. Price, and me (1979–80) show that the bedtime hour has shifted over the years to a later clock time. The cause of this shift is not known.

BEDTIME HOUR (P.M.) BY YEAR

Age	1974	1979	1979–80	1986	2004–08
1 year	7:08	7:41	8:00	8:16	8:00 (2004) (10–12 months)
2 years	7:08	—	8:30	7:46	—
3 years	7:35	7:53	8:15	8:07	8:15 (2006)
5 years	7:46	7:56	8:10	8:11	8:15 (2008)

After about 1980, the trend toward a later bedtime plateaued among children around 1 year and younger, perhaps because increasingly later bedtimes would eventually be significantly disruptive to the child and the family. But the trend for ever-later bedtimes for 3- and 5-year-olds continued through 2006 to 2008. Although the wake-up times were a little later in children 1, 3, and 5 years old (three, seventeen, and four minutes, respectively), these later wake-up times failed to fully compensate for the later bedtimes, resulting in less night sleep than in the past. When the bedtime is always too late, then you should expect behavioral, emotional, and academic problems, even if your child gets up a little later or takes longer naps. *When* your child sleeps at night is as important as *how long* your child sleeps, and longer naps are not a substitute for less night sleep (chapter 2).

A possible contributing factor to the trend of later bedtimes over time might be that, over the same time frame of Dr. Iglowstein's survey (1974 through 1986), other data show that between 1975 and 1985 the percentage of women in the labor force who had children under age 18 dramatically increased, by 14.7 percent. Afterward, this began to taper off: Between 1985 and 1995, the increase was only 7.6 percent, and between 1995 and 2005, it was only 0.8 percent. More mothers in the workforce might be associated with more center-based daycare (also associated with shorter naps) and later bedtimes so that parents could enjoy the company of their children after work. In support of this suggestion, families using child care in centers as their primary child care arrangement more than doubled (13 percent to 28 percent) between 1977 and 1990. By 1995, the increases in the percentage of children age 3–6 enrolled in center-based care began to taper off.

In addition to later bedtimes (1974–86), many more mothers entering the workforce (1975–85), and increased use of center-based daycare (1977–90), another trend occurred: The number of first births among women age 35–39 started to increase in the mid-1970s and rose sixfold from 1973 to 2006. Sleep issues in children appear to be more common among older parents (chapter 6).

The trend of having televisions in the bedroom, causing later bedtimes, began in the later 1980s, after Dr. Iglowstein's survey, but this trend has dramatically increased among children with the addition of newer screen-based technology. Television and other electronic screen-based devices in the bedroom have recently become even more popular (page 681). These intrusive objects cause later bedtimes, which, as we have seen, are associated with less sleep and with sleep problems (chapter 11).

A British study, among 16-month-olds, showed that *late* bedtimes are associated with short sleep durations; separately, short night sleep duration, but not total sleep, was linked to increasing BMI in children age 3–6 years (pages 135 and 722). Also, *late bedtimes alone* at about 5 years predict a higher risk for obesity at age 15 years. Research on 5- and 6-year-old children in Japan and Germany has also shown a connection between short sleeping hours and obesity. In the Japanese study, the later the bedtime, the greater the risk for obesity. In both studies, the shorter the duration of sleep, the more likely the children were obese. The researchers controlled for many of the variables, such as parental obesity, physical inactivity, long hours watching TV, and so forth. Maybe some of these overtired children felt stressed and dealt with it by eating. We know that American society is becoming more overweight; maybe our modern lifestyle is causing us to become more overtired, and this sleep loss is directly causing more obesity. In addition to prevention of obesity, many other benefits from healthy sleep are discussed in chapter 3.

BEDTIME

For younger children, time cues can be used as stimulus control to enforce the bedtime hour. Use a digital clock and a matching picture or photo and say, "Oh, look, it's 7:00 [say "seven, zero, zero"]—time for your bath." After the bath, hugs, stories, and kisses, say, "It's now 7:30 [say "seven, three, zero"]—time to go to sleep." Or use a timer to control the duration of the soothing bedtime routine. Then turn out the lights and close the door. No returning or peeking. Your child learns that after a certain hour, no one will come to play with her, so she falls asleep and stays asleep until the morning. She learns to amuse herself with crib toys or other toys in her room until the wake-up time. For older children, Sleep Rules with silent return to sleep work well. Chapters 4 and 5 give more information regarding how to establish parent-set bedtimes and maintain them without bedtime battles.

One study showed that between the ages of 5 and 12 years, on weekdays, children whose parents *enforced* rules about their bedtime slept longer than children whose parents *encouraged* their child to go to bed at a specific time. "One possible explanation for this finding is that 'encouraging one's child to go to bed at a specific time' is a parent's reaction to their child's already-established poor sleep habits. In other words, encouragement may lend itself to being a reactive behavior, while other behaviors—such as rule-setting— may be more proactive . . . family rules have been shown to be associated with earlier bedtimes and greater total sleep on weekdays for older children (12 to 19 years old) . . . *parent-set bedtimes* had the greatest positive correlation with sleep duration [among adolescents; emphasis added]." It seems like there is a real benefit in being strict about bedtime before adolescence on weekdays, but realistically, parents have to be more flexible on weekends and during adolescence (chapter 11).

BEDTIME BATTLES AND NIGHT WAKING (SIGNALING)

In one study of children between 1 and 2 years of age, about 20 percent woke up at night five or more times a week, while in another study of 3-year-old children, 26 percent experienced night waking at least three times a week. If your child behaves this way, consider this behavior to be worth changing. Unfortunately, you simply cannot assume that difficulty returning to sleep unassisted will magically go away. Returning to sleep unassisted is a learned skill; you should expect problems to persist in your child until she learns how to soothe herself back to sleep without your help.

Also in the study of 1- and 2-year-old children, those children who woke up frequently were much more likely to have an injury such as a broken bone or a cut requiring medical attention than those who slept through; while only 17 percent of good sleepers had injuries, 40 percent of the night wakers were injured! The reason is that fragmented night sleep causes daytime drowsiness and inattentiveness and, maybe, impulsiveness that can lead to injury (chapter 12).

Surveys have shown that the majority of children between the ages of 1 and 5 years have a bedtime routine less than thirty minutes long, go to sleep with the lights off, and fall asleep within about thirty minutes after lights out. Night waking occurs in the older children in this group once a week; only a few wake more than once a night. If your child's pattern between the ages of 1 and 5 is substantially worse (longer latency to sleep or more night wakings), consider the possibility that your child is among the 20 percent of children in this group with disturbed sleep. If so, you might also notice later the excessive daytime sleepiness that has been observed in about 5 to 10 percent of children between the ages of 5 and 14 years.

If your child has had a long history of resistance to falling asleep or of night waking, then reread chapter 5 and work on establishing a healthy sleep pattern in general.

Q: *Does this mean that after my baby falls asleep I can never peek in and never go in to soothe or comfort her?*

A: No. Only during the period when you are establishing a new sleep pattern is it important to avoid reinforcement. After your child is sleeping better and becomes well rested, there is nothing wrong with going in to check on her at night.

Q: *I took her older sisters out of their bedroom so her crying wouldn't disturb them. When can they go back into their old bedroom?*

A: Allow several days or a couple of weeks to pass before making changes. The more rested the baby becomes, the more flexible and adaptable she will be. Changes then will be less disruptive.

Q: *My 2.5-year-old daughter understands what I'm saying; why can't I discuss these problems with her?*

A: You want to avoid discussions or lectures at the time the problem is taking place because your reasoning at that time calls attention to the problem and thus reinforces it. It's like shining a flashlight on a problem. Instead, choose some low-key casual playtime to gently voice your concerns regarding her lack of cooperation. Now she is more likely to be in a better mood to reflect on what you are saying. But when there *is* some cooperation, make sure to praise the *specific behavior*: "Thank you for staying in bed" or "Thank you for trying to sleep." Praising your child ("Thank you for being a good girl") but not the behavior fails to tell her exactly what it is that you want her to do again.

If there has been long-standing ambivalence or inconsistency regarding putting your child to bed at night, then naturally occurring separation anxiety will only aggravate or magnify bedtime problems. The same is true for the naturally occurring fears of darkness, death, or monsters that children often express around age 4. In order to deal with separation anxiety or fears at night, we must understand that all children experience them, and that they can learn not to be overwhelmed by them at the bedtime hour with the help of the consistent, calm resolve of their parents. The routine of a set pattern in a bedtime ritual reassures the child that there is an orderly sequence: Sleep will come, night will end, the sun will shine again, and parents will still be there smiling.

There is not one "right" way to help your child sleep well. What works for one child and one parenting style might not be right for you. Try "no-cry" sleep solutions (page 332) if you feel that ignoring crying is neglectful or insensitive and, in doing so, you might feel shame or guilt, or crying will disturb other children or neighbors, or you fear that crying will harm your child or your relationship with your child. Alternatively, because small amounts of extra sleep have a big impact (page 102), continue to do everything the same with one small modification: Just move the bedtime slightly earlier (five to ten minutes) every three to four nights. Even a little extra sleep will make it easier for your baby to fall asleep and stay asleep at night (pages 240 and 361). If you have symptoms of anxiety or depression, they might worsen because new parents become short on sleep; if so, perhaps have a frank discussion with your child's care provider or seek professional counseling. Consider having your husband, wife, or partner read chapter 1 and take charge of helping your baby sleep. If your symptoms or sleep deprivation interfere with putting your baby on the path to healthy sleep, a child sleep consultant in your community or online might be helpful.

COMMON NIGHT SLEEP ISSUES

When your child starts to walk, babble, and show more personality, you will naturally begin to treat her less as an infant and more like a person. Please try to avoid the trap of endlessly explaining, negotiating, or threatening when it comes to sleep times. Save your breath; let your behavior do the talking.

Teaching self-soothing during the first year may or may not have been easy, but the benefits become clearer as your child grows older. Here is how one parent described her journey:

> My friends and family look at me in disbelief when I tell them my 14-month-old daughter goes to bed around 6:30 on her own (without a bottle or rocking or crying) and sleeps soundly until 7:00 the next morning. The training exercise of putting the baby to bed drowsy but awake so they can learn self-soothing is the key. The crib, her bedroom, naps, and bedtime are a place and time of relaxation and enjoyment for our daughter and for us! No crying, no anxiety. I will admit it wasn't always easy and there were trials and tribulations . . . but once you get over whatever humps are your challenges, it's relatively smooth sailing. My experience this past year can be described as follows: 0-3 months is unnerving and exhausting, especially for the first-time parent; 3-6 months is anxious, wondering if you are doing the right thing; 6-9 months is more rewarding as you start to see your efforts really paying off; 9-12 months brings a sense of satis-

*faction and accomplishment; and 12 months and over makes
all the training worth it.*

Your child's developing personality and awareness of herself as
an individual means that her second and third years will be a time
of testing, noncooperation, resistance, and striving for independence. Your child has stronger self-agency. Sleep problems in 12- to
36-month-olds are related to this normally evolving stubbornness
or willfulness in children, who now want to do their own thing. For
example, they may want to get out of their crib or bed at night, not
take naps, get up too early to play, and, of course, resist falling
asleep and wake up at night. This last problem might have started
during the first year and may now continue during the second year
as an ingrained habit.

Don't confuse these issues:
- **Needs versus wants**
- **A sad cry versus a protest cry**
- **Being abandoned versus being alone**

Fears
Nightmares, monsters, fear of separation, fear of darkness, fear of
death, fear of abandonment . . . don't fears cause disturbed sleep at
this age? Many experts tell us that night fears are common among
children between 2 and 4 years old. Thunderstorms, shadows, barking dogs, loud trucks, and many other events over which we have no
control can frighten our children.

If your child has been a good sleeper up to now, you should expect any disturbed sleep triggered by these events to be short-lived.
Reassurance, frequent curtain calls, open doors, or a longer bedtime routine will help your child get over her fears. Night-lights
might help, but a closet light or even a conventional night-light
might keep a sensitive baby from sleeping well. Instead, try a .03-
watt guide light that produces a faint yellow glow; this will usually

provide sufficient illumination. A new teddy bear, to serve as a protector, might help fight off fears. A parent might walk around the room and capture the "monsters" and put them into a bag or box and then remove them from the room. Guardian angels, charms, or dream catchers may help make your child feel more secure.

My recommendation is to spend extra time soothing your child to sleep or go to her once for reassurance, but use a kitchen timer to control the duration of the extra soothing time. The timer is set to the number of minutes you want to spend with your child, and is then placed under a pillow or cushion to muffle the noise. Tell your child that when the buzzer or bell sounds, you will kiss her and leave. The child learns to associate the sound of the timer with your departure and learns that this signals the end of your hugging, massage, or lullabies. This is called *stimulus control*. Just as you know the play is really over when the final curtain call ends, or just as you know to slow down when the green light turns to yellow, your child learns to associate the sound with the end of your soothing effort. Because crying will not bring you back, the crying ends.

An older child might be given a bell to summon her mother or father with the understanding that she can use it only once, or a pass that allows her to leave her room once at night (page 320). Knowing that she can have some attention at night gives the child confidence, and she will sleep better. The goal is to provide extra attention at night without it becoming open-ended or a ploy to fight sleep. If you are uncertain whether your child is fearful or willful, it may be useful to meet with a child psychologist. Also, if your child now appears during the day to be extremely frightened, withdrawn in new surroundings, shy, or fearful, then it is very difficult for parents to give less attention at night, even if the goal is to enhance consolidated sleep. If this is the case with your toddler, a child psychologist can give you good advice on where to draw the line between supporting the child and encouraging her to learn to overcome her fears.

Some child care experts believe severe sleep disturbances are commonly caused by night fears, because they tend to see mostly children with long-standing sleep issues and fears. These children with serious sleep problems and fears who did not sleep well at younger ages then have their current situation misinterpreted as caused by an age-appropriate concern or "stage."

Q: *My 15-month-old child shows separation anxiety during the day, and at night she wants me to hold her and sit with her on the sofa until she falls asleep. How can I leave her alone at bedtime, when she is most anxious?*

A: Separation anxiety, stubbornness, or simply exhibiting a preference for parents' company over a dark, boring room might separately or in combination cause your child to behave this way. Please understand that it is normal for children to feel some anxiety, and learning to deal with anxiety and not be overwhelmed by it is a healthy learning process. Let's not use separation anxiety as an excuse for our own problems in dealing with a child's natural disinclination to cooperate at bedtime. On the other hand, anxiety issues can occur in your children, and if you suspect that this might be the case with your child, discuss this with her primary care provider.

If your child has not been a good sleeper up to now, increasing cumulative sleepiness might contribute to increasing fearfulness. It's time to review chapters 2 through 4, because sleep problems do not go away on their own. Some parents misattribute their child's sleep problems first to gastroesophageal reflux, then to teething, then to separation anxiety, and lastly to fears, but not to their own behaviors.

Getting Out of the Crib or Bed

It's quite natural for social and curious 2- and 3-year-olds to repeatedly climb out of the crib or bed to check out the interesting things they think their parents are up to. Or maybe they just want to watch the late late movie or have a bite to eat! This is the jack-in-the-box syndrome. Of course, what these children like to do best is to come visit with their parents and get into their bed. This not only disrupts their parents' sleep but also harms the child. For a young child who does not understand consequences, consider a crib tent (page 306) to protect sleep and prevent the development of sleep problems. You may have to use duct tape to keep the child from getting to the zipper. Parents are often reluctant to use a crib tent because they imagine their child will feel like a caged animal in a zoo, restricted, or abandoned. Of course, there might be some protest crying for a few days. However, many children quickly come to enjoy the comfort zone, treating it like a tepee or fort; they do not appear sad or angry.

Some parents do not want to use a crib tent but feel more comfortable putting up a gate or latch lock on the door. If you stand at the door preventing your child from leaving the room, she will fight sleep all the more because she is getting attention from you. If parents want to put a lock on the door, I ask that they have the child watch them put the lock on. One parent felt that the additional step of bringing her 3-year-old to the store where she purchased the lock for the door helped convince him that she was serious. The child is told that if she leaves the room, she will be put back in and the door will be locked. Almost all the time, the child picks up on the parents' serious demeanor and does not even attempt to leave the room in the first place. If, however, the child tests the rules and leaves the room, and the parents place her back into the room and lock the door, although there may be loud and long protest crying, it is usually only for one night, because the child is now highly motivated to prevent the door from being locked in the future.

Sleep Rules and silent return to sleep are used for the older child, about 2.5, who will not stay in bed and understands consequences. Here, too, some parents know that they cannot be consistent at night with silent return to sleep, so they want to put a latch lock on the door. These treatments and others are discussed in chapter 5.

A Regular Bed and the Arrival of a New Baby

One rearrangement is moving your child to a big-kid bed. There is no special age when you should make this change. As long as the crib is large enough, you should not feel that your child must be placed in a regular bed by a certain age. Many parents make the switch around the second or third birthday. Let your child ask for a big bed. One mother described feeling that she had made the move too soon; she thought the big bed must have seemed "oceanic" compared to the crib, because her son always slept curled up in one corner of the bed—that is, when he slept. He slept much better when returned to his crib. Before she made the move back to the crib, his mother wondered whether this would cause a "regression" in her child. It did not. But it did result in a better-rested family.

If the move to a regular bed is needed because of a new baby brother or sister, consider making the move when your newborn is about 4 months old. By then, your newborn has regular sleeping habits. Before your baby reaches this age, there is a constant shifting of household routines due to her naturally irregular sleep pattern. This may cause confusion or insecurity in your older child because he does not know when Mom or Dad will be available, or why he has to wait when he wants to go outside and has gotten used to doing just that. When your newborn is 4 months old and her sleep pattern is stable, events in the house are much more predictable. Your older child now becomes adjusted to the new family arrangements. Your baby goes to the crib and the older child graduates with pride to the big bed for big kids. He does not feel displaced. Before your newborn is actually moved from the bassinet to the crib, feel free to leave the crib up and empty for a while with the understanding that if your older child gets out of bed once, then it's back to the crib.

Moving to a big bed too early—for example, in anticipation of the birth of a new baby—often invites a problem: the commotion and excitement surrounding the arrival of your new baby may create confusion or insecurity in your older child, who may call out or cry at night. The more difficult situation is when your older child starts to get up every night to visit her parents.

If the move to a regular bed prompts frequent nocturnal visits, curtain calls, calls for help going to the bathroom, or calls for a drink of water, think before you act. A habit may slowly develop in which your child learns to expect you to spend more time with her, putting her to sleep or returning her to sleep. Imagine what would occur if a babysitter gave your 2-year-old candy every day instead of a real lunch. Once you discovered this, you would immediately stop the candy for meals. Your child might protest and cry, but would you give in and let her have the candy? No. If you are spending too much time at night with your child when she should be sleeping, consider what you are doing to be giving "social candy"—not needed and not healthy for the child. Be firm in your resolve to ignore the expected protest from your child when you change your behavior.

In addition to moving to a big bed too early causing sleep problems, some families with children with preexisting sleep problems imagine that their child will fight sleep less at bedtime by "promoting" her to a "big girl's" bed. This rarely works. One study of about two thousand infants, between 18 and 36 months, compared those who were still sleeping in a crib versus a bed, in a room separate from the caregivers. "Crib sleeping [compared with bed-sleeping] was significantly associated with an earlier bedtime, shorter sleep onset latency, fewer night wakings, longer stretches of time asleep, increased sleep duration, and decreased bedtime resistance and sleep problems."

Day Sleep

DAY SLEEP DURATION BY AGE

Here are data from my nap study (for children born between 1984 and 1986) regarding the percentage of children taking naps and the total duration of naps. The nap durations are greater than in other reports, presumably because I followed these children since birth and gave the parents advice about sleeping at every visit. So my data might represent optimal naps.

NAP STUDY, 1984–86

Age (months)	Percentage of Children Taking Naps	Average Duration, Total Hours per Day	% in Range: Total Hours	Minimum– Maximum Hours
12	100%	3.0	94%: 2.0–4.0	1.5–5.5
15	100%	2.7	91%: 1.5–3.5	1.0–5.5
18	100%	2.5	98%: 1.5–3.5	1.0–4.0
21	100%	2.4	97%: 1.5–3.5	1.0–4.0
24	100%	2.3	99%: 1.5–3.5	1.0–4.0
36	92%	2.1	80%: 1.5–2.5	1.0–3.5
48	57%	1.9	80%: 1.5–2.5	0.5–5.0
60	27%	1.7	89%: 1.0–2.0	1.0–3.0
72	12%	1.6	90%: 1.0–2.0	0.5–2.5

At every age, the vast majority of children have nap durations within a narrow time frame, but the actual range of nap durations among all children is very wide because a few children have extremely short or long naps. Between 2 and 6 years, the most common duration of day sleep is about two hours for those children still taking naps. All children are taking naps every day until about age 3 years. But naps start to disappear around that age: 8 percent of 3-year-old children are not napping, and among those who continue to nap, they nap, on average, six days per week. In Japan, it is customary to have naps in nursery school, and in one study of 441 children 3–6 years of age, the authors thought that the naps caused the children to go to sleep later at night. Of course, the alternative conclusion is that a bedtime that is too late caused the children to nap more.

Looking at these numbers may reassure you that your child's naps are appropriate for her age, but due to the variability at every age, it is more important to look at your child's mood and behavior than at these numbers.

Individual Stability of Naps

In my nap survey, I divided 6-month-old children into five nap duration groups (chapter 9). Children typically remained in their initial nap duration group until 21–24 months; this individual stability of nap durations probably reflects a *genetic* influence over sleep. In other words, the group of babies whose average nap duration was 3 hours at 6 months of age had nap durations of 2.9 hours by 9 months, 2.8 hours by 12 months, 2.6 hours by 15 months, 2.5 hours by 18 months, and 2.4 hours by 21 months. The babies did not move to a track of much shorter or longer naps. Stated another way, children with long naps at 6 months of age continue to take long naps until 21–24 months; the same is true for children with short or intermediate nap durations. Also, infants' nap durations, for the vast majority of children, remained within a narrow range despite variations in caretaking and social activities, suggesting that *biological* processes affect naps. Nevertheless, considering the actual wide range of nap durations among all the children as a group (shown above) and the fact that many children move away from their initial nap duration group after 21–24 months, it does seem likely that *parents* play an important role regarding naps as well.

Although studies on large groups of children show no consistent relationship between the duration of daytime sleep and nighttime sleep, I think it is likely that most of the children who sleep near the minimum number of hours for naps have problems with night sleep, naps, or both. This may also be true for some of the children who sleep near the maximum number of hours, although I have encountered some very well-rested children, subsequently determined to be very intelligent, who had very long naps at these young ages.

But very long naps might develop as a result of a bedtime that is too late even though night sleep duration seems normal; in this case, despite the long naps, the child is impaired. Long naps are not a substitute for a bedtime that is too late (chapter 2).

NUMBER OF NAPS PER DAY BY AGE

Here are some data from my nap study for children born between 1984 and 1986 regarding the disappearance of naps:

CHILDREN TAKING 1 OR 2 NAPS PER DAY

Age (months)	1 Nap	2 Naps
12	17%	82%
15	56%	44%
18	77%	23%
21	88%	12%
24	95%	5%
36	100%*	0%

* One hundred percent of those still napping take only one nap, but 8 percent are not napping.

As you can see, the majority of children switch to a single nap between 15 and 21 months of age; Dr. Iglowstein observed the transition age to be 18 months. If your child is substantially less than 1 year old and taking one nap, or more than 2 years old and taking two naps, there might be an unappreciated sleep problem.

DAY SLEEP DURATION TRENDS OVER TIME

In addition to the trend over time for bedtimes to become later, causing less night sleep, data are available from studies by Dr. Price and me (1979–80) that show a partial trend over time for less day sleep. The cause of this shift is unknown.

NAP TRENDS, 1979–80 TO 2004

Age	Average Day Sleep Duration	
	1979–80	2004
	3.2 hours (4–11 months)	3.0 hours (4–6 months)
		2.8 hours (7–9 months)
		2.6 hours (10–12 months)
1 year	2.3 hours (12–17 months)	2.5 hours (13–15 months)
3 years	1.4 hours (30–41 months)	1.2 hours (29–33 months)
		1.0 hours (34–39 months)

TRENDS OVER TIME: PERCENTAGE OF CHILDREN TAKING NAPS AND NUMBER OF NAPS PER WEEK

Comparing my data with Dr. Foster's study from 1927, it appears that in the past, between the ages of 4 and 6 years, a higher percentage of children took naps, but they had fewer naps per week.

NAP TRENDS, 1927 AND 1984–86

Age (years)	Percentage of Children Who Nap		Number of Naps per Week	
	1927	1984–86	1927	1984–86
1	100%	100%	Daily	Daily
2	100%	100%	Daily	Daily
3	90%	92%	5	6
4	75%	57%	3.5	5
5	49%	27%	1.7	5
6	20%	12%	0.5	3

Dr. Foster wrote in 1927, "Up to the age of five (the usual age for entering kindergarten) more than half of the children [nap]. The drop from 68 percent at 4½–5 years to 30 percent at 5–5½ years" reflects entry into school. This 38 percent decrease is similar to the decrease noted in 1984–86 of 35 percent between 3 years (92 percent) and 4 years (57 percent), but it is occurring a year earlier! Perhaps this earlier decrease reflects a trend toward earlier involvement in preschool, daycare, or scheduled activities. In other words, more scheduled activities during the day now, compared with 1927, might interfere with naps. But also, later bedtimes today might be driving more naps per week in those children who are given the opportunity to nap. Whatever the cause or causes for these trends, it is clear that parents influence nap behavior and, over time, parenting practices change.

But for the moment let's ignore my nap study (1984–86), because it might represent optimal napping. Other studies, by Drs. Foster, Iglowstein, and Lavigne, still report a trend toward fewer naps per week, and fewer children napping.

NAP TRENDS: NAPS PER WEEK

Age (Years)	Number of Naps per Week	
	1927	1990s
1	7	—
2	7	5
3	5	3

NAP TRENDS: PERCENTAGE OF CHILDREN NAPPING

Age (Years)	Percentage Taking Naps	
	1927	1974–93
1	100%	100%
2	100%	87%
3	90%	50%

Comparing these data on the number of naps per week and the previously discussed data on duration of naps with my nap study and the experience of caring for many children over forty years leads me to the conclusion that many children today are being denied the opportunity to take a nap, and to take a long nap when they do nap. The developing famine in sleep may be a direct contributor to the spreading epidemic of obesity and attention deficit hyperactivity disorder.

However, as previously discussed, taking long naps or more frequent naps might also be an attempt to partially compensate for a bedtime that is too late. In Dr. John Lavigne's study of children 2–5 years old, the lowest-SES group of children went to sleep later, woke later, and took longer and more frequent naps compared with children in all other SES groups. Total sleep duration was similar to the other SES groups, but the children with later bedtimes had more externalizing problems (page 130). Dr. Seog Ju Kim showed that when older children's bedtimes are too late during the school week, there is more catch-up sleep on weekends, and those children with the largest amount of weekend catch-up sleep have the poorest performance on objective attention tasks (chapter 11).

So sleeping later in the morning, taking more naps or longer naps, or trying to catch up on sleep on the weekend does not fully compensate for the harm done by a bedtime that is too late.

> If the bedtime is often too late, sleeping later in the morning and sleeping more during the day does not fully compensate. *When you sleep is as important as how long you sleep.*

COMMON DAY SLEEP PROBLEMS

Specific prevention and treatment strategies for common day sleep problems are discussed in chapters 4 and 5.

Routines and Schedules

Although most 2- to 3-year-old children in my survey went to sleep between 7:00 and 9:00 P.M. and woke between 6:30 and 8:00 A.M., I think that an earlier bedtime is better. A single nap between one and three hours occurs in over 90 percent of children. Try to be *reasonably* regular about nap time and bedtime, and be consistent in your bedtime rituals. There are no absolute, rigid, or firm rules, because every day is somewhat different. Reasonable regularity and consistency imply reasonable flexibility.

How about scheduled, organized activities that take place when your child needs to take her midday nap? If your child is unable to take her midday nap two or three times each week and you are able to get an extra-early bedtime on those days, then there may be no problem, as long as your child is sleeping well in general. But if your child is not sleeping well, for whatever reason, frequently losing a few naps can be quite problematic. Also keep in mind that children are likely to pick up minor illnesses from one another in group settings, and these minor illnesses may disrupt your child's sleep and push her into an overtired state. In general, be cautious regarding preschool classes during the flu season. Have fun with your child, but occasionally take what my wife called a "declared holiday." Missing a swim class, gym class, or any other preschool event now and then because your child is tired and needs to nap, or leaving a class soon after you arrive because some other children look sick, will not jeopardize your child's college plans!

Be aware that your lifestyle helps or hinders your child's sleep patterns, and remember that there will be changes due to growth and rearrangements in relationships within the family such as the arrival of a new baby.

Refusal to Take a Nap

Playtime in the park or shopping together is so much fun; who wants to take a nap? Ask yourself whether not napping is *your child's* problem or *your* problem. Some parents simply find it too inconvenient to hang around the house to enable their child to get her needed daytime sleep. But reflect on how inconvenient it is to drag a tired child around while shopping. Please review chapters 2 and 3 if you feel that naps are not that important.

Refusal to take a nap often occurs after a special event, such as a holiday, party, or vacation. There was so much excitement the day before; your child doesn't want to miss anything again! Sometimes the refusal to nap develops because of unappreciated chronic fatigue due to an abnormal sleep schedule, brief night sleep duration, or sleep fragmentation. If these problems are present, work on them as you work on day sleep. Refusal to take a nap might take place "all of a sudden" after a slow buildup of *cumulative sleepiness,* such as might occur from a bedtime that is only slightly too late during long summer days. Another common cause of cumulative sleepiness occurs when the child drops the midmorning nap but the parents do not make the bedtime a little earlier. For whatever reason, if your child develops cumulative sleepiness, she becomes way overtired and "suddenly" hits a wall. In this state, it is difficult for her to nap because her body is geared up to fight the fatigue.

If your child is substantially under 3 years old and you want to help her nap, try a temporarily super-early bedtime so that she wakes up better rested. For four or five nights, put her to sleep when she is drowsy at 5:00 or 5:30 P.M. That might set things right. However, be aware that it might also backfire and cause her to wake up too early. If this happens, for those four or five mornings, ignore her until 6:00 A.M. Often the early bedtime will help erase her sleep debt, so she is more able to relax and take a nap. Also, to help reestablish the nap habit, you might want to have intense morning stimulation and an extra-long and extra-soothing nap time ritual. Leaving her alone in her crib for no more than one hour, even if she cries, often will allow the nap to occur because she is tired and not receiving any stimulation from her parents. Or you might have to lie down with her in your bed to help induce sleep. If successful, then you would very slowly and gradually transition her back to her crib. Once the nap has been reestablished, the bedtime can be made a little later. Children who slip in and out of good sleeping patterns are usually those who are always going to bed slightly too late. They don't usually have major problems, but they are always on the edge of becoming overtired and they easily and quickly become very overtired whenever there is a disruption of sleep routines. Getting naps back on track is also discussed in chapters 5 and 9.

If your child is close to or past her third birthday, trying to reestablish the nap may not make sense because some children are now naturally outgrowing naps, but trying to establish an earlier bedtime might help your child sleep better anyway.

Keep a sleep chart, log, or diary; pick a time interval that you think is right, and put your child down in the crib at that time. *You* are controlling the nap time. Spend as much time as you want—ten, twenty, or thirty minutes—hugging, kissing, rocking, and nursing to soothe your child. Then down is down—leave her alone for one full hour.

If your child has been quite well rested up to now, the crying may be brief. But if your child has a history of chronic fatigue, prepare yourself for a full hour of crying.

The more rested your child is, the quicker you'll see improvement. A very tired child might require several days of training before she relearns how to nap.

Your goal is to establish an age-appropriate nap routine so your child associates being left alone in a certain place and a familiar soothing routine with feelings of being tired and taking a nap. No more playtime, no more games, just sleep. If your child is young, then every day at about 9:00 A.M. and 1:00 P.M. you should put her down to nap; older children may be put down only at midday. I call this *nap structuring;* we are trying to use natural sleep rhythms to help your child sleep best. After one hour, if there is no nap, then we go to the next sleep period, but a little earlier.

Parents who would rather hold their child in a rocking chair or let her catnap in the stroller are robbing their child of healthy sleep.

This lighter, briefer, less regular sleep is less restorative—it's not as effective in returning your child's energy and attentiveness to its best levels. Remember, sleep is also measured in *quality*, not just *quantity*.

Q: *My problem is not that my child refuses to nap or resists naps, but that her nap schedule is very irregular. What's wrong?*

A: If your child is well rested, it may be that you are in fact very sensitive to her need to sleep and are placing her in an environment conducive to sleep when she needs it. Differences in daily activities produce differences in wakeful intervals and differences in the duration and timing of naps. Perhaps you have unrealistic expectations regarding the regularity of naps according to clock times. If your child is very tired, however, she might be crashing at irregular times when she is totally exhausted. A common problem here is a bedtime that is slightly too late. Early bedtimes appear to regularize and lengthen naps.

Q: *My problem is that my baby takes such long naps that we don't have much time to play together. Are long naps a problem?*

A: There may be a problem if your child snores or mouth-breathes when asleep (chapter 12). These are symptoms of respiratory allergies or large adenoids or tonsils and should be discussed with your child's physician. Another possible problem is that the bedtime is too late and the long naps are attempts to compensate for the lost sleep. In the long run, this compensation will fail because the too-late bedtime causes cumulative sleep deficits (page 82). Or maybe your child needs long naps; long sleep durations are associated with higher intelligence levels, so protect her long naps! Don't worry: You will have more playtime together in the future when your child's naps naturally become shorter.

Getting Up Too Early (page 295)

Getting up too early is another major problem in toddlers. The first question to ask is, how early is too early? If your child gets up at 5:00 or 6:00 A.M. and is well rested, perhaps this pattern is not changeable. You may try encouraging her to sleep later by making the room darker with opaque shades. Getting everyone together in a family bed at that hour may also allow all of you to get some more snooze time. Often families give their baby a bottle at this early hour, after which she returns to sleep for a variable period of time.

While bottles given early in the morning may help your child return to sleep, be aware that if your baby is allowed to fall asleep with a bottle of milk, formula, or juice in her mouth, the result is decayed teeth. This will not occur if the bottle contains only water. Unfortunately, some parents go to their child at 4:00 or 5:00 A.M. with a bottle of milk and then let the baby feed herself.

Treatment for the well-rested child who has a habit of taking an early-morning bottle is to first switch to juice, and then gradually, over about a week, dilute the juice more and more until it is only water. Once your child is drinking only water, place a water bottle at either end of the crib, point them out to her at bedtime, and stop going in.

One mother used to allow her child to watch a video every morning as soon as she woke up. This allowed the mother to have some free time to take care of herself. But her child started waking up earlier and earlier in order to enjoy the video. Stopping the routine of watching videos in the morning was part of the solution.

If your child wakes up too early and is not well rested, work hard to establish a healthy sleep pattern. In the morning, don't go to her until the wake-up hour.

REMEMBER
Getting up too early may be caused by going to sleep too late.
Earlier bedtimes often prolong night sleep and prevent early
wake-ups. *Sleep begets sleep.*

For a 3-year-old child, you can try a variation of controlling the
wake-up hour using *stimulus control*. We previously used a digital
clock as a signaling device to indicate bedtime. Now we are going to
use a digital clock to signal the wake-up time. Place a digital clock
in her room and set the alarm for 6:00 or 7:00 A.M., which may be
after the expected spontaneous wake-up time. Draw a picture of the
clock face showing 6:00 or 7:00—the time that corresponds to when
the alarm will go off. Or you might use a clock radio set to turn on
at the designated time with quiet classical music or a color-changing
bunny light programmed to change color at the desired clock time.

Do not respond to her cries before this wake-up time. Then, at
the wake-up time *you* have picked, you bounce into her room, exclaim how the clock matches the picture or the music is on or the
color has changed, and exclaim, "Oh, see, it's time to start the day!"
Shower her with affection, open the curtains, turn on the lights,
bring her into your bed, or give a bath. Be dramatic, wide-eyed, and
happy to see her. The child learns that the day's activities start at
this time. The pattern on the digital clock, the quiet music, or the
color change in the light acts as a cue, just as a green traffic light tells
you to start moving. Before the wake-up time, the child has her
water bottles but no parental attention.

Sleep Recommendations

Lisa Matricciani's 2013 review of the literature concluded that published recommendations for children's sleep are not based on empirical evidence (chapter 2). She points out that differences exist

among individuals to cope with less sleep: "Interestingly, children from different parts of the world have radically different habitual sleep durations. At any given age, children from Asia sleep 60–120 minutes less each day than children from Europe, and 40–60 minutes less each day than children from the United States. Either there are genetic differences in sleep needs, or sleep needs can be modified by sociocultural context, or Asian children are catastrophically sleep deprived."

She adds that "*sleep timing* [the time when sleep occurs] may be even more important than sleep duration." In a separate 2013 paper titled "Sleep Duration or Bedtime?" the authors studied twenty-two hundred children 9–16 years old and concluded that "*late bedtimes and late wake up times* are associated with poorer diet quality *independent of sleep duration* [emphasis added, page 65]."

Months 12–15

NIGHT SLEEP

Dr. Jacqueline Henderson reported that among a group of 12-month-old children whose average bedtime was 8:30 P.M., many were not sleeping through the night (chapter 9). Based on my research and experience, I think that 8:30 P.M. is too late a bedtime for many, if not most, 12-month-old children.

The percentage of children who were not sleeping uninterrupted between midnight and 5:00 A.M. was 13 percent, and 14 percent were not sleeping uninterrupted for eight hours minimum between sleep onset and time awake in the morning, while 27 percent were not sleeping uninterrupted from at least 10:00 P.M. to 6:00 A.M. I suspect that the factors that caused these children to be unable to sleep uninterrupted at night at 12 months are primarily associated with a failure to learn self-soothing well during the first year of life; the bedtime may also have been too late. The main reasons for not learning self-soothing are post-colic sleep problems and the parent issues described in chapter 4. Because these may be difficult challenges for some parents, if your child is not sleeping through the night at 12 months, I urge you to consider just a simple change that might make a huge difference: Move the bedtime a little earlier, as described in chapter 5.

NAP #1 (MIDMORNING) BEGINS TO DISAPPEAR

How do I know when to drop the midmorning nap? Looking for *drowsy signs* and/or providing nap opportunities in the midmorning may inform you whether your child actually needs a midmorning nap. Another variable is the *bedtime* and whether or not there are bedtime problems. If the bedtime is too late and/or there are bedtime problems, your child might wake up too tired in the morning and be unable to get to a healthy restorative single midday nap and instead crash in the midmorning. Fixing the bedtime erases the need for a midmorning nap. *Daycare policies* may complicate this issue because some children in daycare, starting at 12 months, are moved into a single nap group even though they might need two naps. Here, too, an earlier bedtime might help smooth the transition until the child matures into a single nap mode. As described below, the *age* of your child might help you decide whether a midmorning nap is needed or not.

At 12 months of age, 82 percent of children have two naps and 17 percent take only a single midday nap. But by 15 months of age, 44 percent of children are taking two naps and 56 percent take a single midday nap. This is a dramatic change occurring over a short time period. By 21 months of age, only 12 percent of children nap twice a day and 88 percent nap once a day. The majority of children make the shift from two naps to one nap between 12 and 21 months (page 642).

This transition, however, may not be smooth. You might have a few rough months when one nap is not enough but two are impossible. Here are some ideas for making the transition easier.

Move the Bedtime Earlier

The midmorning nap is always the first nap to naturally disappear. If the bedtime is moved a little earlier, most parents will notice that their child's midmorning nap becomes briefer or turns into a quiet playtime without sleep. Most of these children do not appear to become very tired in the morning, because more sleep at night eventually erases the need for a midmorning nap.

Other children take longer and longer midmorning naps and then appear to actively resist or be unable to take the second midday nap. Often, because this second nap was short anyway, many parents forget it. The result is a child who is overtired late in the afternoon or early evening and who quickly becomes way overtired by bedtime. Instead of, or in addition to, an earlier bedtime, you might want to shorten the midmorning nap by waking your child after about one or one and a half hours so she will be more tired around the midday nap time. But truthfully, very few mothers like the idea of waking their sleeping child to help set a better schedule; sleep is so precious! However, if you do try this, also try to get out of the house immediately following this parent-shortened midmorning nap to provide fun-filled intense stimulation to manage sleep inertia; but tone it down as you get to the middle of the day. Provide extra-long and relaxing soothing to sleep for the midday nap. Maybe also consider moving the midday nap to a slightly later hour so your child is a bit more tired. But what if your child continues to take a midmorning nap and none of the above causes her to take a midday nap? Here's another plan.

Move Back the Midmorning Nap and Skip the Midday Nap

At the usual time of the midmorning nap, delay its onset by ten or twenty minutes. This might require more intense and prolonged soothing to sleep. Anticipate that the late afternoons might be a bit rocky for a while. Slowly, over many days or weeks, continue to delay the midmorning nap until it is occurring near the middle of the day. During this transition, the bedtime might have to be temporarily ultra-early because your child gets pooped every afternoon. After the shift of the midmorning nap to the midday is accomplished, the bedtime might now be moved a little later. However, this new slightly later bedtime (associated with a single, midday nap) should be earlier than the original bedtime that was based on having two naps every day. The earlier bedtime means that a working parent coming home late might not see their child then. If that is the case, that parent can get up extra early to have a longer morning playtime with their child before going off to work.

BE FLEXIBLE

Another solution to getting through the transition from two naps to one nap is to declare some days as two-nap days and other days as one-nap days, depending on when the baby wakes, how long the midmorning nap lasts, scheduled group activities, or the time you want your baby to go to sleep at night. Flow with your child and arrange naps and bedtimes to coincide with her need to sleep as best you can. Be sensitive to the growing need for earlier bedtimes. Eventually, the midmorning nap disappears.

Sleep problems around 1 year of age might involve first attempting to establish two naps with the understanding that it might not succeed; if so, after several days regroup and try a plan that involves a single nap.

Obviously, any combination of parents' scheduling for their convenience and the baby's need to sleep can shape nap patterns as long as the biological nap rhythms are respected (chapter 2). If you love naps for yourself, you may protect your child's nap schedule differently from the parent who does not customarily take naps.

HELPFUL HINT

Some children appear to hate their bedroom in the afternoon and scream as you approach it. One mother solved this by doing all the pre-nap soothing in the living room and then quickly went into her child's room.

Q: *How long should my child nap?*

A: Does your child appear well rested? You be the judge. All of us have good days and bad days, but if you notice a progression toward more fussiness, brattiness, or tantrums, your child may need longer naps.

Months 15–21

NAP #1 (MIDMORNING NAP) DISAPPEARING

The midmorning nap is on its way out (page 653). At 18 months, 77 percent of children take a single midday nap; by 21 months, 88 percent of children sleep only in the midday. Sometimes the child is taking only the midmorning nap and the plan discussed above does not work because the general recommendation of an early bedtime backfires. You try an early bedtime, and all you get is an earlier wake-up time, which makes your child more tired in the morning and makes her need the midmorning nap all the more (see "The 5:30 P.M. Bedtime Rut" in chapter 5). Under these circumstances, you might temporarily put your child to bed a little later at night with the hope that she will sleep in later. It may take several days or a few weeks to build up enough sleep pressure to cause the later wake-up time. Be careful to avoid a second wind (page 43), because if you put her to bed much too late she will have difficulty falling asleep and staying asleep. So this will require some patience and trial and error. Still, wake her, if she is asleep, at 7:00 A.M. and then proceed with one of the plans previously described to get a midday nap.

Q: *What do I do if my child is healthy but cries at night, and the crying stops as soon as I pick her up?*

A: Ask yourself if there is anything you can do to regularize the total sleep pattern, such as timing naps better or making the bedtime earlier. Was there anything that recently disrupted her schedule to cause her to become overtired? Does she snore or mouth-breathe during sleep, or might she be starting to become ill? Look at the big picture, not just the night crying. In general, you will not want to attend to the night crying, because you want to encourage consolidated sleep. If you go to your child, you will cause fragmented sleep, which is poor-quality sleep. If your head says that not going to your child is the right thing to do, but your heart won't let you do it, try some of the following suggestions. One mother tied a ribbon around her ankle and her husband's ankle so that she did not shift into autopilot mode at night and go to her child when he cried. Another mother waited for her husband to go away on business for a few days so she could ignore the crying without having her husband undercut the plan. Sleep temporarily farther away from your child; use earplugs, earphones, pillows over the head; take a shower. Do what is best for your child, but don't torture yourself.

Months 21–36

The midday nap usually lasts until about 3 years of age and then gradually disappears. If drowsy signs are present in the day, offer a nap opportunity. If the midday nap disappears too soon, your child may become overtired in the late afternoon and have difficulty falling asleep at night. Either reestablishing the midday nap (if your child is substantially under age 3) or moving the bedtime earlier (if your child is substantially over age 3) should help. If the midday nap persists in much older children, the bedtime might progressively get later and later, causing bedtime battles to develop. Eliminating the midday nap will permit an earlier bedtime and help erase bedtime battles.

SINGLE MIDDAY NAP BEGINS TO DISAPPEAR

The majority (80 percent) of children between the ages of 2 and 3 years have a nap length in a narrower band from one and a half to two and a half hours. The most common nap duration between the ages of 2 and 6 years is two hours. The stability of the two-hour nap over different ages is another argument for a strong biological influence over sleep, but it does not necessarily mean that your child needs a two-hour nap. Some children need less and some need more daytime sleep.

Q: *When do I transition my child from a crib to a bed?*

A: As she approaches her third birthday, let your child ask for a big bed. If you move her too soon, she may not stay in her bed because she is curious and wants to see what's going on elsewhere in the house.

Years 3–7

The list of new concerns for older children is long: school start times, organized weekend and after-school activities, and enrichment classes or lessons (music, dance, math, or religious). Health habits may appear to be less important to parents than the development of children's academic, social, athletic, or artistic skills. But the contribution of healthy sleep habits to a child's well-being does not diminish with age.

Some of the subjects to review for the prevention and treatment of sleep problems in this age range, discussed in chapters 4 and 5, are: bedtime routines, early bedtimes, parent-set bedtimes, parent issues, no television in the bedroom, sleep log, Sleep Rules and silent return to sleep, control the wake-up time, day correction of bedtime problems, fading, pass system, and choose a sleep solution.

Here are some simple ways to help your child settle down for day or night sleep. Consider them to be a sleeping routine for preschool children. Choose those items that work best for your child and do them at all sleep times.

Slow down activity.
Close physical contact.
Gentle massage or mild stretching.
    Cuddle up with the child in a chair.
    Nestle or snuggle in her bed.
Quiet voices.
    Share a fun event.
    Tell a story, talk about your family.
    Read a book.
    Sing or hum a song.
    Chat about the day.
    Say good night to everyone and everything in the room.
    Play a favorite recording, maybe grandparents singing or say-
       ing good night, sounds of nature.
Comfortable room.
    Photos of family and pets.
    Favorite stuffed animals or dolls.
    Night-light or flashlight.
    Dream catcher or guardian angel for protection.

Please don't think that it is all right to have a late bedtime just because there is a late wake-up time and a long nap. In a study of 1,105 Japanese 3-year-olds, it was observed that half fell asleep at 10:00 P.M. or later. For all children, the later they went to sleep, the later they woke up in the morning and the longer they napped. However, the later bedtime was associated with less total sleep compared with those with an earlier bedtime. The later wake-up time and longer nap did *not* compensate for the later bedtime.

My research and experience suggests that among *well-rested* young children with early bedtimes, in general, there is no strong association between the duration of night sleep and day sleep. After a special occasion that causes a late bedtime, they might sleep in later or have a longer nap the next day only. In contrast, *overtired* children usually have chronically late bedtimes, and the later the bedtime, the later the wake-up time and the longer the naps. But they may still be short on total sleep, and, even when not, the late bedtime causes problems in the child.

Let's look at the issues that may occur in this age range and some of the strategies we can use to deal with them.

NIGHT SLEEP

Three-year-olds may no longer have tantrum behaviors, but they may call parents back many times and clearly express their feelings of love for their parents or fears of the dark. How to reassure your older child without reinforcing undesirable behavior?

In an English study of children about 3 years of age, a *fade* procedure was particularly effective: 84 percent of the children who displayed difficulty in going to bed, night waking, or both, improved. Not surprisingly, the two factors that most likely predicted success were both parental: the absence of marital discord and the attendance of both parents at the consultation sessions. (The important role of the father is discussed in detail in chapter 4.) And although half of the mothers in this study had current psychiatric problems requiring treatment, this did *not* make failure more likely. Another study from England (described in chapter 5) that used a fade procedure included children who took at least an hour to go to bed, who woke at least three times a night or for more than twenty minutes at a time, or who went into their parents' bed. Among those families who completed four or five treatment sessions, 90 percent showed improvement. "Once some success was obtained, the *morale and confidence of the parents rose* and they were reinforced in their determination to persist by the more peaceful nights [emphasis added]."

I have seen this over and over again: When you see even partial improvement, you gain confidence and no longer feel guilty or rejecting when you are firm with your child.

Your 4-year-old might be helped to sleep better if you make a schedule and post it in her room: time for bath, time for sleep routine, lights off, and so on. Regularity helps, but the times might include a range, because not all days are the same. Try to engage or enlist cooperation with your child by doing something together such as singing, reading out loud, or doing artwork as part of a bedtime routine.

It appears that sharing your plans with your older child is more likely to lead to cooperation. In office consultations, it often seems that the child is listening to the treatment plan discussed, because parents often report back that their child slept better that very night!

Regular Bedtimes

Q: *How important are regular bedtimes?*

A: In general, the bedtime should reflect your child's needs. With decreasing naps and increasing physical activity, her night sleep needs may increase. Therefore, the bedtime often needs to be a little earlier, and not later simply because she is older. To maintain orderly home routines such as meals and baths, you might want to keep the bedtime within a narrow range.

Dr. John Bates's study of 204 children 4–5 years old examined in great detail the home environment, behavior at preschool, and sleeping patterns. The researchers noted that a *more variable bedtime,* as well as lateness of bedtime, predicted poor adjustment in preschool, even after considering the roles of family stress and family management/discipline practices. This study provides evidence that sleep problems directly cause behavioral problems in children at preschool. Other research suggests that when older children are overtired, they learn to no longer bother their parents, but instead bother their teachers.

Regularizing the sleep/wake schedule has also been shown to reduce daytime sleepiness and promote long-lasting improvements in alertness. It appears that regularity itself improves the ability of sleep to reverse daytime drowsiness. But some children are so excited at the end of the day, they have trouble unwinding whether they are overtired or not. Hot lavender bubble baths may help make the transition to sleep easier.

Some previously well-rested children who slip into a night-waking mode need only gentle reminders to return to sleep. As related in chapter 5, my wife used to teach the "dolphin game" to one of our sons. She would read a story about how the dolphin swims deep in the water but sometimes has to come up for air before returning to a deep underwater sleep. Then she told our son to pretend that he was a dolphin at night and that it was perfectly all right to come up from sleep, but that he had to go back by himself. It worked.

Some previously very overtired children are so unmanageable at night that the family resources are stretched to the limit. In such cases, the idea of more extreme measures such as extinction, using gates, or locking the door may come up (chapter 5). But before trying these measures, some parents try to avoid bedtime issues altogether by keeping their child up very late, until she crashes, in the hope that she will sleep in later in the morning and be all right during the day. Unfortunately, this only makes matters worse.

Q: *Why can't I just keep my child up later at night to see if she will sleep in later in the morning?*

A: If your child has been well rested up to now, then slowly try a slightly later bedtime. If you move it too late, she might just become more overtired and have difficulty falling asleep and staying asleep in the morning. If your child has always been a problem sleeper and overtired, a later bedtime will only make matters worse, because sleeping later in the morning or taking a longer nap usually does not make up for the lost sleep from a later bedtime. It just throws the rest of your child's sleep schedule out of whack.

Most children between 3 and 6 years of age, according to my survey, still go to sleep between 7:00 and 9:00 P.M. and wake between 6:30 and 8:00 A.M. As previously discussed, I think that these bedtimes, derived from survey studies, are too late for many children. Going to bed too late may cause bedtime battles, night waking, or early-morning wake-ups, or it may mess up the nap schedule. One mother described her son as turning into a "crank monster" at 4:00 P.M. every day because he was going to bed too late, waking up tired, and taking a midmorning nap, which prevented a midday nap and so caused cumulative sleepiness by late afternoon. Another mother described her child's new early bedtime as "a rescue maneuver to get back the old good pattern he fell out of."

THE SLEEP-TEMPERAMENT CONNECTION

I studied a group of sixty children at about 4 months old and again at 3 years old. At both ages, children with easy-to-manage temperaments slept longer than children with difficult-to-manage temperaments. Easier children were more regular, approaching, adaptable, mild, and positive in mood than the more difficult children. Which came first, the temperament traits or the sleep?

I don't think sleep habits, temperament, and fussing or crying are independent; rather, I believe they are all interrelated. However, we name and measure items such as sleep duration, temperament traits, or fussiness in the same way we might describe different features of a rose: its color, its smell, or its texture. But the rose is still a rose and a baby is still a baby; even though we give names to different features, none of them could exist without the whole.

It seems to me that after about 4 months of age, parenting practices such as loving attention during wakeful periods and encouraging good-quality sleep during sleep times can modulate or influence those features we call temperament (page 491). At age 3 years, among those children who had been easy-temperament infants at 4 months, some remained easy and were sleeping a total of 12.4 hours, while some became more difficult and slept less, 11.8 hours. So to help keep easy infants easy when they arrive at toddlerhood, protect their sleep.

What about those difficult infants? Some of them remained difficult at age 3 years and slept only 11.4 hours, but others became easy and slept 12.0 hours. I think part of the reason why some difficult infants mellowed into easy 3-year-olds is that they were handled in a more structured and regular fashion, learning more social rules and becoming better rested. The power of sleep to modulate temperament is reflected, at age 3 years, in the rank order of hours of total sleep durations: 12.4, 12.0, 11.8, and 11.4, respectively.

TEMPERAMENT AND SLEEP DURATION

Temperament at 4 months	Temperament at 3 years	Total Sleep Duration at 3 years (hours)
Easy	Remained Easy	12.4
Difficult	Became Easy	12.0
Easy	Became Difficult	11.8
Difficult	Remained Difficult	11.4

Adaptability, the ease with which children adjust to new circumstances, was the only temperament trait that showed individual stability over the three-year study. Remember, temperament traits are not like fingerprints, which are completely biologically based, unchanging over time, or unique identifiers. Temperament traits are more like hair. Our hair has a biological basis, but it changes over time; texture, length, curliness, and color can change naturally or at our will. How we care for our hair affects its health and appearance. And how we care for our children, including how we care for their sleep, influences temperament. Helping your fussy baby sleep better will make her less of a fussy child when older. Between 4 months and 3 years, there was *no individual stability* regarding the durations of total sleep, night sleep, or naps, which means this time is the window of opportunity for parents to teach healthy sleep habits.

You shouldn't be surprised if your colicky 3-month-old has a difficult temperament at 4 months, but that doesn't predict anything for the future, not even for 5 months. A fussy nature may persist when colic and parental mismanagement together cause enduring post-colic sleep deprivation, or it may vanish when the child develops healthier sleep habits. You cannot change the fundamental personality of your child, but you can modulate it.

As previously described (page 142), sleep problems and benefits tend to persist. At 4 months of age, infants described at temperamentally easy slept 15.6 hours, and those with a difficult temperament slept 12.3 hours (page 499). But there was no individual stability or maintaining rank order regarding sleep durations (night, day, or total sleep) over the next three years. However, looking at those two groups of easy temperament 3-year-olds, *infants at 4 months of age with a difficult temperament* (and shorter sleep durations) who developed an easy temperament at age 3 years slept 12.0 hours. But *infants at 4 months with an easy temperament* (and longer sleep durations) who retained their easy temperament at age 3 years slept longer, 12.4 hours, suggesting some individual stability of sleep durations. This data was derived from parent reports in 1981. Now we have more objective data from 2018.

Measurements of sleep, using wrist-worn motion sensors were performed on a single group of children at 2, 3, and 4 years of age.

"Children who slept less or less well than their peers at 2 years did not catch up with them over the 2.5-year-study period . . . The persistence of these differences suggests that early sleep patterns may set children on a trajectory that could have significant long-term consequences." So there is a tendency for children to maintain their rank order relative to other children regarding sleep, *starting at age 2 years*. But I think that parents, especially when starting at a much younger age, can have both a positive and negative effect on how well their child sleeps—for example, by maintaining early bedtimes and, as discussed below, protecting naps.

Another example of the importance of *parents* influencing sleep, as previously mentioned, among the children I studied were three children between the ages of 2 and 3 who stopped napping during a period of marital discord or problems with caretakers. When they stopped napping, they underwent what looked like a personality transplant! Fatigue masked their sweet temperaments. But after resolution of the conflicts, all three resumed napping and continued to nap for years. The resumption of napping restored their original or "natural" temperament.

Reestablishing naps was discussed earlier, but it is worth restating that in this study the kinds of stressful events that tend to disorganize home routines—the death of a parent, divorce, a move to a new home, the birth of twin siblings, or the death of a sibling—did not cause any napping problems in 90 percent of the children. It appears that when parents and caretakers maintain nap routines, children continue to nap despite disruptive and stressful events.

After the publications of my original discovery on the association between sleep patterns and temperament—in infants in 1981 and in toddlers in 1984—many other studies in preschool children have confirmed and extended my findings. In adults, sleep loss has been shown to affect mood more than cognitive or motor performance; we all get a bit testy or cranky when we are tired, but we can still learn and perform reasonably well. For children it may be a different story, because the developing brain may be more sensitive to sleep loss than the mature brain. Evidence to support this suggestion comes from animal studies, which have shown that less light was needed to affect the sleeping and behavior of young animals. In other words, the developing brain may suffer more, and in more ways, than the adult brain from the harmful effects of insufficient sleep.

Q: *Is it ever too late to see benefits from better sleep quality?*
A: No. It is never too late—nor too early—to help *healthy* children sleep better. In addition, some neurologically impaired children can be helped to have fewer seizures by becoming better rested. Sadly, other children have neurological diseases or medicine requirements that directly disrupt sleep. And tragically, recent research suggests that children who were severely traumatized by abuse or neglect beginning in infancy might not respond to ordinary sleep training like healthy children.

THE SLEEP-BEHAVIOR AND SLEEP-EMOTION CONNECTION (PAGE 127)

Many research studies have shown that there are more daytime behavioral problems in preschoolers who are poor sleepers. In some studies, "externalizing" problems such as aggression, defiance, noncompliance, oppositional behavior, acting out, and hyperactivity were associated with less sleep. When parents listed the types of daytime behavior problems their children were expressing, it became apparent that the less sleep they had, the longer the list! In other studies, there was an association between sleep and "internalizing" problems such as anxiety or depression. A recent study by Dr. Wendy Troxel showed a direct relationship between sleep problems at 36 months and internalizing problems at 54 months.

So sleep duration is clearly a factor associated with behavior and emotional problems. Still, we do not have absolute scientific proof on whether (1) less sleep directly causes daytime behavior/emotion problems, (2) parenting or biological forces cause both the daytime behavior/emotion and nighttime sleep problems, or (3) daytime behavior/emotion problems cause the nighttime sleep problems. However, as mentioned earlier, research by Dr. John Bates on 202 children 4–5 years old shows that sleep does have a direct effect on daytime behavior in children, in support of the first theory. My impression is that parents who are somewhat regular, consistent, and structured—in terms of both meeting the child's need to sleep and helping the child learn social rules—enable the child to have fewer behavior problems. In contrast, circumstances such as a parent who works late and keeps the child up too late in order spend time with her produce an overtired child; then behavioral problems will be more frequent.

Another study of preschool children noted that the poor sleepers who had more behavioral problems did not get up more frequently than good sleepers, but that the poor sleepers were unable to soothe themselves back to sleep unassisted. They always disturbed their parents' sleep with signaling behaviors. I think the ability to return to sleep unassisted to avoid fragmented sleep (and to avoid upsetting parents!) is learned behavior. So consolidated sleep doesn't just mean longer sleep: It helps to avoid behavior problems.

Regular bedtimes also seem to be important, maybe even when the total amount of sleep is not quite enough. There were fewer school adjustment problems in Dr. Bates's study where a regular bedtime was maintained by the parents.

One study of 499 children showed that sleep problems at age 4 years predicted behavioral and emotional problems, such as depression and anxiety, when the same children were age 15. Another study of 817 children, also at age 4 years, showed that short sleep durations then predicted more attention-deficit hyperactivity disorder symptoms later, at age 7.

Previously (page 127), a study was described how only *thirty minutes* less sleep was associated with behavioral and emotional problems in children 6 and 8 years old when the children were re-examined two years later. A strength of this paper is that common method variance was avoided by objectively measuring the children's sleep and clinical interviews were conducted instead of relying on the mother as the single source for both types of information. Although not included in this paper, the lead author shared with me the mean group sleep durations and bedtimes of these children. At age 6, 8, and 10 years, the sleep durations were 9.7, 9.3, and 9.0 hours, respectively, all of which are shorter than reported for year 2008 (page 678); the bedtimes were 9:35 P.M., 9:50 P.M., and 10:12 P.M., respectively, all of which are later than reported for years 2009–13 (page 679). These data raise the possibility that in a large group of children where some children tend to go to bed *very late,* and thus not get enough sleep, there is a higher risk of small chronic additional sleep deficits (for example, *thirty minutes* less sleep) producing major adverse outcomes. But the same chronic sleep deficits in children who are better rested, because of bedtimes that are only a little late, might not be so harmful. I think this illustrates why it is more important to watch your child for drowsy signs (page 167) than published numbers of sleep durations or bedtimes: The numbers might have been derived from a group of children who were not truly well rested.

Please be mindful that if you struggled with sleep issues when your child was younger, although your older overtired child may not bother you as much as he did when he was younger, that does not mean that the sleep problems have gone away. Sleep issues in young children may be somewhat hidden, only to resurface later in different forms, much like too little calcium in our diet causes weak bones when we are older.

PREVENT AND SOLVE SLEEP PROBLEMS

Chapters 4 and 5 cover the prevention and treatment of sleep problems in the preschool age range. The emphasis is on reasonably early bedtimes and no screen-based media in the bedroom.

Difficulty Falling Asleep (page 693)

In one survey of about one thousand children, where the average age was between 7 and 8 years, about 30 percent resisted going to bed at least three nights per week. This was the most common sleep complaint of the parents. About 10 percent of the children had difficulty falling asleep once they were in their beds. Many took up to an hour to fall asleep on more than three nights per week. Some children *both* resisted going to bed and had difficulty falling asleep, and these children had a host of other problems: fears, anxiety, night wakings, need for reassurance, closeness of parents, complaints of fatigue, and a *history of not being able to successfully self-soothe*. Please review chapters 4 and 5 regarding how to help your child learn self-soothing.

Another study emphasized the distinction between bedtime resistance (bedtime battles) and difficulty falling asleep. If your child resists bedtime and does *not* have difficulty falling asleep, then treatments such as an earlier or more regular bedtime, Sleep Rules, and other solutions described in chapter 5 are likely to help. But if your child has no bedtime resistance and instead has difficulty falling asleep, has never slept well, and exhibits chronic mild anxiety-related symptoms, then consulting with a child psychologist or other mental health professional may be needed. This study also confirmed other observations that night wakings in early childhood tend to persist. Persistence of sleep problems is a theme in many reports, and it is only ignorance among some professionals that leads to the advice "Don't worry, she'll outgrow the problem."

Bedtime Becomes Later

Preschool- and school-aged children appear to be sleeping less today than in the past as the bedtime hour has gradually became later and later. If healthy sleep habits are not maintained, the result is increasingly severe daytime sleepiness.

Recurrent Complaints

Some children complain of aches and pains for which no medical cause can be found: abdominal pains, limb pains, recurrent headaches, and chest pains. Children who suffer from these pains often have significant sleep disturbances. Stressful emotional situations thought to cause these complaints include real or imagined separation of or from parents, fear of expressing anger that might elicit punishment or rejection, social or academic pressures, or fear of failing to live up to parents' expectations.

These are real pains in our children, just as real as the tension headaches adults get when we work too hard or sleep too little. All laboratory tests or studies during these episodes of tension headache will have normal results. All tests will also show normal results in children who have similar somatic complaints if the cause is sleep deprivation. Unless there is a strong clinical sign pointing toward organic disease, performing laboratory tests to rule out obscure diseases should be discouraged, because of the pain of drawing blood, the risks of irradiation, the expense, and, most important, the possibility of creating in the child's mind the notion that she is sick. Also, a slightly abnormal test result might lead to more and more tests, all of which, in the end, are likely to show basically normal results.

No Apparent Solution

Parents with older children have more scheduled activities to attend, and they are more likely to have more than one child requiring attention. What happens if the parent is a shift worker, or works in a bakery or restaurant with extremely early or late hours, or travels a lot for the job, or has irregular hours built into the job like some physicians? In these cases, it can be hard to arrange to be present when your children participate in an important scheduled school, music, or sports event. I have met some mothers and fathers who are absolutely dedicated to their children and try very hard to strike a balance between the time requirements of child care and their work outside the home. Usually there is a sharing of responsibilities regarding putting the children to sleep at night. However, what do you do if both parents have work schedules that make it difficult to be home reasonably early at night for bedtimes? To further complicate matters, one parent alone cannot easily manage different bedtimes for two or more children. To make it even more of a problem, what if the parents are blinded by their love for their children and their own subjective blindness to sleep loss (page 101) and cannot see that the late-afternoon tiredness, headaches, or developing academic problems are connected to unrelenting mild sleep deprivation in their child? For some parents, it appears impossible to change their lifestyle or work schedule in order for their children to have a reasonably early bedtime.

When the children were much younger, as infants and preschoolers, morning times were available to enjoy being together as a family, but now mornings are a frantic blur trying to get ready for out-of-the-house activities. So the night is the only quiet and relaxed time the family has together. These factors converge into a too-late bedtime. It may seem that there is no solution to this problem, but in fact it's not that the solution isn't apparent. The problem is that the solution is not easy. But many worthwhile things are not easy. And as parents, we often have to place the welfare of our children above our own desires and comfort. This is such a time. An earlier bedtime, even at the cost of less family time at night, is the solution.

Major benefits accumulate even when the bedtime is moved just a few minutes earlier (page 102).

DAY SLEEP

Naps naturally become less common after the third birthday (page 657). Some parents stop their child from napping, but as a group, the children whose parents stopped naps did not have different nap patterns from those children who naturally outgrew naps. In other words, naps were not stopped because they were too short or too long. There were three reasons why parents stopped their children from napping. First, among 3- to 6-year-old children, scheduled preschool or school activities conflicted with the nap (60 percent of families). Second, parents of 5-year-olds wanted their child to go to sleep earlier, because their children were fighting going to sleep around 9:00 to 10:00 P.M. (30 percent of families). Finally, stressful events that disorganized home routines caused an additional 10 percent of parents to stop naps.

Summary and Action Plan for Exhausted Parents

If you are too tired to read much and just want to do *something* to help your child sleep better, read chapter 1.

1. *Sleeping through the night* may be defined in different ways, but if the bedtime is too late, if there are unnecessary feedings, or if you attend to your child too often, fragmented sleep will be the result, which in turn will cause your child to wake up at night, even when older. This will lead to earlier wake-up times in the morning, leaving your child in the position of always playing catch-up when it comes to sleep needs. This a recipe for chronic sleep deprivation, with the network of negative consequences we have seen.

2. There are trends over time for the bedtime hour to become later, for children to sleep less during the night, and for some children to sleep less during the day. Pay attention to your

own child's mood and behavior to determine what's best for your child. Ignore advice from others or what you read.

3. There is enormous variation at specific ages for bedtimes and sleep durations for night sleep and day sleep. Don't compare your child's sleep with other children's sleep.

4. Transitions from two naps to one nap may require trial and error, a temporarily earlier bedtime, and patience.

5. Difficulty in falling asleep, as distinct from resistance to bedtime, might require a referral to a mental health professional.

What a Parent Can Do

Encourage your partner to help care for the baby daytime and nighttime.

Encourage self-soothing; the earlier, the better.

Put to sleep drowsy but awake, then leave the room.

Enforce rules about your child's bedtime (parent-set bedtimes).

Set an early bedtime based on drowsy signs; practice consistent bedtime routines, including massage; be emotionally available at bedtime.

Ignore nighttime non-distress vocalizations.

Provide opportunities for naps based on drowsy signs.

When the morning and/or the midday nap disappear, consider moving the bedtime slightly earlier.

Avoid irregularity of sleep schedules, including between weekdays and weekends.

No TV or screen-based media in your child's room; limit screen time.

Take breaks; try to get more sleep for yourself.

Appreciate the individuality of your child's temperament and sleep needs.

Seek help if your child is not sleeping well, especially if she has difficulty falling asleep (from the child's primary care provider or a community sleep consultant), or for yourself or your partner, especially if there are symptoms of anxiety or depression or significant *risk factors, parent issues,* or *adverse concerns.*

Chapter 11 Outline

TOTAL SLEEP DURATION TRENDS OVER TIME

BEDTIME HOUR TRENDS OVER TIME

Television and Screens in the Bedroom

WAKE-UP HOUR TRENDS OVER TIME

SLEEP RECOMMENDATIONS

YEARS 7–12

Prevent and Solve Sleep Problems
Optimal Wakefulness
Recurrent Complaints

ADOLESCENCE

Sleep Recommendations Revisited
Prevent and Solve Sleep Problems
Sleep Spa and Beauty Sleep
Difficulty Falling Asleep
Shifting Sleep Schedules
Delayed Sleep Phase Syndrome
Chronotherapy
Not Enough Time to Sleep in the Morning
Social Jet Lag
Weekend Recovery Sleep
Irregular Bedtimes
Drugs and Diet for Sleep
Parents' Advice

SUMMARY AND ACTION PLAN FOR EXHAUSTED PARENTS

Healthy Sleep Habits in Older Children: Age 7-Adolescence

Total Sleep Duration Trends over Time

HEALTHY SLEEP HABITS IN OLDER CHILDREN: AGE 7–ADOLESCENCE

Total Sleep Duration Trends over Time

Dr. Ivo Iglowstein showed that total sleep durations decreased from 1974–79 to 1986 from age 6 months to 16 years. For example, among 5-year-olds, sleep decreased from 11.5 to 11.2 hours. Adding Dr. Anna Price's (2008 data) with my own data (1979–80) indicates that this trend, for 5- and 9-year-olds, has continued past 1986. Other studies have shown similar trends. In one study, for 10- to 15-year-olds, night sleep duration on school days decreased between 1985 and 2004, due largely to later bedtimes. Sleep durations decreased from 9.2 hours to 8.7 hours because the bedtime went from 9:47 P.M. to 10:12 P.M.

AVERAGE TOTAL SLEEP DURATION: HOURS PER DAY

Age (Years)	1974–79	1979–80	1985–86	2004	2008
5	11.5	11.4	11.2		11.1
9		10.5			10.0
10–15				9.2	8.7

Also, Dr. Katherine Keyes documented the trend over time for less night sleep among adolescents between 1991 and 2012. A 2012 review by Lisa Matricciani found that "over the last 103 years, there has been consistent rapid declines in the sleep duration of children and adolescents." However, in 2017, she noted that while high-SES children age 13–16 had decreased their sleep duration between 1985 and 2004, the trend between 2004 and 2013 reversed; that is, they had an increase in sleep duration. Children age 10–13 and low-SES children did not show this improvement. The cause(s) of the long-term decline and recent improvement for some children is not known. In contrast, among a nationally representative survey of over three hundred adolescents, "Compared to 2009, adolescents in 2015 were 16%–17% more likely to report sleeping less than 7 hours a night on most nights." The authors attributed this to electronic device use, social media, and reading news online, not TV. Small nightly deficiencies in sleep—as little as nineteen minutes (page 298)—may cumulatively (page 51) have major consequences.

Bedtime Hour Trends over Time

In the history of parenting, it is only recently that children have been able to stay up late at night, as discussed in chapter 9. But now it is so common that we don't even think about it. Data collected by Drs. Iglowstein, Anna Price, Jennifer Falbe, and me (1979–80) document how the bedtime hour has shifted over time to a later clock time. The cause of this shift is not known.

BEDTIME HOUR (P.M.) BY YEAR

Age	1974	1979	1979–80	1986	2004–08	2012–13
5 years	7:46	7:56	8:10	8:11	8:15 (2008)	—
10 years	8:45	8:50	8:50	8:59	9:00 (9 years)	9:15 (grade 4)*
14 years	9:43	9:47	9:54	10:02	—	10:12 (grade 7)*
10–15 years				9:47	10:12	

* = lower SES.

After about 1980, the trend toward a later bedtime plateaued in children 1 year old and younger, perhaps because an increasingly later bedtime would eventually be significantly disruptive to the child and the family. It is possible that the trend of ever-later bedtimes has continued in older children because of increasing viewing of television and other screen-based media in the bedroom. For 5-year-olds, the wake-up time was a little later (four minutes), but the later wake-up time failed to fully compensate for the later bedtime. The wake-up time for the 10-year-olds did not change over time, and for the 14-year-olds it was eleven minutes earlier! The take-home message is that because of later bedtimes, children are getting less night sleep now than in the past.

Older surveys of sleep durations by age (but not newer surveys) showed that the gradual decline in total hours of sleep flattened out around age 13 or 14, and it even appeared that some 14- to 16-year-olds actually slept more before the gradual decline with age resumed! There might be an increased biological need for sleep during a portion of adolescence, but modern life makes it more difficult to satisfy this need.

In the past, it appears that some teens 14–16 years old needed more sleep to maintain optimal daytime alertness.

TELEVISION AND SCREENS IN THE BEDROOM
(PAGES 87, 216, AND 323)

The growing popularity of television and other electronic screen-based devices in the bedroom is directly associated with less sleep and with sleep problems. Here are some data from different studies to illustrate this trend:

1981: No correlation between TV viewing and duration of evening sleep.

1999: 26 percent of 4- to 10-year-old children have TV in the bedroom. More TV viewing is associated with less sleep and more sleep problems.

2005: 40 percent of 3- to 6-year-old children and 18 percent of children under 2 years old have TV in the bedroom.

2012: 75 percent of fourth and seventh graders (mean age, 10.6 years) sleep with a TV in the bedroom and 54 percent sleep near a small screen (smartphone or iPod Touch). It appears that sleeping near a small screen is worse than having a TV in the bedroom: Children sleeping near a small screen reported twenty-one minutes less night sleep (eighteen minutes less for those with a TV in the bedroom), the bedtime was thirty-seven minutes later (thirty-one minutes later for those with a TV in the bedroom), and they reported perceived insufficient sleep—that is, symptoms of daytime sleepiness.

2018: In students 11–20 years old, "Using social media for at least one hour a day was associated with greater odds for short sleep duration in a dose-response manner." That is, the more time using social media, the more likely the child is to have a short sleep duration.

2019: Children 6–17 years have shorter sleep duration and more irregularity (page 78) of bedtimes associated with increases in digital screen time.

2019: Objective actigraph measurements of preschoolers between about 3 and 6 years showed that children who had TV in the bedroom compared with those who did not, "displayed significantly shorter sleep duration and worse sleep . . . watched TV later at night, and watched more adult TV programs, and had higher negative affect." They also fell asleep later and had more irregular sleep durations, later sleep onset times, and later wake onset times. Overall, about 36 percent of families had a TV in the child's bedroom. "Among children without TVs in their bedroom, 80% of their mothers have a college degree or higher-level education." But among the families with a TV in the child's bedroom, 33 percent of the mothers had a college degree or higher education level!

Another study of even younger children, age 1–6 years, asked the parents to respond to a twenty-six-item questionnaire about possible sleep disturbances. The group with an abnormal score (more sleep disturbances such as sleep terrors, nightmares, sleep talking, and tired when waking up) were more likely to have a TV in the child's bedroom. Similar to the previously described study showing that maternal higher education level is a questionable protective factor, in this study, overall, 51 percent had a TV in the child's room and among these mothers, 73 percent had a university education. In the subgroup with more sleep disturbances plus a TV in the bedroom, 84 percent had a university education.

It appears that the American Academy of Pediatrics recommendation to keep the TV out of the bedroom (page 150) has not reached a high level of public awareness.

Furthermore, two studies have been published that suggest the trend toward more screen viewing has now reached infancy. One study, from England in 2017, analyzed touchscreen viewing in children 6–36 months. They found that increased viewing was associated with increased time to fall asleep, reduced night sleep duration, increased day sleep duration, and a net reduction of total sleep even in the age range of 6–11 months. The other study, from Singapore, in 2019, analyzed screen viewing and showed that the greatest reductions in sleep associated with increased viewing was in the group aged 6 months and younger. In both studies, the results were independent of the mother's education level.

Television and media viewing may cause the bedtime to be too late, or the content might make it more difficult for the child to fall asleep. Alternatively, among infants and young children, more viewing may be a parental response to their child not sleeping well. As described in Dr. Jenny Radesky's 2014 paper, parents might be allowing more screen time as a coping strategy:

> Our findings demonstrate that, longitudinally, infants with regulatory problems [excessive fussiness, poor self-soothing, difficulties in falling asleep and staying asleep and modulating their emotional state] do watch more TV and videos later in their toddler years. However, the relationship is probably not unidirectional: child self-regulation abilities and media habits likely influence each other through a transactional process whereby parents might try to soothe fussier infants through screen time, which reduces the amount of enriching parent–infant interactions and other developmental activities, exposes infants to potentially inappropriate content, and contributes to continued regulatory difficulties, which in turn predict greater media exposure, and so on.

Wake-Up Hour Trends over Time

A trend toward earlier wake-up times was also observed by Dr. Iglowstein for 14-year-olds between 1974, 1979, and 1986: 6:41, 6:39, and 6:30 A.M., respectively.

Sleep Recommendations

Lisa Matricciani's 2013 review of the literature concluded that published recommendations for children's sleep are not based on empirical evidence (chapters 2 and 10). She found that "sleep timing [the time when sleep occurs] may be even more important than sleep duration." In a separate 2013 paper titled "Sleep Duration or Bedtime?" the authors studied twenty-two hundred 9- to 16-year-old children and concluded that "late bedtimes and late wake up times are associated with poorer diet quality independent of sleep duration."

> **Commonly occurring sleep patterns among your relatives, friends, and neighbors might not be what is right for your child. Ignore what they recommend and what you read about bedtimes and total sleep needs and instead watch your child. Don't be surprised if he needs an earlier bedtime than other children.**
>
> **When your child sleeps might be more important than how long your child sleeps.**

Years 7–12

The contribution of healthy sleep habits to a child's well-being does not diminish with age even though parents have many new concerns: school assignments, organized after-school activities, individual lessons, parties, more homework, dating, and riding with teens who are driving cars. Healthy sleep habits may appear to be less important to parents than the development of their children's social, athletic, artistic, or academic skills. But healthy sleep does interact with skill development. Two sleep surveys of about one thousand preadolescents, one from Belgium and the other from Taiwan, show that school achievement difficulties were encountered significantly more often among poor sleepers than good sleepers. For those children on a college path, the more academic pressure they felt, the fewer hours they slept.

Young children who have difficulty sleeping become older children with more academic problems. But children who are academically successful risk not getting the sleep they need!

PREVENT AND SOLVE SLEEP PROBLEMS

Chapters 4 and 5 cover the prevention and treatment of sleep problems in the school-aged range, with an emphasis on reasonably early bedtimes, no screen-based media in the bedroom, relaxation training, and stimulus control/temporal control. For issues related to difficulty in falling asleep, please see chapter 10. Parent-set bedtimes that are a little earlier (page 297) might, over time, have a dramatic cumulative benefit. For example, a Canadian school-based program, Sleep for Success, covered topics such as barriers to proper sleep, the consequences of poor sleep, and the benefits of proper sleep. The children were 7–11 years old. These students' "report card grades in mathematics and languages improved significantly compared to a control that did not receive the program. "Objective measurements (actigraphy) of nighttime sleep showed that "in the intervention group, true sleep was extended by *18.2 minutes* [emphasis added]." This small number of extra minutes of sleep highlights the power of small sleep increases to produce major improvements (page 102).

Optimal Wakefulness

School-aged children are sleeping less and less as the bedtime hour gradually becomes later and later. In my study (1979–80), most 12-year-olds went to sleep around 9:00 P.M.; the range was from about 7:30 to 10:00, and the range for total sleep duration was about nine to twelve hours. These findings are in close agreement with those from a study at Stanford University where researchers found that the prepubertal teenager needs nine and a half to ten hours of sleep in order to maintain optimal wakefulness during the day (page 120). This finding has been cited often as a recommendation for how much sleep is needed, but the sleep duration needed at any given age varies from child to child, and the time when the sleep occurs is important for sleep quality. As children get older, it appears that impairments from short sleep become more common. About one thousand children were studied in 2004, 2008, and 2010 at age 10, 12, and 15 years, respectively. "Frequent daytime sleepiness occurred in 13% of children at age 10 and increased to 24% at the age of 15." As mentioned above, instead of paying close attention to published recommendations about bedtime hours and sleep duration, watch your child (page 196).

Recurrent Complaints

Many children in this age range complain of aches and pains for which no medical cause can be found: abdominal pains, limb pains, recurrent headaches, and chest pains. Children who suffer from these pains often have significant sleep disturbances (page 671).

Adolescence

In addition to increased use of screen-based electronic media in the bedroom, there are worrisome new trends in high schools that place more pressure on our teens. Some high schools have scheduled activities that start before the regular school day or allow students to opt out of the lunch period to take an additional class (honors or Advanced Placement courses) or electives (band, choir, or foreign language). Further, some high schools require a twelve-month commitment to sports such as volleyball or football that is incompatible with other regularly scheduled elective activities such as drama or debate. These trends and the decrease in sleep durations from 1974 to 2008 as a result of later bedtimes are a recipe for mental health problems. A report by Dr. Jean Twenge showed that symptoms of depression (trouble sleeping, thinking, and remembering; shortness of breath) among high school students have increased from the 1980s to 2010: "More than twice as many 2010–2012 teens (8%) reported having trouble sleeping on 20 or more days a month compared to 1982–1984 (3%). . . . Apparently, the pressures, lifestyle, and social forces of modern life have led people to experience more psychosomatic issues such as sleeping issues and difficulty concentrating." As will be discussed later, the salient role of insufficient sleep, as a cause of or contributing factor to depression in adolescents, is highlighted in the American Academy of Pediatrics 2014 recommendation for later start times for high schools.

Chronic sleep deficits were observed in 13 percent of teenagers in a Stanford University study that included more than six hundred high school students. These poor sleepers attributed their sleep problems to worry, tension, and personal, family, and social problems. The students appeared to be mildly depressed. Of course, we don't know which came first, disturbed sleep or the mood changes. Perhaps both the mood changes and the sleep disturbance develop from the same endocrine changes that occur naturally during adolescence or which might be a result of the pressure in school to perform well both academically and athletically. But healthy lifestyle habits, including sensible sleep patterns, might prevent or lighten the depression seen in so many adolescents.

How do you know if your teenager has disturbed sleep? Here is how the Stanford University sleep researchers defined chronic and severe sleep disturbances in adolescents:

- Forty-five or more minutes required to fall asleep on three or more nights a week

or

- One or more awakenings a night followed by thirty or more minutes of wakefulness occurring on three or more nights a week

or

- Three or more awakenings a night on three or more nights a week

So if your teenager exhibits any of these sleep patterns, don't dismiss it as a "normal" part of growing up.

In New Zealand, as in California, about 10 percent of teenagers had sleep problems. They appeared anxious, depressed, and inattentive, and they had conduct disorders more often than those without sleep problems. Anxiety and depression were also common symptoms of poorly sleeping teenagers in Italy, where about 17 percent of all teens met research criteria for sleep problems. A separate survey study of 3,136 children between age 11 and 17 showed that 17 percent were experiencing sleep that wasn't sufficiently restorative, just as in the Italian study.

Solid research, published in 1991, has documented that adolescents' sleep time has decreased one hour over the past twenty years. The evidence is clear, whether it's from Belgium, Taiwan, China, South Africa, New Zealand, or Italy: Teenagers are increasingly at risk for becoming overtired. (See "Sleep Recommendations" in chapters 2 and 10.)

In two separate studies of experimental sleep restriction in children 10–14 years of age, the researchers limited night sleep either to seven hours for three days or to five hours for a single night. Although rote memory task performance and routine performance were maintained, higher cognitive functions such as verbal creativity and abstract thinking were impaired. This highlights an important point: that our children can and do perform quite well even when mildly sleep-deprived—as long as they are not challenged to write or be creative. Mild sleep deprivation is often trivialized or overlooked because more routine memorization tasks and athletic performances are successfully accomplished.

Another experimental sleep restriction study was performed on 11- and 12-year-olds. Comparisons were made between sleeping ten hours on six nights versus six and a half hours on six nights. The sleep restriction caused measured inattentiveness, irritability, noncompliance, and academic problems. Two additional experimental studies and a large survey study (page 128) all agree that sleep restriction has a powerful negative effect on the mood of teenagers.

Sleep Recommendations Revisited (page 696)

The National Sleep Foundation recommendation for school-aged children 6–13 years is nine to eleven hours (previously, it was ten to eleven hours); for teenagers age 14–17 years it is eight to ten hours (previously, it was eight and a half to nine and a half hours). For both age groups, less than seven hours is "Not Recommended." But many children are not getting enough sleep. A large study (about twenty-eight thousand children) in Fairfax County, Virginia, in 2015, examined all students in the eighth, tenth, and twelfth grades. The high school start time was 7:20 A.M. "To provide context, Fairfax County . . . is ranked second nationally in terms of highest median household income . . . is the 13th largest school system in the US, with the largest fleet of school buses in the nation." Only 3 percent of high schoolers reported having the then-recommended eight and a half to nine and a half hours of sleep per night. The average for the high school students was six and a half hours of sleep per school night, and 20 percent slept five or fewer hours; the average for middle-school students was seven and a half hours. "Just one hour less of weekday sleep was associated with significantly greater odds of feeling hopeless, seriously considering suicide, suicide attempts, and substance use . . . our study shows the difference a mere hour of sleep can make in terms of increasing the odds of adverse outcomes in adolescents [author's emphasis]."

In 2017, another report, by a different group of researchers, also in Fairfax County, was published regarding eighth-grade students (about ten thousand). The results were similar to the previous report: About 18 percent reported six hours or less of sleep and 44 percent reported seven hours or less. They observed a dose-response effect for each hour less sleep; for example, for those sleeping less than seven hours, there was increased likelihood of early initiation of antisocial behavior or drug use and for those sleeping less than five hours there was increased likelihood of gang involvement. "There are now a number of studies assessing health outcomes related to adolescent sleep duration which have suggested that 7 hours of sleep may be the 'tipping point' below which negative outcomes are more likely to occur."

For middle school students, sleep duration of less than seven hours is associated with increased risky behaviors.

A third study in Fairfax County, published in 2019, showed that among about one thousand 13-year-olds, a thirty-minute school start time advance (earlier school start time) was associated with a decreased sleep duration of fifteen minutes, which was associated with a 2 percent increased prevalence of low mood. But among about two thousand 15-year-olds, a school start time delay of fifty minutes caused an increased sleep duration of thirty minutes, which was significantly associated with an almost 5 percent reduced prevalence of low mood (page 103), and a reduction of skipping breakfast and drowsy driving. Drowsy driving causes distraction-related crashes. A 2020 report from Fairfax County showed that implementation of the school start time delay of fifty minutes caused a significant reduction in the crash rate for 16- to 18-year-olds unlike every other county in the state. So school start times (page 696) have a real impact on sleep durations, academic, and health outcomes.

PREVENT AND SOLVE SLEEP PROBLEMS

Chapters 4 and 5 cover the prevention and treatment of sleep problems in the school-aged range, and the emphasis is on reasonably early bedtimes (page 65), no screen-based media in the bedroom, relaxation training, and stimulus control/temporal control. An analysis of adolescent sleep patterns by Dr. Megan Hagenauer concluded that teens would be well served by falling asleep earlier, a goal that could be "enhanced by the incorporation of greater physical activity into the school day and [the time of falling asleep] could be shifted earlier by parental restrictions on screen time in the evenings and a reduction of evening light exposure." While recommendations for increased physical activity to promote sleep are common, objective data show that there is a bidirectional effect between physical activity and sleep duration, and the effect size is small.

Studies on the role of parenting and adolescent sleep, in the Netherlands, showed that parents' general monitoring of their adolescents' whereabouts and daily activities was associated with subjective earlier bedtimes, longer time in bed, better sleep quality, and less sleepiness. These were young adolescents, age 12–15, and of course the relationship between parent monitoring and sleep may be coincidental and not causal. Nevertheless, the authors "concluded that general parenting behavior may contribute to better adolescent sleep over time (page 142)."

Sleep Spa and Beauty Sleep

Sometimes I have recommended to teenagers who are short on sleep that they take a five-day "sleep spa" treatment. No, that doesn't mean having their parents book them into an expensive resort! It simply means dedicating five days to going to sleep earlier than usual. Afterward, I ask the teenagers to reflect on whether the earlier sleep made a difference. Usually they report, rather sheepishly, that it did. Also, for some teenagers, I point out how important it is for models, musicians, and other performers to have radiant skin and glowing dispositions, and how important beauty sleep is to maintain their appearance. Of course, that is not a suitable incentive for all teens, but in the battle for sleep, one must pick one's weapons carefully! One mother reported to me after her daughter's sleep spa:

> I asked Sophia to make a list of how extra sleep helped her feel, and she wrote: "After getting the new routine I feel a lot better. I'm in a way better mood and feel more positive and have a ton more energy. I feel more willing to do things and feel more active and happier in general. I perform better in sports and am able to strategize and process things faster. I enjoy music more. I am ready to do more things throughout the day and feel more social because before I wasn't up to doing much. I wake up earlier in the morning and have more time to do things throughout the day."

Another teenager who went to bed earlier during the summer so she could accompany her father to work in the early morning compared her new lifestyle with that of her two older sisters, who liked to stay up later and sleep in: "By the time they get up, they've killed half the day." This echoes a comment made by a father who, because his professional career (1st Special Forces Operational Detachment-Delta) involved periods of severe sleep restriction or complete sleep deprivation in life-or-death situations, was aware of sleep banking (page 245) and fatigue countermeasures (page 328), and appreciated the importance of early bedtimes: "Most people certainly have cluttered lives and have become overextended. If they understood this or had the frame of reference of valuing good sleep, more people would begin to prioritize life a little better, and eliminate some activities or habits (TV, web surfing, et cetera) that steal their evenings."

For babies, children, and Delta Force Operators, expert agree (chapter 13), good sleep, especially early bedtimes, produces specific benefits for everyone.

DIFFICULTY FALLING ASLEEP (PAGE 670)

As your child gets older, it becomes harder to determine what is cause and what is effect regarding disturbed sleep and problems of mood and performance because of the development of mental health problems and increasing pressure to perform academically during adolescence. It is possible that chronically disturbed sleep causes children to grow up experiencing excessive daytime sleepiness, low self-esteem, or mild depression in adolescence. In one study, about 13 percent of teenagers with disturbed sleep were reported to be like this. They usually took longer than forty-five minutes to fall asleep or woke frequently at night. As previously mentioned, about 10 percent of 7- and 8-year-olds took up to an hour to fall asleep, and difficulty falling asleep in younger children was associated with anxiety. Trouble falling asleep or staying asleep (insomnia) or waking up feeling tired (unrestful sleep), but not sleep duration, in 16-year-olds with anxiety symptoms strongly predicted depressive symptoms 13 years later. Some of these preteens and teenagers may simply have never learned self-soothing skills to fall asleep easily when they were much younger. As adults, they are described as insomniacs. Consider seeking professional help if your child takes a long time to fall asleep.

Many school-aged children have difficulty falling asleep because they worry about their grades, test scores, appearance, or sports skills. Anxiety about not doing well academically or athletically might lead to impaired performance. This is called performance anxiety. Impaired sleeping likewise occurs when there is too much worrying or nagging about not getting enough sleep. Worrying too much about not sleeping well creates anxiety or stress, interfering with the relaxation needed to successfully perform the task, which is to fall asleep. The solution to this vicious circle might be relaxation training. If your child, at any age, appears to need more sleep, and he wants to sleep but cannot easily fall asleep, please consider working with a professional to help your child learn to relax and avoid performance anxiety. Working with a therapist, older children can learn to sleep better through relaxation training techniques as a stand-alone strategy or in combination with stimulus control and temporal control (page 325). The attempt is to reduce the level of arousal, therefore permitting the sleep process to surface.

SHIFTING SLEEP SCHEDULES

In 1913, Dr. Lewis Terman noted that adolescents shifted toward a later bedtime and later wake-up time. This shift toward delayed sleep patterns occurs in all adolescents, in all countries and cultures. So although electronic screen-based technology use at night among children is new and tends to cause bedtimes to be even later, there appears to be a biological shift that predates modern times. He also suggested that early start times for school may cause sleep deprivation in these children. Now, more than a hundred years later, there is a trend toward shifting the start time for school later (chapter 3 and page 696).

Delayed Sleep Phase Syndrome

In addition to problems associated with falling asleep and staying asleep, there are normal shifts in sleep patterns that begin in preadolescence or adolescence. Do you notice that your teenager is going to bed later and later? A biological process associated with the development of puberty might cause a shift to a later bedtime. Eventually your child might consider himself to be a night person, an owl. This tendency of your teenager to delay going to sleep may be normal, and so, too, may be his need to wake up later. If this is the case, then the late bedtime is not the problem; rather, it's the too-early start of the school day that's causing problems. Alternatively or additionally, what may be occurring is the development of cumulative sleepiness, causing an inability to fall asleep at a socially and biologically appropriate time.

In healthy adolescents, the trend toward a later bedtime and later wake-up time is called the delayed sleep phase syndrome: Your child has no difficulty falling asleep or staying asleep, but only when sleep onset is delayed, maybe to 1:00, 2:00, or 3:00 A.M. When he tries to go to sleep earlier, he can't. On weekends and vacations, he'll sleep later, so his total sleep time is about normal. But on school days it's always a struggle to get him up for those early classes.

As a consequence of delayed sleep phase syndrome or an unhealthy sleep schedule, schoolwork suffers and your child's mood may swing widely—the long-term result of brief sleep on school days or a chronically abnormal sleep schedule. Some teenagers try to combat the fatigue with internal stimulation (anger or elation) or external stimulation (sports or exercise).

Chronotherapy

Treatment for delayed sleep phase syndrome is called chronotherapy, or delaying the internal sleep clock. Let's say your child can easily fall asleep at 2:00 A.M. The therapy consists of forcing him to stay up until 5:00 A.M. and then letting him sleep as long as he wishes. (Obviously, we don't do this during the school year!) The next night, his sleep is allowed to start at 8:00 A.M. the following day and at 11:00 A.M. the day after that. In other words, you are allowing sleep to occur about three hours later every cycle. Over the next few days, sleep begins at 2:00 P.M., 5:00, 8:00, and finally 11:00. Sleep onset, the bedtime, has been shifted from 2:00 A.M. to 11:00 P.M. by delaying the sleep period. Now, keeping careful watch over clock time, always try to have your child go to sleep at 11:00 P.M. You have shifted the sleep clock around to a more conventional time, and usually this can be maintained by sustaining a regular nighttime sleep schedule. Advancing the internal sleep clock by moving the bedtime a bit earlier on successive nights might also work. Exposure to bright light in the morning and avoidance of light (especially from electronic screens) at night might also be helpful.

Not Enough Time to Sleep in the Morning (page 99)

Research has shown that most teenagers would probably be much better rested if they were allowed to sleep longer in the morning. Starting school or practice times for sports early in the morning often causes teenagers to have to nap in the afternoon, which interferes with going to bed at a reasonable time or may force them to get up too early in the morning to finish homework. In Israel, starting times for school were examined for children 10–12 years of age. One group started school at 7:10 A.M. at least two times a week and the other group always started school at 8:00 A.M. The children in the early-start-time group had less total sleep, suffered more daytime fatigue and sleepiness, and complained more about difficulties in attention and concentration compared with the later-start-time group.

A report by Dr. Julie Boergers on 15- and 16-year-olds showed that when the school start time was delayed from 8:00 A.M. to 8:25 A.M., there was a twenty-nine-minute increase in sleep duration on school nights. The researchers measured significant improvements in daytime sleepiness (including less falling asleep in the classroom, less tardiness, and less napping), mood (less depression), and less caffeine use. While the twenty-nine-minute improvement may seem trivial, small changes, as little as nineteen minutes, can cumulatively make a big difference (page 102). In fact, in this study the percentage of students getting eight or more hours of sleep on a school night dramatically increased from 18 percent to 44 percent! Dr. Judith Owens co-authored that study, and in another report, she described how "students reported going to bed earlier after start times were delayed, resulting in a greater-than-expected increase in average school night sleep duration. . . . [A]necdotal student comments suggest that the perceived benefits of additional sleep motivated students to further modify their sleep–wake behavior to optimize sleep duration. It appears that the later classes start, the more academic performance improves."

Here is a short list of studies demonstrating the powerful effect of a shift to a later school start time with an emphasis on how even a small increase in sleep time helps teens.

Among 15-year-olds, the intervention school delayed the school start time by only fifteen minutes. These students woke up later and five months later, compared with the control school students, demonstrated improved mental health along with better prosocial behavior, peer relationships, and attention level. Teachers observed improved concentration, reduced dozing off, and reduced tardiness rates. The average difference in night sleep duration between the pre-intervention and the five-month follow up was only *2.4 minutes*! "Although it is reasonable to question whether a few minutes difference in sleep could have any clinical significance, our study demonstrated such a sleep gain could readily benefit adolescents' sleep, mental, behavioral, and daytime functioning."

Among 15-year-olds, a school delayed its start time from 7:30 to 8:15 A.M. Actigraphy objectively measured sleep, and after one month, time in bed was delayed by nine minutes while rise times were delayed by thirty-two minutes, resulting in an increased time in bed of twenty-three minutes. This time in bed remained stable when reassessed nine months later, and then total sleep time was measured to have increased by just *ten minutes*. Students reported at both one- and nine-month follow-ups lower levels of subjective sleepiness and improvements in alertness and well-being.

Also, in another study among 12- to 15-year-olds, "Attending a school starting 37 minutes later was associated with an average of *17 additional minutes* of sleep per weeknight, despite an average bedtime 15 minutes later. Students attending late starting schools were less sleepy than their counterparts in early starting schools, and more likely to be wide awake [emphasis added]."

Among 15-year-olds, starting school fifty minutes later was associated with a *thirty-minute* longer sleep duration and significantly lower prevalence of low mood, drowsy driving, and skipping breakfast.

Delaying a high school start time from 7:50 to 8:45 A.M. was associated with "an increase in the daily median sleep duration of

34 minutes [objectively measured by actigraphy] associated with a 4.5% increase in the median grades of the students and an improvement in attendance [emphasis added]."

Dr. Mary Carskadon, a pioneer in adolescent sleep research, points out that earlier start times for school are a fairly recent development, and their impact on sleep deprivation for older children is only now being appreciated. Dr. Carskadon "compares sleep deprivation to walking at the edge of a cliff on a path that gets narrower and narrower until you are balancing on a rail. Sleep usually gives you a healthy buffer zone, but when you're seriously sleep-deprived, if the wind blows, you've got nothing. Take one false step and you're done."

According to Dr. Judith Owens,

When schools start too early, students are being asked to wake up and function at a time when their circadian rhythm is telling them to stay asleep. Changing school start times not only allows students to get more sleep but allows them to sleep at the optimal time. When they sleep may be equally important, if not more so, than how much sleep they get [emphasis added].

These and other studies showing that later bedtimes are associated with lower grade point averages and that short sleep durations are associated with more car and pedestrian accidents (see chapter 3 for other problems with teenagers) led to a 2014 policy statement from the American Academy of Pediatrics that schools should not start before 8:30 A.M. "Delaying school start times is an effective countermeasure to chronic sleep loss and has a wide range of potential benefits to students with regard to physical and mental health [such as lower rates of obesity and depression], safety [for instance, crashes caused by drowsy driving] . . . academic performance, and quality of life." Here is the AAP's list of the impacts of chronic sleep loss in adolescents:

Physical Health and Safety
    Increased obesity risk
    Metabolic dysfunction (elevated cholesterol and Type 2 diabetes)
    Increased risk for hypertension or stroke
    Increased rates of motor vehicle crashes
    Higher rates of caffeine consumption
    Use of stimulant medication for diversion
Mental Health and Behavior
    Increased risk for anxiety, depression, suicidal ideation
    Poor impulse control and self-regulation; increased risk-taking behaviors
    Emotional dysregulation, decreased positive affect
    Impaired interpretation of social/emotional cues in self and others
    Decreased motivation
    Increased vulnerability to stress
Academic and School Performance
    Cognitive deficits
    Impairments in executive function (organization, time management, persistence)
    Impairments in attention and memory
    Deficits in abstract thinking, verbal creativity
    Decreased performance efficiency and output
    Lower academic achievement
    Poor school attendance
    Increased dropout rates

Starting school later is an effective countermeasure to chronic sleep loss in adolescents. An early bedtime is an effective countermeasure at any age. A slightly earlier bedtime may cumulatively have a big impact, but children may be blind to their own sleep deprivation, so parents have to enforce bedtimes.

A study supporting the AAP guidelines showed that when high school start times are stratified (before 7:30, 7:30–7:59, 8:00–8:29, and 8:30 or later), employing objective measurements from actigraphy, "Adolescents starting school at 8:30 or later exhibited significantly longer actigraphically-assessed 24-hour sleep duration (by *21–34 minutes*) . . . when compared with the adolescents grouped by earlier school start times [emphasis added]."

Another study also using actigraphy showed that compared with a baseline measured during ninth grade when all schools started about 7:30 A.M., teens in both tenth and eleventh grades who attended schools with later start times (fifty to sixty-five minutes later) slept forty minutes longer than teens who attended schools that maintained their original early start times. "Furthermore, concurrent with the increase in school night sleep duration, those attending delayed-start schools had a decrease in weekend night sleep duration, suggesting lesser accumulated sleep debt with the later start times."

Starting school later will help adolescents get more sleep, but if parents continue to allow the bedtime to be later and later because of screen-based media, then the trend toward more problems associated with sleep deprivation, such as somatic complaints or depression, might continue.

Naps after school usually do not fully compensate either for bedtimes that are too late or for a wake-up time that is too early. For example, in a study of about ten thousand Japanese junior high and high school students, 50 percent napped after school at least once a week. Because the late naps made the bedtime later, the result was less sleep at night. My impression is that when teenagers are almost exhausted after school or around dinnertime, it is better not to nap then; instead, they should eat, do a little homework, go to bed early, and wake up much earlier to complete the unfinished homework. I think doing homework very late at night or way after midnight, after a late-afternoon or early-evening nap, is much more inefficient because the brain is in sleep mode. It might take two hours to finish an assignment between 1:00 and 3:00 A.M. after an after-school nap, but only one hour to finish the same assignment between 5:00 and 6:00 A.M. with no after-school nap, an earlier bedtime, and several hours of night sleep.

Dr. Michelle Stone studied sleep and physical activity in 856 children between 10 and 12 years separately for school weekdays and weekends and related her findings to weight status. Obese children sleep less throughout the week and are less likely to experience weekend catch-up sleep.

SOCIAL JET LAG

School-aged children may experience short sleep duration during the week because they stay up too late at night and use an alarm clock to get up early, but on the weekend, they might get more sleep because, even though they might stay up later, they are able to sleep in much later in the morning (delayed sleep phase syndrome). This chronic cycling between weekday sleep restriction and weekend delayed sleep phase is called social jet lag.

Social jet lag is common among teenagers but it may also occur in some very young children attending daycare who might alternate between different sleep schedules on weekdays and weekends. The symptoms (problems in sleep and performance) that occur with travel-induced jet lag are transient, but with social jet lag they may be chronic. According to Dr. Till Roenneberg, social jet lag may directly cause obesity. Another study by Dr. Malone agreed with this finding and noted that the association between social jet lag and obesity was independent of night sleep duration. Separately, in a recent review by Dr. Alison Miller, in early childhood, "late bedtimes (after 9:00 P.M.) magnified and independently predicted the association between short sleep duration and obesity." So late bedtimes (page 67), short night sleep duration, and social jet lag might be independent risk factors for the development of obesity.

One study of over ten thousand adolescents age 13–18 years showed that on weekends, on average, they stayed up 1.8 hours later and woke up 1.2 hours later. Children who tended to stay up later during the weeknight had shorter weeknight sleep duration, and they tended to stay up later on weekends. Independent of whether they sleep in a little or a lot more on weekends, these children were more likely to have "mood disturbances, anxiety, substance abuse, and behavioral disorders, as well as suicidality, tobacco smoking and poor perceived mental and physical health." The researchers discussed the connection between social jet lag and these issues in the context of bidirectionality. One possibility is that the sleep disturbance is a precursor to the full development of a mental health problem, or perhaps, the teenager is biologically shifting toward becoming a "night owl." For example, a Canadian study surveyed almost thirty thousand teenagers and found that "A later chronotype [night owl] was associated with poorer mental health, independent of sleep duration and school start time across internalizing and externalizing mental health domains." Alternatively, the irregular sleep pattern may cause the mental disorder. Evidence supporting this view comes from studies showing that delaying high school start times causes an increase in sleep duration, which in turn is associated with improvements in mood (page 696). Also, a school-based sleep education program successfully helped children sleep better and improved the mental health for seventh graders.

WEEKEND RECOVERY SLEEP

Social jet lag syndrome is a cycling between late bedtimes plus short sleep on weekdays and even later bedtimes with later wake-up times and long sleep on weekends. The long sleep on weekends is often viewed as "catch-up" or weekend recovery sleep. Does catch-up sleep work?

An experimental catch-up sleep study was performed on young

adults: "Our findings show that muscle- and liver-specific insulin sensitivity were worse in subjects who had weekend recovery sleep . . . [this] shows that weekend recovery sleep is not likely [to be] an effective sleep-loss countermeasure regarding metabolic health when sleep loss is chronic." Chronic sleep loss chronically damages the body, and the damage is not repaired over a weekend of extra sleep.

Similarly, regarding academic performance, catch-up sleep on weekends probably does not fully compensate for grueling school schedules. A study of almost three thousand Korean 17-year-olds showed that on weekdays they slept an average of five hours forty-two minutes; on weekends it was eight hours twenty-four minutes, a difference of two hours forty-two minutes. But the greater the weekend catch-up sleep, the greater the number of errors of omission and commission observed on attention tasks. "Increased weekend catch-up sleep as an indicator of insufficient weekday sleep is associated with poor performance on objective attention tasks," concluded Dr. Kim.

We do not know, in a well-rested child, whether occasional sleep loss coupled with weekend sleep extension is harmless. When thinking about helping your child recover from overtiredness, try to distinguish between reestablishing his habitual state of mild sleep deprivation, which might be restored over a weekend of catch-up sleep, versus setting a new optimal sleep duration pattern that might take weeks to establish.

We see excessive tiredness, daytime sleepiness, or decreased daytime alertness in many adolescents—there simply are not enough hours in the day to do everything. The time demands for academics, athletics, and social activities are enormous. Even without worrying about sex, drugs, alcohol, and loud music, parents worry that their teenagers may become burned out from lack of sleep.

Social pressures and early start times for schools cause reduced sleep times and chronic sleep deficits.

IRREGULAR BEDTIMES

Dr. Carskadon also identified irregular sleep times at night to be a significant problem independent of short sleep duration. Her research showed that the more irregular the bedtime hour, the more impairment of grades, the more injuries associated with alcohol or drugs, and the more days missed from school. Previous research among preschool children also focused on the importance of bedtime regularity regarding school adjustment behaviors (page 77).

DRUGS AND DIET FOR SLEEP

Prescription drugs and over-the-counter sleeping medicines don't solve sleep problems (page 328). There are no scientific data on nutrition in children that could be translated into a sleep-promoting diet.

PARENTS' ADVICE

I asked the same parents that I surveyed in chapter 3 if they continued later to put forth the effort, with age-appropriate modifications, to encourage healthy sleep in their preteen or teenager, or whether they were forced to abandon trying to help their older child sleep well because it was an impossible task. To summarize their responses: Helping preteens and teenagers to sleep well continues to be a part of parenting, but there are many challenges, individual variations, and no guarantees. Here are some reports from different parents.

Guidance and Suggestions, but Not Mandates

Battles with teens are many. I have consciously decided not to make sleep one of them. We provide guidance and suggestions, but not mandates.

Ellen is in eleventh grade. For her, we try to encourage sleep without bludgeoning. Alice is now a freshman in college. At this point, when it comes to Alice's sleep, we offer advice when solicited but feel it is no longer our place to comment. Our approach with the girls has always been to treat them, first and foremost, with respect. As they have gotten older, we recognize that when they choose to go to sleep is their decision, but as their parents, we are still in a position to help them see their options.

Work Backward from the Bedtime

Broadly, I would say that the challenges during the preteen and teen years are the pushback, or resistance, from the child, who is developing independence, and the difficulty of saying no to an overscheduled lifestyle that burdens the children and the whole family. I work with our son and daughter to decide on a reasonable bedtime for them. They are actually in their school and have a better understanding of what they need to do and how much time they need to do it. Preteens and teens want to develop independence, so working together to come to an agreement is both instructive and age-appropriate. We sort of back into the bedtime. What I mean is that once the bedtime is agreed upon, we work backward to get everything finished in time in order to respect the bedtime. So set the bedtime. Work back and set the dinnertime. How much time is needed in between? Work back to include all activities and homework. Work back to the time the child arrives home.

Our children are limited in the number of activities they are allowed to do because we feel this is the number one obstacle to reasonable bedtimes. What we know, plain and simple in our family, is that our children function better in every aspect of their young lives when they are rested. They are happier, kinder, work harder, are more focused, and generally our family functions better. The drama and stress of tween and teenage years are inevitable. We can't control those outside influences, but we can influence what we believe helps our children navigate these challenges. Over the years, without question, we believe our children can self-regulate and cope much better when they are rested. The key for us is to find the right bedtime and prioritize. Our focus has always been to "work backward" from the time we wanted the children to be in bed—with enough downtime to allow for reading. That means planning dinner, homework, projects, and outdoor time to be finished early enough so that the bedtime isn't compromised. What we learned very early on was to stick to a schedule a majority of the time, and when the exceptions happen, the healthy habits are still intact.

Naps After School: Pro, Con, and Compromise

Doing homework following a long nap after school means exercising the brain around the middle of the night, when, theoretically, learning should be less efficient because of circadian rhythms. Additionally, falling asleep after midnight means that the student is likely to be in a sleep-deprived fog at school the next morning. I usually recommend that adolescents not take a nap after school; instead, they should do a little homework, go to bed early, and set the alarm clock early in the morning to finish the homework. I think that studying early in the morning after a good night's sleep should be more efficient.

When they came home after school, if they were exhausted, I would insist that they take a nap to refresh before starting their homework if at all possible. Usually they fell right asleep and awakened refreshed. This nap was maybe only thirty to forty-five minutes, but it helped.

Up until about age 14 or 15, I tried to enforce what I thought were healthy sleep habits, meaning come home from school or sports, eat dinner, do homework, go to bed at a reasonable hour (by eleven or twelve). But Sam, age 17, was so tired after he got home that sometimes he would fall asleep after dinner, or before dinner. For a while, I'd wake him up from these evening naps, insisting that he finish his homework and then go to bed at a more reasonable hour. One day, his patience came to an end, and he said it really bothered him that I kept waking him up. He pointed out that he was managing his grades, his activities, his job, and his family chores just fine. He just wanted to do it his way. So I stopped. He continued to be successful at school, in sports, and in his community.

Sleep-in Days

The saving grace for both our children was that we strictly adhered to a one-day-per-week, non-negotiable, no-exceptions sleep-in day. Once high school began, in addition to exponentially more homework, sports occurred both before and after school. The sleep-in day became a lifeline.

We declare a sleep-in "holiday" on the mornings following a late night.

Sleepovers

Through the years, we felt pressure to skip naps and have sleepovers from our relatives and friends, rather than from our boys. Neither of our boys loved sleepovers; they didn't love staying up late and feeling horrible the following day. One sleepover experience for them was enough to not want to have another.

I would say it gets more difficult each year to maintain healthy sleep habits because of the added demands on the child's time. We only allowed a few sleepovers a year.

The preteen years, when sleepovers and slumber parties became part of the landscape, posed some challenges since they always resulted in loss of sleep and, often, crabbiness the following day. While we did not want to deprive them of the social aspect (we hosted quite a few sleepovers and slumber parties ourselves), we did feel that it would be best if they took more responsibility for their behavior as they got older. We gently reminded them that the grumpiness induced by inadequate sleep is unpleasant for everyone, the perpetrators especially! After a few years, the novelty wore off and the girls realized that they didn't miss out much if they came home and slept in their own beds. I believe that their cognizance of their sleep needs—a direct result of their early sleep "training"—was at the heart of their decision.

Individual Variation

There is individual variation in the need for early bedtimes, duration of night sleep, and the ability to cope with less-than-optimal sleep. Please don't expect all your children's sleep needs to be the same as or similar to those of their classmates.

It was important to recognize that the twins had different sleep patterns. John likes early to bed, early to rise. Elizabeth prefers staying up and sleeping in. Naps for Elizabeth are more important due to her sleep patterns. She also sleeps much later and longer on her sleep-in day, compensating for the fewer hours of sleep during the week.

Performance

We try to hold tight with a 9:00 P.M. weekly bedtime. Trystan (age 13) knows he swims better after a good night's sleep, so he will head to bed at 8:00–8:30 P.M. on the night before a meet so as to offset the 5:30 A.M. wake-up. We know that Trystan does as well as he does in school because of his dedication to a regular sleep schedule that gives his brain time to rest and really learn all that he has taken in each day.

The point that hit home for my three sons (ages 17, 19, and 22) is that sleep can improve sports performance, test performance, and, really, performance in all aspects of their lives.

Summary and Action Plan for Exhausted Parents

Over the years, bedtimes have become later, resulting in less sleep, especially in light of early start times for school and sports activities. A later bedtime in itself is not necessarily a problem; after all, there is a normal shift among adolescents to later bedtimes and correspondingly later wake-up times. But when children are allowed to stay up too late or early school start times prevent sleeping later, sleep deficits accumulate. Depending on the cumulative sleep debt, catch-up sleep on weekends may or may not compensate for lost sleep on weekdays. One concrete step that parents can take to protect their child's sleep is to eliminate all electronic screen-based media in the bedroom after bedtime.

Bedtime resistance is more common than difficulty falling asleep. But difficulty falling asleep may be associated with anxiety and depression, and consultation with mental health professionals may be indicated. Many children who are short of sleep complain of aches and pains (headaches, stomachaches, chest pain, and limb pain), so if your child has any of these complaints, don't neglect to look beyond the immediate somatic symptoms and take sleep patterns into account.

What a Parent Can Do

Encourage or establish early bedtimes or parent-set bedtimes.

Avoid irregularity of sleep schedules, including between weekdays and weekends.

No TV or screen-based media in your child's room; limit screen time.

Appreciate the individuality of your child's temperament and sleep needs.

Seek help from your child's primary care provider if your child is not sleeping well, especially if the sleep duration is less than seven hours during the week, or there is difficulty in falling asleep. Seek help for yourself or your partner if there are symptoms of anxiety or depression in a parent or child, or significant *risk factors, parent issues,* or *adverse concerns.*

Chapter 12 Outline

SLEEP PROBLEMS

Poor-Quality Breathing
Allergies
Snoring
Atopic Dermatitis and eczema

SPECIAL CONCERNS

Injuries
Overweight and exercise
Overweight
Exercise
Child Abuse

Solving Sleep Problems and Special Concerns

Sleep problems may occur at different ages, and you should read the earlier age-specific sections of this book to determine whether your child's sleep pattern is appropriate for his age.

One medical problem, severe and chronic snoring, may be especially hazardous to a child's health. Please read the section on poor-quality breathing even if your child has no specific sleep problems or if you think she does not snore. Snoring is sometimes not appreciated as a problem because the child has always snored, or because allergies developed when she was older—an older child is usually in her own bedroom and the parents are unaware of how much snoring is occurring every night because they do not go into her bedroom after she has fallen asleep.

Sleep Problems

POOR-QUALITY BREATHING: ALLERGIES AND SNORING

When you have a cold, you can't breathe easily during sleep, and you can't sleep easily, either. In turn, this makes you sleepy during the day, which can affect your mood and performance. When the cold finally disappears, you feel like your old self again, and your mood improves, as does your performance. Some children experience the same type of disrupted sleep *every night* because of allergies or snoring.

ALLERGIES

Allergies may cause difficulty breathing during sleep. Here's a partial list of symptoms among children with difficulty breathing during sleep.

Snoring
Stopping breathing during sleep
Restless sleep
Breathing through the mouth when awake
Sweating when asleep
Excessive daytime sleepiness
Chronic runny nose
Frequent colds

Perhaps the chronic runny nose and the frequent colds are due to allergies—for example, to dust or the protein in cow's milk. Allergists have long associated food sensitivities or sensitivity to environmental allergens with behavioral problems, such as poor ability to concentrate, hyperactivity, tension, or irritability. Terms such as *tension-fatigue syndrome* or *allergic-irritability syndrome* are used by allergists to describe children who exhibit nasal or respiratory allergies, food allergies, and behavioral problems. Perhaps allergies cause behavioral problems in children by producing swollen respiratory membranes that partially obstruct breathing during sleep. The difficulty these children experience in breathing during sleep causes them to lose sleep and thus directly causes fatigue, irritability, and tension.

SNORING

Two of the world's leading sleep researchers, Dr. Christian Guil-leminault and Dr. William C. Dement, published a landmark paper in 1976 that was the first careful study of how impaired breathing during sleep destroys good-quality sleep in children. They studied eight children age 5–14 years, all of whom snored. All eight children snored loudly every night, and snoring had been present for several years. Snoring started in one child at 6 months, and while the snoring in most of the children was originally intermittent, it eventually became continuous. Here's how their symptoms were described:

Daytime drowsiness: The report noted that "the children, particularly at school, tried desperately to fight it off, usually with success. To avoid falling asleep, the children tended to move about and gave the appearance of hyperactivity."

Bed-wetting: All the children had been completely toilet-trained, but seven started to wet their beds again.

Decreased school performance: The teachers reported lack of attention, hyperactivity, and a general decrease in intellectual performance, particularly in the older children.

Morning headaches: Headaches occurred only when they woke in the morning; the headaches lessened or disappeared completely by late morning.

Mood and personality changes: Half the children had received professional counseling or family psychotherapy for "emotional" problems. The report noted that "three children were particularly disturbed at bedtime; they consistently avoided going to bed, fighting desperately against sleepiness. They refused to be left alone in their rooms while falling asleep and, if allowed, would go to sleep on the floor in the living room."

Weight problems: Five of the children were underweight, and two were overweight.

Not all children who snore have all of the problems described above, and these differences may be explained by differences in the severity and duration of the underlying problem. But overall we have a picture here of impaired mood and school performance, which deteriorated as the children grew older or as the snoring became more continuous or severe. Sleep is definitely not bliss for these children! After surgery to remove enlarged adenoids, tonsils, or both, these symptoms were quickly—and often dramatically— reduced or eliminated. For example, in one report, a 13-month-old boy was assessed as having the developmental level of an 11-month-old baby before surgery, but five months after surgery, his developmental level had jumped past his real age, to the level of a 20-month-old! So the good news is that these problems are reversible when the sleep deficits are corrected. One word of caution: If the problem has been long-standing, then once children are cured of their snoring or their allergies are under control, bad social or academic habits or chronic stresses in the family or school will still require the attention of professionals, such as psychologists, tutors, or family therapists. The treated child is now a more rested child, however, and is in a better position to respond to this extra effort.

But was this a new discovery? Not really. Medical texts written as early as 1914 acknowledged that snoring can disrupt sleep and cause behavior problems. As Dr. William Ballenger noted over one hundred years ago:

> Restlessness during the night is a prominent symptom; the patient often throws the covers off during the unconscious rolling and tossing which is so characteristic. . . . Daytime restlessness is also a characteristic sign. The child is fretful and peevish, or is inclined to turn from one amusement to another . . . the mental faculties are often much impaired . . . difficult attention is very often present. The child is listless and has difficulty in applying himself continuously to his play, studies, or other tasks, of which he soon tires. He has fits of abstraction.

A 1925 study identified enlarged adenoids and tonsils as a physical cause of poor sleep. Even a major pediatric professional journal cited "difficulty in breathing, such as seen with extreme enlargement of the adenoids," as a common cause of "infantile insomnia" as far back as 1951.

Why, then, has kids' snoring particularly been ignored? In part, this is another example of a medical concern that has taken a long time to be recognized by physicians and parents as a real problem (chapter 3). But also, could it be that there are more snorers around today? Perhaps yes, because although surgical removal of tonsils and adenoids is much less common today, it was for many years in the past a very popular procedure for recurrent throat infections; it also happened to "cure" snoring in children. And perhaps yes, because the air we breathe is increasingly polluted and our processed foods increasingly allergenic; this may cause reactive enlargement of adenoids or tonsils in more children.

Children with documented obstruction of breathing generally sleep less than normal children. At about age 4, the average duration of night sleep was only eight and a half hours in affected children, compared with ten and a quarter hours in healthy children.

In another study I performed, the total sleep duration for snorers was about half an hour less than that of children who did not snore. They also had night wakings that lasted longer, they went to bed later, and they took longer to fall asleep after going to bed. These affected children exhibited snoring, difficult or labored breathing, or mouth breathing when asleep. Parents described problems such as overactivity, hyperactivity, a short attention span, an inability to sit still, learning disabilities, or other academic difficulties in their snoring children.

Even in infants, snoring might be a problem. I studied a group of 141 normal infants between 4 and 8 months of age. In these infants, 12 percent exhibited snoring and 10 percent exhibited mouth breathing when asleep. These snoring infants slept one and a half hours less and woke twice as often as infants who did not snore.

And as we have seen, a chronic sleep deficit of only *nineteen minutes* per night might cause impaired development (pages 102 and 298).

Although snoring reflects difficulty breathing during sleep, it is not related to sudden infant death syndrome (SIDS).

The night waking in these snoring infants and the restless light sleep in older children probably represent protective arousals from sleep: The child wakes or sleeps lightly in order to breathe better. When awake, the child breathes well, but the brain's control over breathing is blunted during deep sleep stages. So to prevent asphyxiation, the child wakes frequently, cries out at night, and has trouble maintaining prolonged, consolidated deep sleep states. Here the crying and waking at night and resistance to falling asleep are caused by a valid medical problem—not a behavioral problem, not nightmares, not a parenting problem.

All children snore a little, and frequent colds or a bad hay fever season might cause more snoring, which usually does no harm. Consider snoring a problem when it gets progressively worse, is chronic or continuous, disrupts your child's sleep, and affects daytime mood or performance. About 10 to 20 percent of children snore frequently.

The term *sleep-related breathing disorders (SRBDs)* was coined to describe those children who had snoring or heavy or loud breathing while sleeping, or who appeared to be struggling to breathe while sleeping, or who made a snorting sound and woke up. One research study conducted in 1997 directly connected SRBDs to attention deficit hyperactivity disorder (ADHD). They calculated that about 25 percent of children with ADHD would have their symptoms eliminated by correcting their habitual snoring or SRBD. In 1998, two studies showed that SRBD was associated with extremely poor academic performance in first grade (improvement occurred upon removal of tonsils and adenoids) and also that SRBD was associated with difficulties with behavioral sleep disorders such as fighting sleep at night or bedtime battles. By 2002, the terminology had changed to *sleep-disordered breathing (SDB)*, but the message was the same. Inattention, hyperactivity, and behavioral and emotional difficulties are more common in children with SDB. However, the relationship between ADHD and SDB was controversial until a 2014 review by Dr. Karim Sedky, who concluded that "ADHD symptoms are related to SDB and improve after adenotonsillectomy." A survey of about four thousand almost-11-year-olds showed that "Daytime sleepiness mediated the relationship between SDB symptoms and depression, loneliness, and poor school performance."

If snoring appears to be disrupting your child's sleep, consult with your physician. Your child's doctor may have to do some tests to determine how serious the problem really is. Most children's hospitals have sleep centers to help diagnose and treat these problems.

ATOPIC DERMATITIS AND ECZEMA

Atopic dermatitis is a chronic skin condition that causes severe itching. Itching of the skin can cause restlessness during sleep because a lot of the scratching goes on during light and REM sleep. As a result, children wake frequently throughout the night. Some studies have shown that these children have difficulty waking up for school, difficulty staying awake in the afternoon, and major discipline problems. However, one study that used sleep lab recordings and video recordings during sleep of atopic children showed that the sleep abnormalities of frequent arousals actually did not occur with the act of scratching. This study was performed when the skin condition was in remission, so it is possible that during flare-up there might be more intense itching that interfered with sleep consolidation. Another study followed almost five thousand children with atopic dermatitis between 2 and 16 years of age. At each of the eight time points they studied, compared with controls, the researchers observed more early-morning awakenings, difficulty falling asleep, and nightmares, but there were no differences in sleep duration. Other studies have objectively documented increased time spent awake after sleep onset (page 91) in these children. If your child is often scratching her skin, talk to your pediatrician or ask for a referral to a dermatologist.

Special Concerns

Special concerns, such as frequent injuries, may well be the result of unhealthy sleep habits. Here are some examples.

INJURIES (PAGE 131)

Injuries occur to children of all ages. Some can be prevented, but some cannot. Examples of preventable injuries include leaving a 4-month-old infant alone on a changing table from which she falls, poisonings occurring when safety seals are not used or medicines are left lying around, or electrical shocks from uncovered wall sockets. A non-preventable injury is truly an accident—for example, those resulting from an earthquake or a lightning bolt.

The truth is, though—and I realize this sounds harsh to many parents' ears—that most so-called childhood accidents are really preventable injuries that occur because of parental neglect or the lack of parental forethought. These injuries can be one consequence of home routines that create tired children—and tired *families*.

But is there such a thing as an accident-prone child? To determine if traits within a child can cause her to suffer frequent injuries, various studies have examined babies before injuries start to occur. (After a child has had several injuries, a "halo" effect develops, and adults are more likely to perceive traits in the child—clumsiness, lack of self-control, and so on—that "explain" why she has had so many injuries.)

One study included two hundred babies between 4 and 8 months of age. Some of the infants were difficult to manage. As we saw earlier, these infants were called "difficult" because they were irregular, not very adaptable, initially withdrawing, and negative in mood. During the next two years, difficult babies were much more likely to have cuts requiring sutures than were babies with easy-to-manage temperaments. This study showed that during the first two years of life, about one-third of the difficult children had cuts deep or severe enough to require stitches, while only 5 percent of easy babies had similar cuts.

Remember also my data: At 4–8 months of age, difficult babies slept about three hours less than easy babies, and at age 3 years, the difference was about one and a half hours. By age 3, the briefer the sleep, the more active, excitable, impulsive, inattentive, and easily distracted the child appeared—the perfect description of an accident-prone child. Little wonder, then, that these tired children fell more often, sustaining deep cuts.

Obviously, for both the "difficult" kids and all other children, chronic fatigue can lead to more injuries, such as cuts and falls. More sleep is the remedy.

Another study that supports this connection between fatigue and injury included more than seven thousand children who were 1–2 years old. Researchers compared children who frequently woke up at night with those who slept through the night. Among the night wakers, 40 percent had injuries requiring medical attention, compared with only 17 percent of the good sleepers. The parents of the children who were night wakers reported that they immediately went to their child when they heard a cry in order to prevent further crying. There was a tendency for the mothers of night wakers to feel more irritable in general and "out of control." One sign of family tension was that these mothers felt unable to confide in their husbands; the association of marital difficulties with disturbed sleep has been mentioned in many studies (chapter 4).

Maybe the parents who don't supervise sleep patterns so that their child can have her sleep needs met are the same ones who don't supervise children at play in order to protect their physical safety. The message is clear: If your child is often injured, it's not necessarily because she is careless or clumsy—she may be exhausted instead.

I have seen many children who were so overtired that they fell down only a stair or two or fell from a very low height. But because they hit their head and were later noted to be sleepy or wobbly, the parents worried about a head injury or concussion. In fact, it was the overtired state that produced both the fall and the wobbliness. What these children needed was more sleep, not a head CT scan!

OVERWEIGHT AND EXERCISE

Overweight (pages 77 and 135)

Difficult-to-manage children fuss and cry a lot. One way to quiet them is to put food in their mouths. One theory is that fussiness might have some evolutionary value, ensuring survival in times when food is scarce. This was shown to be the case among the Masai of East Africa during drought conditions in 1974, when babies who cried more, and were perceived to be stronger, were fed more. But in a 1985 study by Dr. William Carey, conducted in a white, middle-class Pennsylvania pediatric practice, the babies with a more difficult temperament (who tend to have short sleep durations) tended to be fatter. Perhaps this connection between fussiness and being fed sets the stage for obesity in later years.

In my own pediatric practice, fat babies are almost always over-tired babies. That's because their mothers have incorrectly attributed their babies' crying to hunger instead of fatigue. These mothers are always feeding their babies, then telling me that their babies can't sleep because they're always hungry! The major point here? Overfeeding the crying child to keep her quiet could cause unhealthy weight gain or obesity.

This overfeeding habit may actually begin innocently enough in some children at 3–4 months of age, when nutritional feedings in the middle of the night give way to recreational feedings. Later, the bottle or breast is used as a pacifier and the frequent sipping and snacking causes excessive weight gain. Please try to become sensitive to the difference between nutritive and non-nutritive feeding.

Overdoing milk or juice bottles is a common way babies learn to not "like" eating solids. After all, they are getting calories, so they have no appetite to motivate them to eat solid foods when they are older. For children between 5 and 7 years, we now have direct evidence that the more tired the child is, the more likely it is that she will be overweight or obese.

Q: *If I give my child a bottle at naps or at bedtime, will I make her fat? When should I not include a bottle in the bedtime ritual?*

A: Sucking or sipping a bottle before falling asleep comforts most babies and even older children. There is no harm in doing this, and there is no particular age when you should stop as long as (1) you prop the baby, not the bottle, so she drinks in your arms, (2) the rate of weight gain is not too fast, and (3) frequent or prolonged feedings are not part of a sleep problem.

A 2012 paper by Dr. E. de Jong showed that a late bedtime causing short sleep duration was associated with being overweight among 4- to 8-year-old boys and among 9- to 13-year-old boys and girls. For all children, short sleep duration was strongly associated with more television viewing and computer use.

Exercise

Recent research has shown that adolescents with high levels of physical activity have longer total sleep time, fewer wakings at night, fewer symptoms of insomnia, and higher sleep quality. Additionally, it is possible that exercise reduces anxiety. On the other hand, strenuous exercise, especially common among teenagers, might mask an underlying problem of chronically insufficient sleep. The chronically or severely overtired adolescent is sometimes described as living in a "twilight zone": frequent episodes of drowsiness, "micro-sleeps," lethargy, depression, apathy, cognitive impairment, and proneness to accidents. Counteracting measures that fight the fatigued state are internal stimulation (heightened emotionality, such as anger or elation) or external stimulation such as exercise. So exercise may be helpful, but it will not solve an underlying sleep problem.

CHILD ABUSE

Let's get one ugly fact out in the open: When we are very, very tired of hearing our baby cry to fight sleep at night, we might like to shut her up. We don't act on our feelings; we don't harm our baby. But at nighttime, the thought might have occurred to us: "What if I weren't in so much control? Might I . . . ?"

The tired, difficult-to-manage infant whose howling at night will not stop can become a target for abuse or infanticide. Crying is the behavior that seems to trigger child abuse in some parents, and crying at night instead of sleeping is the historical context for infanticide.

So when your baby gets all cranked up late at night with desperate, angry, or relentless screaming when she should be asleep, and you feel like a tightly wound spring, don't be surprised if you feel you want to "get even" or "shut her up for good." If you and your child don't get the sleep you need, you may have experienced these intense feelings of anger, resentment, or ill will toward your child. That doesn't make you a bad person. The important thing is to be aware of what you are feeling and why. If you feel the need for help, contact your pediatrician, social workers at local hospitals, or the following organizations.

Prevent Child Abuse America
preventchildabuse.org
1-800-422-445

Parents without Partners
parentswithoutpartners.org

When we ourselves are extremely sleep-deprived, it can be difficult for us to see that the sleep problems in our family are solvable. There is no shame or failure in calling for help.

CHAPTER 13

Conclusion

Like the rest of the body (muscles, skin, and internal organs), the brain has physiological needs for food, water, and oxygen—basic needs that must be met not only to ensure proper brain functioning, but also to sustain life itself. However, unlike the rest of the body, the brain has one additional physiological need: sleep. *The brain requires sleep to maintain normal function.* Sleep is necessary to sustain not only alertness, but also higher order cognitive abilities such as judgment, decision making, and situational awareness. In short, sleep makes children better children. *Sleep is the critical requirement for brain health and function.* To achieve optimal readiness, children must have sleep and the more sleep obtained the better (extra sleep can make a difference, even small amounts). Inadequate sleep weakens children's performance and jeopardizes their success in life. Healthy sleep consists of four components:

1. Duration

Cognitive ability and readiness vary as direct functions of the amount of sleep obtained. *The more sleep children get, the greater their mental acuity, with faster response times, fewer errors, and fewer lapses in attention. Also improved are judgment, problem solving, situational awareness, mood, resilience, and general well-being.*

2. Timing

Human beings are designed to be awake during the daytime and to sleep during the nighttime. A portion of the brain that serves as an *internal clock*—sensitive to the timing of sunrise in the morning and sunset in the evening—largely controls these sleep–wake tendencies. Maintaining a consistent sleep–wake schedule on both school days and weekends has the benefit of strengthening and reinforcing the internal wake- and sleep-promoting processes controlled by the brain's internal clock. However, children can only achieve such benefits if they get adequate sleep on a regular basis. If they get less sleep, then a *"sleep debt"* accrues.

3. Continuity

The restorative value of sleep is determined not only by the duration of the sleep period, but also by the continuity of the sleep period—that is, the extent to which the sleep period is continuous and uninterrupted.

4. Regularity

Ultimately, the promotion of sleep for health in the home, school, or playground entails optimizing each child's sleep duration, timing, and continuity to the greatest extent possible, given existing family circumstances.

Sleep Fundamentals

The brain needs sleep to restore and repair itself, to work efficiently, to fix new memories, and to process new information appropriately. Prioritizing sleep, and ensuring that opportunities for children's sleep are maximized serves to optimize brain, psychological, and immunological health. Sleeping properly after learning improves the ability to both remember and appropriately utilize newly acquired skills and information. Although some children may require a little more or a little less sleep, for the vast majority of children, a steady diet of sleep every twenty-four hours is needed to sustain normal levels of brain function and health indefinitely. Most children who regularly obtain less sleep every twenty-four hours pay a price: They unwittingly (subjective blindness to sleepiness) but steadily accrue a significant sleep debt, characterized by increasingly suboptimal alertness, reduced mental sharpness, and an impaired ability to recover from stress. These children typically believe that they are fine and may perform most basic duties adequately. From an objective standpoint, their alertness and mental acuity is significantly (and invariably) impaired. As sleep duration increases, so does the likelihood of success in school tests, athletic events, and performances. *Insufficient sleep degrades the brain's function.* The effects of inadequate sleep on brain function and performance are well documented:

- Reduced ability to concentrate, impaired judgment, problem solving, and decision making
- Increased irritability and reduced mood
- Reduced motivation level
- Reduced ability to effectively cope with stress
- Increased risk of physical injury

Insufficient sleep negatively affects not only cognitive performance, but emotional and social functioning. Adequate sleep promotes an optimistic outlook and social acuity. *In short, the brain has a physiological need for sleep, and sleep promotes and sustains the ability to think* and maintain mental toughness. Although obtaining enough hours of nightly sleep generally results in the ability to sustain normal levels of alertness and performance during the daytime, obtaining *even more sleep results in greater brain readiness*—enhanced mental sharpness and resilience.

Promoting Healthy Sleep

PRE-SLEEP ROUTINE

Bedtime routines and soothing to sleep promote winding down and tend to facilitate the transition to sleep. These routines will maximize sleep duration. Conversely, activities such as watching television, playing videogames, chatting online, and similar interesting or engaging activities tend to arouse the brain and delay sleep onset.

SLEEP SCHEDULE

Adequate performance is best achieved by children who consistently get adequate sleep on a schedule aligned with the brain's natural circadian rhythm of alertness. Both sleep duration and sleep continuity are maximized on such schedules. However, life is influenced by random and unpredictable events, such as illnesses. Sleep opportunities are sometimes unpredictable for virtually all children. The following situations commonly contribute to sleep loss and decrements in waking performance:

• Late bedtimes

The human brain is biologically hard-wired to be alert during the daylight hours and asleep during the nighttime and early morning hours. Because of this, poor quality sleep results from late bedtimes even when children spend adequate time in bed during the daytime; long naps do not fully compensate for short night sleep.

Although such a schedule is unnatural for the human brain, some adaptation to less night sleep and more daytime sleep does occur over time, but such adaptation is *never* complete. Children always pay a cost in their waking performance.

• Irregular sleep schedules

Parents should always aim to optimize the child's sleep to the extent possible given the existing family circumstances. Toward this end, parents should strive for sleep regularity.

Parent's Role

• Strive to create an optimal sleep environment by controlling noise, light, and temperature. The brain's internal clock is very sensitive to light, and any amount of light that reaches the brain through the eyes at night can be harmful. Even dim lights emitted from electronics such as a smart phone, computer, or television can have a negative impact. Parents need to strictly enforce the lights-out policies.

• Address school-related and other sources of stress for children that may be interfering with sleep.

• Implement schedules that optimize nighttime sleep and daytime alertness.

Individual Differences

No one can maintain alertness and performance indefinitely without sleep, but some individuals are more impacted by sleep loss than others. Individual differences are determined by both genetics and habitual sleep duration. As a rule, sleep-deprived children will overestimate their own capabilities.

Unhealthy Sleep and Performance

The greatest impacts from unhealthy sleep are seen in sleep disturbances, deficits in self-assessment, risk of errors and accidents, and degradation of efficiency and productivity. The following strategies assist children coping with unhealthy sleep, and school tests, athletic events, and performances:

- Before a special event, children pay down sleep debt and *bank sleep* by getting more hours of sleep per night.
  Increasing the amount of sleep prior to an event improves performance. Children best accomplish sleep extension by *going to bed earlier.*
- Avoid over-the-counter sleep aids. These compounds do *not* improve sleep.
- Avoid over-the-counter melatonin (marketed as a sleep aid) since it does *not* increase actual sleep time.
- *Naps* will improve alertness and performance.
- *The notion that one can adapt to sleep loss is a myth.*

Although chronically sleep-restricted children do become accustomed to a reduced level of alertness, which they think is normal (subjective blindness to sleepiness), objective assessments to reveal deficits show that there is *no* evidence of habituation or adaptation to sleep loss.

- When children's alertness is compromised, there is an increased risk of lapses in attention and even brief, uncontrolled sleep episodes.
- The restorative effects of sleep accrue primarily to the brain and are primarily manifested as improved cognitive performance.

Accordingly, it is especially important that parents and others engaged in higher-order cognitive tasks—such as planning, decision making, risk assessment, and problem solving—are afforded and take full advantage of opportunities to obtain adequate sleep for themselves. Parents need sleep, too!

The above conclusion is supported by material in *Healthy Sleep Habits, Happy Child*. In fact, it is a paraphrase of the United States of America Department of the Army Field Manual No. 7–22 titled "Holistic Health and Fitness," wherein I substituted the word "Children" for "Soldiers" and "Parents" for "Leaders." This manual is based on trustworthy and scientifically verified data and was published after the completion of my book. To illustrate the importance and power of sleep, here are some brief samples from this manual:

> Holistic Health and Fitness establishes the Army's doctrine for the readiness training of Soldiers. The H2F System formalizes the way the Army trains, develops, and cares for Soldiers. To achieve optimal readiness, Soldiers must have sleep and the more sleep obtained the better. Inadequate sleep weakens Soldier performance and jeopardizes the mission. Ultimately, the promotion of sleep health in the operational environment entails optimizing each Soldier's sleep duration, timing, and continuity to the greatest extent possible, given existing mission constraints. As sleep duration increases, so does the likelihood of mission success.
>
> Adequate performance is best achieved by Soldiers who consistently get adequate sleep on a schedule aligned with the brain's natural circadian rhythm of alertness. However, military operations are influenced by random and unpredictable events and requirements. Sleep opportunities are sometimes unpredictable for virtually all Soldiers. Leaders should always aim to optimize the Soldier's sleep to the extent possible given the

existing operational constraints. Toward this end, commanders should strive for consistency for individual Soldiers. *Think of sleep as an item of logistical resupply, like beans and bullets,* and plan accordingly. Planning for sleep in training and tactical environments is a leader competency. Sleep management optimizes Soldiers' performance in austere conditions. *Sleep is a force multiplier.* The goal in all operational scenarios should always be to maximize sleep duration because *more sleep always results in greater alertness, resilience*—greater readiness. *Effective leaders consider sleep an item of logistical resupply like water, food, fuel, and ammunition.*

In short, healthy sleep will make your child healthier, stronger, smarter, happier, and more successful:

A healthy child needs a healthy brain.

A healthy brain needs healthy sleep.

References for the 5th Edition

Further references can be found online at marcweissbluth.com.

Aatsinki, A-K., Lahti, L., Uusitupa, H-M., Manukka, E., Keski-talo, A., Nolvi, S., O'Mahoney, S., Pietila, S., Elo, L. L., Eerola, E., Karlsson, H., and Karlsson, L. (2019). Gut micro-biota composition is associated with temperament traits in infants. *Brain, Behavior, and Immunity, 80,* 849–858.

Acosta, J., Garcia, D., and Bagner, D. M. (2019). Parent-child inter-action therapy for children with developmental delay: the role of sleep problems. *Journal of Developmental and Behavioral Pediatrics, 40,* 183–191.

Alexander C. P., Zhu, J., Paul, I.M., and Kjerulff, K.H. (2017). Fa-thers make a difference: positive relationships with mother and baby in relation to infant colic. *Child: Care, Health, and Development, 43,* 687–696.

Altof, T., Horvitz, E., White, R. W., and Zeitzer, J. Harnessing the web for population-scale physiological sensing: a case study of sleep and performance. (2017). arXiv:1701.07083v2[cs. HC].

Anderson, S. E., Andridge, R., and Whitaker, R. C. (2016). Bedtime in preschool-aged children and risk for adolescent obesity. *Journal of Pediatrics, 176,* 17–22.

Anderson, S.E., Sacker, A., Whitaker, R.C., and Kelly, Y. (2017). Self-regulation and household routines at age three and obesity at age eleven: longitudinal analysis of the UK Millennium Cohort Study. *International Journal of Obesity, 41,* 1459–1466.

Arnal, P. J., Sauvet, F., Leger, D., van Beers, P., Bayon, V., Bougard, C., Rabat, A., Millet, G. Y., and Chennaoui, M. (2015). Benefits of sleep extension on sustained attention and sleep pressure before and during total sleep deprivation and recovery. *Sleep, 38,* 1935–1943.

Asarnow, L. D., McGlinchey, E., and Harvey, A. G. (2014). The effects of bedtime and sleep duration on academic and emotional outcomes in a nationally representative sample of adolescents. *Journal of Adolescent health, 54,* 350–356.

Ashworth, A., Hill, C. M., Karmiloff-Smith, A., and Dimitriou D. (2014). Sleep enhances memory consolidation in children. *Journal of Sleep Research, 23,* 304–310.

Bakermans-Kranenburg, M. J. and van IJzendoorn, M. H. (2006). Gene-environment interaction of the dopamine D4 receptor (DRD4) and observed maternal insensitivity predicting externalizing behavior in preschoolers. *Developmental Psychology, 48,* 406–409.

Barr, R. G. (1998). Crying in the first year of life: good news in the midst of distress. *Child: Care, Health and Development, 24,* 425–439.

Batra, E. K., Teti, D. M., Schaefer, E. W., Neumann, B. A., Meek, E. A., and Paul, I. M. (2016). Nocturnal video assessment of infant sleep environments. *Pediatrics, 140,* e20170122.

Bat-Pitault, F., Sesso, G., Deruelle, C., Flori, S., Porcher-guinet, V., Stagnara, C., Guyon, A., Plancoulaine, S., Adrien, J., Da Fonseca, D., Patural, H., and Franco, P. (2017). Altered sleep architecture during the first months in infants born to depressed mothers. *Sleep Medicine, 30,* 195–203.

Beebe, D. W., Field, J., Miller, M. M., Miller, L. E., and LeBlond, E. (2017). Impact of multi-night experimentally induced short sleep on adolescent performance in a simulated classroom. *Sleep, 40,* doi:10.1093/sleep/zsw035.

Belanger, M-E., Bernier, A., Simard, V., Desrosiers, K., and Carrier, J. (2018). Sleeping toward behavioral regulation: relations between sleep and externalizing symptoms in toddlers and preschoolers. *Journal of Clinical Child & Adolescent Psychology, 47,* 366–373.

Bell, G., Hiscock, H., Tobin, S., Cook, F., and Sung, V. (2018). Behavioral outcomes of infant colic in toddlerhood: a longitudinal study. *Journal of Pediatrics, 201,* 154–159.

Belmon, L.S., van Stralen, M. M., Busch, V., Harmsen, I. A., and Chinapaw, M. J. M. (2019). What are the determinants of children's sleep behavior? A systematic review of longitudinal studies. *Sleep Medicine Reviews, 43,* 60–70.

Berger, A. T., Wahlstrom, K. L., and Widome, R. (2019). Relationships between sleep duration and adolescent depression: a conceptual replication. *Sleep Health, 5,* 175–179.

Bernier, A., Beauchamp, M. H., Bouvette-Turcot, A-A., Carlson, S. M., and Carrier, J. (2013). Sleep and cognition in preschool years: specific links to executive function. *Child Development, 84,* 1542–1553.

Bilgin, A. and Wolke, D. (2020). Parental use of "cry it out" in infants: no adverse effects on attachment and behavioural development at 18 months. *Journal of Child Psychology and Psychiatry,* doi:10.1111/jepp.13223.

Bin-Hasan, S., Kapur, K., Rakesh, K., and Owens, J. (2020). School start time changes and motor vehicles crashes in adolescent drivers. *Journal of Clinical Sleep Medicine,* DOI: 10.5664/jcsm.8208.

Bouvette-Turcot, A-A., Pluess, M., Bernier, A., Pennestri, M-H., Levitan, R., Sokolowski, M. B., Kennedy, J. L., Minde, K., Steiner, M., Pokhvisneva, I., Meaney, M. J., and Gaudreau, H. (2015). Effects of genotype and sleep on temperament. *Pediatrics, 136,* e914–921.

Bruni, O., Baumgartner E., Sette, S., Ancona, M., Caso, G., Di Cosimo, M. E., Mannini, A., Ometto, M., pasquini, A., Ulliana, A., and Ferri, R. (2014). Longitudinal study of sleep behavior in normal infants during the first year of life. *Journal of Clinical Sleep Medicine, 10*, 1119–1127.

Buchanan, L., Yeatman, H., Kelly, B., and Kariippanon, K. (2018). A thematic content analysis of how marketers promote energy drinks on digital platforms to young Australians. *Australian & New Zealand Journal of Public Health, 42*, 530–531.

Burnham, M. M., Goodlin-Jones, B. L., Gaylor, E. E., and Anders, T. F. (2002). Nighttime sleep-wake patterns and self-soothing from birth to one year of age: a longitudinal intervention study. *Journal of Child Psychology and Psychiatry, 43*, 713–725.

Carter, B., Rees, P., Hale, L., Bhattacharjee, D., and Paradkar, M., S. (2018). Association between portable screen-based media device access or use and sleep outcomes. A systematic review and meta-analysis. *JAMA Pediatrics, 170*, 1202–1208.

Castelnovo, A., Lopez, R., Proserpio, P., Nobili, L., and Dauvilliers, Y. (2018). NREM sleep parasomnias as disorders of sleep-state dissociation. *Nature Reviews, Neurology, 14*, 470–481.

Chan, N. Y., Zhang, J., Yu, M. W. M., Lam, S. P., Li, S. X., Kong, A. P. S., Li, A. M., and Wing, Y. K. (2017). Impact of a modest delay in school start time in Hong Kong school adolescents. *Sleep Medicine, 30*, 164–170.

Chen, B., van Darn, R. M., Tan, C. S., Chua, H. L., Wong, P. G., Bernard, J. Y., and Muller-Riemenschneider, F. (2019). Screen viewing behavior and sleep duration among children aged 2 and below. *BMC Public Health*, doi.org, /10.1186/s12889-018-6385-6.

Cheung, C. H. M., Bedford, R., De Urabain, I. S., Karmiloff-Smith, A., and Smith, T. (2017). Daily touchscreen use in infants and toddlers is associated with reduced sleep and delayed sleep onset. *Scientific Reports, 7*, doi;10.1038/srep46104.

Chiesa, A. E., Kallechey, L., Harlaar, N., Ford, C. R., Garrido, E. F., Betts, W. R., and Maguire S. (2018). Intimate partner violence victimization and parenting: a systematic review. *Child Abuse & Neglect, 80,* 285–300.

Conway, A., Modrek, A., and Gorroochurn, P. (2018). Maternal sensitivity predicts fewer sleep problems at early adolescence for toddlers with negative emotionality: a case of differential susceptibility. *Child Psychiatry Human Development, 49,* 86–99.

Cooney, M. R., Short, M. A., and Gradisar, M. (2018). An open trial of bedtime fading for sleep disturbances in preschool children: a parent group education approach. *Sleep Medicine, 46,* 98–106.

Cook, F., Giallo R., Petrovic, Z., Coe, A., Seymour, M., Cann, W., and Hiscock, H. (2017). Depression and anger in fathers of unsettled infants: a community cohort study. *Journal of Paediatrics and Child Health, 53,* 131–135.

Cook, F., Conway, L. J., Garland, D., Giallo, R., Keys, E., and Brown, S. (2019). Profiles and predictors of infant sleep problems across the first year. *Journal of Developmental and Behavioral Pediatrics, 13,* 1–13.

Cook, F., Conway, L. J., Giallo, R., Gartland, D., Sciberras, E., and Brown, S. (2020). Infant sleep and child mental health: a longitudinal investigation. *Archives of Diseases of Childhood,* 10.1136/archdis child-2019-318014.

Cook, F., Giallo, R., Hiscock, H., Mensah, F., Sanchez, K., and Reilly, S. (2019). Infant regulation and child mental health concerns: a longitudinal study. *Pediatrics, 143,* e20180977.

Cremone, A., Kurdziel, L. B. F., Fraticelli-Torres, A., McDermott, J. M., and Spencer, R. M. C. (2017). Napping reduces emotional attention bias during early childhood. *Developmental Science,* DOI:10.1111/desc.12411.

Cremone, A., McDermott, J. M., and Spencer, R. M. C. (2017). Naps enhance executive attention in preschool-aged children. *Journal of Pediatric Psychology, 42,* 837–845.

Cremone, A., deJong, D. M., Kurdziel, L. B. F., Desrochers, P., Sayer, A., LeBourgeois, M. K., Spencer, R. M. C., and McDermott, J. M. (2018). Sleep tight, act right: negative affect, sleep, and behavior problems during early childhood. *Child Development, 89,* e42–e59.

Darwin, Z., Galdas, P., Hinchliff, S., Littlewood, E., McMillan, D., McGowas, L., and Gilbody, S. (2017). Fathers' views and experiences of their own mental health during pregnancy and the first postnatal year: a qualitative interview study of men participating in the UK Born and Bred in Yorkshire (BaBY) cohort. (2017) *BMC Pregnancy and Childbirth, 17,* doi:10.1 186/s12884-017-1229-4.

De Bruin, E. J., Bogels, S. M., Oort, F. J., and Meijer, A. M. (2018). Improvements of adolescent psychopathology after treatment: results from a controlled trial over 1 year. *Journal of Child Psychology and Psychiatry, 59,* 509–522.

Dejong, K., Olyaei, A., and Lo, J., O. (2019). Alcohol use in pregnancy. *Clinical Obstetrics and Gynecology, 62,* 142–155.

De Ruiter, I., Olmedo-Requena, R., Sanchez-Cruz, J-J., and Jimenez-Moleon, J-J. (2016). Change in sleep duration in Spanish children aged 2–14 years from 1987 to 2011. *Sleep Medicine, 21,* 145–150.

Depner, C.M., Melanson, E. L., Eckel, R. H., Snell-Bergeon, J. K., Perreault, L., Bergman, B. C., Higgins, J. A., Guerin, M. K., Stothard, E. R., and Morton, S. J. (2019). *Ad. Libitum* weekend recovery sleep fails to prevent metabolic dysregulation during a repeating pattern of insufficient sleep and weekend recovery sleep. *Current Biology, 29,* 957–967.

Dewald-Kaufmann, J. K., Oort, F. J., and Meijer, A. M. (2014). The effects of sleep extension and sleep hygiene advice on sleep and depressive symptoms in adolescents: a randomized controlled trial. *Journal of Child Psychology and Psychiatry, 55,* 273–283.

Dollman, J., Matricciani, L., Booth, V. B., and Blunden, S. (2017).

Secular trends in Australian school children's sleep and perceived importance of sleep between 1985 and 2013. *Acta Paediactrica, 106,* 1341–1347.

Dunster, G. P., de la Iglesia, L., Ben-Hamo, M., Nave, C., Fleischer, J. G., and Panda, S. (2018). Sleepmore in Seattle: later school start times are associated with more sleep and better performance in high school students. *Science Advances, 4,* doi: 10.1126/sciadv.aau6200.

Finan, P. H., Quartana, P. J., and Smith, M. T. (2015). The effects of sleep continuity disruption on positive mood and sleep architecture in healthy adults. *Sleep, 38,* 1735–1742.

Finan, P. H., Quartana, P. J., Remeniuk, B., Garland, E. L., Rhudy, J. L., Hand, M., Irwin, M. R., and Smith, M. T. (2017). Partial sleep deprivation attenuates the positive affect system: effects across multiple measurement modalities. *Sleep, 40,* 1–9.

Fu, K., Ho, F. K. W., Rao, N., Jiang, F., Li, S. L., Lee, T. M., Chan, S. H., Yung, A. W., Young, M. E., and Ip, P. (2017). Parental restriction reduces the harmful effects of in-bedroom electronic devices. *Archives of Diseases of Children, 102,* 1125–1131.

Galbally, M., Watson, S. J., Teti, D. and Lewis, A. J. (2018). Perinatal maternal depression, antidepressant use and infant sleep outcomes: exploring cross-lagged associations in a pregnancy cohort study. *Journal of Affective Disorders, 238,* 218–225.

Galland, B. C., Sayers, R. M., Cameron, S. L., Gray, A. R., Heath, A. M., Lawrence, J. A., Newlands, A., Taylor, B. J., and Taylor, R. W. (2017). Anticipatory guidance to prevent infant sleep problems within a randomized controlled trial: infant, maternal, and partner outcomes at 6 months of age. *British Medical Journal Open, 7,* e014908.

Gao, B., Dwivedi, S., Milewski, M. D., and Cruz. A. I. (2019). Lack of sleep and sports injuries in adolescents: a systematic review and meta-analysis. *Journal of Pediatric Orthopedics, 30,* e324-e333.

Gariepy, G., Riehm, K. E., Whitehead, R. D., Dore, I., and Elgar, J. (2019). Teenage night owls or early birds? Chronotype and the mental health of adolescents. *Journal of Sleep Research*, e12723.

Giallo, R., Cooklin, A., Zerman, N., and Vittorino, R. (2013). Psychological distress of fathers attending an Australian early parenting service for early parenting difficulties. *Clinical Psychologist, 17*, 46–55.

Giallo, R., Dunning, M., and Gent, A. (2017). Attitudinal barriers to help-seeking and preferences for mental health support among Australian fathers. *Journal of Reproductive and Infant Psychology, 35*, 236–247.

Giesbrecht, G. F., Letourneau, N., Campbell, T., Hart, M., Thomas, J. C., Tomfohr-Madsen, N., and the APrON Study team. (2020). Parental use of "cry out" in a community sample during the first year of infant life. *Journal of Developmental & Behavioral Pediatrics, 41*, 379–387.

Giganti, F., Fagioli, I., Ficca, G., and Salzarulo, P. (2001). Polygraphic investigation of 24-h waking distribution in infants. *Physiology and Behavior, 73*, 621–624.

Godinho-Silva, C., Domingues, R. G., Rendas, M., Raposo, B., Ribero, H., da Silva, J. A., Viera, A., Costa, R. M., Barbosa-Morais, N. L., Carvalho, T., and Viega-Fernades, H. (2019). Light-entrained and brain-tuned circadian circuits regulate ILC3s and gut homeostasis. *Nature, 574*, 254–258.

Goodrich, J. K., Waters, J. L., Poole, A. C., Sutter, J. L., Koren, O., Blekhaman, R., Beaumont, M., Van treunen, W., Knight, R., Bell, J. T., Spector, T. D., Clarm, A. G., and Ley, R. E. (2014). Human genetics shape the gut microbiome. *Cell, 158*, 789–799.

Gradisar, M., Jackson, K., Spurrier, N., J., Gibson, J. G., Whitham, J., Williams, A. S., Dolby, R., and Kennaway, D. J. (2016). Behavioral interventions for infant sleep: a randomized controlled trial. *Pediatrics, 137*, e20151486.

Gruber, R., Somerville, G., Enros, P., Paquin, S., Kestler, M., and Gillies-Poitras, E. (2014). Sleep efficiency (but not sleep duration) of healthy school-age children is associated with grades in math and languages. *Sleep Medicine, 15,* 1517–1525.

Gruber, R., Somerville, G., Bergmame, L., Fontil, L., and Paquin, S. (2016). School-based sleep education program improves sleep and academic performance of school-aged children. *Sleep Medicine, 21,* 93–100.

Guadagni, V., Burles, F., Ferrara, M., and Iaria, G. (2014). The effects of sleep deprivation on emotional empathy. *Journal of Sleep Research, 23,* 6, 57–663.

Guadagni, V., Burles, F., Valera, S., Hardwicke-Brown, E., Ferrara, M., Campbell, T., and Iaria, G. (2017). The relationship between quality of sleep and emotional empathy. *Journal of Psychophysiology, 31,* 158–166.

Guerrero, M. D., Barnes, J. D., Waksh, J. J., Chaput, J-P., Tremblay, M. S., and Goldfield, G. S. (2019). 32-hour movement behaviors and impulsivity. *Pediatrics, 144,* e20190187.

Gulenc, A., Butle, E., Sarkadi, A., and Hiscock, H. (2018). Paternal psychological distress, parenting, and child behavior: a population based cross-sectional study. *Child Care Health Development, 44,* 892–900.

Gustafsson M-L., Laaksonen, C., Salantera, S., Loyttyniemi, E., and Aromaa, M. (2019). Changes in the amount of sleep and daytime sleepiness: a follow-up study of school children from ages 10 to 15 years. *International Journal of Nurse Practioners, 25,* e12689.

Habard, E., Allen, N. B., Trinder, J., and Bei, B. (2016). What's keeping teenagers up? Prebedtime behaviors and actigraphy-assessed sleep over school and vacation. *Journal of Adolescent Health, 58,* 426–432.

Hatch, B., Galland, B. C., Gray, A. R., Taylor, R. W., Sayers, R., Lawrence, J., and Taylor, B. (2019). Consistent use of bedtime parenting strategies mediates the effects of sleep education on child sleep: secondary findings from an early-life randomized controlled trial. *Sleep Health, 5,* 433–443.

Hauck, J. L., Zoot, G. R., Felzer-Kim, I. T., and Adkins, C. M.

(2018). A comparison of low-intensity physical activity, growth, and sleep behavior in 6-month old infants. *Infant behavior and Development, 53*, 18–24.

Heinrichs, C., Munson, P. J., Counts, D. R., Cutler, G. B. Jr., and Baron, J. (1995). Patterns of human growth. *Science, 268*, 442–446.

Helms, A. F., and Spencer, R. M. C. (2019). Television use and its effect on sleep in early childhood. *Sleep Health, 5*, 241–247.

Hiscock, H., Bayer, J., Gold, L., Hampton, A., Ukoumunne, O. C., and Wake, M. (2007). Improving infant sleep and maternal mental health: a cluster randomized trial. *Archives of Diseases of Childen, 92*, 952–957.

Hiscock, H., Bayer, J. K., Hampton, A., Ukoumunne, O. C., and Wake, M. (2008). Long-term mother and child mental health effects of a population-based infant sleep intervention: cluster-randomized, controlled trial. *Pediatrics, 122*, e621–627.

Honaker, S. M., Schwichtenberg, A. J., Kreps, T. A., and Mindell, J. A. (2018). Real-world implementation of infant behavioral sleep interventions: results of a parental survey. *Journal of Pediatrics, 199*, 106–111.

Horvath, K. and Plunkett, K. (2016). Frequent daytime naps predict vocabulary growth in early childhood. *Journal of Child Psychology and Psychiatry, 57*, 1008–1017.

Horvath, K., Hannon, B., Ujima,P., Gombos, F., and Plunkett, K. (2018). Memory in 3-month-old infants benefit from a short nap. *Developmental Science, 21*, e12587.

Huang, Y. A., Ye, Y., Huang, X. N., Feng, W. W., Chen, Q., He, C. Y., Li, Z., and Wang, N. R. Association of maternal nocturnal sleep throughout pregnancy with the early nocturnal sleep of infants. *Zhonghua Erke Zazhi, 57*, 606–613.

Huhdanpaa, H., Morales-Munoz, I., Aronen, E. T., Polki, P., Saarenpaa-Heikkila, O., Paunio, T., Kylliainen, A., and Paavonen, E. J. (2019). Sleep difficulties in infancy are associated with symptoms of inattention and hyperactivity at the age of

5 years: a longitudinal study. *Journal of Developmental & Behavioral Pediatrics, 40,* 432–440.

Hupbach, A., Gomez, R. L., Bootzin, R. R., and Nadel, L. (2009). Nap-dependent learning in infants. *Developmental Science, 12,* 1007–1012.

Hysing, M., Harvey, A. G., Torgersen, L., Ystrom, E., Reichborn-Kjennerud, T., and Sivertsen, B. (2014). Trajectories and predictors of nocturnal awakenings and sleep duration in infants. *Journal of Developmental and Behavioral Pediatrics, 35,* 309–316.

Hysing, M., Reichborn-Kjennerud, T., Markestad, T., Elgen, I., and Sivertsen, B. (2019). Sleep duration and nocturnal awakenings in infants born with gestational risk. *Journal of Developmental and Behavioral Pediatrics, 40,* 192–199.

Inderkum, A. P. and Tarokh, L. (2018). High heritability of adolescent sleep-wake behavior on free, but not school days: a long-term twin study. *SleepJ., doi: 10.1093/sleep/zsy004.*

Izawa, S., Chowdhury, S., Miyazaki, T., Mukai, Y., Ono, D., Inouw, R., Ohmura, Y., Mizoguchi, H., Kimura, K., Yoshioka, M., Terao, A., Kilduff, T. S., and Yamanaka, A. (2019). REM sleep-active MCH neurons are involved in forgetting hippocampus-dependent memories. *Science, 365,* 1308–1313.

Janssen, K. C., Phillipson, S., O'Connor, J., and Johns, M. V. (2017). Validation of the Epworth Sleepiness scale for children and adolescents using Rasch analysis. *Sleep Medicine, 33,* 30–35.

Jian, N. and Teti, D. M. (2016). Emotional availability at bedtime, infant temperament, and infant sleep development from one to six months. *Sleep Medicine, 23,* 49–58.

Kahn, M., Bauminger, Y., Volkovich, E., Meiri, G., Sadeh, A., and Tikotzsky, L. (2018). Links between infant sleep and parental tolerance for infant crying: longitudinal assessment from pregnancy through six months postpartum. *Sleep Medicine, 50,* 72–75.

Kahn, M., Ronen, A., Apter, A., and Sadeh, A. (2017). Cognitive-behavioral versus non-directive therapy for preschoolers with severe fears and sleep-related problems. (2017). *Sleep Medicine, 32,* 40–47.

Karr J. L., Schmiege, S. J., Vadiveloo, M., Simon, S. L., and Tovar, A. (2018). Sleep duration mediates the relationship between health behavior patterns and obesity. *Sleep Health, 4,* 442–447.

Kellams, A., Hauck, F. R., Moon, R. Y., Kerr, S. M., Heeren, T., Corwin, M. J., and Colson, E. (2020). Factors associated with choice of infant sleep location. *Pediatrics,* 2020;145(3): e20191523.

Kobayashi, K., Yorifuji, T., Yamakawa, M., Oka, M., Inoue, S., Yoshinaga, H., and Doi, H. (2015). Poor toddler-age sleep schedules predict school-age behavioral disorders in a longitudinal survey. *Brain and Development, 17,* 572–578.

Konrad, C., Herbert, J. S., Schneider, S., and Seehagen, S. (2016). Gist extraction and sleep in 12-month-old infants. *Neurobiology of Learning and Memory, 134,* 216–220.

Konrad, C., Seehagen, S., Schneider, S., and Herbert, J. S. (2016). Naps promote flexible memory retrieval in 12-month-old infants. *Developmental Psychobiology, 58,* 866–874.

Konrad, C., Dirks, N. D., Warmuth, A., Herbert, J. S., Schneider, S., and Seehagen, S. (2017). Sleep-dependent selective imitation in infants. *Journal of Sleep Research, 28,* e12777.

Kurdziel, L. B., Kent, J., and Spencer, R. M. C. (2018). Sleep-dependent enhancement of emotional memory in early childhood. *Scientific Reports, 8,* 12609.

Lam, P., Hiscock, H., and Wake, M. (*2003*). Outcomes of infant sleep problems: a longitudinal study of sleep, behavior, and maternal well-being. *Pediatrics, 111,* e203–207.

Lampl, M., Veldhuis, J. D., and Johnson, M. L. (1992). Saltation and stasis: a model of human growth. *Science, 258,* 801–803.

Leach, L. S., Mackinnon, A., Poyser, C., and Fairweather-Schmidt, A. K. (2015). Depression and anxiety in expectant and new fathers: longitudinal findings in Australian men. *British Journal of Psychiatry, 206,* 471–478.

Lee, S., Hale, L., Chang, A-M., Nahmod, N. G., Master, L.,

Berger, L, M., and Buxton, O. M. (2018). Longitudinal associations of childhood bedtime and sleep routines with adolescent body mass index. *SleepJ*, doi: 10.1093/sleep/zsy202.

Lee, Y. J., Park, J., Kim, S., Cho, S-J., and Kim, S. J. (2015). Academic performance among adolescents with behaviorally induced insufficient sleep syndrome. *Journal of Clinical Sleep Medicine, 11,* 61–68.

Lemura, A., Iwasaki, M., Yamakawa, N., Tomiwa, K., Anji, Y., Sakakihara, Y., Kakuma, T., Nagamitsu, S., and Matuishi, T. (2016). Influence of sleep-onset time on the development of 18-month-old infants: Japan Children's cohort study. *Brain & Development, 38,* 364–372.

Leocadio-Miguel, M. A., Carneiro, B. T., Ximenes-da-Silva, A., Caumo, W., Grassi-Kassisse, D., and Pedrazzoli, M. (2018). PER3 gene regulation of sleep-wake behavior as a function of latitude. *Sleep health, 4,* 572–578.

Li, Y. I., Starr, L. R., and Wray-lake, L. (2019). Insomnia mediates the longitudinal relationship between anxiety and depressive symptoms in a nationally representative sample of adolescents. *Depression and Anxiety, 35,* 583–591.

Lin,Y., Tremblay, M. S., Katzmarzyk, P. T., Fogelholm, M., Hu, G., Lambert, E. V., Maher, C., Maia, J., Olds, T., Sarmiento, O. L., Standage, M., Tudor-Locke, C., and Chaput, J-P. (2018). Temporal and bi-directional associations between sleep duration and physical activity/sedentary time in children: an international comparison. *Preventive Medicine, 111,* 436–441.

Liu, J., Liu, X., Ji, X., Wang, Y., Zhou, G., and Chen, X. (2018). Sleep disordered breathing symptoms and daytime sleepiness are associated with emotional problems and poor school performance. *Psychiatry Research, 242,* 218–225.

Lo, J. C., Lee, S. M., Lee, X. K., Sasmita, K., Chee, N. I. Y. N., Tandi, J., Cher, W. S., Gooley, J. J., and Chee, M. W. L. (2018). Sustained benefits of delaying school start time on adolescent sleep and well-being. *SleepJ*, doi:10.1093/sleep/zsy052.

Macknin, M. L., Medenhorp, S. V., and Maier, M. C. (1989). Infant sleep and bedtime cereal. *American Journal of Diseases of Childhood, 143,* 1066–1068.

Makela, T. E., Peltola, M. J., Paavonen, E. J., Saarenpaal-Heikkila, O., Paunio, T., and Kylliainen, A. (2018). Night awakening in infancy: developmental stability and longitudinal associations with psychomotor development. *Developmental psychology, 54,* 1208–1218.

Malone, S. K., Zemel, B., Compher, C., Souders, M., Chittams, J., Thompson, A. L., Pack, A., and Lipman, T. H. (2016). Social jetlag, chronotype, and body mass index in 14 to 17 year old adolescents. *Chronobiology International, 33,* 1255–1266.

Marinelli, M., Sunyer, J., Alvarez-Pedrerol, M., Iniguez, C., Torrent, M., Vioque, J., Turner, M.C., and Julvez, J. (2014). Hours of television viewing and sleep duration in children. S multicenter birth cohort study. *JAMA Pediatrics, 168,* 458–464.

Martini, J., Petzoldt, J., Knappe, S., Garthus-Niegel, S., Asselmann, E., and Witchen, H-U. (2017). Infant, maternal, and familial predictors and correlates of regulatory problems in early infancy: the differential role of infant temperament and maternal anxiety and depression. *Early Human Development, 115,* 23–31.

Massignan, C., Cardoso, M., Porporatti, A. L., Aydinoz, S., Canto, G, D., Mezzomo, L. A., and Bolan, M. (2016). Signs and symptoms of primary tooth eruption, a meta-analysis. *Pediatrics, 137,* e20153501.

McDonald, L., Wardle, J., Llewellyn, C. H., van Jaarsveld, C. H. M., and Fisher, A. (2014). Predictors of shorter sleep in early childhood. *Sleep Medicine, 15,* 536–540.

McMakin, D. L., Dahl, R. E., Buysse, D. J., Cousins, J. C., Forbes, E. E., Silk, J. S., Siegel, G. J., and Franzin, P. L. (2016). The impact of experimental sleep restriction on affective functioning in social and nonsocial contexts among adolescents. *Journal of Child psychology and Psychiatry, 57,* 1027–1037.

McQuillan, M. E., Bates, J. E., Staples, A. D., and Deater-Deckard, K. (2019). Maternal stress, sleep, and parenting. *Journal of Family Psychology, 33*, 349–359.

Melaku, Y. A., Appleton, S., Reynolds, A. C., Sweetman, A. M., Stevens, D. J., Lack, L., and Adams, R. (2019). Associations between childhood behavioral problems and insomnia symptoms in adulthood. *JAMA Network Open.* 2019:e1910861. doi:10.100/jamanetworkopen.2019.10861.

Meijer, A. M., Reitz, E., and Dekovic, M. (2016). Parenting matters: a longitudinal study into parenting and adolescent sleep. *Journal of Sleep Research, 25,* 556–564.

Meltzer, L. J. and Mindell, J. A. (2014). Systematic review and meta-analysis of behavioral interventions for pediatric insomnia. *Journal of Pediatrics, 39,* 932–948.

Mennella, J. A. and Garcia-Gomez, P. L. (2001). Sleep disturbances after acute exposure to alcohol in mothers' milk. *Alcohol, 25,* 153–158.

Miller, A. L., Seifer, R., Crossin, R., and Lebourgeois, M. K. (2015). Toddler's self-regulation strategies in a challenge context are nap-dependent. *Journal of Sleep Research, 24,* 279–287.

Mindell, J. A., Li. A. M., Sadeh, A., Kwon, R., and Goh, D. Y. T. (2015). Bedtime routines for young children: A dose-dependent association with sleep outcomes. *Sleep, 38,* 717–722.

Mindell, J. A., Leichman, E. S., and Walters, R. M. (2017). Sleep location and parent-perceived sleep outcomes in older infants. *Sleep Medicine, 39,* 1–7.

Mindell, J. A., Leichman, E. S., DuMond, C., and Sadeh, A. (2017). Sleep and social-emotional development in infants and toddlers. *Journal of Clinical Child & Adolescent Psychology, 46,* 236–246.

Mindell, J. A., Leichman, E. S., Lee, C., and Williamson, A. A. (2017). Implementation of a nightly bedtime routine: How quickly to things improve? *Infant Behavior and Development, 49,* 220–227.

Mindell, J. A., Lee, C. I., Leichman, E. S., and Rotella, K. N. (2018). Massage-based bedtime routine: impact on sleep and mood in infants and mothers. *Sleep Medicine, 41,* 51–57.

Mindell, J. A. and Williamson, A. A. (2018). Benefits of a bedtime routine in young children: Sleep, development, and beyond. *Sleep Medicine Reviews, 40,* 93–108.

Mireku, M. O., Barker, M. M., Mutzm J., Dumontheil, I., Thomas, M. S. C., Roosli, M., Elliot, P., and Toledano, M. B. (2019). Night-time screen-based media device use and adolescents' sleep and health-related quality of life. *Environmental International, 124,* 66–78.

Molfese, V. J., Rudasill, K. M., Prokasky, A., Champagne, C., Holmes, M., Molfese, D. L., and Bates, J. E. (2015). Relations between toddler sleep characteristics, sleep, problems, and temperament. *Developmental Neuropsychology 40,* 138–154.

Morales-Munoz, I., Saarenpaas-Heikkila, O., Kylliainen, A., Polkki, P., Porkka-Heiskanen, T., Paunia, T., and Paavonen, J. (2018). The effects of maternal risk factors during pregnancy on the onset of sleep difficulties in infants at 3 months old. *Journal of Sleep Research, 27,* e12696.

Mullins, E. N., Miller, A. L., Cherian, S. S., Limeng, J. C., Wright Jr, K. P., Kurth, S., and Lebourgeois, M. K. (2017). Acute sleep restriction increases dietary intake in preschool-age children. *Journal of Sleep Research, 26,* 48–54.

Nahmod, N. G., Lee, S., Master, L., Chang, A-M., Hale, L., and Buxton, O. M. (2019). Later high school start times associated with longer actigraphic sleep duration in adolescents. *SleepJ,* doi: *10.*1093/sleep/zsy212.

Olsen, A. L., Ammitzboll, J., Olsen, E. M., and Skovgaard, A. M. (2019). Problems of feeding, sleeping, and excessive crying in infancy: a general population study. *Archives of Diseases of Children, 104,* 1034–1041.

Owens, J., Wang, G., Lewin, D., Skora, E., and Baylor, A. (2017). Association between short sleep duration and risk behavior factors in middle school students. *Sleep, 40,* doi.org/10.1093/sleep/zsw004.

Paavonen, E. J., Ralkkonen, K., Lahti, J., Komsi. N., Heinonen, K., Pesonen, A-K., Jarvenpaa, A-L., Strandberg, T., Kajantie, E., and Porkka-Heiskanen, T. (2009). Short sleep duration and behavioral symptoms of attention deficit/hyperactivity disorder in healthy 7- to 8-year-old children. *Pediatrics, 123,* e857–e864.

Paavonen, E. J., Morales-Munoz, I., Polkki, P., Paunio, T., Porkka-Heiskanen, T., Kylliainen, A., Partonen, T., and Saarenpaa-Heikkila, O. Development of sleep-wake rhythms during the first year of age. (2019). *Journal of Sleep Research,* doi.org/10.1111/jsr.12918.

Paine, S. and Gradisar, M. (2011). A randomized controlled trial of cognitive-behaviour therapy for behavioral insomnia of childhood in school-aged children. *Behaviour Research and Therapy, 49,* 379–388.

Pallesen, S., Gunderson, H. S., Kristoffersen, M., Bjorn, B., Thun, E., and Harris, A. (2017). The effects of sleep deprivation on soccer skills. *Perceptual and Motor Skills, 124,* 812-829.

Palmstierna, P., Sepia, A., and Ludvigsson, J. Parent perceptions of child sleep: a study of 10,000 Swedish children. (2008). *Acta Paedictrica, 97,* 1631–1639.

Pattinson, C. L., Smith, S. S., Staton, S. L., Trost, S. G., and Thorpe, K. J. (2018). Investigating the association between sleep parameters and the weight status of children: night sleep duration matters. *Sleep health, 4,* 147–153.

Paul, I. M., Savage, J. S., Anzman-Frasca, S., Marini, M. E., Mindell, J. A., and Birchm L. L. (2016). INSIGHT Responsive parenting intervention and infant sleep. *Pediatrics, 138,* e20160762.

Pearson, R. M., Carnegie, R. E., Cree, C., Rollings, C., Rena-Jones, L., Evans, J., Stein, A., and Tilling, K. (2018). Prevalence of prenatal depression symptoms among 2 generations of pregnant mothers. A longitudinal study of parents and children. *JAMA Network Open,* doi:10.1001/jamaopennet work.0725.

Pennestri, M-H., Moss, E., O'Donnell, K., Lecompte, V., Bouvette-Turcot, A-A., Atkinson, L., Minde, K., Gruber, R., Fleming, A. S., Meaney, M. J., and Gaudreau, H. (2015). Establishment and consolidation of the sleep-wake cycle as a function of attachment pattern. *Attachment & Human Development, 17,* 23–42.

Pennestri, M-H., Laganiere, C., Bouvette-Turcot, A-A., Pokhvisneva, I., Steiner, M., Meaney, M. J., and Gaudreau, H. (2018). Uninterrupted infant sleep, development, and maternal mood. *Pediatrics, 142,* e20174330.

Peralta, G. P., Forns, J., de la Hera, M. G., Gonzalez, L., Guxens, M., Lopez-Vicente, M., Sunyer, J., and Garcia-Aymerich, J. (2018). Sleeping, TV, Cognitive stimulating activities, physical activity, and Attention-Deficit Hyperactivity Disorder symptom incidence in children: a prospective study. *Journal of Developmental & Behavioral Pediatrics, 39,* 192–199.

Perkin M. R., Bahnson, H. T., Logan, K., Marrs, T., Radulovic, S., Craven, J., Flohr, C., and Lack, G. (2019). Association of early introduction of solids with infant sleep. A secondary analysis of a randomized clinical trial. *JAMA Pediatrics, 172,* e18 0739.

Petzoldt, J., Wittchen, H. U., Einsle, F., and Martini, J. (2016). Maternal anxiety versus depressive disorders: specific relations to infants' crying, feeding and sleeping problems. *Child: Care, Health & Development, 42,* 231–245.

Petzoldt, J. (2018). Systematic review on maternal depression versus anxiety in relation to excessive infant crying: it is all about the timing. *Archives Women's Mental Health, 21,* 15–30.

Philbrook, L. E. and Teti, D. M. (2016). Bidirectional association between bedtime parenting and infant sleep: parenting quality, parenting practices, and their interaction. *Journal of Family Psychology, 30,* 431–441.

Philbrook, L. E. and Teti, D. M. (2016). Associations between bedtime and nighttime parenting and infant cortisol in the first year. *Developmental Psychology, 58,* 1087–1100.

Philip, P. and Guilleminault, C. (1996). Adult psychophysiologic insomnia and positive history of childhood insomnia. *Sleep, 19,* S16–22.

Phillips, A. J. K., Clerx, W. M., O'Brien, C. S., Sano, A., Barger, L. K., Picard, R. W., Lockley, S. W., Klerman, E. B., and Czeisler, C. A. (2017). Irregular sleep/wake patterns are associated with poorer academic performance and delayed circadian and sleep/wake timing. *Scientific Reports, 7,* 3216

Pisch, M., Wiesemann, F., and Karmiloff-Smith, A. (2019). Infant wake after sleep onset serves as a marker for different trajectories in cognitive development. *Journal of Child Psychology and Psychiatry, 60,* 189–198.

Plancoulaine, S., Lioret, S., Regnault, N., Heude, B., and Charles, M-A. (2015). Gender-specific factors associated with shorter sleep duration at age 3 years. *Journal of Sleep Research, 24,* 610–620.

Plancoulaine, S., Reynaud, E., Forhan, A., Lioret, S., Heude, B., and Charles, M. H. (2018). Night sleep duration trajectories and associated factors among preschool children from the EDEN cohort. *Sleep medicine, 48,* 194–201.

Plomin, Robert. (2018). Blueprint. How DNA makes us who we are. Cambridge, Massachusetts: MIT Press.

Poroyko, V. A., Carreras, A., Khalyfa, A., Khalyfa, A. A., Leone, V., Peris, E., Almendros, I., Gileles-Hillel, A., Qiao, Z., Hubert, N., Farre, R., Chang, E. B., and Gozal, D. (2016). Chronic sleep disruption alters gut microbiota, induces systemic and adipose tissue inflammation and insulin resistance in mice. *Scientific Reports,* 6:35405.

Price, A. M. H., Wake, M., Ukoumune, O. C., and Hiscock, H. (2012). Five-year follow-up of harms and benefits of behavioral infant sleep intervention: Randomized trial. *Pediatrics, 130, doi10.1542.*

Price, A. M. H., Wake, M., Ukoumunne, O. C., and Hiscock, H. (2012). Outcomes at six years of age for children with infant sleep problems: longitudinal community-based study. *Sleep Medicine, 13,* 991–998.

Przybylski, A. K. (2019). Digital screen time and pediatric sleep: evidence from a preregistered cohort study. *Journal of Pediatrics, 205,* 218–223.

Pyper, E., Harrington, D., and Manson, H. (2017). Do parents' support behaviors predict whether or not their children get sufficient sleep? A cross-sectional study. *BMC Public Health, 17,* 432–442.

Quach, J., Price, A. M. H., Bittman, M., and Hiscock, H. (2016). Sleep timing and child and parent outcomes in Australian 4-9-year-olds: a cross-sectional and longitudinal study. *Sleep Medicine, 22,* 39–46.

Quach, J. L., Nguyen, C. D., Williams, K. E., and Sciberras, E. (2018), Bidirectional associations between child sleep problems and internalizing and externalizing difficulties from preschool to early adolescence. *JAMA Pediatrics,* doi:10.1001/jamapediatrics.2017.4363.

Ramires, F. D., Chen, S., Langan, S. M., Prather, A. A., McCulloch, C. E., Kidd, S. A., Cabana, M. D., Chren, M-M., and Abuabra, K. (2019). Association of atopic dermatitis with sleep quality in children. *JAMAPediatrics,* doi:10.1001/jamapediatrics.2019.0025.

Ranum, B. M., Wichstram, L., Pallensen, S., Falcj-Madsen, J., Halse, M., and Steinsbekk, S. (2019). Association between objectively measured sleep duration and symptoms of psychiatric disorders in middle childhood. *JAMA Network Open.* doi:10.100/jamanetweorkopen.2019.19281.

Reader, J., M., Teti, D. M., and Cleveland, M. J. (2017). Cognitions about infant sleep: interparental differences, trajectories across the first year and coparenting quality. *Journal of Family Psychology, 31,* 453–463.

Reddy, R., Palmer, C. A., Jackson, C., Farris, S. G., and Alfano, C. A. (2017). Impact of sleep restriction versus idealized sleep on emotional experience, reactivity and regulation in healthy adolescents. *Journal of Sleep Research, 26,* 516–525.

Reynaud, E., Forhan, A., Heude, B., de Lauzon-Guillain, B., Charles, M., and Plancoulaine, S. (2016). Night-waking trajectories and associated factors in French preschoolers from the EDEN birth-cohort. *Sleep Medicine, 27-28,* 59–65.

Reynaud, E., Vecchierini, M-F., Heude, B., Charles, M-A., and Plancoulaine, S. (2018). Sleep and its relation to cognition and behaviour in preschool children of the general population: a systematic review. *Journal of Sleep research, 27,* 1–13.

Richter, D., Kramer, M. D., Tang, N. K. Y., Montgomery-Downs, H. E., and Lemola, S. (2019). Long-term effects of pregnancy and childbirth on sleep satisfaction and duration of first-time and experienced mothers and fathers. *SleepJ,* doi:10.1093/sleep/zsz015.

Rudnicka, A. J., Nightingale, C. M., Donin, A. S., Sattar, N., Cook, D. G., Whincup, P. H., and Owen, C. G. (2017). Sleep duration and risk of Type 2 Diabetes. *Pediatrics, 140,* e20170338.

Rupp, T. L., Wesensten, N. J., Bliese, P. D., and Balkin, T. J. (2009). Banking sleep: realization of benefits during subsequent sleep restriction and recovery. *Sleep, 32,* 311–321.

Richter, D., Kramer, M. D., Tang, N. K. Y., Montgomery-Downs, H. E., and Lemola, S. (2019). Long term effects of pregnancy and childbirth on sleep satisfaction and duration of first-time and experienced mothers and fathers. *SleepJ,* doi:10.1093/sleep/zsz015.

Sadeh, A., De Marcas, G., Guri, Y., Beger, A., Tikotzky, L., and Bar-Haim, Y. (2015). Infant sleep predicts attention regulation and behavior problems at 3–4 years of age. *Developmental Neuropsychology, 40,* 122–137.

Sadeh, A., Judah-Handel, M., Livne-Karp, E., Kahn, M.,

Tikotzky, L., Anders, T. F., Calkins, S., and Sivan, Y. (2016). Low parental tolerance for infant crying: an underlying factor in infant sleep problems? *Journal of Sleep Research, 25,* 501–507.

Sampasa-Kanyinga, H., Hamilton, H. A., and Chaput, J-P. (2018). Use of social media is associated with short sleep duration in a dose-response manner in students aged 11–20 years. *Acta Paediatrica, 107,* 694–700.

Santangeli, O., Lehtikuja, H., Palomaki, E., Wigren, H-K., Paunio, T., and Porkka-Heiskanen, T. (2016). Sleep and behavior in cross-fostering rats: development and sex aspects. *Sleep, 39,* 2211–2221.

Scott, N., Blair, P. S., Emond, A. M., Fleming, P. J., Humphreys, J. S., Henderson, J., and Gringas, P. (2013). Sleep patterns in children with ADHD: a population -based cohort study from birth to 11 years. *Journal of Sleep Research, 22,* 121–128.

Shen, L., van Schie, J., Ditchburn, G., Brooks, L., and Bei, B. (2018). Positive and negative emotions: differential associations with sleep duration and quality in adolescents. *Journal of Youth and Adolescence, 47,* 2584–2595.

Short, M. A., Blunden, S., Rigney, G., Matriccini, L., Coussens, S., Reynolds, C., and Galland, B. (2018). Cognition and objectively measured sleep duration in children: a systematic review and meta-analysis. *Sleep Health, 4,* 292–300.

Simard, V., Nielson, T. A., Tremblay, R. E., Boivin, M., and Montplaisir, J. Y. (2008). Longitudinal study of preschool sleep disturbances. *Archives of Pediatric and Adolescent Medicine, 162,* 360–367.

Skorucak, J., Arbon, E. L., Dijk, D-J., and Achermann, P. (2018). Response to chronic sleep restriction, extension, and subsequent total sleep deprivation in humans: adaptation or preserved sleep homeostasis. *SleepJ,* doi:10.1093/sleep/zsy078.

Smarius, L. J. C., Strieder, T. G. A., Loomans, E. M., Doreleijers, T. A. H., Vrijkotte, T. G. M., Gemke, R. J., and van Eijsden, M. (2017). Excessive infant crying doubles the risk of mood and behavioral problems at age 5: evidence for mediation by maternal characteristics. *European Child Adolescent Psychiatry, 26*, 293–302.

Smith, R. P., Easson, C., Lyle, S. M., Kapoor, R., Donnelly, C. P., Davidson, E. J., Parikh, E., Lopez, J. V., and Tartar, J. L. (2019). Gut microbiome diversity is associated with sleep physiology in humans. *PLoS ONE, 14*, e0222394.

Sockol, L. E, and Allred, K. M. (2018). Correlates of symptom of depression and anxiety among expectant and new fathers. *Psychology of Men & Masculinity, 19*, 352–372.

Spencer, R. M. C., Campanella, C., deJong, D. M., Desrochers, P., Root, H., Cremone, A., and Kurdziel, L. B. F. (2016). Sleep and behavior of preschool children under typical nap-promoted conditions. *Sleep Health, 2*, 35–41.

St. James-Roberts, I., Roberts, M., Hovish, K., and Owen, C. (2016). Video evidence that parenting methods predict which infants develop long night-time sleep periods by three months of age. *Primary Health Care research & Development, 18*, 212–226.

St. James-Roberts, I., Robert, M., Hovish, K., and Owen, C. (2016). Descriptive figures for differences in parenting and infant night-time distress in the first three months of age. *Primary Health Care Research & Development, 17*, 611–621.

Taveras, E. M., Rifas-Shiman, S. L., Bub, K. L., Gillman, M. W., and Oken, E. (2017). Prospective study of insufficient sleep and neurobehavioral functioning among school-age children. *Academic Pediatrics, 17*, 625–632.

Tay, R. Y., Wilson, J., McCormack, C., Allsop, S., Najman, J. M., Burns, L., Elliott, E. J., Jacobs, S., Olsson, C. A., Mattick, R. P., and Hutchinson, D. (2017). Alcohol consumption by breastfeeding mothers: Frequency, correlates and infant outcomes. *Drug and Alcohol Review, 36*, 667–676.

Taylor, R. W., Gray. A., Heath, A-L. M., Galland, B. C., Lawrence, J., Sayers, R., Healey, D., Tannock, G. W., Meredith-Jones, K. A., Hanna, M., Hatch, B., and Taylor, B. J. (2018). Sleep, nutrition, and physical activity interventions to prevent obesity in infancy: follow-up of the Prevention of Overweight in Infancy (POI) randomized controlled trial at ages 3.5 and 5 y. *American Journal of Clinical Nutrition, 108,* 228–236.

Temkin, D. A., Princiotta, D., Ryberg, R., and Lewin, D. DS. (2018). Later start, longer sleep: implications of middle school start times. *Journal of School Health, 88,* 370–378.

Teti, D. M., Shimizu, M., Crosby, B., and Kim, B. (2016). Sleep arrangements, parent-infant sleep during the first year, and family functioning. *Developmental Psychology, 52,* 1169–1181.

Tetreault, E., Bernier, A., Matte-Gagne, C., and carrier, J. (2018). Normative developmental trajectories of actigraphic sleep variables during the preschool period: a three-wave longitudinal study. *Developmental Psychobiology, 61,* 141–153.

Tham, E. K. H., Richmond, J., Gooley, J. J., Jafar, N. K., Chong, Y-S., Yap, F., Teoh, O-H., Goh, D. Y. T., Broekman, B. F. P., and Rifkin-Graboi, A. (2019). Variations in habitual sleep and relational memory in 6-month-olds. *Sleep Health, 5,* 257–265.

Tikotzky, L. and Sadeh, A. (2001). Sleep patterns and sleep disruptions in kindergarten children. *Journal of Clinical Child Psychiatry, 30,* 581–591.

Tikotzky, L. and Sadeh, A. (2009). Maternal sleep-related cognitions and infant sleep: a longitudinal study from pregnancy through the 1st year. *Child Development, 80,* 860–874.

Tikotzky, L., De Marcas, G., Har-Toov, J., Dollberg, S., Bar-Haim, Y., and Sadeh A. (2019). Sleep and physical growth in infants during the first 6 months. *Journal of Sleep Research, 19,* 103–110.

Tikotzky, L., Sadeh, A., Volkovich, E., Manber, R., Meiri, G., and Shahar, G. (2015). Infant sleep development from 3 to 6 months postpartum: links with maternal sleep and paternal involvement. *Monographs of the Society for Research in Child Development, 80,* 107–124.

Tikotzky, L. (2016). Postpartum maternal sleep, maternal depressive symptoms, and self-perceived mother-infant emotional relationship. *Behavioral Sleep Medicine, 14,* 5–22.

Tkachenko, O. and Dinges, D. F. (2018). Interindividual variability in neurobehavioral response to sleep loss: a comprehensive review. *Neurosciences and Biobehavioral Reviews, 89,* 29–48.

Twenge, J. M., Krizan, Z., and Hisler, G. (2017). Decreases in self-reported sleep duration among U.S. adolescents 2009–2015 and association with new media screen time. *Sleep Medicine, 39,* 47–53.

Urfer-Maurer, N., Weidmann, R., Brand, S., Holsboer, E., Grob, A., Weber, P., and Lemola, S. (2017). The association of mother's and father's insomnia symptoms with school-aged children's sleep assessed by parent report and in-home sleep-electroencephalography. *Sleep Medicine, 38,* 64–70.

Van den Berg, M. P., van der Ende, J., Crijnen, A. A. M., Jaddoe, V. W. V., Moll, H. A., Mackenbach, J. P., Hofman, A., Hengeveld, M. W., Tiemeier, H., and Verhuist, F. C. (2009). Paternal depressive symptoms during pregnancy are related to excessive infant crying. *Pediatrics, 124,* doi:10.1542/peds .2008–3100.

Viner, R. (2018). Ban on sale of energy drinks to children. It's time to legislate. *British Medical Journal,* doi: 10.1136/bmj.k3856.

Viola, A. U., Archer, S. N., James, L. M., Groeger, J. A., Lo, J. C., Skene, D. J., von Schantz, M., and Dijk, D. J. (2007). PER3 polymorphism predicts sleep structure and waking performance. *Current Biology, 17,* 613–618.

Volkovich, E., Bar-Kalifa, E., Meiri, G., and Tikotzky, L. (2018). Mother-infant sleep patterns and parental functioning of room-sharing and solitary-sleeping families: a longitudinal study from 3 to 18 months. *SleepJ,* doi:1093/sleep/zsx207.

Voltaire, S. T. and Teti, D. M. (2018). Early nighttime parental interventions and infant sleep regulation across the first year. *Sleep Medicine, 52,* 107–115.

Walsh, T. B., Davis, R. N., and Garfield, C. (2019). A call to action: screening fathers for perinatal depression. *Pediatrics,* 2020;145(1):e20191193.

Wang, G., Deng, Y., Jiang, Y., Lin, Q., Dong, S., Song, Y., Zhu, L., Zhu, Q., Sun., W., Zhang, Y., and Jiang, F. (2018). Trajectories of sleep quality from late pregnancy to 36 months postpartum and association with maternal mood disturbances: a longitudinal and prospective cohort study. *SleepJ,* doi:10.1093/sleep/zsy179.

Whalen, D. J., Gilbert, K. E., Barch, D. M., Luby, J. L., and Belden, A. C. (2017). Variation in common preschool sleep problems as an early predictor for depression and anxiety symptom severity across time. *Journal of Child Psychology and Psychiatry, 58,* 151–159.

Whitaker, J. C., Dearth-Wesley, T., Herman, A. N., Oakes, J. M., and Owens, J. A. (2019). A quasi-experimental study of the impact of school start times changes on adolescents' mood, self-regulation, safety, and health. *Sleep Health, 5,* 466–469.

Williams, A. A., Mindell, J. A., Hiscock, H., and Quach, J. (2019). Child sleep behaviors and sleep problems from infancy to school-age. *Sleep Medicine, 63,* 5–8.

Winkleman, J. W. (2015). Insomnia disorder. *New England Journal of Medicine, 373,* 1437–1444.

Winsler, A., Deutsch, A., Vorona, R. D., Payne, P. A., and Szklo-Coxe, M. (2015). Sleepless in Fairfax: The difference one more hour of sleep can make for teen hopefulness, suicidal ideation, and substance use. *Journal Youth Adolescence, 44,* 362–378.

Wolke, D., Bilgin, A., and Samara, M. (2017). Systematic review and meta-analysis: fussing and crying durations and prevalence of colic in infants. *Journal of Pediatrics, 185,* 55–64e4.

Wolke, D. (2019). Persistence of infant crying, sleeping and feeding problems: need for prevention. *Archives of Diseases of Children, 104,* 10221023.

Wynter, K., Rowe, H., and Fisher, J. (2013). Interactions between perceptions of relationship quality and postnatal depressive symptoms in Australian, primiparous women and their partners. *Australian Journal of Primary Health,* doi.org/10.1071/ PY12066.

Wynter, K., Wilson, N., Thean, P., Bei, Bei., and Fisher, J. (2018). Psychological distress, alcohol use, fatigue, sleepiness, and sleep quality: an exploratory study among men whose partners are admitted to a residential early parenting service. *Australian Psychologist, 54,* 143–150.

Xiu, L., Ekstedt, M., Hagstromer, M., Bruni, O., Bergvist-Noren, L., and Marcus, C. (2020). Sleep and adiposity in children from 2 to 6 years of age. *Pediatrics, 145,* (3); e20191420.

Ystrom, H., Nilsen, W., Hysing, M., Sivertsen, B. (2017). Sleep problems in preschoolers and maternal depressive symptoms: an evaluation of mother- and child-driven effects. *Developmental Psychology, 53,* 2261–2272.

Ystrom, E., Hysing, M., Torgersen, L., Ystrom, H., Reichborn-Kjennerud, T., and Siversten, B. (2017). Maternal symptoms of anxiety and depression and child nocturnal awakenings at 6 and 18 months. *Journal of Pediatric Psychology, 42,* 1156–1164.

Yu, X-T., Sadeh, A., Lam, H. S., Mindell, J. A., and Li, A. M. (2017). Parental behaviors and sleep/wake patterns of infants and toddlers in Hong Kong, China. *World Journal of Pediatrics, 13,* 486–502.

Zaidman-Zait, A. and Hall, W. A. (2015). Children's night waking among toddlers: relationship with mothers' and fathers' parenting approaches and children's behavioral difficulties. *Journal of Advanced Nursing, 71,* 1639–1649.

Zang, J., Paksarian, D., Lamers, F., Hickie, I. B., He, J., and Merikangas, K. R. (2017). Sleep patterns and mental health correlates in US adolescents. *Journal of Pediatrics, 182,* 137–143.

Zhou, Y., Aris, I. M., Tan, S. S., Cai, S., Tint, M. T., Krishnaswamy, G., Meaney, M. J., Godfrey, K. M., Kwek, K., Gluckman, P. D., Chong, Y-S., Yap, F., Lek, N., Gooley, J. J., and Lee, Y. S. (2015). Sleep duration and growth outcomes across the first two years of life in the GUSTO study. *Sleep Medicine, 16,* 1281–1286.

Zinke, K., Noack, H., and Born, J. (2018). Sleep augments training-induced improvement in working memory in children and adults. *Neurobiology of Learning and Memory, 147,* 46–53.

Index

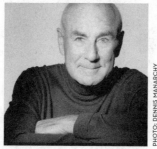

MARC WEISSBLUTH, M.D., has been a pediatrician since 1973. A leading researcher on sleep and children, he founded the original Sleep Disorders Center at Children's Memorial Hospital (now the Ann and Robert H. Lurie Children's Hospital of Chicago) and is a Professor of Clinical Pediatrics, Emeritus, at the Northwestern University Feinberg School of Medicine. Dr. Weissbluth discovered that sleep is linked to temperament and that sleep problems are related to infant colic, and he coined the now familiar phrase *sleep training* to describe his method for helping children learn how to fall asleep. His finding that changing the time a child is put to bed dramatically decreases the number of night awakenings was published in the prestigious journal *Sleep* in 1982. His landmark seven-year study on the development and disappearance of naps, published in *Sleep* in 1995, highlighted the importance of daytime sleep. Since its original publication in 1987, *Healthy Sleep Habits, Happy Child* has sold more than a million copies and, in twelve foreign editions, helped millions of families the world over. Dr. Weissbluth was acknowledged by the American Academy of Pediatrics for his extensive contributions to the chapter "Your Child's Sleep" in their popular book for parents, *Caring for Your Baby and Young Child: Birth to Age 5*. Dr. Weissbluth is also the author of *Your Fussy Baby* and *Healthy Sleep Habits, Happy Twins*, and the producer of a CD, *Sweet Baby: Lullabies to Soothe Your Newborn*. Married to his wife, Linda, since 1965, he is the father of four sons and eight grandchildren— and they are all good sleepers. Dr. and Mrs. Weissbluth live in Chicago.

marcweissbluth.com

About the Type

This book was set in Sabon, a typeface designed by the well-known German typographer Jan Tschichold (1902–74). Sabon's design is based upon the original letter forms of sixteenth-century French type designer Claude Garamond and was created specifically to be used for three sources: foundry type for hand composition, Linotype, and Monotype. Tschichold named his typeface for the famous Frankfurt typefounder Jacques Sabon (c. 1520–80).